IN THE

SHADOWS

OF THE NET

"This is the book we've all been waiting for on cybersex. It explains what computer sex is all about and how to get help if it becomes a problem. The personal stories are excellent for assisting clients in relating to this issue."

—Joseph M. Amico, M.Div., C.A.S., C.S.A.C.
President, National Council on Sexual Addiction and Compulsivity

"The authors provide a simple, effective guide for self-evaluation and recovery if cybersex is causing problems."

—Pia Mellody
Author, *Facing Codependence* and *Facing Love Addiction*
Coauthor, *Breaking Free*

"A much needed resource for professional and lay audiences. An important and timely book about a contemporary problem that is escalating and causing enormous personal, family, and professional distress. The authors are to be commended for clearly articulating how this problem behavior develops and presenting methods for therapeutically addressing it."

—Christine A. Courtois, Ph.D.
Author, *Healing the Incest Wound* and *Recollections of Sexual Abuse*
Clinical director of the CENTER: Posttraumatic Disorders Program,
Psychiatric Institute of Washington

"Once again, Patrick Carnes, with the help of David Delmonico and Elizabeth Griffin, is pushing the frontier of our knowledge of trauma and emptiness, manifesting in addictions. Cybersex addiction is the latest of a myriad of sexual behaviors in our culture where courtship so often goes awry. The authors' gentle approach to the newest compulsive users and their families is realistic, thorough, knowledgeable, practical, and helpful to all who read it, including those whose Internet use is not a problem. Since sexuality is so very powerful an issue, we must learn to use it wisely, safely, and with discretion, lest it destroy us. *In the Shadows of the Net* gives us a way to approach it with integrity."

—Martha Turner, M.D.
Medical director of the STAR (Sexual Trauma and Recovery) Program

IN THE

SHADOWS

OF THE NET

Breaking Free of
Compulsive Online Sexual Behavior

Second Edition

Patrick Carnes, Ph.D.
David L. Delmonico, Ph.D.
Elizabeth Griffin, M.A.
with Joseph M. Moriarity

Hazelden

Hazelden
Center City, Minnesota 55012-0176

1-800-328-0094
1-651-213-4590 (Fax)
www.hazelden.org

Library of Congress Cataloging-in-Publication Data

Carnes, Patrick, 1944–
    In the shadows of the net : breaking free of compulsive online sexual behavior / Patrick
Carnes, David L. Delmonico, Elizabeth Griffin; with Joseph M. Moriarity. — 2nd ed.
        p. cm.
    Rev. ed of: In the shadows of the net. c2001.
    Includes bibliographical references.
    ISBN 978-1-59285-478-3 (softcover)
    1. Sex addiction. 2. Computer sex. I. Delmonico, David L. II. Griffin, Elizabeth,
1958– III. In the shadows of the net. IV. Title.
    RC560.S43I52 2007
    616.85'83—dc22
                                                                                                2007014156
    11   10   09   08   07   6   5   4   3   2   1

Authors' note
Every story in this book is true; however, each has been edited for clarity. Names, locations, and other identifying information have been changed to protect confidentiality.

Editor's note
The Twelve Steps are reprinted and adapted with permission of Alcoholics Anonymous World Services, Inc. (AAWS). Permission to reprint and adapt the Twelve Steps does not mean that AAWS has reviewed or approved the contents of this publication, or that AAWS necessarily agrees with the views expressed herein. AA is a program of recovery from alcoholism *only*—use of the Twelve Steps in connection with programs and activities which are patterned after AA, but which address other problems, or in any other non-AA context, does not imply otherwise.

Cover design by Theresa Gedig
Interior design by Elizabeth Cleveland
Typesetting by Prism Publishing Center

Contents

Illustrations

Figures

Preface

Since 2001, when this book first was published, the issue of cybersex has taken many new twists and turns. Some we imagined and predicted, others caught us completely by surprise. One aspect that was most surprising was how widespread the issue has become and how many professionals are faced with cybersex issues in their office. We expected that counselors, psychologists, social workers, and law enforcement personnel would need to become more aware of cybersex issues. We didn't, however, imagine we would be consulting with human resource managers, divorce attorneys, and people from the religious community about compulsive online sexual behavior.

Regardless of whether we saw the changes coming or not, we realized it was time to create a new edition of this book for the millions of people struggling with their problematic online sexual behavior. For those of you who read the first edition, you will find updated statistics, new thoughts, and a couple new exercises that address problematic cybersex issues. For those who are reading this book for the first time, you will learn how to determine if you or a loved one has a significant problem with online sex, and the steps you can take to address these issues.

It is our hope that this book continues to be a useful resource for both the professional community as well as individuals (and their families) who struggle with cybersex behavior. Just as it was when the first edition of this book was published, it is impossible to predict the nature and course of cybersex over the coming years. All we really know is that cybersex will continue to change the way we relate to others, and for some it will present a lifelong battle for which we hope to bring a small amount of hope and relief.

PATRICK CARNES, PH.D.
DAVID L. DELMONICO, PH.D.
ELIZABETH GRIFFIN, M.A.

I

The Shadow Side
of the Net

THE INTERNET. This worldwide phenomenon has created a communication and information network unlike anything previously seen. Even inventions such as radio and television have not been as far-reaching as or had the impact of the Internet. There are an estimated 322 million active users of the Internet spread over at least 120 different countries throughout the world.[1] Whatever we want—information, goods, connections—we can find it or do it whenever we want via the Internet. Yes, everything . . . even sex. We can have sex on the Internet whenever we want with exactly the kind of person we want.

Sometimes that creates a problem. The opportunity is too enticing, alluring, fulfilling, immediate, and powerful. So much is available. There are so many options, ones we've only dreamed of—or have yet to dream of! So much opportunity and stimulation is available that it's difficult to control. And hard to stop. For some it is seemingly impossible to stop.

No, the Internet isn't all sunshine and progress. There is the shadow side to the Net. For some people, the pull of cybersex can be so powerful that, like alcohol or other drugs, it's hard to put down and control. The shadowy world of cybersex is overtaking and overwhelming far too many people, undermining careers and upending relationships. And the problem is growing. Worse, it is becoming clear that for some, cybersex becomes a compulsive or an addictive disorder. No one could have forecast that cybersex would have had such an impact.

KEVIN'S STORY

Kevin, a married thirty-seven-year-old manufacturing company executive with two children, gives his account of what it's like to be hooked on cybersex:

It is 3:30 A.M. and I'm still online. Pornographic images of women stream onto my computer screen. Earlier tonight, after putting my two kids to bed, I watched the evening news with my wife, Jeneen. Since my wife was tired after a long day at work, she soon went to bed. Though I, too, was exhausted, primarily from too many late nights on the computer, I, as usual, told her I was still not tired and would stay up late and read for a while.

Once I was sure that Jeneen was asleep, I turned off the bedroom light and headed for the den and the family computer. "OK, tonight I'm just going to stay online for an hour," I promised myself. "It'll be midnight when I'm done, and that's enough time. I really just can't stay up half the night again. Today at work I actually caught myself nodding off during Alan's important sales plan presentation. I haven't been able to really focus lately, either."

Once I sat down, I arranged my chair and the screen so that if Jeneen should awaken and come in, I'd have a moment to switch the screen view over to a work-related document. I'm more careful now, since a few months ago my wife surprised me and saw the photo of a naked woman I was viewing.

I talked myself out of that embarrassing situation with the excuse that while trying to finish a work project, I'd opened an e-mail from one of my colleagues. In it was a link to a site that the guy had said I would find interesting. It was a porn site, and I told my wife that I'd never seen anything like it and was just looking at it out of curiosity.

I remember only too well how I'd felt at that moment. Heart pounding in my chest. My mouth instantly parched. Feelings of fear, shock, embarrassment, and panic coursing through my body as, in those very, very long moments, I searched for a plausible explanation. I didn't ever want to go through that again. Besides, I knew there would be no good excuse if my wife caught me again.

I'd actually sworn off porn sites after that night. I deleted the bookmarks and told myself that it wasn't worth it. I realized that I loved my wife and children and didn't want to jeopardize these relationships over some nude photos.

That promise was broken in less than a week. After a particularly hard day at work, I told myself that I deserved a reward. I'd take just thirty minutes to masturbate, and then I'd go off to bed with Jeneen.

For several evenings, I kept to this thirty-minute ritual. Feeling more confident now with my control over my Internet usage, I decided to give myself an hour each evening. A few weeks passed, and before I knew it, I was online for hours on end again each evening—until two, three, even four o'clock in the morning. I just didn't know where the time was going. What felt like an hour just suddenly turned into three or four. I was searching for just the right woman, just the right look to masturbate to before going to bed. At times, I felt like this Internet thing was spiraling out of control.

I felt extreme anticipation and excitement when I first went online in the evening, the concentration and thrill increasing as I searched various Web sites and found new ones. But after I masturbated, I felt awful. I had so many harsh feelings and was angry for wasting so much time. I felt ashamed and guilty that I had done this again. And worst of all, I felt helpless and full of despair because I realized I didn't know how or when I would be able to stop. Exhausted and beaten down, I quietly slipped into bed, wondering how I was going to make it at work again on just three hours of sleep.

CAN YOU RELATE TO KEVIN'S STORY?

Kevin isn't alone in his problems with sex and the Internet. Countless others, men and women alike, also find themselves in what seems to be a futile struggle with online sexual behavior. Of the estimated 322 million individuals who actively use the Internet, an estimated 40 million adults admit to regularly visiting pornographic Web sites. Pornography accounts for an estimated 4.2 million Web sites generating a hefty $2.5 billion annually.[2] Many people struggle alone and in silence, too embarrassed or guilt-ridden to seek help, not knowing where they can find help, believing that no one else would really understand anyway. Just like Kevin, they experience a roller coaster of emotions each day. Perhaps you are in a similar predicament. Have you ever done any of the following?

- kept sexual activity on the Internet a secret from family members
- carried out sexual activities on the Net at work
- frequently found yourself erasing your computer history files in an effort to conceal your activity on the Net
- felt ashamed at the thought that someone you love might discover your Internet use
- found that your time on the Net takes away from or prevents you from doing other tasks and activities
- found yourself in a kind of online trance or time warp during which hours just slipped by
- frequently visited chat rooms that are focused on sexual conversation
- looked forward to your sexual activities on the Net and felt frustrated and anxious if you couldn't get on it when you planned
- found yourself masturbating while on the Net
- recognized the people in the interactive online video while they recognized your screen name when you signed on
- had sexual chat room friends who became more important than the family and friends in your life
- regularly visited porn sites
- downloaded pornography from a newsgroup
- had favorite porn sites
- visited fetish porn sites
- taken part in the CuSeeMe sexual video rooms
- viewed child pornography online

Discovering the Net's potential for sexual activity may have at first felt very exciting. After all, a new world was opening up for you, ready for exploration. It may have seemed like a harmless one in which to play, to fulfill fantasies, to occasionally find sexual gratification. It may have felt like a dream come true. But eventually you may have found, as Kevin did, that there was a downside—a very powerful one that seemed difficult, if not impossible, to control. Even as resolutions are made to limit or stop using the Net for sex, they are rendered hollow by the echoes of previous vows and promises. "How could this be happening to me?" you may wonder. Again, you are not alone in these feelings. The power and attraction of the Internet in general, and its use for sexual activity in particular, have entered and permeated our culture subtly and with blinding speed.

A DIFFERENT WORLD

It's almost impossible to imagine it now, but only ten short years ago, most of us knew little, if anything, about this mysterious creation for communication called the Internet. Today, however, its burgeoning growth and wide accessibility are altering patterns of social communication, business activity, and interpersonal relationships. Internet users spend an average of ten hours per week online. This includes both adult men and women. Teenagers often spend far more time online than adults: an estimated fifteen to twenty hours per week. This demographic is second only to computer professionals for their average amount of time spent online per week.[3]

Given the dramatic pace at which this remarkable and powerful technology has entered our lives, few of us are aware that the Internet has profoundly changed many aspects of our lives. Telephones, computers, and television, once separate technologies, are merging. Our schools, work environments, and even our social lives are becoming more and more centered around computers. Ten years ago, you probably could not have imagined doing your holiday shopping online, sending an RSVP to a wedding invitation via e-mail, being able to send letters and photos in seconds to a friend on the other side of the world, or "chatting" online with five, fifty, or five hundred people simultaneously. That these activities now seem commonplace indicates just how quickly we adapt to and take for granted technologies that a few years ago lived only in the realm of science fiction.

While it's not difficult to recognize technological changes, anticipating how pervasive and profound an effect they will have is a far greater challenge. Numerous authors, including Lynn White in a classic book on the Middle Ages, *Medieval Technology and Social Change,* and Alvin Toffler in *Future Shock,* have argued that new technological developments can actually create changes in human thinking patterns and in how we see the world—changes that are known as paradigm shifts.[4] Who would have imagined when the Wright brothers discovered how to build an airplane that only seventy-five years later, national and international flight would be commonplace? That a world without electricity, telephone, radio, and television is almost unimaginable today is testimony to the profound effect these technologies have had on the human race in less than a century. Our world is absolutely dependent on them. Yet at the time of their discovery, these inventions seemed little more than oddities developed by eccentric inventors.

What effect has the Internet had on society since it came into use by the general public in the early 1990s? It's difficult to know now, but the speed at which it has penetrated our culture is an indication of its power. As you know, sexuality is one important aspect of our lives that is being dramatically affected by the Internet. Mention "cybersex" and the response you'll receive will be, more often than not, a chuckle and a lewd comment. Such reactions do not, however, come from anyone who is familiar with the reality of sex and the Internet. Access to the Internet, and more specifically sex on the Internet, is on the rise. Access to sex-related online activities by children and teens also appears to be on the rise. Hundreds of thousands of adult-oriented Web sites are readily accessible to online users by simply typing the word "sex" in one of the many search engines available to Internet users. In fact, the word "sex" is one of the most frequently typed words in search engines. (The only words more common than "sex" are "and" and "the.")

The statistics are as remarkable as they are surprising:

- An estimated 72 million unique individuals visit pornography Web sites each year.
- Approximately 25 percent of all search engine requests are pornography related.
- Of all daily e-mails, it is estimated that 2.5 billion contain pornography. This represents 8 percent of all daily e-mails.
- Ten percent of adult Internet users believe they are cybersex addicts.
- The average age of first exposure to online pornography is eleven years old.
- Seventy percent of teenagers report they have seen pornographic images online.

- Twenty percent of all United States adults admit having intentionally visited a pornographic Web site.
- Thirty percent of visitors to adult pornography sites are believed to be women.
- The Playboy Web site averages 5 million hits each day.
- An estimated $320 billion per year is spent by consumers on Internet pornography.

It is easy to categorize online sexual behaviors as either all good or all bad. The Internet, however, is a communications tool that is inherently neither good nor bad. It is, rather, the interaction of the content offered by its creators (those who host Web sites, post to newsgroups, organize chat rooms, and so on) and the ways Internet users of these electronic meeting sites react and respond to these messages, images, and sounds that result in "good" or "bad" outcomes.[5] Some social scientists have noted the educational potential of the Internet, citing the greater availability of information about sexuality and the potential for more candid discussions of sexuality online. The Internet can also offer the opportunity for forming online or virtual "communities" in which isolated or disenfranchised people can communicate with one another about sexual topics.

Far more often, however, an increasing and rapidly growing number of people find that using the Internet for sexual purposes is fraught with risks and, at the very least, interferes with many aspects of their lives, including family relationships, work life, and financial security.

Three people share their experiences here. (Please note that while the stories used in this book are true, they have been altered as needed to protect individual anonymity.)

Carl, a parole officer, tells his story:

I had worked for several years as a parole officer and recently I'd been seeing more sex offenders, some of whom had been using the Internet in their crimes. I hadn't really known of or thought about the Internet's potential for sexual activity or encounters until I talked with my clients and their caseworkers. Curious about the cybersex scene, I went online a few times at work just to see what sexual content was actually available on the Net. My superiors were aware of my sex activities on the

Net and accepted them as necessary for my job. After a few months passed, I was still surfing sex-related sites at work. What's more, the time I spent online had been inching up. One day, I'd been online exploring sex-related sites for nearly an hour. My boss noticed and commented to me about it. I reiterated that it was work-related and that I needed to know what my guys were doing. My boss said, "OK," but suggested that maybe I was spending a bit too much time doing this, I'd best watch myself more closely, and I'd better make sure none of my other responsibilities were being neglected.

Jake, a wealthy twenty-five-year-old single man, narrowly escaped being arrested:

I seemed to have it all: a well-off family, hot new car, and nice apartment. But I had never really taken charge of my life; supported by my parents, I was unemployed, spoiled, a heavy drinker, and lacked ambition. However, I did have one area of expertise—computers. My computer knowledge developed as a young adult while being holed up in my bedroom at home as punishment for my many transgressions. I had spent endless hours on the computer during this time and was truly skilled at programming, games, and surfing the Net.

I discovered chat rooms fairly quickly, and eventually I decided that I wanted to set up sex with a young girl. Soon, I was regularly in online conversations with a particular fifteen-year-old girl. Thanks to my superior computer skills, however, I discovered that there was another older guy who was also trying to arrange to have sex with this girl. I e-mailed this man and asked him how it was going with her. By maintaining regular communications with him, I eventually discovered that the girl had finally agreed to meet him to have sex.

I discovered that the two had arranged to meet at a restaurant in town. Since I knew the time and place and was curious to see what the two looked like, I decided to anonymously observe the rendezvous, but not participate. By this time, I had given up my frequent online conversations with this girl.

On the appointed evening, I was sitting in my car in a parking lot adjacent to the restaurant where I expected to have a great view of the action. Soon, the other man showed up—and seemingly out of nowhere three police squad cars and a half dozen FBI agents appeared. Before the man knew what had happened, he'd been arrested, handcuffed, and dumped in the back of a police car.

My heart was in my mouth, pounding like a jackhammer. I could hardly breathe. I couldn't move a muscle. I'd heard of guys being busted for trying to hook up with teen girls for sex, but I thought I was clever enough to avoid such a trap. Now I knew how close I had come to being in the back of that squad car on the way to jail. I realized I had a problem, and I sought help the very next day.

Marcy, a middle-aged social worker, with a history of relationship infidelity:

I had been married thirteen years—and unfaithful the whole time. In fact, when I married, I was actually having an affair with one of the groomsmen in my wedding party. My husband never had a clue about what was going on. Finally, I started going to counseling, as my behavior began to bother me. Very soon into therapy, my therapist told me, "I think you have a problem with sex addiction." My response, however, was that the real problem was a "problematic marriage."

At this time, I discovered the Internet—more specifically, chat rooms. My husband regularly went to bed around 9:30 or 10:00 P.M. That's when I would get on the computer and head straight into one of my favorite chat rooms, where I would converse with various men. These "chats" became increasingly sexual and seductive, and eventually I was staying up very late, until three or four in the morning. I realized that my Internet use was getting out of hand, and each night I promised myself that I'd be in bed by eleven. But I just couldn't meet that goal. Despite my efforts at control, I became even more infatuated with my online life. The conversations became more and more sexual and tantalizing. Eventually, I became more and more daring. I began giving out my phone number to men I'd met online. They would call me and then together we would have phone sex. All the while, my husband was asleep in an adjacent room.

Finally, I encountered a guy who seemed irresistible, and crossing yet another boundary, I arranged an in-person meeting for sex with the

guy, who lived in Dallas. We agreed to meet at a Dallas hotel. We had
sex, and then I was attacked, beaten unconscious, and left for dead. I
awoke days later in a hospital with no clue as to where I was, how I'd
gotten there, or how much time had passed. The hospital staff had no
way to identify me, since my purse had been stolen along with all my
identification and money. And my husband? He knew nothing about
what had happened. Since I was not at the hotel I claimed to be staying
at, he was frantic with worry and had called the police to file a missing
person report.

When I was finally able to use a phone at the hospital, my first call
was to my therapist. I said, "OK, you're right. I have a problem. I need
help."

WHAT IS CYBERSEX?

Internet sex can be accessed and experienced in many different ways. Each
has the potential to cause users problems and to lead them into risky or
dangerous situations. In the following section, we outline these new avenues of sex to give you an idea of the breadth of the cybersex world.

The term "cybersex" has become a catchall to address a variety of sex-
related behaviors when using your computer. They fall into several general
categories:

1. ACCESSING ONLINE PORNOGRAPHY AND AUDIO, VIDEO, AND TEXT STORIES

The kind of pornography available on the Internet varies widely, just as it
does in the non-cyber-world, ranging from photographs of models posing in
bathing suits or lingerie to young children being sexually abused. It can be
found in various forms, including photos and audio, video, and text stories.
Its variety and ease of access, however, is much greater than offline access
since many of the sexual content and activity laws that exist in the United
States are difficult to enforce or don't apply in other countries (which can be
easily accessed via the Internet).

Pornographic materials can be found on personal and commercial Web
pages, with access just a mouse click away. Pornographic pictures, video,
audio, and text can also be exchanged via e-mail and discussion or newsgroups. These forums allow participants to use their e-mail to post stories,

ideas, photographs, or software related to the topic of the group. These messages can then be stored for other group participants to read or retrieve. Literally thousands of sex-related newsgroups exist on the Net and, as such, accommodate the highest volume of traffic of all newsgroups—so much so that they are often excluded from Internet statistics because of their extremely high usage.

Video- and photo-sharing Web sites have recently become a common area for exchanging online pornographic material. Many amateurs use this venue to post pornographic pictures and videos of themselves online. It is also an area where users can find videos and photos that meet their particular arousal interests.

2. Real Time with a Fantasy Partner

The second form of cybersex takes place in what is known as "real time"—though time may be the only aspect of the interaction that is real. Real-time chatting can be likened to a computerized version of citizens band (CB) radio. Internet chat rooms resemble CB channels in that they offer varying numbers of people the opportunity to listen to and discuss specific topics. The number of CB radio channels is relatively small and is limited to available broadcast frequencies. At any one time on the Internet, however, there are typically about ten to twenty thousand "channels" available to "join." In addition, while Federal Communications Commission (FCC) laws limit the types of communication that can take place over the airwaves, most of these laws do not apply to international cyberspace.

After reviewing the chat room topic areas, it is not difficult to understand how one may engage in sexual conversation with others online. Advanced technology has also provided ways to exchange images and files online during a live conversation. In addition, "virtual locations" exist in which you can engage in online chatting with others. You may, for example, start in the virtual "dining area" and talk with someone over "virtual coffee" and later be invited to a "virtual bedroom" where "one thing often leads to another."

Current technology also allows for the exchange of voice and video images via the Internet. By simply providing a credit card number, you can take advantage of live video cameras that capture and transmit images of males or females engaged in everything from everyday activities to explicit sexual acts. Though a fee is common, some of these sites can be accessed for free. Some live video sites accept requests for specific sexual behaviors from online users, thus enabling an individual to create and fulfill personal fantasies. Thanks to live video feed technology, it is even possible to chat online while viewing pornography. Such virtual video booths are steadily growing in number and allow cybersex users to have nearly complete control over the "object" at the other end of the phone line, even though the "object" happens to be a human being. For a relatively small fee, you can also link to X-rated video feeds without any interaction or, with CuSeeMe software and camera, watch others masturbate or engage in other sexual activities while they watch you do the same.

Special sex toys for both men and women can now be connected to the Internet and allow remote control of the devices during chat sessions. Each partner has the ability to manipulate the other partner's sex toy. These new sex toys seek to add another dimension to the online cybersex encounter.

3. OTHER CYBERSEX VENUES

Internet users have recently begun using several new online technologies such as social networking sites, Internet-based dating services, and portable Internet devices for cybersex purposes.

Social networking sites (such as MySpace) allow users to post individualized Web pages about themselves, post photos of themselves and others, and interact with their group of online "friends." Such Web sites have become extremely popular with both adults and teens. Like all Internet-related venues, there are many entertaining and enjoyable ways people can use these resources to meet and communicate with others, and share information about themselves with people they know or would like to meet. However, these same characteristics that attract users to social networking sites also present vulnerabilities for their users. Many teens lack the ability to make good judgments about risky behaviors and when and what is appropriate to share with others online. As a result, online sex offenders flock to these areas to meet both adults and teens for possible exploitation.

Internet-based dating services and online personal ads help Internet users meet new people either online or in the real world. Many people use these services to meet others in the hopes of intimate and romantic relationships, while others simply use them to find sex partners.

Originally, accessing the Internet was possible only through the use of a desktop or laptop computer. These days there are many portable devices such as cell phones, Blackberries, and gaming systems that can access the Internet through a wireless connection. Many of these portable devices can access the same types of cybersex discussed in the previous paragraphs, and in some cases, they provide additional ways to engage in cybersex behavior. For example, the pornography industry publishes material that can be downloaded directly onto a cell phone—an extremely lucrative business. "Podnography" refers to pornography specifically designed to be downloaded onto iPods and similar video/music devices. Most gaming systems that connect to the Internet allow for "chat sessions" during games. Many times this chat conversation can turn sexual and lead to further cybersex behavior with a gaming partner.

4. MULTIMEDIA SOFTWARE

The final category of cybersex does not take place online at all. With the invention of more sophisticated multimedia systems, people can play X-rated movies, engage in sexual games, or view the latest issues of erotica magazines on a desktop or laptop computer. Compact disc read-only memory (CD-ROM) technology allows companies to release software titles with sound and video clips. Such multimedia productions can also include erotic information. Studies estimate that erotica CD-ROMs account for 20 percent of all CD-ROM business, with sales in 1994 reported at $260 million. Others report that the CD-ROM market has helped turn X-rated cyberspace into a billion-dollar-plus business.

WHY CYBERSEX?

With all the different forms of media available in our culture, what is it that attracts people to the Internet to engage in sexual activities in such a high-tech fashion? David Delmonico, Elizabeth Griffin, and Joe Moriarity developed a model called the CyberHex for understanding the reasons why the Internet is so attractive and powerful for individuals.[6] The CyberHex was named because it contains six components (a hexagon) that combine to create a "hex-like" or trance state for online users. The

CyberHex components include integral, imposing, isolating, interactive, inexpensive, and intoxicating.

CyberHex

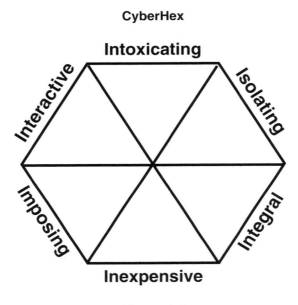

Figure 1.1

INTEGRAL

In just a few short years, the Internet has become an integral part of most people's personal and work lives. On the Internet we can acquire a home mortgage, shop for groceries, trade on the stock market, check the weather anywhere in the world, e-mail friends or business colleagues, create and conduct business, do research for school assignments, and so much more. The prices of computers and Internet access continue to fall and are within the budget for many families. What's more, the Internet is available publicly in a variety of settings (public libraries, coffee houses, and college campuses, for example) and has simply become a way of life. Such integration allows convenience, but it also makes avoidance of the Internet difficult. The more the Internet becomes a part of our lives, the more indispensable—or "integral"—it becomes. The option not to use it becomes less viable.

Without the Internet, access to various forms of sex-related materials and sexual experiences has limitations. Most strip clubs and X-rated theaters are not open twenty-four hours a day. Buying a porn magazine requires walking or driving to a store that sells them, and most stores aren't open all the time either. Another limitation is distance/location. Stores, theaters, strip clubs, and areas where prostitutes ply their trade cannot be conveniently found in every neighborhood of every city, suburb, or rural community, thus requiring those who wish access to them to have time and transportation. The Internet changed all of this. It offers incredibly broad and easy access to sex of all kinds. Twenty-four hours a day, seven days a week, anyone with the use of a computer with an Internet connection—be it at work, a cybercafé, the public library, a school, a university, or at home—can choose from literally millions of sex-related Web sites offering whatever type of sexual experience is desired.

IMPOSING

While related to the integral aspect of the Internet, this "imposing" attribute suggests that the Internet is not simply available for use on an everyday basis for a variety of reasons, but that its use is becoming more and more often a necessity. Because of the extent to which the Internet is being integrated into our lives, its use is, in a sense, being externally imposed on us by society. Ironically, while the interactive nature of the Internet offers us control over what we access, this imposing factor suggests a loss of control in that we have fewer options to decline using the Net. To understand the difference between "integral" and "imposing," let's compare the telephone and the Internet. The telephone has long played an integral role in our lives, but it has never been imposing in the sense we're speaking of with the Net. People don't habitually spend three, five, or eight hours at a time on the phone, three or more times a week—though this a not an uncommon occurrence for far too many people with the Internet.

In addition, the very breadth of the Internet's content is, in and of itself, formidable and imposing. While choice may be good in many circumstances, having too much from which to choose can be overwhelming. Think of the Internet as a Thanksgiving dinner. There are so many enticing "dishes" and "desserts" from which to choose that you want to sample every one. You know that if you do, however, you'll feel awful afterward. It's so hard to say no, and despite our best efforts at control, we often overindulge. The Internet offers us so many enticing opportunities that it's difficult to decline. Soon, some people find themselves overindulging to the detriment of their health, families, relationships, and work. And still, stopping seems impossible.

ISOLATING

Perhaps the most powerful component of cybersex is isolation. The Internet allows for the aforementioned intoxication to occur quickly and privately. It provides a perfect opportunity to separate yourself from others and to engage in whatever fantasy you prefer without risk of sexually transmitted infections or the distraction of reality. Previous methods of obtaining pornography involved (at a minimum) a trip to an adult bookstore or corner market. Now, those same images can be obtained with the click of a mouse button and appear on the screen with absolutely no contact with the outside world, which allows the user to remain anonymous. Separated from the outside world, users can create the justifications and rationalizations needed to convince themselves and others that their behavior is both victimless and harmless.

While on the Internet, people have no physical contact with others. Time spent on the Net is time not spent in "real time" interacting with those who are important in our lives. A fast-growing complaint of men and women in couple relationships is that Net use has taken a partner away from them. The complaining partner is less and less a physical part of the using partner's life because the using partner spends so much time at the computer on the Net.

This CyberHex attribute also points to the paradoxical nature of the Internet: it separates and isolates us from others and the world as never before, while at the same time, it connects us to the world as never before.

INTERACTIVE

Unlike other forms of media, the Internet is truly interactive. Shout or cajole as we might at the faces on our television screen or at the writer of a magazine or newspaper editorial, those people cannot respond. The Internet, however, lets us interact with others and form a pseudo-intimacy with others from around the world. We guide our browsers to the locations, people, and information of our choice. Some interactive sex sites allow viewers to choose the person they want to interact with and the activity that will take place. With the right equipment and software, conversations can be in real time.

The Internet gives us a sense of control over what we see and receive as well as a sense of an interactive community where we belong.

INEXPENSIVE

For anyone on a budget, cybersex provides a low-cost alternative means to a sexual high. Hard-core pornography magazines run fifteen to fifty dollars each. However, for the cost of Internet access, anyone can find hundreds of photographs, stories, chat channels, and more. In addition, the user can choose to retrieve and view only the information that is of interest; there's no need, for example, to purchase an entire magazine full of mostly un-wanted advertisements and articles.

Online sex: what you want, when you want it, at low cost, minus the "messiness and hassles" of a person-to-person relationship, and with anonymity. It should not be surprising that online sexual activities are ex-ploding along with the number of people accessing and using them.

INTOXICATING

Some may believe that comparing the Internet to a drug is absurd. Individuals who use the Internet for cybersex, however, often report feeling euphoria while preparing for or engaging in cybersex. It is this "rush" that lures individuals back to cybersex after they have sworn off such behavior. The combination of all the prior facets of the CyberHex creates a powerful force that many cybersex compulsives compare to drug addicts' seduction by their substance.

The Internet also provides immediate access to a staggeringly immense information base. Live in Nebraska and want to read a German newspaper? No need to go to a bookstore to buy one (assuming you could find a book-store that carried them). You need only jump online, and with a few clicks of the mouse, you are reading *die Zeitung*. It's even possible to log on to NASA's Web site at any time and access live video footage from space. No matter what our interest may be, we can easily and quickly find information about it on the Net. This immediate access plays directly into our society's demand to have desires gratified instantly. We want to get what we want immediately, and everything that's available on the Internet can be reached very quickly—not just information, but communication via instant messag-ing, chat rooms, and e-mail.

The Internet's ease of use further adds to its seductive and intoxicating nature. Surfing the Net requires only a computer and Internet access; one can find access at home, at work, in libraries, in cybercafés, and at the homes of friends and neighbors. Need a Net "fix"? Access can be quickly at hand.

Take this inherently intoxicating nature of the Net and add to it access to sex—an obviously powerful force in people's lives—and its draw is even stronger. Having the easy and immediate access the Net provides to whatever kind of sexual experiences, information, pictures, and videos you want is enormously alluring. Once online, hours can slip by unnoticed, almost as though one is in an intoxicating trance.

In addition, cybersex provides a perfect opportunity for people to develop sexual fantasies and objectify others without the fear of rejection. In fact, the CD-ROM versions of adult sexual material often let the user choose the ideal partner and ideal situation—one step beyond noninteractive magazines. The computer user may choose a partner's gender, age, hair, skin, body type, and eye color, as well as whatever sexual scenario he or she wants to engage in. Some sexual CD-ROM titles are disguised in the form of a game. Perhaps a sexual mystery must be solved or an adventure taken in which users have to solve puzzles or find clues that lead them to their next sexual "conquest." The common factor among all cybersex material is that the user is free to become part of the fantasy without responsibility, consequence, or rejection. What's more, the variety of possibilities on the Internet is truly mind-boggling: whatever kind of sexual activity or depiction you can think of, you can likely find it on the Net.

These six components of the CyberHex increase the chances that the Internet will become a problem for those who already struggle with sexual compulsivity and for those who are emotionally or psychologically vulnerable to such sexual availability.

While research in the area of cybersex usage is only beginning, a recent survey by Al Cooper, David L. Delmonico, and Ron Burg of 9,265 Internet users describes three categories of people who use the Internet for sexual pursuits:[7]

- Recreational users access online sexual material more out of curiosity or for entertainment purposes and are not typically seen as having problems associated with their online sexual behaviors.

- At-risk users may never have developed a problem with online sexuality if not for the availability of the Internet. These individuals use the Internet a moderate amount of time for sexual activities, and if their pattern of use continues, it could become compulsive.
- Sexually compulsive users, due to a propensity for pathological sexual expression, use the Internet as a forum for their sexual activities. For people in this group in particular, the power of isolation, fantasy, anonymity, and affordability interacts with certain underlying personality factors to increase their use of the Internet for sexual activities to the point where it becomes difficult, if not impossible, for them to control it. We also want to note here that compulsion is a sign of an addictive disorder. In the addiction field, one of the signs of addiction to alcohol or another drug is that someone uses the substance compulsively.

The study also found that while 84 percent of the respondents did not meet criteria for cybersex compulsivity, 6 percent scored in a way that suggested cybersex compulsivity. A third group of approximately 10 percent of the entire sample also emerged as those at-risk users who may not be exhibiting all signs of cybersex compulsion, but who are in a potentially dangerous stage with their behavior. According to a 2006 Nielsen survey, there are 322 million active Internet users. Extrapolating from the cybersex use percentages in the study by Cooper, Delmonico, and Burg, approximately 20 million people (6 percent of 322 million) need intervention for their sexually compulsive use of cybersex. In addition to these 20 million, there are 32 million individuals (10 percent of 322 million) who are using cybersex moderately and show beginning signs of sexual compulsivity. Their continued use can predictably be a significant danger to many of them. It is also important to note that the above approximations are thought to be conservative estimates.

There is little doubt that use of the Internet will continue to explode. As people spend more time online and look to the Internet to fulfill an ever greater number of sexual needs and fantasies, the problems associated with online sexuality will become increasingly prevalent.

2

Do I Have a Problem with Cybersex?

IN THIS CHAPTER, we will help you examine your own use of sexually explicit material on the Internet. You may have many questions about when or even if using the Internet for sex is a real problem for you. By reading the stories of others, you'll be able to look more closely at your own Internet behavior and determine whether it's a problem or not.

In chapter 1, we looked at the many ways people use the Internet for sex. Reading about these people may have left you wondering about how you and others view your use of the Internet. You might now be asking yourself, "Do I have a problem with my sexual use of the Internet?" "How would I know if there's a problem?" "Am I at risk for sexually problematic behavior on the Internet?" or "Just what *is* 'problematic' sexual behavior on the Internet?"

Let's take a moment to clarify our use of the word "problematic." When a particular behavior or a set of behaviors begins to interfere with other aspects of your life, psychologists, psychiatrists, and counselors call them problematic. This simply means that these behaviors are causing problems and jeopardizing important areas in your life. Let's say, for example, that you've been using the Internet for sex more than ever lately. You've gone online with the intention of staying there for thirty minutes only to suddenly realize that two or three hours have slipped by. On more than one occasion, this "slipup" had some consequence—once you missed an important business appointment and another time you were late picking up your daughter from soccer. Perhaps you learned of some consequence only later. It's not unusual for people to be unaware of the consequences their actions are having in their own and other people's lives.

When isolated instances like this occur, they probably are not an indication of a problem. However, if they continue or increase, it may be a signal to pay more attention to what is happening. As these behaviors increase and we become aware of them, we may try to avoid or minimize consequences by attempting to control the problematic behavior. Unfortunately, during this time it also becomes more and more difficult to clearly see what is happening to us and more difficult to control our behaviors.

INDICATORS OF PROBLEMATIC BEHAVIOR

Three criteria are often used as indicators of problematic behavior. They are compulsivity, continuation despite consequences, and obsession.[1] A detailed description of each follows.

COMPULSIVITY

This is the loss of the ability to choose freely whether to stop or continue a behavior. In our daily lives, we establish habit-forming routines. We often get up at the same time every day, brush our teeth in the same way, keep a workbench or cupboard arranged in a particular order, put the same arm into a shirt first when getting dressed, or shop at the same grocery store week after week. We repeat many behaviors, often to the point where they become habits. We could even say that habits serve a useful function in that they free us from having to actually think about what we're doing all the time. Imagine if every single time you put on your shirt or brushed your teeth, you had to think about how you were going to do it.

Compulsive behavior is altogether different from simple daily or rigid habits. It is out-of-control behavior marked by deeply entangled rituals and obsessions along with overwhelming feelings of frustration, self-blame, powerlessness, and hopelessness. Sean experienced these feelings and shares his story about what life is like when using cybersex compulsively:

> I had long fantasized about going to a strip club, but had never followed through because I was worried about being recognized by someone I knew when entering or leaving the club. I knew I would die of embarrassment if my wife or friends found out. One day at home, I was surfing porn sites when I discovered a link to a site that offered live

video feeds from a strip club—twenty-four hours a day, no less! Here was the answer to my dreams.

That first time, I stayed online for a couple hours . . . until I heard the garage door opening when my wife and kids arrived home. Forced to quickly jump offline, I was already wondering when I could find a way to get back to "the club."

That opportunity came the following evening when everyone in my family was tired after a busy weekend and headed to bed. Though I was tired too, I made an excuse about needing to finish a report for work and headed into my home office, where I again logged on to the live feed from the strip club. Riveted to the screen, I watched for hours until I could no longer stay awake. The next day at work, I began obsessing again about this new discovery and decided that perhaps during my lunch hour, I could just jump on to that site for a few minutes—which I subsequently did.

Soon, I found myself visiting "the club" more and more often. So often, in fact, that I became concerned about the amount of time I was spending online. I was staying up at night more and more often. I was visiting more and more often at work, and for longer periods of time. So I made a promise to myself that I'd just set some rules up for my use. I made a commitment to stop visiting while at work altogether and to visit at home only every other day for thirty minutes.

That promise to myself was broken only two evenings later when I was online at home for two and a half hours. I rationalized by saying, "Well, everyone is gone, so what difference does it make?" Slowly, my time online at the strip club steadily increased. It became an obsession for me. I just couldn't stay away from it.

CONTINUATION DESPITE CONSEQUENCES

It is common to continue the behavior despite adverse consequences, such as loss of health, job, relationships, marriage, or freedom. All behaviors have consequences—some positive and some negative. At a relatively basic level, if we brush and floss our teeth regularly, we'll have a more positive experience at the dental office. If we neglect our teeth, the consequences will include painful dental procedures and costly dental bills. We learn how to work cooperatively and meet expectations on the job, thus avoiding being fired. Most of the time, we are able to look at our behavior and make the appropriate changes to reduce negative consequences. Unfortunately, this isn't always the case.

At first, Sean didn't see any negative consequences resulting from his Internet use. But it was only a matter of time before he was discovered.

One weekend afternoon, my wife and kids were out visiting my wife's sister. Not expecting them home for a couple more hours, I was deeply engrossed in a new online strip club I'd recently located and I never heard her car pull up in the driveway. Walking past my home office window, my wife inadvertently glanced in and saw me sitting at the computer screen masturbating. She bolted into the house and said, "Sean, my God, what were you doing? What if one of the children had seen you? How often do you do this? Whenever I'm not around? And why? Why?"

I made up a string of apologies and promised to behave myself in the future. I didn't dare visit the online strip club at home anymore. Instead, I began spending more time at work visiting sexually explicit sites. One day, however, a company memo was circulated warning all employees that our Internet usage was now being monitored during work hours and that visiting porn sites was expressly forbidden. I knew that the company was serious. In fact, I'd heard of another employee who'd been caught surfing porn sites, and he was warned that if he did it again, he'd be fired on the spot.

Realizing I'd better be careful, I decided that I'd only go to "the club" before or after hours when almost no one was around, and I'd only stay online for ten or fifteen minutes. I convinced myself that I wouldn't really be violating company policy if I wasn't surfing the porn sites during actual working hours. After a week, I found this regimen too difficult and began trying to find a way to go to my "club" more often. I started believing that maybe visiting during my lunch hour would be safe. I sincerely thought that by now enough time had passed since my wife discovered my computer activity and it was OK to start visiting the "club" again on my home computer, too, as long as I was careful.

Despite Sean's attempts at control and potentially dire consequences, he continued his behavior and no longer thought about how he could stop it.

Instead, he tried to find a way to visit his "club" without incurring any negative consequences. Sean's experience also reveals the indirect consequences of his behavior—and how he is unaware of them. By calculating the number of hours Sean spent online in his "club" at work and multiplying that by his hourly wage, it is easy to see that his employer lost thousands of dollars in productivity. What might have—or should have—Sean accomplished for his company in the hours he was "missing" at work?

OBSESSION

Obsession means being so preoccupied, you focus exclusively on a particular behavior (in this case, sex) to the exclusion of other parts of your life and without care for the consequences of that behavior. You are obsessed with something when you just can't stop thinking about it. It occupies much of your mental energy most of the time. In our example, Sean had become obsessed with using the Internet to visit particular Web sites, especially the strip clubs.

By this point, Sean really lived in one of three states of mind: planning his next visit to an online strip club, being online, and coming down from a visit. In one way or another, online strip clubs were always on Sean's mind. When he was at work in a meeting, for example, Sean was thinking about how long it was going to last. He was trying to figure out whether he'd have ten minutes or so during a break to go online.

Sean became very creative about finding additional time for cybersex activities:

> One day, a great idea came to me. Occasionally, my wife and I would have wine with our dinner. This usually made her pretty tired and she'd go to bed earlier than usual and sleep pretty soundly on those nights. So, I fabricated a story about how I had decided we ought to try some better wines and have them with dinner more regularly, "like the Europeans do." Shelly agreed and was actually quite excited about this. Pretty soon, we were drinking a bottle of wine with nearly every dinner, and as a result, my wife was often in bed and sound asleep by nine. Looking back, I'm embarrassed to say that I was proud of myself for coming up with this idea and actually carrying it out.

TEN CRITERIA OF PROBLEMATIC ONLINE SEXUAL BEHAVIOR

Earlier we talked about the difficulty in deciding how to determine whether a given online sexual behavior is actually problematic. Taking into consideration Sean's account of his online sexual behavior, do you think he has a problem? To help you evaluate your own online behavior, we've developed the following set of ten criteria. As you read through them, pay close attention to those that seem to apply to your life.

1. Preoccupation with sex on the Internet

This is more than just thinking about online sex; it's not being able to *not* think about it. At some level, these thoughts are always with you. You find yourself regularly wondering how you can orchestrate your life in ways that will allow you time online. You think about past online sexual experiences or about what future online experiences will be like. You can't seem to get away from thoughts about online sex. You may even find yourself dreaming about sex on the Internet. It's there in both your conscious and unconscious life.

2. Frequently engaging in sex on the Internet more often or for longer periods of time than intended

When you look at the amount of time you're spending online, you see that it has been increasing. You decided, for example, to go online for sex for just an hour, but when you looked at the clock, you realized you'd been on for more than two hours. You don't know where the time went. Perhaps you told yourself you could be online for just two hours from midnight to 2:00 A.M., but suddenly you discover it's 4:00 A.M. and you're still online. You had originally been going online for sex-related activities a couple days a week. Now you're on daily and not just once, but four, five, six, or more times per day. You keep track of your time for a few days and discover that you're actually spending five hours a day online for sex-related activities.

In a sense, you are developing a "tolerance" to Internet usage. The concept of tolerance is common in the field of drug and alcohol addiction. When people begin drinking, for example, they may feel intoxicated after only one or two beers. Over time, however, their bodies develop a tolerance to alcohol, and they find that they need six, eight, or twelve bottles of beer to achieve that same high. This concept applies to Internet sex too. Many people have discovered that they have a psychological need to be online more and more over time to achieve the same high.

3. Repeated unsuccessful efforts to control, cut back on, or stop engaging in sex on the Internet

Once you realized that the amount of time you'd been spending for sex online was excessive, you decided to set some limits. Perhaps you promised yourself that you would go online only once a day or week and only for thirty minutes at a time. Or maybe you decided to quit cold turkey for a week or to go online only on weekends. But whatever promise you made to yourself, you couldn't keep it. Maybe your attempts at control worked for a few days, a week, several weeks, or even a month, but eventually something happened and you "needed" to go back online. No matter what you tried, you eventually returned to the Internet for sexual activities.

4. Restlessness or irritability when attempting to limit or stop engaging in sex on the Internet

When you've attempted to stop or limit your online sexual activity, you've found that you become nervous and irritable. If you haven't noticed this yourself, think about what others who know you—family members, friends, work colleagues—would say if you asked them about this. Often these people will recognize changes in your behavior before you yourself can see them. Do you know someone who has recently quit smoking? If so, how did this person act in the first days and weeks without a cigarette? Is this similar to how you act when you try to stop or limit your online activities?

5. Using sex on the Internet as a way of escaping from problems or relieving feelings such as helplessness, guilt, anxiety, or depression

Everyone has feelings of helplessness, sorrow, worry, depression, and anger. There are many ways to address or cope with these feelings. When you are just feeling down and would like a little boost or pick-me-up, do you turn to the Internet for a sexual release so you can feel better and function at home or work?

6. *Returning to sex on the Internet day after day in search of a more intense or higher-risk sexual experience*

Your expectations of what you want out of the Internet continue to increase and become more elaborate. You might hope to find your true love via the Internet. At first, you may drop into chat rooms, remaining anonymous, just to see whether you could find a potential mate online. Eventually, being anonymous no longer does it for you. Your search of various chat rooms becomes more intense, frantic, and time-consuming. After connecting with one man in particular, you begin corresponding privately with him via e-mail. Eventually, you arrange a meeting with him for sex in a hotel. The excitement and hope you feel in your search lead to more risky behavior both on and off the Internet.

What have you been looking for on the Internet? How has that changed from when you first started going online? Are you moving into areas you once told yourself you'd never explore?

7. *Lying to family members, therapists, or others to conceal involvement with sex on the Internet*

In our culture, most people are secretive about their sex lives, regardless of whether their behavior is normal or problematic. What is of concern is being dishonest about it when asked. When Sean was questioned by his wife about his late nights on the computer, he regularly answered by saying that it was a work-related project with a tight deadline. When initially confronted about his use of the Internet for sexual purposes, Sean lied to his wife and told her it was his first time.

Have you lied about using the Internet for sex-related activities? Have you downplayed your involvement or failed to be honest about your involvement to a spouse, partner, boss, or therapist? Have you used the "just curious" excuse?

8. *Committing illegal sexual acts online (for example, sending or downloading child pornography or soliciting illegal sex acts online)*

Certain activities on the Internet have been declared illegal in many, if not all, states. As people use the Internet for sex-related activities, and as they increase their time on the Net, some also move closer and closer to engaging in illegal behaviors. A forty-year-old male who'd fantasized about having sex with a teenager for several years eventually began visiting a teen chat room. He engaged in a conversation with a thirteen-year-old female for some time before moving the relationship to a point where he asked where he could meet her to have sex. Soliciting sex acts with minors online is illegal, just as sending, exchanging, or downloading child pornography is illegal. These are felony offenses that, in many states, will result in mandatory prison time. Have you engaged in or are you thinking about such actions?

9. Jeopardizing or losing a significant relationship, job, or educational or career opportunity because of online sexual behavior

Online sex-related activities can have serious consequences. Ray downloaded a child pornography image to a chat room. As a result, he was arrested through an undercover operation. The shame of being charged with felony counts for sexual exploitation of a minor became overwhelming, and the consequences rippled through every aspect of his life. Because of escalating legal fees, he lost most of his savings and retirement funds. He was closing on his new home the day the search warrant was served. Consequently, he lived in his new home for only two days before he had to sell it as a result of this crime. He lost a well-paying, prestigious job with tremendous advancement potential in an excellent corporation. He endured house arrest and faced a potential prison term of 220 years. Ray had been respected in his community and was on numerous boards and committees. This all ended with his arrest.

What parts of your life are being affected by your online sexual behavior? Have you jeopardized or lost a significant relationship? What about a job, a career, or your health and well-being?

10. Incurring significant financial consequences as a result of engaging in online sexual behavior

While basic Internet access can be fairly inexpensive, many cybersex sites charge a monthly access fee. A thirty-two-year-old male client was shocked when he opened his credit card bill one day to find charges totaling more than twelve hundred dollars. He'd been registering to enter various cybersex sites and had completely lost track of how many he'd paid for. A twenty-three-year-old female client received an Internet server bill for hundreds of dollars. She'd spent six or so hours per day in chat rooms and had sailed miles past her free-minute limit without having any idea of the charges that were accruing. Another male client spent forty thousand dollars in one month dating high-priced call girls and using cocaine. He'd arranged for both through an online prostitution service.

Have you felt the financial consequences of your time online? How many memberships are you paying for each month? What are your monthly Internet fees? Have you lost job or educational opportunities because of your time online?

WHAT IT MEANS FOR YOU

We assume that you are reading this book because you or someone who cares about you is concerned about your use of the Internet for sex-related activities. The most important step you can take now is to look honestly at your Internet behavior *and* the consequences of that behavior. Perhaps you're spending more time than you really want in sex-related Internet activities. This should sound an alarm indicating that something is out of balance and that you need to take action and seek help.

If you can relate to three or more of the ten criteria for problematic online sexual behavior, your online activities are probably a problem. This is not something you should ignore, and the sooner you act to make changes in your life, the easier it will be for you to overcome this problem.

Complete the following Internet Sex Screening Test to further examine your online behavior:

INTERNET SEX SCREENING TEST
Read each statement carefully and answer honestly. If it is true or mostly true for you, mark the blank with a T. If it is false or mostly false, mark the blank with an F. After answering all thirty-four questions, add the number of statements you marked true in part 1 and part 2.[2]

Part 1

_____ 1. I have some sexual sites bookmarked.

_____ 2. I spend more than five hours per week using my computer for sexual pursuits.

___ 3. I have joined sexual sites to gain access to online sexual material.

___ 4. I have purchased sexual products online.

___ 5. I have searched for sexual material through an Internet search tool.

___ 6. I have spent more money for online sexual material than I planned.

___ 7. Internet sex has sometimes interfered with certain aspects of my life.

___ 8. I have participated in sexually related chats.

___ 9. I have a sexualized username or nickname that I use on the Internet.

___ 10. I have masturbated while on the Internet.

___ 11. I have accessed sexual sites from computers in locations other than my home.

___ 12. No one knows I use my computer for sexual purposes.

___ 13. I have tried to hide what is on my computer or monitor so others cannot see it.

___ 14. I have stayed up after midnight to access sexual material online.

___ 15. I use the Internet to experiment with different aspects of sexuality, such as bondage, homosexuality, or anal sex.

___ 16. I have my own Web site that contains some sexual material.

___ 17. I have made promises to myself to stop using the Internet for sexual purposes.

___ 18. I sometimes use cybersex as a reward for accomplishing something such as finishing a project or enduring a stressful day.

___ 19. When I am unable to access sexual information online, I feel anxious, angry, or disappointed.

___ 20. I have increased the risks I take online, such as giving out my name and phone number or meeting people offline.

___ 21. I have punished myself when I use the Internet for sexual purposes, such as arranging a time-out from my computer or canceling Internet subscriptions.

___ 22. I have met face-to-face with someone I met online for romantic purposes.

___ 23. I use sexual humor and innuendo with others while online.

___ 24. I have run across illegal sexual material while on the Internet.

___ 25. I believe I am an Internet sex addict.

Part 2

___ 26. I repeatedly attempt to stop certain sexual behaviors and fail.

___ 27. I continue my sexual behavior despite it having caused me problems.

___ 28. Before my sexual behavior, I want it, but afterward I regret it.

___ 29. I have lied often to conceal my sexual behavior.

___ 30. I believe I am a sex addict.

___ 31. I worry about people finding out about my sexual behavior.

___ 32. I have made an effort to quit a certain type of sexual activity and have failed.

___ 33. I hide some of my sexual behavior from others.

___ 34. When I have sex, I feel depressed afterward.

Total number of statements marked true for part 1: _____

Total number of statements marked false for part 2: _____

Scoring the Internet Sex Screening Test

For part 1 (items 1 through 25), total the number of items you indicated were true for you. Use the chart below to determine if Internet sex may be problematic for you.

1 to 8 items marked true = You may or may not have a problem with your sexual behavior on the Internet. You are in a low-risk group, but if the Internet is causing problems in your life, seek a professional who can conduct further assessment.

9 to 18 items marked true = You are at risk for your sexual behavior to interfere with significant areas of your life. If you are concerned about your sexual behavior online, and you have noticed consequences as a result of your online behavior, you should seek a professional who can further assess and help you with your concerns.

19 or more items marked true = You are at the highest risk for your behavior to interfere with and jeopardize important areas of your life (social, occupational, and educational, for example). You should discuss your online sexual behaviors with a professional who can further assess and assist you.

Part 2 (items 26 through 34) is an abbreviated version of the Sexual Addiction Screening Test (SAST). These items should be reviewed for general sexual addiction behavior, not specifically for cybersex. Although there are no cutoff scores calculated for these items, a high number of true items in part 1 paired with a high number of true items in part 2 should be seen as a greater risk for sexual acting-out behavior on the Internet. Please note: part 2 should not be calculated in the total score for part 1.

You've taken an important, positive first step by beginning to read this book and showing a willingness to begin exploring and addressing the problem. Be assured that you can find help here to better understand and regain control over your online sex-related behavior.

On the other hand, you may not recognize yourself as having a problem. If you see a pattern in your Internet behavior that seems similar to the problematic behavior we've explored thus far, this may be an indication that you are at risk for problems and that you would do well to learn more about your behavior and your reasons for using the Internet for sexual activities. If you can relate to only some examples or feel that a partner might have a problem with online sexual behavior, read on.

Remember that no set of criteria or test is an absolutely accurate measure or indication of a problem. Tests do not deal well with individual differences and behaviors. Screenings are based on the behavior of many people; they are not capable of measuring individual differences or of addressing every kind of behavior. Scoring between 9 and 18 could indicate that you do have some behaviors that may be problematic or that will eventually become problematic.

Once again, if you are reading this book because you are concerned about your use of the Internet for sex-related activities, pay attention to that, regardless of your score on the screening test.

If you don't feel you have a problem and you scored below nineteen on the screening, but are reading this book at the suggestion of someone who cares about you, pay attention. As you likely know, those who know us can often see our lives and our behavior in ways we cannot. It's difficult to be objective with ourselves. It's important to realize that others may see you having a problem that you do not see.

We also want to point out that sex-related activity on the Internet covers a broad range of activities, as indicated in chapter 1. Problematic behaviors lie on a continuum, from those that are relatively harmless to those that are compulsive or addictive and pose serious health, relationship, and legal risks.

In chapter 3, we will more closely examine problematic sexual behavior on the Internet. You'll learn more about why people use the Internet for sex, how problems develop and manifest themselves, and the potential consequences of sex-related behavior on the Internet.

3

Understanding Problematic Sexual Behavior on the Internet

IN THIS CHAPTER, we will look in greater detail at the types of problematic online sexual behavior, and show you how that behavior can become so compulsive that it seems impossible to control. Not everyone who is using the Internet for sexual activities does so for the same reason or to the same extent. We can divide those who are engaging in sexual behavior on the Internet into five groups: recreational users, sexual harassers, discovery, predisposed, and lifelong sexually compulsive. The diagram on page 35 illustrates these five groups. Recreational users of cybersex as a rule have little, if any, problem with compulsive or addictive cybersex use. Sexual harassers are individuals who use material on or from the Internet intrusively with others. Although people in any of the five categories could become compulsive with their Internet sex behavior, the individuals most likely to develop problems at this level are the lifelong sexually compulsive. It should be noted that the term "sex offender" may apply to any of these categories. Sex offender is a legal term indicating that someone has broken a law with regard to a sexual behavior—on or off the Internet. Therefore, this term may be applicable to any cybersex user category since even recreational users may commit illegal sexual behaviors online.

RECREATIONAL USERS

The people in the recreational users category seem to be able to explore sex on the Internet without any sign that their behavior is becoming problematic. They may, in fact, use cybersex as a way to enhance their sexual experiences

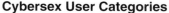

Cybersex User Categories

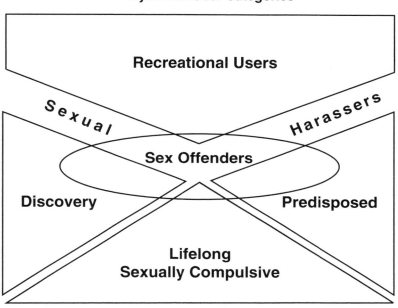

Figure 3.1

in a positive way. The recreational users category tends to be the largest group of Internet sex users and may account for as much as 80 percent of all cybersex users. These users tend to report few, if any, consequences as a result of their behavior and do not admit to any life area (social, occupational, educational, or others) being in jeopardy as a result of their cybersex behaviors.

SEXUAL HARASSERS

The sexual harasser uses information, photos, or other items found on the Internet in sexually intrusive or exploitive ways. The individual may, for example, show a photograph, joke, or Web site he or she discovered on the Internet to others, such as work colleagues, family members, or friends who may be offended or embarrassed by it. Typically, sexual harassers do so not as a means of intentionally hurting or embarrassing others, but simply because they think such information is funny. However, sometimes the sexual harasser shares inappropriate information from the Internet as a way to shock others or become covertly aroused by the power they feel or by the sexualized content of the material.

PROBLEMATIC CYBERSEX USERS

People who have problematic sexual behavior on the Internet tend to fall into one of three groups:

1. Discovery Group: those who have no previous problem with online sex nor any history of problematic sexual behavior
2. Predisposed Group: those who have had their first out-of-control sexual behavior on the Internet after years of obsessing over unacted-on sexual fantasies and urges
3. Lifelong Sexually Compulsive Group: those whose out-of-control sexual behavior on the Internet is part of an ongoing and severe sexual behavior problem

DISCOVERY GROUP

People in this group have no previous problem with online sex and no history of problematic sexual behavior. Shania's story is typical of this group:

> In my mid-twenties, I led quite a conservative life when it came to sex. I'd never had a sexual relationship or even kissed anyone before. It wasn't that I didn't have an interest in men. I just hadn't found a good way to approach and meet eligible guys. One day while surfing the Net, I discovered the realm of Internet sex, and it rocked my world. I suddenly felt free to explore relationships and my own sexuality. I spent hours and hours online visiting sexually oriented chat rooms and writing ads for online personal columns. Soon I discovered I was attracted to men from other countries. After finding one seemingly very attractive man, I made arrangements to meet him on a cruise ship. How did it turn out? The cruise was fine, but the guy was anything but. He was crude, physically not at all how he'd depicted himself, and he had the personality of a dead fish. But despite this and other so-so experiences, I've continued to rendezvous with other guys. I'm sure I'll find "Mr. Right" one of these times.

There is, in a sense, a healthy aspect to Shania's story in that she had wanted to have sexual relationships and the Internet freed her to do so. She discovered and explored her ideas about relationships and sexuality through the Internet. On the other hand, Shania became completely carried away with her online activities, spending countless hours at her computer and avoiding reality. By courting and meeting strangers about whom she actually knew nothing, Shania also put herself in great danger. She could have chosen instead to use one of the many dating services available that carefully screen their members.

Gerry is another person who had no history of problematic sexual behavior before discovering the realm of cybersex. He had had no previous arrests or any history of compulsive sexual behavior. In his mid-forties, Gerry came to treatment as part of a sentencing agreement after he had been arrested for trying to meet a teenage girl whom he'd first contacted online. Here is Gerry's story:

> I was a man whose children were grown up and out of the house. I was unhappy in my marriage and dissatisfied with my job. I felt that, given my age, I should have had more responsibility and been making more money in my career. One night, I stumbled upon a cybersex site. I began playing around just to see what was out there, and in a matter of weeks I couldn't stay away. Gradually, my Internet use increased from thirty minutes to an hour, then two hours or more every night. I began spending fifteen to twenty hours a week online, surfing porn sites and visiting chat rooms where I tried to hook up with young girls. Before I knew what had happened, I was obsessed with cybersex activities. After my arrest, I admitted that I knew the "girl" I was trying to meet (who was actually an adult male FBI agent) was under eighteen, but I was so flattered by the thought of her wanting to meet me that I arranged the rendezvous anyway. I knew I was taking a chance but just couldn't stop myself.

Predisposed Group

This group comprises people who had never acted out sexually—though they had thought about it—until they discovered cybersex. They might have fantasized about exposing themselves or had the urge to see a prostitute or go to strip clubs. Until the arrival of cybersex they were, however, able to control those fantasies and urges. They might have been afraid of being recognized at a strip club or being busted in a prostitution sting. Perhaps they simply were healthy enough and possessed adequate coping skills to recognize and resist acting impulsively.

When it comes to Internet use, people in this group may use the Net for sexual purposes—perhaps looking at pornography, occasionally visiting a chat room or a voyeur site—but not too often . . . five, six, or seven hours a week at most.

They are, however, at risk for more problematic online sexual behavior. With the Internet, sex is just a click away. And at some point, they discover sexually explicit activities that they just can't resist. They may become attracted to live-feed strip clubs or live video of women having sex. At first, the consequences of doing these activities may seem minimal. After all, no one will see them or recognize them online.

Sharon's story is an excellent example of this behavior:

> I had often wondered about what it would be like to have sex with another woman. I was thirty-four, happily married with two children, and generally happy with my life. Over the past few years, I'd heard more about bisexuality and realized that I had bisexual tendencies. I didn't know how to explain the sexual feelings I'd have for other women as well as those for my husband. I was more curious than ever now, but I'd always been a little afraid to act on these feelings. And I didn't know, really, how I could go about meeting a woman who had similar feelings. Besides, I wasn't interested just in sex. I wanted a real relationship where I could feel some connection to her too. Since I'd occasionally visited chat rooms in the past, one night I decided to search for one focused on lesbianism. To my surprise, I found one quickly. I was instantly intrigued and began spending more time online in lesbian-oriented chat rooms. While my online explorations were initially positive experiences and helped me sort out my feelings, I began to spend so much time online that other aspects of my life became affected. My work life suffered as a result of too many late nights on the computer. And I had less time and energy for my family too.

Don provides another excellent example of this behavior:

After twelve years of marriage, I felt that there just had to be more to a relationship. I'd never been unfaithful to my wife and didn't intend to because I felt that it was simply morally wrong. But I was becoming more and more frustrated with my marriage as time passed. Over the years, I had spent much time fantasizing about having affairs with other women. Almost by chance, I found a chat room in which there were others like me with similar feelings about their relationships. I "met" and began conversing with a woman, and soon we both found that we had much in common. Our conversations were fun, interesting, and progressively more sex-related. I loved how I felt after my time online—energized, happy, supported, and satisfied. Eventually, we began having sex online. Was I being unfaithful? I decided I wasn't because I wasn't really having actual sex with anyone. In fact, I wasn't even physically with this woman. I didn't even know her real name. After a few months, however, online sexuality wasn't fulfilling enough for me. I wanted to meet this woman I'd been conversing with online in person. She lived fairly close to me, as it turned out, so we met at a local hotel for dinner and sex—and in so doing, I crossed my own boundary into infidelity. Since I had already crossed the line, I had nothing more to lose by continuing this behavior. And it had all been so easy—easy to arrange meeting women online who were interested in sex; easy to meet them in person; and easy to have sex with them. My illicit liaisons increased in frequency. Before I knew what was happening, I was becoming involved with more and more women.

Part of the power of cybersex is that it's one step removed from reality. Having thoughts and urges and fantasies and then acting on them via the Internet seems different from acting on them in real time. We are not face-to-face, literally, with another human being. We can't look into their eyes, feel their touch, read their emotions, or in any other way physically interact with them. Cyber-interactions feel more remote, safer. The "other" is out there somewhere, at arm's length. We tend to view the computer as a magical place where everything is safe and secure. We can be whoever we want to be, with no apparent consequences.

This distance, this step apart, however, also makes it easier to cross lines that we would not otherwise cross—something that's not uncommon for people in this group. Don, for example, swore he'd never have an affair, but that is exactly what he was doing, albeit initially without actual physical contact. That "step apart" made it very easy for him to rationalize and excuse his behavior when meeting women in hotels for offline sexual encounters. People in this group often have clear boundaries around their urges or fantasies—until they encounter the cyber-world where they feel OK about pushing beyond them. Once that boundary is stretched or breached, little may be left to control behavior.

LIFELONG SEXUALLY COMPULSIVE GROUP

People in this group have been involved in problematic sexual behavior throughout most, if not all, of their lives. They might compulsively masturbate, use pornography, practice voyeurism or exhibitionism, or frequent strip clubs and prostitutes. For these people, while cybersex provides a new option for acting out sexually, it fits within their already existing patterns of problematic behavior.

Gene's story is typical of people in this group:

As a child, I was sexually abusive to my younger brother. During adolescence, I frequently exposed myself to others. This behavior began as a bit of a joke at first. I would "streak" through a sporting event or beach, for example. There was a dark side too. I had a history of molesting children, but in more discreet and subtle ways. I would invite a young child to sit on my lap and then fondle her—but always in the context of trying to move the child off my lap. During my mid-thirties, I was finally arrested for exposing myself to teenage girls. When I came into treatment, I revealed that I had a lengthy history of exposing myself at a well-known department store as well as a long history of using pornography and compulsive masturbation.

As a skilled computer programmer, I discovered sex online before most people had even heard of the Internet. I primarily ventured into cybersex while on the job. When I was at work, I couldn't expose myself and I couldn't have pornographic magazines lying around my office, so I instead visited porn sites. I spent hours each day in nudist, exhibitionist, and voyeuristic sex sites, with a particular preference for nudist sites with pictures of children.

How was it that I was never caught? Since I provided computer and Internet tech support for employees, I arranged my computer in such a way that I could still talk on the phone and provide support and yet keep my computer monitor screen hidden from anyone who just happened by. I was very savvy at multitasking. I could be surfing sex sites and at the same time provide help to others over the phone. Thanks to my computer skills, I was able to thwart any site blockouts or attempts by my company's tech information services staff to monitor my online behavior.

My preferred behaviors were exposing myself and window peeping. I entered treatment after being arrested for exposing myself to two girls at a department store. I initially denied this behavior, and then claimed it wasn't sexual. The truth was that I used cybersex merely as a stopgap measure while I was at work because I didn't dare expose myself there.

Gene's story shows the intensity of what it's like to have out-of-control sexual behavior and how it is fueled by accessing sex online. There are three separate subgroups within the lifelong sexually compulsive group. First, there are those people who use the Internet as an additional way of acting out with the same behaviors they use offline. A person may have long used pornography and compulsively masturbated. The advent of the Internet now provides this person with a new source of pornography. Someone like Gene, who exposes himself regularly, can do so now on the Net using a Webcam with far less risk than doing so in public.

A second group of people includes those who see the Internet as a less risky way of acting out. Sean, whom we met in chapter 2 and who enjoyed frequenting live video feeds from strip clubs, could now spend time in teen chat rooms communicating with young girls. As long as he didn't try to meet them, he felt he was being safe with his behavior. Cybersex allows these people to feed their compulsion—in virtual anonymity—and receive the rush of doing so with less risk than if they were interacting face-to-face with another person.

The final group includes people whose sexual behavior is out of control already and who use the Internet to further increase the danger associated with their sexual behavior. Mark's fascination with young girls accelerated after using the Internet:

> I loved to cruise past school yards during recess and other places where children congregated, but I never went so far as to risk actually talking to any of them. Instead, I'd drive by and fantasize about stopping, picking up a young girl, talking to her, and fondling her. Through the Internet, I found that I could easily have personal conversations with young girls. By actually communicating with children online, I had unknowingly crossed a line into more dangerous territory. This moved me another step closer to illegal behavior. It heightened my arousal and excitement, because I was actually doing what I had been afraid to do all the years when I had only been cruising for children.

SEX OFFENDERS

A sex offender in the cybersex user categories is someone who uses the Internet to commit an illegal sexual act. This includes viewing or distributing illegal images or videos, or using the Internet to have sexual conversations with minors and/or arranging to meet minors offline for sexual activity. Sex offenders can fall into other existing categories since sex offenses can occur in a variety of circumstances by individuals regardless of their history.

VIEWING A PROBLEMATIC SEXUAL BEHAVIOR AS AN ADDICTION

The people's stories contained in this book all involve a problem with their use of the Internet for sexual behavior, ranging from relatively minor to very serious. We would like to go one step further and help you to understand how these problematic sexual behaviors can, in some cases, actually be addictive behaviors.

A way to understand the behavior of someone like Gene is to compare his behaviors with those of alcohol and drug addicts. A common definition of alcoholism, for example, is that a person has a pathological relationship with this mood-altering chemical. The alcoholic's relationship with alcohol becomes more important than family, friends, and work. The relationship progresses to the point where alcohol use is necessary to feel normal. To feel "normal" for the alcoholic is also to feel isolated and lonely, since the primary relationship he or she depends on to feel adequate is with a chemical, not with other people.

A parallel pattern can be found among those people who have problematic sexual behaviors, including cybersex activities. Again, an addict substitutes a sick relationship with an event or a process for a healthy relationship with others. An addict's relationship with a mood-altering "experience" becomes central to his or her life. Gene, for example, routinely jeopardized all that he loved for the sake of his cybersex activities. His attempts to stop his behavior were lost against the power of his behaviors. According to this definition, Gene is addicted to cybersex.

Addicts progressively go through stages in which they retreat further from the reality of friends, family, and work. Their secret lives become more real than their public lives. Eventually, what other people know is a false identity. Only the person knows the shame of living a double life—the real world and the addict's world.

Leading a fantasy double life is a distortion of reality. Marcy, the middle-aged social worker whom we discussed in chapter 1, was so caught up in the thrill and fantasy of meeting men that she never considered the danger she was placing herself in until she was nearly murdered. An essential part of sanity is being grounded in reality. One thing is certain: addiction warps one's sense of reality.

THE ADDICT'S BELIEF SYSTEM

Addiction is a system, one with its own momentum. The more often you engage in the addictive behaviors, the more momentum your addiction has. The addictive system also has various component "parts," the first of which is a belief system. Addiction begins with delusional thought processes, which are rooted in the individual's belief system. That is, these people begin with core beliefs about themselves that affect how they perceive reality. This belief system is very important, and for now we will point out only its role in addicts' impaired thinking.

Each of us has a belief system that is the sum of the assumptions, judgments, and myths that we hold to be true. It contains potent family messages about our value or worth as people, our relationships, our basic needs, and our sexuality. It includes beliefs about men and women and having a secret life. Within it is a repertoire of what options—answers, solutions, methods, possibilities, and ways of behaving—are open to each of us. In short, it is our view of the world.

On the basis of that view, we plan and make decisions, interpret other people's actions, make meaning out of life experiences, solve problems, pattern our relationships, develop our careers, and establish priorities.

For each of us, our belief system is the filter through which we conduct the main task of our lives: making choices.

Core Beliefs

An addict's belief system contains certain core beliefs that are faulty or inaccurate and, consequently, provide a fundamental momentum of problematic behavior and addiction. Simply put, these are the four core beliefs:

1. I am basically a bad, unworthy person.
2. No one would love me as I am.
3. My needs are never going to be met if I depend on others.
4. Sex is my most important need. (For an alcoholic, it would be alcohol.)

Generally, addicts do not perceive themselves as worthwhile human beings. Nor do they believe other people would care for them or meet their needs if everything was known about them, including the addiction. Finally, those who have problems with sexual behavior believe that sex is their most important need. Sex is what makes isolation bearable. Their core beliefs are the anchor points of sexual addiction.

Our core beliefs are formed as we are growing up and are primarily developed within our families. Healthy families have the capacity to organize and reorganize as they grow and change. Children are supported and nurtured. Above all, children get the message that, despite mistakes and inappropriate behavior, they are worthwhile human beings who deserve love—and they are indeed loved.

In unhealthy families, however, children are abused and neglected. When parents don't nurture and support their children, these children make the assumption that they are not good human beings, that they are not worthy of love and affection, and they carry these attitudes into adulthood.

As adults, they do not perceive themselves as worthwhile, nor, again, do they believe other people would care for or love them. This extends into another core belief. Someone with this perception might state, "Since you will never love me anyway because of my innate badness, there's no reason for me to think you would want to do anything for me. I can't count on you to help, assist, support, or take care of me." This thinking destroys trust in others and leaves only one option: to survive, you must be in control. An equation is created: an increased level of distrust equals more controlling behavior. Sex becomes a source of nurturing that they believe they have control over. Finally, these people come to believe that sex is their most important need.

These core beliefs have become the anchor points of what, by our definition, is sexual addiction. Sex is what makes their isolation bearable. They believe that sex will fill the loneliness and that it will make them feel good. They have, however, mistaken sex for intimacy, a true connection with another. What they want and need is intimacy, but what they seek instead is sex. Without intimacy, sex will never fulfill their needs, no matter how much they get.

INTERNET AND DETACHMENT

The Internet and cybersex can be so powerful because the actual online experience can reinforce unhealthy coping mechanisms learned in childhood. When children experience traumatic situations, they often cope by dissociating (mentally and emotionally detaching) themselves from the traumatic situation. For children in such circumstances, this can be a useful strategy.

Such childhood coping mechanisms can, however, easily be carried forward into adulthood. But that causes problems. If, as children, they never learned how to be in a relationship, they will lack the interpersonal skills to interact with others on an emotional level. Additionally, when people encounter situations that remind them, even unconsciously, of childhood trauma, they automatically switch off. In other words, they dissociate, and by so doing they are not really in the present any longer. When this happens in relationships, it creates distance and prevents intimacy.

The Internet is a way to interact with others while keeping a barrier between you and other people. It is especially useful if you never learned healthy ways to engage with or relate to other people or if you don't trust or feel safe with them. You can remain anonymous and distant and never have to reveal your true identity or anything else about yourself. Sex in real time, no matter how impersonal, still requires some physical contact or proximity to another human being. For example, you have to tuck money into a stripper's G-string. Exposing yourself requires another person seeing you. Having some form of sex with a prostitute requires physical contact.

Cybersex provides the ultimate pseudo-connection with another person—the perfect impersonal personal relationship—with no hassles or demands or connection. Cybersex enables users to truly objectify the person on the other side of that computer connection. In real time, you are still forced to confront, at some level, the fact that you are interacting with a human being. He or she is there in front of you, moving, breathing, talking, and so on. On the Internet, nothing is really there, save a flickering image on a computer monitor.

In many ways, the Internet allows people to create a kind of cyber-dissociation. They remain detached from those with whom they are interacting. The ineffective coping mechanisms learned as a child can come into play seemingly without negative consequences. The cyber-world offers the ultimate form of detachment.

IMPAIRED THINKING

Out of the belief system—the set of interacting faulty beliefs—come distorted views of reality. Denial leads the list of ways addicts distort reality. They use many devices to deny to themselves and to others that there is a problem. Ignoring the problem, blaming others, and minimizing the behaviors are part of the addict's defensive repertoire. Consequences such as venereal disease, lost jobs, arrests, and broken relationships are either overlooked or attributed to factors other than their problematic sexual behavior.

> Arrest: "I wasn't really going to do anything with that girl; I just wanted to talk to her."

> Job loss: "My boss had it in for me anyway. Other guys were e-mailing hot pictures around too, and nothing happened to them."

> Relationship: "She's been looking for an excuse to dump me for years."

When these people believe in defensive rationalizations, the result is denial that a specific incident or behavior is part of an overall pattern.

Arguments, excuses, justifications, and circular reasoning abound in the person's impaired mental process:

"If I don't go online for sex every few days, the pressure builds up."

"I just have a high sex drive."

"What he doesn't know won't hurt him."

"If only my wife (or husband or partner) would be more responsive."

"We men are like animals—we're just more sexual than females."

"With the stress I am under, I deserve this."

"It doesn't hurt anyone because . . ."

"It's my way of relaxing."

"It's just on the computer."

"No one knows but me, and no one would care anyway."

No matter what rationalization is used, people who use statements like these are further cut off from the reality of their behavior. The people who make a commitment to themselves and others to change, quit, or follow through on a behavior are often sincere in their intentions. They may even experience a great deal of emotion—painful tears, expressions of tenderness, or anger when someone doesn't believe in their good intentions. When their behavior simply doesn't match up to their commitment, they begin defending a lie that they believe is true. This is an example of seriously impaired thinking. For those caught up in addictive sexual behaviors, there is tremendous delusion, and that delusion is just part of a much larger rationalization they use to justify all their behaviors. For example, a man who has been confronted by his partner because he was not at work when he was supposed to be tells a lie regarding his whereabouts. His partner doubts he is telling the truth. The man becomes incensed at his partner's distrust. He assumes that she would act this way even if he were telling the honest truth. His emotions about her distrust are real, and he's even angrier now. His lies and sincerity become fused.

Making declarations of love just to seduce the other person, becoming incensed at the behavior of an arresting officer just to obscure your own behavior, and protesting that something "happened only once" to cover up—these all are types of delusion and rationalization.

Ironically, these people *know* that they are not really trustworthy. In their isolation, they are also convinced that most people cannot be trusted. Further, they are certain that if anyone found out about their secret life of sexual experiences, there would be no forgiveness, only judgment. To complicate matters, they have placed themselves in so many precarious situations that they live in constant fear of the eventual discovery that they are being untrustworthy. Suspicion and paranoia heighten their sense of alienation.

Blaming others for all their problems is another way they protect their secret life. Fault lies with others who are critical, self-righteous, and judgmental. There is no acceptance of personal responsibility for mistakes, failures, or actions. This appearance of integrity further insulates their world from reality. The blame dynamic provides further justification for their behaviors. Ungrateful children, demanding spouses, and hard-nosed bosses create an unfair world in which they deserve a reward. To be honest about their limitations would bring the wall crumbling down and, in turn, jeopardize the one source of nurturing and care that can be counted on: their sexual behaviors and compulsions.

Each of these delusional thought processes—denial, rationalization, sincere delusion, paranoia, and blame—closes off an important avenue of self-knowledge and contact with reality for those struggling with problematic sexual behavior. Their world becomes closed off from the real world. Within their closed-off world, the addictive cycle is now free to work.

THE ADDICTIVE CYCLE

The addictive experience progresses through a four-step cycle that intensifies with each repetition:

1. Preoccupation—the trance or mood wherein the person's mind is completely engrossed with thoughts of sex. This mental state creates an obsessive search for sexual stimulation.
2. Ritualization—the person's own special routines that lead up to the

sexual behavior. The ritual intensifies the preoccupation, adding arousal and excitement.

3. Compulsive sexual behavior—the actual sexual act, which is the end goal of the preoccupation and ritualization. The person is unable to control or stop this behavior.
4. Unmanageability and despair—the feeling of utter hopelessness and powerlessness the person has about his or her sexual behavior.

The pain felt at the end of the cycle can be numbed or obscured by sexual preoccupation that reengages the addictive cycle.

PREOCCUPATION

Sex addicts are hostages of their own preoccupation. Every passerby, every relationship, and every introduction to someone passes through a sexually obsessive filter. More than merely noticing sexually attractive people, there is a quality of desperation that interferes with work, relaxation, and even sleep. People become objects to be scrutinized. A walk through a crowded downtown area is translated into a veritable shopping list of "possibilities."

To understand the trancelike state of preoccupation, imagine the intense passion of courtship. We laugh at two lovers who are so absorbed in one another that they forget about their surroundings. The intoxication of young love is what these people attempt to capture. It is the pursuit, the hunt, the search, the suspense heightened by the unusual, the stolen, the forbidden, and the illicit that are so intoxicating to them. The new conquest of the hustler; the score of the exposer, voyeur, or rapist; or the temptation of breaking the taboo of sex with a child—in essence, they are variations of a theme: courtship gone awry.

People with addictive sexual behavior use—or, rather, abuse—one of the most exciting moments in human experience: sex. Sexual arousal becomes intensified. Their mood is altered as they enter the obsessive trance. The metabolic responses are like a rush through the body as adrenaline speeds up the body's functioning. The heart pounds and the person focuses on his or her search object. Risk, danger, and even violence are the ultimate escalators. One can always increase the dosage of intoxication. Preoccupation effectively buries the personal pain of remorse or regret. They do not always have to act. Often just thinking about it brings relief.

Their excitement-seeking parallels preoccupation found in other addictions. In that sense, there is little difference between the voyeur waiting for hours by a window for a minute of nudity and the compulsive gambler taking a hunch on a long shot. What makes those with sexual addictions different is that they draw on the human emotions generated by courtship and passion.

RITUALIZATION

The trance is enhanced by the sexual addict's ritualization. Professionals have often wondered why sex offenders use the same "MO" (modus operandi, or method) each time when it only makes apprehension easier. Why would someone visit sexually explicit Web sites while at work, knowing full well that all employee Internet activity is being electronically monitored, making his or her discovery inevitable?

The answer is simple: a ritual helps induce the trance. Like a yogi in meditation, people caught up in compulsive sexual behavior do not have to stop and think or disrupt their focus. The ritual itself, like preoccupation, can start the rush of excitement. In that moment, they have become oblivious to external factors, consequences, and environmental cues that say, "Stop, this is not the time." When you study techniques of meditation, one step is learning how to focus, how to avoid distractions. Online rituals put people into a trancelike state that has incredible focus. The ritual becomes another way to further distort perception and distance cybersex users from reality.

Sex addicts often talk about their rituals. The compulsive masturbator and his surroundings, the incestuous father and his elaborate preparations, the exposer's regular routes, the hustler's approach and cruising area, the cybersex user's favorite chair, lighting, time of day, and Web sites—all involve complex rituals. The rituals contain a set of well-rehearsed cues that trigger arousal.

The preoccupation trance supported by extensive rituals is as important as—or sometimes more important than—sexual contact or orgasm. The intoxication of the whole experience is what they seek in order to move through the cycle from despair to exhilaration. One cannot be orgasmic all the time. The search and the suspense absorb their concentration and energy. Cruising, watching, waiting, and preparing are part of the mood alteration.

The first two phases of the addictive cycle (preoccupation and ritualization) are not always visible. Those in the addictive cycle struggle to present an image of normalcy to the outside world. The public self is a false ego, since they know the incongruity of their double lives. Compulsive sexual behavior, the third phase of the cycle, however, leaves a trail despite the protective public image.

COMPULSIVE SEXUAL BEHAVIOR

As you may recall, chapter 1 included a story about Kevin. He promised himself and his wife that he'd stop going online for sex. Yet that promise was broken in less than a week. Kevin could not control his behavior even though he wanted to. Like Kevin, addicts are powerless over their behavior. They have lost control over their sexual expression, which is exactly why they are defined as addicts. The failure of their efforts to control their behavior is a sign of their addiction. Sexual addicts often describe the process of picking a day—a child's birthday, a change of jobs, a holiday—as "the last day." Usually, this marks a time when "it" will never happen again. Sometimes, addicts will set goals—a year, a month, or a week. It could be forever or a shorter period of time, but addicts betray themselves, buying into the delusion that they are in control of their behavior. When they fail, yet another indictment of self-control and morality is added to ever increasing shame. For recovering addicts who have acknowledged powerlessness, there is hope. They know that they might get through one day free from their addiction—with a lot of help.

The despair that addicts experience after being compulsively sexual is the "low" phase of the four-step cycle. The letdown combines the sense of failure at not having lived up to resolutions to stop with hopelessness about ever being able to stop. If the behavior was particularly degrading, humiliating, or risky, the addict's self-pity grows. If the behavior violated basic personal values or exploited them, the addict experiences self-hatred as well. Addicts often report suicidal feelings along with their despair and shame.

Standing in the wings, however, is the ever-ready preoccupation that can pull the addict out of despair. The cycle then becomes self-perpetuating. Each repetition builds on the previous experiences and solidifies the reiterative pattern of the addiction. As the cycle fastens its grip on the addict, the addict's life starts to disintegrate and become unmanageable. The addict is similar to the hamster running around the wheel in a cage; he or she runs around and around through the addictive cycle, unable to escape and becoming more and more physically, emotionally, and mentally exhausted.

UNMANAGEABILITY AND DESPAIR

Addicts are caught up in the task of keeping their secret lives from affecting their public lives. Even so, the consequences come: arrests, unmasked lies, disruption, unmet commitments, and attempts to explain the unexplainable. The addiction surfaces in addicts' inability to manage their lives. For a moment, mental process blurs reality with euphoric recall of sexual successes. They face yet again the ultimate seduction: a unique opportunity that, of course, will be "the last time."

This unending struggle to manage two lives—the "normal" and the addictive—continues. The unmanageability takes its toll. Family relationships and friendships are abbreviated and sacrificed. Hobbies are neglected, finances are adversely affected, and physical needs are unattended. The lifestyles of addicts become a consistent violation of their own values, compounding their shame. The impaired mental processes result in faulty problem solving in all areas of their lives. These decisions add to further unmanageability.

Nowhere is this clearer than in the workplace. Faulty problem solving and diversion of energy require the addict to devote extra time and effort to hold down a job. Extra hours at work further the unmanageability at home. Worse, if the addiction is connected with the work environment, it becomes even more precarious.

Addicts often point to the connection between their addiction and the stress of high-performance demands involving an important personal investment. Graduate school, for example, is often the time when people first encounter compulsivity. New jobs, promotions, and solo business ventures are also good examples. The stress of proving oneself in an area where every inadequacy is evaluated is a potent flash point for the ignition of problematic sexual behavior and sexual addiction. Unstructured time, heavy responsibility for self-direction, and high demands for excellence seem to be the common elements that are easy triggers for compulsive or addictive behaviors. Procrastination becomes a daily nemesis for these addicts. Once ignited, the compulsion and addiction make work easy to put off. One of the worst consequences of such behavior is isolation. The intensity of the double life affects relationships with family and friends. The more intensely involved addicts become in their compulsive sexual life, the more alienated they are from their parents, spouses, and children. Without those human connections, addicts paradoxically lose touch with their own selves. The unmanageability stemming from the addiction has run its course when there is no longer a double life. When there are no longer friends or family to protect or a job to hold or pretenses to be made—even though some things are valued enough to at least have a desire to stop—the addiction is at its most destructive and violent point. The addict's world has become totally insulated from real life. As we have already noted, the Internet and cybersex feed perfectly into the need for isolation. Even when online in a chat room or using a video feed, the addict is essentially still alone. The reality is that he or she is sitting alone in front of a computer monitor. No one else is there.

THE ADDICTIVE SYSTEM

As people move from healthy relationships to sexual compulsion and addiction, their internal processes combine to form an addictive system. The addictive system—as with all systems—contains subsystems that support one another. Often this support occurs in repetitive, predictable cycles.

To picture the addictive system with its subsystems, consider the human body. It is a complex system with many subsystems—the nervous system, digestive system, immune system, and so on. Clearly, when one subsystem, such as the digestive system, is upset, all the other bodily systems are affected and must adjust in some way.

The addictive system starts with a belief system containing faulty assumptions, myths, and values that support impaired thinking. The resulting delusional thought processes insulate the addictive cycle from reality. The four-phase addictive cycle (preoccupation, ritualization, sexual compulsivity, and despair) can repeat itself unhindered and take over the addict's life. All the other support systems, including relationships, work, finances, and health, become unmanageable. The negative consequences from the unmanageability confirm the faulty beliefs that the addict is a bad person who is unlovable. In turn, revalidated beliefs allow further distortion of reality. Diagrammed, the addictive system looks like this:

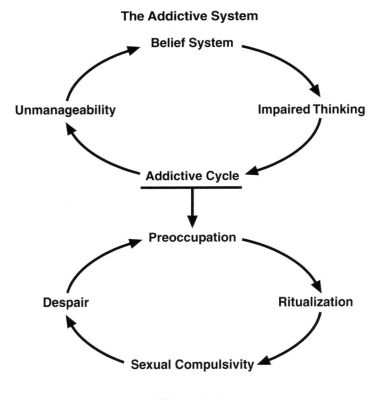

The Addictive System

Figure 3.2

Within the addictive system, sexual experience becomes the reason for being—the primary relationship for the addict. The sexual experience is the source of nurturing, focus of energy, and origin of excitement. It is the remedy for pain and anxiety, the reward for success, and the means for maintaining emotional balance. Outsiders, especially those who care about the addict, witness the unmanageability and maybe even the behavior. They see the addict's personal loss, the self-degradation, and the abandoned hope and values. It would seem so simple to just stop, even for a while. For the cybersex user, for example, who may spend up to seven hours a day online and another four thinking about it, the task is not so easy. The addiction is truly an altered state of consciousness in which "normal" sexual behavior pales by comparison in terms of excitement and relief from troubles.

In the addict's world, there is an ongoing tension between the person's normal self and the addicted self. A Jekyll-and-Hyde struggle emerges. The addictive system is so compelling that the addict feels it would be deadly to stop it. Yet, as the system continues, the person's values, priorities, and loved ones are attacked. Sometimes, only a major crisis can restore perspective.

Twenty-five years ago, one of the authors of this book, Patrick Carnes, first proposed the existence of the addictive system for sex addicts. Over the years, this hypothesis has been verified by literally millions of people who have used it to help them understand their recovery from sex addiction. The Internet has a profound effect on this system in that it dramatically intensifies the system, in turn making it all the more difficult to break and stop. The Internet is "the great amplifier." People who never experienced problematic or compulsive sexual behavior before now find themselves seemingly inextricably trapped. Such was the case for Kevin, whom you met in chapter 1. Kevin tells more of his story:

> I was a highly respected executive in my company. I was admired by my peers, and my innovative ideas regularly contributed to my company's success. I loved my wife and children dearly and made sure that my work demands did not take time away from them. But I had another, hidden side. My growing obsession with Internet sex was beginning to take its toll. I didn't really know why this obsession was so powerful. My productivity at work was beginning to suffer. Others hadn't noticed, but I knew. The time I wasted on the Internet bothered me, since I could have instead been spending time with my family. I began using work as an excuse to come home later in the day and for more late nights on the computer.
>
> My sexual behavior was also taking a toll on my health. I wasn't sleeping enough, and the stress of making excuses, of covering for work not completed, of keeping more and more of my life hidden was exhausting.
>
> I didn't like what I was doing. In the morning, looking at the trusting faces of my wife and children, I would feel the profound incongruity

of what I'd been doing late into the night. They were happy and loving, ignorant of my secret life. Still, I knew.

I finally asked for help with my sex addiction when I had an unexpected heart attack. The short nights and increased stress had been taking their toll on me. Finally, sitting in a hospital bed, I told my story to a chaplain. Amid deep sobs, I disclosed my loneliness and my love of family and work. Through my conversations with the chaplain, I acknowledged and took responsibility for what I'd been doing.

Kevin, like any other addict, lived in two worlds. One was a world of business challenges and accomplishments, family gatherings, and love for his wife and children. The other world was filled with isolation as he spent hours glued to a computer monitor, his face lit by dancing images of naked women. The coexistence of these two worlds continued until Kevin's body refused to live up to the strain.

All types of compulsive behavior can be woven into the scenario of addiction. Shoplifting, gambling, and spending are frequent counterparts. Sexually abused families often report that sexual addicts use physical violence to release pent-up energy. The workaholic who gets high on the excitement of a new deal or a new breakthrough finds professional life even more exhilarating when coupled with sexual addiction.

By far the most common combination of addictions is when the sexual addict is also dependent on alcohol or another drug. Many people attribute sexual excesses and some instances of incest to the power of alcoholism. The reality, however, is that alcoholism is often a concurrent illness with, rather than the cause of, sexual addiction. Emotional illness also flourishes within the addict's world. Depression, suicide, obsessive-compulsive behavior, and paranoia are common companions.

GETTING HELP

Recovery from compulsive online sexual behavior is possible by reversing the alienation that is integral to the addiction. With the proper help, you can integrate new beliefs and discard dysfunctional thinking. Without the mood-altering insanity to insulate you from knowledge about your own self, you become a participant in the restoration of your own sanity.

All forms of addiction are vicious because they reinforce the inability to trust others. Yet without help from others, you cannot regain control because the addiction feeds itself. Compulsive online sexual behavior is especially virulent because few forms of fixation or excitement are as supercharged with social judgment, ridicule, and fear. Consequently, seeking help is especially difficult for anyone with compulsive online sexual behavior.

One proven path to recovery, though by no means the only one, is the Twelve Steps of Alcoholics Anonymous. Many people suffering from compulsive disorders have translated the Steps for their own use, such as Overeaters Anonymous, Gamblers Anonymous, and Emotions Anonymous. This book proposes the Twelve Steps as one way for people with compulsive online sexual behavior to emerge from their double lives. Across the country, Twelve Step groups are available for the sexually compulsive. The Twelve Steps of Alcoholics Anonymous Adapted for Sexual Addicts is listed in the appendix (page 226).

Twelve Step programs can help people restore the living network of human relationships, especially in the family. The program asks addicts to first accept their problem by looking at their addictive cycle and the consequences of it. A first step is to admit that they are powerless over their sexual behavior and that their lives have become unmanageable. With that admission, the sexual addicts, called program members, are then able to start rebuilding relationships by taking responsibility for what they have done and by making amends where possible. Values and priorities are reclaimed. Throughout the program, members explore basic spiritual issues as a way of understanding and facing their anxiety. As members live by the program's tenets, the double life, with all its delusion and pain, can be left behind.

In chapters 7 and 8, we will talk in greater detail about various interventions, including the Twelve Step approach, therapy, medication, support groups, and spiritual guidance, that you can use to break out of the world of compulsive cybersex. In the next chapter, we will examine how we learn about sex, what makes people sexually aroused, and the impact the Internet is having on sexual stimulation.

4

What Turns You On? The Arousal Template

WHAT AROUSES YOU SEXUALLY? Lingerie? Certain words or images? Role playing? Romantic dinners? Dancing?

Each of us has different preferences for what turns us on sexually, and this is what we call an arousal template—the total constellation of thoughts, images, behaviors, sounds, smells, sights, fantasies, and objects that arouse us sexually. While most of us, if we're asked, can describe what turns us on, we generally react unconsciously to these sexual stimuli. They are just a part of us.

Humans are pattern seeking and pattern creating. For example, when young children are learning how to speak English, they might use the wrong past tense for some verbs: "I see'd it" rather than "I saw it" or "I go'd to the store" rather than "I went." This mistake actually demonstrates that the child has discovered a pattern in English; generally past tenses are formed by adding "ed" to the present-tense form—"change" becomes "changed," "follow" becomes "followed," and so on.

Our tendency and ability to create patterns is why, for example, metaphors are such useful tools for conveying ideas. In a discussion about a problem at work, for example, a person might say, "Well, we'd been having trouble with our new online ordering system. We thought we had solved the problem, but today, more incidents cropped up and then, suddenly, the dam burst." The idea of a bursting dam creates a visual image of an uncontrollable flow of water pouring through a gap and spreading chaos and destruction far and wide. With only three words, the speaker instantly conveys the scope of the problem. Of course a dam didn't really burst in the office, but you can imagine, thanks to that image, the extent of the disaster. You recognize the "pattern" and respond to it. When encountering new situations or ideas, your brain immediately searches for connections, for ways to make that information fit within already existing structures. You will see how this process is important when we look at the influence of Internet sex on arousal templates.

Sexual arousal works on the same principle in that it is pattern based. You have an arousal template that is essentially a pattern you created unconsciously as you were growing up—one that determines what you find sexually arousing—whether or not you are now aware of its existence.

HOW AROUSAL TEMPLATES ARE FORMED

While it's not absolutely certain how arousal templates are established, we do know that their formation is a complicated process involving many factors, including:

- physiology, biology, and genetics
- culture, including religious and ethnic background
- family history
- experiences of physical, emotional, or sexual abuse or exploitation, if any
- general life experiences
- sexual history

Much discussion exists within the scientific community about what determines an arousal template. Part of it is likely biologically "hardwired," but even our brain may be less hardwired than originally thought. Until recently, brain scientists accepted as a matter of faith that the neurons, or brain cells, you were born with were all the brain cells you would ever possess. In 1998, however, neurobiologist John Gage revealed in a groundbreaking experiment that neurons are constantly being born, particularly in the learning and memory centers.[1] Gage now believes that changes in behavior—like exercising more—can affect the growth of brain cells and alter the brain's "wiring." He speculates that what you do can actually change the structure of your brain.

It's also clear that what humans find sexually attractive and arousing is affected by their environment, culture, and upbringing. Some cultures, for example, regard heavier women as extremely attractive. Others hold the opposite view. In cultures where women's bodies must be nearly completely covered, the glimpse of a wrist, a forearm, or an ankle is extremely erotic.

THE THREE PRIMARY EMOTION SYSTEMS

Helen Fisher, an anthropologist and research professor at Rutgers University, has done remarkable work studying the neurochemistry of sex.[2] Humans and other mammals, she says, have evolved three primary emotion systems: one for reproduction, one for mating, and one for parenting. The first to evolve was the sex drive (lust or libido). Characterized by a craving for sexual gratification, it is associated primarily with the estrogens and androgens. The sex drive evolved principally to motivate people to seek sexual union with any appropriate member of the species to continue the survival of the species.

The second emotion system is attraction, which we call passionate love, obsessive love, or infatuation. It is characterized by feelings of exhilaration, intrusive thinking about the object of our attraction, and a craving for emotional union with this partner or potential partner. Attraction is associated primarily with high levels of dopamine and norepinephrine and low levels of serotonin. This emotion system evolved primarily to facilitate mate choice, enabling people to select between potential mating partners, conserve their mating energy, and focus their attention on genetically superior individuals.

The third emotion system is attachment, usually termed "companion love" in humans. It is characterized in birds and mammals by mutual territory defense or nest building (or both), mutual feeding and grooming, staying physically close to one another, feelings of anxiety when separated, shared parental chores, and other affiliation behaviors. In humans, attachment is also characterized by feelings of calm, security, social comfort, and emotional union. Attachment is associated primarily with the neuropeptides oxytocin and vasopressin. This emotion system evolved to motivate people to engage in positive social behaviors and to sustain their relationships long enough to raise their children.

Fisher concludes that during the course of our evolution, these three emotion circuits—lust, attraction, and attachment—became increasingly independent from one another and have a physiological component.

The Internet can significantly affect these three emotion systems as well as the neurochemical reactions that underlie them. As "the great amplifier," the Internet allows you to quickly access and stimulate these emotions in a powerful way. "But," you may be thinking, "everything on the Net is virtual, so how could it really affect me physically?" Do you recall watching a particularly scary movie scene in a theater? What was going on in your body at that moment? Maybe your heart was racing, your stomach was in a knot, and you tightly gripped the arm of your seat. Why did you react this way? Nothing was "really" happening. You were just sitting in a comfortable seat in a large room with a lot of other people simply watching images projected on a large white screen accompanied by dubbed-in voices. What you were watching and hearing was completely fictitious, unreal, and virtual. It was created one scene at a time over a long period of time. Nevertheless, this virtual experience had a profound impact on your emotions and an obvious physical effect. This is also true of the Internet and cybersex.

Cybersex can produce a trancelike state, capturing you and drawing you in just as a good movie does. It becomes all the more powerful and captivating because you can control your experience. What you can do is virtually limitless. Interested in romance and relationships? Countless chat rooms are waiting just a mouse click away. Seeking sex and lust? Again, it's right there. While these experiences are virtual, they do affect you emotionally and physically (just like watching a horror movie). In addition, you have the opportunity to be exposed to activities you've never before engaged in or perhaps never even thought of. And you can do that repeatedly whenever you want and for as long as you want. As we have already seen, these seemingly wonderful experiences can, and often do, lead to dire consequences.

TRIGGERING THE AROUSAL TEMPLATE

Lingerie. A cute butt. Nylons and garters. Underwear. Small breasts. Large breasts. Full, wavy hair. Well-cut pecs and abs. An erotic message on your answering machine. There are situations, thoughts, actions, places, and images that trigger your arousal template. Often, however, you're not very aware of them, but you find yourself sexually aroused anyway. These triggers can and often do date back to your childhood and adolescence.

IDENTIFYING THE TRIGGERS

As a set of well-rehearsed cues that trigger arousal, the special routines we call rituals lead up to the sexual behavior and work together with triggers. Some actions may not initially seem to be sexual triggers, but they can become so under certain circumstances. For example, taking your dog for a walk could be an arousal trigger for you if you had been a voyeur who used to peep in other people's windows while walking your dog. Going into a bar was the trigger for Barry because he had, in the past, gone to bars to pick up a sexual partner and wouldn't leave until he'd found someone. For someone who regularly practices online sex, just the sound of a modem dialing and connecting, or touching the keyboard, could be an erotic trigger. For some people, watching young girls smoke is very erotic. Certain Web sites provide just these types of photos for that reason. Feelings such as anger and sadness can also become erotic triggers.

THE CONNECTION BETWEEN AROUSAL AND CHILDHOOD ABUSE

It may seem impossible that sexual or physical abuse could be part of a person's arousal template, but it can and does happen. If as a child, for example, you felt both fear and pleasure during an act of sexual abuse, often you will have similar feelings as an adult—to the point of actually putting yourself in abusive relationships. In a sense, trauma becomes connected, even fused, to the arousal template. If you were abused as a child, then trauma, though painful, can become comforting too. Repeating the familiar trauma, you experience a complex biological reaction that includes a neurochemical component that is biologically the same as when you were a child. Jacquelyn's story helps to illustrate this:

> As a young girl, I became erotically aroused, scared, and filled with shame and contempt when my father had sex with me. In addition, however, I felt very powerful because he would do anything I wanted after he had sex with me. In my late teens, I ran away from home and ended up on the street as a prostitute. When I walked into the hotel room with a trick, I knew I had to gain control of the situation. I felt both shame and pleasure—the same feelings I experienced as a child

during sex with my father. In my mind, I was in control too, because these guys paid me a lot of money. I felt strong and powerful as well because to me these men were contemptible scum.

THE ROLE OF HIERARCHIES

Arousal templates can include a variety of activities and situations. Not all parts of the arousal template are triggered every time. There is a hierarchy among the arousing activities and situations. In fact, many people with compulsive/addictive sexual behavior have very clear and changeable hierarchies out of which they operate. James, for example, travels often for business and is turned on by just walking into a hotel room—primarily because he has a long history of illicit sexual behavior in hotel rooms. Upon arriving at a new hotel, James first goes to the Yellow Pages to look for escort services or massage parlors. If the phone book is missing the Yellow Pages, he goes to option two—walks down to the hotel bar to see if any hookers are hanging around or perhaps even a lonely woman to hustle. If James strikes out again, he returns to his hotel room, opens his laptop computer, hoping to log on to the Internet and start searching for cybersex Web sites. Should he discover that his battery is dead, he locates a nearby bookstore where he buys a copy of the latest *Penthouse*. James has a set of sexual options—sex with a prostitute, sex with a woman he picks up, cybersex, and pornography—as well as a clear order of preference.

THE "EROTIC MOMENT"

Most people assume that the goal of sex is intercourse, orgasm, and ultimately intimacy. Often, however, this is not so. Many people instead seek what we call the "erotic moment." A stripper, for example, may find her erotic moment when she takes off her clothes and then watches the men pull out their wallets to give her money. She feels that she has humiliated them and that she is the winner in this exchange. Her arousal template is tied to aspects of sexuality that are related to money and power rather than to intercourse, orgasm, or intimacy.

Cybersex can become part of a person's arousal template. Many people find eroticism in the trancelike state previously mentioned. Internet chat rooms can be captivating, particularly for women, because they provide opportunities for romantic intrigue, manipulation, seduction, and power.

The erotic moment for these women is not found in actually physically having sex with men, but rather in seduction.

Teresa, a woman who grew up in an incestuous family, for example, will often find it very erotic to bring a man to the point of being sexually aroused—and then refuse to have sex with him. The act of flirtation is so powerful that it becomes her erotic moment. Internet chat rooms provide a perfect way for Teresa to create erotic moments at the expense of others, hence the incredible allure and power of cybersex for her.

There are many other examples of erotic moments being quite removed from the actual sex act or orgasm. Voyeurs can experience their erotic moments by finding on the Internet an endless supply of erotic pictures taken through windows or by small hidden cameras in locker rooms or department store dressing rooms.

In a sense, it's the chase rather than the actual capture that is arousing. Many cybersex users talk about the excitement of finding a sex site that has the particular images they really like. For others, the erotic moment comes as a given photo slowly downloads onto their screen.

The Internet is a perfect tool for supplying many kinds of erotic moments, and it can do so endlessly. Those moments are always there, just waiting to be called up. For the voyeur, the Internet creates a new opportunity. No longer is there any need to sit for hours outside the home of a young woman waiting for ninety seconds of nudity. His desires can be met for hours on end in the safety of his home.

Exploring the Forbidden

The Internet can also provide a way to explore long-held fantasies and discover unacknowledged parts of the arousal template. Clyde tells his story:

> I had long fantasized about watching in person two women have sex with one another. Since I'm a man who takes my marriage and religion seriously, I thought this fantasy would never come true. One day while messing around on my computer, I discovered an interactive pornography site where I could request just such a scenario. In no time, however, I was hooked on this fantasy. I'd spend countless hours watching women have sex with one another.

Most of us have a part of our sexuality that lies unacknowledged, unexplored, and without a voice, and the Internet offers a way to explore that sexuality. These sites, however, can quickly take on a larger role in people's lives. Some people, like Clyde, lose control once they enter the cybersex world. After years of suppression, the floodgates are opened and they don't know how to close them again.

The Greek myth of Pygmalion and Galatea provides a useful analogy for understanding the role of cybersex and the Internet in the fulfillment of sexual fantasies. In this myth (upon which the musical *My Fair Lady* was based), Pygmalion carves a statue of what he thinks is the perfect woman. He names her Galatea and falls in love with her. This desire of men to create perfect women is deeply embedded in Western culture, and the Internet provides the opportunity for a reenactment of this ancient Greek myth. Thanks to live-feed video sites and interactive sex sites and their kin, it's possible to log on and describe the woman or man you want to see and what that person should be doing. It's a kind of "instant Galatea."

CHANGING AROUSAL TEMPLATES

Historically, the arousal template has been regarded as quite rigid and fixed, but in recent years, research has shown it to be more flexible and malleable, almost amoeba-like in its ability to grow and incorporate new information as time passes. Much of the original research and writing on arousal templates was based on work with pedophiles, people who were severely damaged as children and who, as a result, had rigid and narrow arousal templates that deviated dramatically from normal behavior. It is extremely difficult for these people to make significant changes in their arousal templates because the damage they suffered is so deep and came so early in life. Their behavior has been in a set groove for a long time.

SPONTANEITY, FLEXIBILITY, AND THE AROUSAL TEMPLATE

For the majority of people, however, arousal templates have a great deal of spontaneity and flexibility. Food can be used as an analogy for the arousal template. Your sexuality is, of course, far more complex than your relationship to food, but the analogy does have similarities that will help make our message clearer.

There are many sexual activities and arousal triggers from which you can choose, akin to a smorgasbord of foods. Consider some of the people in this chapter who have been damaged. Let's say they lived for many years with only hamburgers to eat. Maybe they've had lettuce and tomato on them sometimes, and perhaps an occasional side of French fries, but they've still never seen mashed potatoes and gravy or vegetables, let alone the dessert cart.

We first learn about food likes and dislikes as children in our families. All of us carry our food background, together with our likes and dislikes, into adulthood. As adults, we are exposed to a wider variety of foods. There are many people who, as adults, just aren't particularly interested in exploring new foods and tastes. They like what they grew up with and are content to stick with what they know.

We begin to learn about sex in our childhood, with the process intensifying as we enter our teen years. As a part of that process, we develop a sense—a "taste," if you will—for what turns us on sexually, and this becomes our arousal template. As we've said, its creation is influenced by physiological, biological, and genetic factors; our culture; our religious and ethnic background; and any experiences of physical, emotional, or sexual abuse or exploitation.

John Money has described the template as a kind of "love map."[3] We follow the trails and roads on our love map to sexual arousal. From our point of view, however, the arousal template is much more dynamic than a map. A map describes a territory that is basically unchanging, with set roads and trails. We see the template as more of a fluid matrix in which decisions are made regularly.

As adults, most of us begin to have more sexual experiences. We may, for example, have a partner who introduces us to oral sex, role playing, or sex toys. We may find this new experience erotic and pleasing and add it to our sexual repertoire. It then becomes part of our arousal template.

For many people, however, the arousal template seems to have a static quality to it because they never examine it. Most people never really think about what turns them on and why it does so, just as we don't really think about why we like certain foods and dislike others. In addition, until recently many of us simply didn't have the opportunity to explore the broader landscape of sexual possibilities. Because of the myriad sexual materials and activities available online, it's now possible to access the entire sexual landscape from home (or office or library) with the click of a mouse.

Through our research and work with people who are having problems with their sexual behavior, we see more and more people whose arousal templates are being altered as a result of cybersex experiences. We are also seeing obsessions forming—sometimes very quickly—that ultimately affect all aspects of their lives.

The Internet allows people to discover new sexual interests, as they find that the things that used to arouse them in the past no longer do so. The new interests often take on a power and a focus that have an almost obsessional quality. Thanks to the Internet, people are being sexually stimulated in ways that have nothing to do with culture or any of their previous experiences. Our arousal templates seem to be much more fluid than originally thought.

For centuries, humans have been looking at sex as though through a magnifying glass. We have focused on a small range of activities and ideas. This view has been further narrowed by the taboos fostered by religion and culture. Polygamy, for example, was more commonly practiced in Asia, Africa, and the Middle East many centuries ago than it is now. Some cultures forbade (and still do today) women to interact with men who were not their relatives. Public male or female nudity has long been unacceptable in many cultures. And sex before marriage has also been widely considered immoral for centuries. The Internet, however, acts like a wide-angle lens that instantly gives us a view of the whole sexual landscape.

We now have access to a worldwide sexual smorgasbord. Sex via the Internet is accessible, affordable, and anonymous—a powerful combination. These factors are changing arousal templates, and changing them rapidly.

The Internet allows a new and novel way for people to explore sexuality, and in some respects, this can be a positive experience. People can find other people who have similar tastes, no matter how unusual. Discovering that you are not alone in having a particular desire or fantasy can reduce shame and reinforce positive feelings about yourself, and it can offer a means for exploring these areas of sexuality.

We like to say that one of the best things about the Internet is that you can find others who have interests similar to yours. At the same time, one of the worst things about the Internet is that you can find people who have interests similar to yours.

Web sites can be educational, not only allowing people to learn about and experience particular sexual desires or fantasies, but also pointing the way to new and related areas. In areas and activities that are illegal or unhealthy, the Internet makes it possible for people to reinforce that undesirable behavior and strengthen an unhealthy arousal template.

The Internet also connects people, making it possible to compare notes and exchange materials. Child pornography is an example of illegal activity that is rampant on the Internet. An active and sophisticated child-porn black market exists there, one that has been difficult to infiltrate and control.

HOW CRAVINGS AND OBSESSIONS BEGIN

Given a look at the sexual smorgasbord available on the Internet, people may want to sample some of the new offerings they've seen. More and more people are experimenting sexually in areas that were previously unavailable to them—and not only do they like what they're finding, they now crave it. People can develop new sexual obsessions very rapidly. It is not unusual to see people become absolutely fixated on a new sexual idea—one they've never before imagined—literally within days of discovering it. It's amazing how suggestible people can be and how quickly a previously unknown behavior can become part of a person's arousal template. This reality further points out how complex our templates are.

There's yet another reason why cybersex can create such a powerful hold on people so quickly. When a person goes to a strip club, views a porn movie in a theater, or takes part in some other kind of voyeuristic or exposing activity, it's usually not possible to have an orgasm at the moment that the activity is taking place. People generally return to a car or their home and masturbate to the memory of the event. One of the attributes of the Internet that makes it so powerful is that it's possible to have an orgasm while watching a stripper or "spying" on a woman via a voyeur cam in the safety of your own surroundings. The sexual activity and orgasm suddenly become linked. In addition, the computer and its location become sexualized too. Going to the computer, turning it on, logging on to the Net, taking part in online sexual activities, and orgasm all become fused into a very powerful ritualized activity.

MODIFYING UNHEALTHY BEHAVIORS

The malleability of arousal templates runs the gamut of inflexible to fairly loose and free-floating. Depending on the person, it may be fairly easy or quite difficult to modify unhealthy behaviors in the template. Some individuals become obsessed with certain activities quickly, while others seldom, if ever, do so.

Why do some people become hooked, or hooked so quickly, and others do not? A number of factors seem to play a role. One has to do with a person's innate resiliency. For example, in abusive families, we know now that it is not unusual for two children to have different responses to similar traumatic experiences. Often one will be much more damaged than the other. What seems to have the biggest influence in helping those healthier children keep bouncing back is having a healthy relationship with a kind and supportive adult—a teacher, neighbor, relative, or coach, for example, who takes the child under his or her wing. That kind of positive relationship can make an enormous difference in a child's life.

Stress—and the resources we have to cope with it—also plays a significant role. One client, a successful businessman whose company was about to go public, was under tremendous stress the day of his company's initial public offering. How did he cope with the pressure? He went to his office and logged online to have cybersex for more than six hours. He took refuge in cybersex during the most critical moment in his company's history because he simply didn't have the resources to cope in a positive way with this level of stress. He used cybersex as a way to reduce it and to take his mind away from the situation. Fortunately, the initial public offering moved ahead without problems despite his lack of oversight.

Sometimes people break down despite having plenty of coping resources. For example, the death of a loved one or feelings of isolation can leave someone quite vulnerable. A person who is not normally interested in cybersex might, under stress, respond by trying to avoid the outside world and retreating into cybersex. Some might also use cybersex merely as a stopgap measure, but then not be able to turn away from it once the "excuse" for its use is gone. We find that there is no way to predict who will have a problem with cybersex. Those who do come from a broad range of ethnic, social, and economic backgrounds. They can be people who've had trouble with sex before and people for whom it has never been a problem. They may be people with healthy or unhealthy coping responses. This is one of the unique aspects of cybersex. In other sexual problems, it's possible to detect patterns or common points—such as childhood sexual or emotional abuse or a familial history of addictive disorders, for example—among the people who are struggling. Not so with cybersex.

TURNING OFF THE AUTOPILOT MECHANISM

Many people's attitudes toward sex and their arousal templates generally lie unexamined. The same is true for our response to stress—we often just react without thinking about why we did what we did. It's as though we are an airplane on automatic pilot. The Boeing 767 and the French Airbus are enormous machines that use complicated computer programming to monitor much of what is happening during takeoff, flight, and landing. The pilots don't actually do a lot of flying; instead they oversee the system. When everything is running smoothly, the pilots are hardly aware of all the complex adjustments that are being carried out automatically.

Our bodies are far more complex than any airplane, and much of what we do isn't monitored by our conscious mind. We fall into patterns and roles and continue them for years, not realizing that a process is being followed, one that we can both become aware of and change. One of the goals of this book is to help you become aware of some of your unrecognized habits, rituals, and responses to life's events.

You can examine, evaluate, and change the systems and responses you've been using throughout your life. There is hope. Just as the pilot can break in and override the autopilot, you, too, can take greater control over your life and the decisions you make. The first step, of course, is to acknowledge the existence of your unconscious programming and to become aware of its messages.

We have already mentioned the importance of having healthy relationships. One of the factors that consistently plays a role in all addictions, including cybersex addiction, is the inability to develop and maintain healthy, positive relationships. One of the core components of the arousal template is our relationship and courtship experiences and skills. Our arousal template is connected to our relationship and courtship template. In this chapter, we have been looking at the broad picture of arousal. In chapter 5, we will specifically examine what happens during courtship and its connection to relationships and cybersex.

As we conclude this chapter, we would like to help you look more closely at what makes up your arousal template and how it may have been affected by your sexual activities on the Internet. The following exercise will help you do this. Keep in mind that there are no right or wrong answers; what you discover will help you better understand your own sexuality.

1a. List whatever it was that you found sexy *before* you became involved in cybersex:

b. Next, list whatever it was that you found sexy *after* you became involved in cybersex:

2a. List whatever it was that you found romantic *before* you became involved in cybersex:

b. Next, list whatever it was that you found romantic *after* you became involved in cybersex:

3a. List whatever it was that kept you attached in a romantic relationship *before* you became involved in cybersex:

b. Next, list whatever it was that kept you attached in a romantic relationship *after* you became involved in cybersex:

4. Look over your previous answers. What effect has the Internet had in each of the areas on the next page?

Sex:

Romance:

Attachment:

5. What new ideas or activities have you incorporated into these three areas since you became involved in cybersex?

Sex:

Romance:

Attachment:

6. Which changes do you feel good about in these three areas?

Sex:

Romance:

Attachment:

7. Which changes do you feel bad about in these three areas?

Sex:

Romance:

Attachment:

8. Looking back on your experiences and answers to the questions in this exercise, can you create any goals for what you would like in terms of sex, romance, and attachment? Write them in the space below. This exercise will serve as good preparation for the next chapter, and you may find that you will want to refer back to it as you read further in this book.

5

Courtship Gone Awry

WHAT DOES THE TERM "courtship" mean to you? If you are like most people, it's defined as meeting, getting to know, and attempting to gain the affection or love of another person. We would like to suggest that there is a far broader meaning to this term—one that encompasses the process by which we meet and establish all our relationships. In a sense, we "court" our acquaintances, business colleagues, and friends, as well as those with whom we have romantic and intimate relationships. Not all aspects of courtship apply to every relationship, but the basic courtship process is really about creating and building relationships. Keep this wider definition of courtship in mind while reading the rest of this chapter.

We are discussing courtship in this book because we believe that it is one of the most important aspects of being human—and because the Internet is dramatically affecting human interactions and relationships. While the Internet has enhanced communication, it also often contributes to unhealthy patterns of relating to others. Basically, the technology of Internet communication changes the way we relate to others by limiting certain aspects of the courtship process. While there are positive aspects and results in using the Internet to meet and get to know others, there are negative factors that interfere with the courtship process too.

In this chapter, we will introduce you to the twelve components of courtship and explain how the Internet interferes with successfully moving through them. There are three groups of people who have courtship disorders. The first includes those who have had a lifetime of difficulty beginning and establishing relationships. Their problems with Internet-based relationships are a small part of a bigger problem. The second group includes those who have what we describe as "situational" courtship problems. These people have generally, in the course of their lives, been able to develop good relationships. There are times, however, due to stress or a life crisis, that their relationship and courtship skills seem to fall apart. The third group includes people who have not had courtship difficulties until they became involved with the Internet.

UNDERSTANDING COURTSHIP BEHAVIOR AND THE INTERNET

One of the original pioneers of understanding problematic sexual behavior as a courtship disorder was Havelock Ellis, who referred to exhibitionism in 1933 as a "symbolic act based on a perversion of courtship."[1] Over the years, Sigmund Freud and various colleagues elaborated on the concept of courtship disorder. They specified four general examples of courtship distortion that resulted in paraphilic behaviors; that is, sexual behaviors that are outside of what our culture would consider typical and that have negative consequences. First, they pointed to the process of locating a potential partner that, when distorted, becomes voyeurism. During the second phase, which they called "pretactile interaction," exhibitionism and obscene calls served as examples of disordered courtship. The third phase, tactile interaction, is marked by inappropriate touch, such as deliberately brushing against a woman's breasts in a subway train. Finally, they described rape patterns as a distortion of normal efforts to "effect genital union."[2] The concept of courtship disorders has also been useful in understanding various forms of sexual assault. This courtship model can apply, too, to "nonperverse" behaviors such as sexual compulsivity within marriage, compulsive masturbation, or compulsive prostitution, and it also creates a framework to understand problematic cybersex behavior.

Consider the case of Carrie:

> While growing up, I was sexually abused by my father who fondled me regularly until I was fourteen years old. I was also emotionally and physically abused. At one point, I became pregnant and my parents forced me into an abortion. My mother had the doctor place the fetus next to my head after the surgery so I would "learn a lesson." As an adult, I found it very difficult to allow myself to be sexual with a man whom I

cared for. I was always very anxious and was worried about whether the relationship mattered at all. When I was with men I didn't care about and considered "slime," I was very promiscuous. I also was intensely sexual with myself. I would masturbate whenever I got anxious.

Carrie was tremendously relieved when she finally understood that the abuse she suffered as a child created a disordered sense of courtship in which she was unable to be sexual with a man who really mattered. After all, her father mattered and yet he betrayed her. A further legacy of that betrayal was that unreliable men who did not matter were attractive.

The example of Carrie does not include how the Internet could have impacted Carrie's relationship development. Imagine an individual like Carrie logging on to the Internet and feeling the power and protection of the online world. Perhaps she would have discovered chat rooms as a place where she could overcome her difficulties in real life courtship but where her negative promiscuous behaviors would be encouraged and rewarded. Although it is unclear exactly how Carrie's world may have been impacted by online behavior, the possibility that the Internet can alter and affect the courtship process is clear.

Remember the four phases of courtship that were discussed earlier: (a) locating a partner, (b) pretactile interaction (communication), (c) tactile interaction (learning to touch), and (d) genital union (intercourse). Now, think about what you know about the Internet and how it can impact these four phases. While the Internet provides new avenues to meet others and locate partners, as well as new methods for relational communication, it also lacks significant factors in courtship. For example, it often lacks the non-verbal communication necessary to form relationships, and it does not allow for tactile interaction or genital union. The Internet provides a pseudo-courtship world where couples think they can achieve the same relationship goals online as offline. The success stories of online relationships always have one thing in common: the couples figured out early on how to move their courtship process from the online world to the real world.

There is no doubt that online courtship is easier, less risky, and allows for an easy escape if things aren't going well. The truth remains that real relationships are hard work. For some people, the Internet makes relationships appear easier. However, in the real world nothing can make intimate relationships easier. Relationships result from real life interactions and hard work. Imagine teens today whose primary mode of communication, relationship building, and relationship maintenance takes place online. Are they redefining the courtship process, or are they bound to struggle with intimacy issues in their future real-world relationships? We have yet to see.

THE TWELVE COMPONENTS OF COURTSHIP

The courtship process existed long before the Internet. Researchers have identified twelve basic components of the courtship process. Although it is unclear exactly how the courtship process has changed as a result of the Internet, it is clear that change has occurred and will continue to occur as new technologies allow people to meet, date, and relate online.

1. NOTICING

This is the ability to notice attractive traits in others. With an existing partner, this means staying conscious of the desirable traits in that partner. This dimension also requires the capacity to filter out traits that, while desirable, are not a good match for you. This includes the ability to be discriminating.

We communicate at all times on two levels. The basic level of communication contains the words and content of the message. The second level is known as metacommunication. Messages sent at this level qualify and enhance the basic-level message and are delivered through tone of voice, facial expression, body movement, touch, and other nonverbal means. For example, one person might comment to another, "I'm glad we met, and I'll call you soon." Depending on the metamessage being sent, that sentence could communicate two very different messages—that the person really will call, or that he or she isn't at all interested in the other person and has no intention whatsoever of calling.

Noticing is a critical first step in all relationships. When we meet other people for the first time, we are physically in touch with their appearance. We note how they look; their clothes, smile, body type, physicality, tone of voice, and sense of humor; whether they're shy or effusive; and much more. We often have a physical reaction to them. And we get an almost immediate sense as to whether this is a person we might like to know better. (That first impression may turn out to be inaccurate, but regardless, *everyone* forms such impressions.)

The Internet affects the way we notice others in the sense that it doesn't supply any metamessages. Consequently, without nonverbal cues we have no access to the enormous amount of information we normally use when we first meet and interact with another person. As such, the Internet provides people with a completely new and different way to meet. Meeting by phone is similar, but we still have a kind of physical connection—we can hear the other person's voice. Even telephone conversations, then, give us metamessages such as voice expressiveness, sense of humor, and feelings (excitement, nervousness, or boredom, for example). People can communicate with letters, which also contain some metamessages—the style of one's script and the little personal touches and embellishments created by hand—that give nonverbal information about the writer.

By its very nature, the Internet dilutes individuality enormously. Since it is devoid of metamessages, noticing is severely limited. People who meet online have only words on a stark computer monitor upon which to make judgments. Since we are so used to having these metamessages when we meet another person, we unconsciously try to supply them when they're not available. We want to "fill in the blanks." Particularly in romantic relationships, we tend to fill in the blanks in ways that will meet our expectations of what we want a person and a relationship to be like. That information is necessarily speculative, and what we add is based on our projections of what we want that person to be. We don't have the data to really discriminate, which is a critical aspect of noticing.

Misinterpretation of meaning is another problem in Internet communication. In the business world, such problems are commonplace. For example, let's say that an e-mail is sent and the person receiving it feels put down by the message, although the sender meant nothing of the sort. Text alone seldom supplies enough information for accurate message sending and receiving, even when the writer has been very careful. Over time, these misunderstandings actually begin to inhibit communication because they damage the trust on which the relationship depends.

When a message is carried out face-to-face or even on the phone, it has a better chance of being sent and received accurately. We read other people's metamessages—a pause or a questioning tone can indicate misunderstanding—and once we realize what is happening, we can clarify our intent. We might say, "Oh, no . . . don't get me wrong, I was just kidding." Clarification takes just seconds. In person, we can be playful with each other in ways that are simply impossible on the Internet.

When meeting via the Internet, the discriminating process becomes very skewed because we simply don't have the information we need to judge whether the person is a good match for friendship or romance.

2. ATTRACTION

This is the ability to feel attraction toward others and to imagine acting on those feelings. This dimension assumes a functional arousal template in which you select behavior and persons appropriate for you. Attraction involves curiosity about as well as desire for the physical, emotional, and intellectual traits of others. In an existing relationship, it means the ability to maintain an openness to change. In quality relationships, the partners continue to "discover" each other. Attraction is passion's starting point and the basis for relationships that endure.

People find the Internet so attractive for meeting others because it offers complete control over the information we give to other people. We let them discover only the things about us that we want them to know. We can even create a fantasy self. This possibility points out another major problem with Internet relationships: how do we know whether what another person is telling us is true? In the physical world, for example, if you move into your neighborhood, drive an old car, don't go to work every day, seldom dress well, and then tell others you are a successful lawyer making $250,000 a year, others might look at your lifestyle and question your truthfulness. On the Internet, however, you could tell others whatever you want and they would have no other information to help them know whether your statement is true. What's more, when we meet physically, we communicate many messages inadvertently or even unconsciously to others. For example, a woman, Louise, meets a man at a party, a man she finds very attractive. Not wanting to appear too excited, she tries to act a bit aloof, but the look in her eyes clearly reveals her true feelings.

Attraction depends on the ability to notice. In order to discriminate and to be attracted to others, we have to be able to notice them. We need to be able to learn about who they are. The discovery process is what makes attraction real. But in cyber-meetings, what we learn about others is limited to text and, perhaps, a photo or video—and they learn *exactly* what we want them to know. The meeting is devoid of metamessages.

3. FLIRTATION

This is the ability to make playfully romantic or sexual overtures to another person. Everyone needs to know how to flirt. Successful flirting uses playfulness, seductiveness, and social cues to send signals of interest and attraction to the desirable person. This ability also includes noticing and accurately reading the flirtation of others. The critical factor in flirtation is knowing when it is appropriate to send and receive it. In addition, the success of long-term relationships requires ongoing flirtation between partners.

Playfulness and flirtation are relevant to all relationships, not just romantic ones. The critical component of healthy flirtation is the difference between the message sent and the message received—you have to know how to send a message so that what you want to convey is what is actually received by the other person.

When flirting online, however, this task is very difficult to accomplish. Once again, the problem is rooted in a lack of "noticing" information available on the Internet. Without these cues, it is easy to misinterpret the message being sent, and flirtation is derailed. Outside the cyber-world, we can, for example, indicate sarcasm simply by using a particular tone of voice while finishing the phrase or sentence with a chuckle. In e-mail, it is impossible to deliver such complex content.

The Internet does make a kind of pseudo-flirtation possible. If you visit a pay porn site and begin interacting with someone, it's really no different from paying a prostitute. The person with whom you're talking will smile at you (if they have a live video feed) and flirt and say you're wonderful, and so forth. Because that person doesn't know you and because you're paying for his or her time, however, this is not true flirtation. In fact, it's even less "real" than if you were actually with a prostitute, because then you would at least have some sense of who he or she is, and vice versa. On the Net, you can pretend that your partner is flirting with you, but in fact he or she is only flirting with his or her camera and your money. At some level, the buyer knows that this person isn't attracted to and doesn't care at all about him or her. It's merely a business transaction.

Once again, trust is the potential victim. Believing another person's flirtation online requires a great deal more trust because we have so little information on which to base a judgment. People can say anything, and they can choose to disappear at any time. The flirtation suddenly becomes nothing more than electrons now randomly dispersed into space.

4. DEMONSTRATION

Sometimes inaccurately described as "showing off," it is in this step where one demonstrates "prowess" (a physical trait, skill, or capability). Sexually, it's the classic "I will show you mine if you show me yours" scenario. There is, in fact, pleasure or eroticism in having a potential partner show interest in your sexuality. Behaviors include demonstrating a skill such as athletic ability, dressing to attract another person, or doing specific sexual acts that further the partner's interest. It is important that you are aware of what you are doing and that you are being appropriate to the context and to the person.

As we have noted, the Internet allows us to create a persona; we are not restricted to who we actually are. The "rich, attractive attorney" had only to *say* (to write, actually) that this was what he was in order to "demonstrate." On the Net, "saying so makes it so." No actual *physical* demonstration is required—or possible—online. Again, so few cues are available online. In real life, someone can say he's a great athlete, but if he's fifty pounds overweight and breathes hard after a two-block walk, we have some pretty good evidence that this just isn't true! Whoever reads a similar claim on the Net will be none the wiser because there's no reality check there.

In courtship, we must be able to verify demonstration. This stage is, by definition, a way to demonstrate that what you say is true, that you are who you say you are. It's really the first test of one's honesty and integrity. In person, we have information, feelings, and intuition on which to base this judgment, but online there is no way to verify that we are who we say we are.

As you can see, each of the steps of courtship build on one another. At this point, it's very difficult to trust demonstration if you haven't really been able to move through noticing, attraction, and flirtation. If you don't have the first steps in place, your ability to move ahead in the courtship is limited.

5. ROMANCE

This is the ability to experience, express, and receive passion. Romance assumes the ability to be aware of feelings of attraction, vulnerability, and risk. More important, a lover must be able to express these feelings and have sufficient self-worth to accept the expressions of care from a lover as true. Included in romance is the ability to test the reality of our feelings. Are the people we select as romantic partners consistently appropriate or inappropriate choices? Is what we perceive in the other person accurate, or is it instead a *projection* of what we want to be true? Romance may cause us to see others as we *want* them to be, not as they are.

As we've pointed out, the very nature of Internet communication requires us to project onto others our hopes, desires, and fantasies—what we want to be true about them—because our knowledge of them is based only on what they've told us. So much information that we would generally have in a face-to-face relationship is missing that we feel the need to fill in the blanks. We give potential suitors the attributes that we want them to have.

In addition, we assume (or project) *their* responses to *us* too. "She really likes me and thinks I'm hot," or "He really loves me," or "I'm funny and attractive to her." All of us do this to some extent in our relationships, but the Internet requires us to do so even more because we don't have anything solid on which to base our judgments and assumptions. Reality-based judgments are very difficult because we can't easily grasp reality in an Internet-based relationship. It is this factor that contributes so much to online fantasy—and its related problems.

Thirty-nine-year-old Jane describes her experience:

> I had been communicating with this guy for some months, and I was starting to get serious about him. He was a wonderful writer, very expressive and eloquent. He described himself as good-looking with a high-paying job at a major corporation. We seemed to share many interests and values. It was just fun to converse with him. We had both told each other that we were becoming romantically interested in one another. Finally, I proposed that it was time for us to meet in person. He seemed to hesitate a bit, but finally agreed. Well, I was so disappointed. He was very nervous and shy and couldn't hold a conversation. He didn't seem at all like the person I'd been e-mailing all this time. We didn't meet again, and now I wonder if he was really even the one who was actually writing to me. I mean, maybe he had someone help him.

6. INDIVIDUATION

This is defined as the process by which we differentiate ourselves from others. In the midst of courtship and romance, healthy people are able to be true to themselves. They feel no fear of disapproval or control by the other person. They tell the truth and do not feel intimidated. They can ask for their needs to be met, and they do not have to defer to the other person. They trust and believe that people care for them as they are.

Successful individuation depends on the first five steps for its foundation. Individuation depends on truth, trust, and full disclosure. Internet-based relationships, however, are at best only tentatively grounded in reality. The information we have about the other person is severely limited compared with an in-person relationship, and there is absolutely no guarantee that we were told the truth in the first place.

Deep down, we all want to believe that people are honest. In physical, world-based relationships, we have many tools and cues to help us distinguish whether a person is being honest or not. But the Internet takes nearly all of them away and leaves us far less able to make good judgments about others. So we fall back on the desire to believe that others will not deceive us—itself another projection.

Because the Internet interferes with or inhibits the previous five courtship steps, it is nearly impossible to create a foundation strong enough to hold the rest of the courtship. Without the first five steps solidly in place, the sixth step, individuation, is difficult, if not impossible.

7. INTIMACY

As the exhilaration of early passion subsides, partners enter the "attachment" phase, during which the relationship deepens in its meaning and integrity. Intimacy creates a level of profound vulnerability that is ongoing and more difficult than the exhilaration of discovery during early romance. This is the "being known fully and staying anyway" part of relationships.

Internet relationships are not intimate. Intimacy takes work, time, *and* physical connection and interaction. It's very important to understand that people who are hooked on cybersex, regardless of whether they have lifelong or situationally triggered relationship problems, are avoiding intimacy.

The Internet offers a way to get a quick sexual fix with absolutely no requirement of intimacy. Cybersex demands even less intimacy than the most impersonal physical-world relationship. If, for example, you have sex with a prostitute, some intimacy is still required. At the least, you have to be physically in his or her presence; you have to interact face-to-face and body-to-body. Even people who expose themselves must confront a minimal level of intimacy—they have to actually be in the presence of another human being.

The total lack of intimacy on the Internet is the reason why so many people who are avoiding intimacy in their lives get hooked on the Internet in general and cyber-relationships and cybersex in particular. Not only is the cyber-relationship impersonal but ending it is easy. In physical-world relationships, when matters get uncomfortable and too intimate with a friend, lover, or even a prostitute, it's harder to leave. Leaving takes time and communication. It can be difficult and painful because we feel an obligation to respond to that person and explain why we are leaving. Intimate relationships require us to respond to the other's needs.

Online relationships ultimately require no such demands or responsibilities because we can leave with no (apparent) consequences or explanation. We don't have to respond to another's needs. With a click of the mouse, the relationship evaporates.

Can there really be true intimacy without physical connection? Or is this merely "virtual" intimacy?

8. TOUCHING

Physical touch requires trust, care, and judgment. It is important and should not be taken lightly. Touching affirms the other person, but it is respectful of timing, situation, and boundaries. Touching without permission or sexualizing touch betrays trust. While touch can be seductive and misleading, it can also be extraordinarily healing. Adults who were not touched or who were neglected as children often feel extremely touch deprived. They will sacrifice their judgment and their needs simply to be touched.

When touch isn't available in a relationship, again people tend to turn to their own fantasies to replace it. This process can be satisfying in the short term, but not in the long run. Humans simply need to touch and be touched.

We want to reemphasize that touch is essential in all relationships, not just romantic or sexual ones. So much can be communicated by such simple gestures as a pat on the back, a hug, the brush of a hand, or a quick, passing kiss. It's OK to say, "I care about you," "I'm here for you," "I'm thinking about you," and "You matter to me."

In addition, people who spend excessive time on the Internet begin to neglect their own real-world relationships. They have less contact, including the physical contact of touch, and this deprivation can actually bring on depression. Often people involved in cyber-relationships think they're having human contact, but in reality they only have contact with a machine. When we get caught up in cybersex, all other personal relationships ultimately suffer.

9. FOREPLAY

Sometimes referred to as the most important part of sexual contact, foreplay is the expression of sexual passion without genital intercourse. Holding, fondling, talking, kissing, and sexual play build sexual tension and are erotic and pleasurable. As a stage, foreplay includes the verbal expression of passion and meaning. In repeated surveys, most people say it is the best part of sex. Despite this reality, foreplay is often skipped over in our culture because of time pressure and stress.

Cyber-foreplay is necessarily limited to very specific kinds of online behaviors since physical touch is not available online. People think they are having foreplay online by having sex-related conversations and even cybersex, but these activities are really only sex talk. True foreplay must also include other courtship steps such as flirtation, demonstration, and intimacy.

Couples who have had online relationships tend to be sexual more quickly when they meet offline because they feel as though foreplay has already happened. It's not unusual for people who have been "together" online to set out on a date with the intent to have sex. They think they can skip right to this level because they have already formed a relationship—when in fact they haven't formed anything more than a text-connection with one another. And when they do meet in person, many people are surprised at what they discover. Even if both have been honest about themselves, they learn that they are really still in the noticing stage. They don't know one another at all. Jane's experience, described earlier under the "romance" component of courtship, is a typical example of an all-too-common experience among people who try to establish romantic relationships on the Net.

10. INTERCOURSE

Much more than the mere exchange of body fluids, this is the ability to surrender yourself to passion, letting go and trusting yourself and your partner to be vulnerable. Intercourse, while extremely pleasurable, is also an index of the degree to which one is able to give up control. To give oneself over to passion requires true abandonment of expectations. Many people limit themselves or fail in orgasm simply because of trust and control issues.

By definition, intercourse is the physical connection of two people. The closest approximation to intercourse online is mutual masturbation or phone sex—a pseudo-intercourse that doesn't even include the "exchange of body fluids." And since it lacks any of the components of healthy courtship, it can't possibly compare to the more broadly defined act of intercourse that requires complete trust in the other. Online intercourse requires neither commitment nor connection. It is nothing more than one individual satisfying himself or herself with the aid of an online partner.

11. COMMITMENT

Commitment is the ability to bond or attach to another. Some describe addiction as the failure to bond or of not having the capacity to form a deep, meaningful relationship. If someone matters enough, you honor that relationship by your fidelity to it. Being bonded in meaningful relationships, including nonsexual ones, is true commitment.

People who grew up in families where they learned that they couldn't count on others are continually searching for something that they *can* count on—what many addicts refer to as the "black hole" they are trying to fill. Alcohol, sex, drugs, and high risks always deliver what they promise, albeit briefly and ultimately destructively. This pathological relationship with a mood-altering behavior or drug, however, will not fill the void created by the lack of committed relationships.

While one can commit emotionally online, true commitment to an electronic relationship should be questioned. How do people know their partners well enough to be certain that they are, for example, monogamous? Do they have other online—or offline—partners whom they court? Perhaps what we are committing to online are only brief encounters and the pseudo-relationships that result.

12. RENEWAL
The capacity must exist to sustain renewal, as well as all the above dimensions in an existing relationship.

Being in a committed relationship does not mean you stop flirting or expressing passion with your partner. There is a difference between being attached to someone out of habit and being devoted because of the meaning that has evolved in your journey together. Successful couples continue courtship, continue to show the other they are valued, continue to make efforts to attract their mate, and continue to express the caring they have for one another. If a relationship is not working, partners take responsibility to change it. If the relationship is not tenable, they leave. In online relationships, renewal is impossible if the previous dimensions cannot be achieved online.

COURTSHIP AND THE TEN TYPES OF SEXUALLY COMPULSIVE BEHAVIOR

In the original research for *Don't Call It Love,* ten types of sexually compulsive behavior were identified.[3] Over the years, these ten types have been developed as an empirically based model of compulsive sexual behavior. Now that courtship dimensions have been added, there is help for people who have problematic sexual behaviors by identifying specific courtship distortions in each of the ten types of behaviors. This makes understanding compulsive online sexual behavior as an intimacy disorder, as well as a compulsion or an addiction, much easier.

The following list examines types of problematic sexual behaviors and cybersex from the perspective of a courtship problem—that is, courtship gone awry. If you are struggling with compulsive online sexual behavior, there are steps you can take that will offer a new perspective on these problems.

The chart on page 89 summarizes the stages of courtship and the ten compulsive types. It shows how each type of behavior is affected by problems in specific courtship dimensions. For example, people who struggle with voyeuristic behaviors (the second of the compulsive types) have problems in three courtship stages: noticing, attraction, and flirtation. Their problem is rooted in an inability to competently carry out the tasks of these three stages. Likewise, a person struggling with seductive-role sex (the fourth compulsive type) needs help in the courtship areas of flirtation, demonstration, romance, individuation, and intimacy. Studying this chart can help you better understand how compulsive behavior is, in part, a courtship problem. These people's life experiences never allowed the evolution of effective and satisfying courtship skills.

FANTASY SEX

Here, people notice attractive traits in others and feel attracted to them, but they don't move beyond this stage. Staying in the fantasy world feels safer than acting on the fantasy. Romance and sex can flourish when there is no reality testing. These people also can become obsessed. Laurie, a middle-aged female physician, for example, sought counseling for multiple cyber-affairs. Laurie was in e-mail contact with a number of physicians on her hospital's medical staff and, in her mind, was having a cyber-affair with each of them—except that nothing was actually going on. It was all a fantasy. Countless chat rooms are filled with romance junkies like Laurie.

Masturbation to fantasies is how we learn about our own desire. When masturbation becomes compulsive, we make it a way to escape loneliness. It is about fear of rejection, fear of reality, and anxiety reduction. It can also be self-indulgent in the sense of seeking comfort as opposed to risking a relationship. Many people who engage in cybersex find refuge in fantasy sex because other forms of sexuality are simply too complicated, risky, or require too much effort. Fantasy sex is a way to disassociate from reality, including relationships. The noticing and attraction parts of courtship become very skewed in fantasy sex.

Fantasy sex fits very well with the Internet because, as we have seen, so much of Internet relationships are fantasy. Cybersex is all about trying to stay in a fantasy world because it is safe and requires no work, unlike real relationships.

Courtship Disorder and the Ten Compulsive Types

COMPONENTS OF COURTSHIP

SEXUALLY COMPULSIVE BEHAVIOR	Noticing	Attraction	Flirtation	Demonstration	Romance	Individuation	Intimacy	Touching	Foreplay	Intercourse	Commitment	Renewal
Fantasy	•	•										
Voyeurism	•	•	•									
Exhibitionism		•	•	•								
Seductive Role			•	•	•	•	•				•	•
Trading			•	•	•	•	•				•	•
Intrusive						•	•	•	•		•	•
Paying						•	•	•	•	•	•	•
Anonymous						•	•	•	•	•	•	•
Pain Exchange								•	•	•	•	•
Exploitive	•	•	•	•	•	•	•	•	•	•	•	•

Figure 5.1

VOYEURISM

Voyeurs are also nonparticipants in the sex game. They, however, do move beyond fantasy by searching for sexual objects in the real or cyber-world. In today's society, it is normal to enjoy looking at others sexually. Most people want to take the next step of participating.

Often, people who are Internet voyeurs are extremely passive participants whose goal is not to be involved in chat rooms or interactive Web sites, but instead merely to lurk and watch. To put it in childhood terms, it's "you show me yours and I'll watch."

Usually voyeurism involves objectifying the other person, so it is not a personal relationship. This is the crucial aspect of online voyeurism: the whole experience is about objectifying. Noticing and attraction are skewed because they aren't mutually experienced. A pseudo-flirtation takes place because the person being watched doesn't know the viewer and is not truly interacting with him or her either.

EXHIBITIONISM

Exhibitionism is the "I will show you mine" part—a way of introducing oneself in an inappropriate way. It is pleasurable and normal to have others notice you sexually. With a partner, exhibitionism is a significant part of sex play. Those with problematic sexual behavior fixate on just being noticed and have difficulty moving beyond this stage. Eroticism for them is being looked at. For some, it involves the power of realizing that they have captured another's attention. For others, it is being angry and aggressive by forcing their sexuality on someone. From a relationship perspective, exhibitionism means introducing oneself in an inappropriate way or seeking attention from others with no intent of going further, which is teasing. Sometimes it is the pleasure of breaking the rules. When exhibitionism is obsessional and compulsive, it is a significant distortion of normal courtship.

Cyber-exhibitionism is commonly played out by men who use live-video-feed camera sites. Their goal is to go online and masturbate while others can watch them. This becomes their primary, and sometimes exclusive, way to relate sexually to others. Some men, particularly those who have actually exposed themselves in public, believe that cyber-exhibitionism is a safer and legal way to be sexual. Granted, this form of acting out does not create victims and generally is not illegal (breaking into teen chat rooms with such photos would, however, be illegal). This "solution" does not, however, allow them to address or deal with the deeper relationship and courtship issues underlying their behavior. It's merely a way to carry out the same behavior in a way that isn't illegal. What's more, these men often eventually move or return to the real world using this behavior.

SEDUCTIVE-ROLE SEX

In seductive-role sex, relationships are about power and conquest. Flirtation, demonstration, and romance are the erotic keys in this category. These people—most often women—are hooked on winning the attention of others and falling in love. Once they have accomplished this, however, sexual interest usually subsides. While they can quickly gain the confidence of others and be intimate in the early discovery and romantic stage, establishing a deeper relationship eludes them. Others in this group feel trapped and unable to be themselves. So, they have multiple online or offline relationships where they can act in different ways with different people. They have a hard time being themselves or being truthful. Since they fear abandonment, having more than one relationship is a way to prevent the hurt they are sure to receive once the relationship ends.

Online, it's possible to have numerous sexual relationships by taking part in different chat rooms. These online trysts provide a way to feel as though you are in a relationship but, at the same time, ensure that you will not really be abandoned—because you're not really in a relationship in the first place. Some women cruise chat rooms to flirt and seduce, but when a man actually becomes interested and suggests a face-to-face meeting, these women immediately run the other way. These women don't want to actually meet men because their game would instantly lose its power. The game's attraction is to get guys so hooked that they beg to meet the woman. This way, the woman remains in control and can refuse the encounter. People in this group are crippled in their ability to form lasting bonds and enduring relationships.

TRADING SEX

Online trading for sex can be carried out in a number of ways. Exchanging pornography is the most obvious example; however, the Internet has been the greatest boon to prostitution since the invention of the telephone. It is easy to go online to a prostitution service, view the variety of men or women available, choose one, and reserve him or her without speaking to anyone. The Internet makes the whole process easier and "safer," though certainly not legal.

Some sex workers actually do form some attachment to their clients, but typically bartering sex for money is devoid of relationship. The goal is to simulate flirtation, demonstration, and romance. What actually happens in most cases is a replication of childhood sexual abuse in which the child seemingly gains power while being forced to be sexual with a caregiver. If a prostitute is a sex addict—meaning that she or he finds sex more pleasurable with clients than in personal relationships and is "hooked on the life"—the situation represents a significant distortion of normal courtship. Often the money exchanged is a sign of success in the sexual "game." Forging significant, enduring bonds or being true to oneself is not part of the game.

INTRUSIVE SEX
People who carry out intrusive sex, such as touching people in crowds or making obscene calls, are really perverting the touching and foreplay dimensions of courtship. In most cases, they are using others for sexual arousal with little chance of being caught. Their behavior represents both intimacy failure and individuation difficulties. Although their behavior is predatory, they do not see it as such. An implicit anger exists here. They "steal" sex because they believe no one would respond as they want. The goal becomes "taking sex" without the other's knowledge. They become quite expert in their subterfuge. Professionals such as physicians, clergy, or attorneys are capable of intrusive sex just as easily as anyone else. For example, they can use their occupation to appear quite compassionate, when in fact, they use their clients' vulnerability for their own arousal. Sue's story is typical of such abuse:

> I saw Dr. "X," a gynecologist, for the first time because of a Pap smear that showed irregular cells. I chose him because my family physician was concerned about cervical cancer. During his digital exam, this gynecologist, well, he just kept his fingers inside me too long. It felt like something more than just an exam, like he was getting off on it. And then when he talked to me afterwards, he kept touching me. It was

nothing really overt, but I really had an icky feeling when I walked out of that exam room.

Sue felt "icky" for good reason. This doctor was crossing sexual boundaries with her. He was exploiting the power he had as a doctor for sexual gratification in a very covert, yet intrusive, way.

For this type of person, stolen intrusion becomes the obsession, and an ongoing relationship life suffers because of secret shame. These people may try to enter nonsexual realms of the Internet and make them sexual. They may go into nonsexual chat rooms like a game room and have sexual conversations. Or people will occasionally enter live video sites that are clearly nonsexual (such as online "coffeehouses" where the discussions focus on philosophy, politics, books, and so forth) and try to turn the conversation to sex or even expose themselves to others with a live video cam. Some men will go into teen chat rooms, pretend they are a teen, ask for a photo exchange, and then send in photos of themselves naked. This is very intrusive, and illegal, since they know that the teens are underage.

Some people keep sexually explicit screen savers on their work computers that may intrude on others. Public libraries currently have a problem with people who view or download and print pornographic material just so other library patrons will see it. Again, this is intrusive and harassing. It is intentionally crossing a boundary by confronting people with a sexual image that they did not agree to see.

Paying for Sex

These people are willing participants in simulated intimacy. They may pay for sex using a credit card on live video feeds and have someone perform the sexual acts they want to see. They may pay for porn, often spending hundreds of dollars a month for membership in many Internet porn sites. And today there are increasing numbers of prostitution rings online, sites through which you can schedule the time and place where your offline meeting will take place. This system bridges the gap between online and offline prostitution, since payment and arrangements take place online, with the meeting happening offline in the physical world. For those who obsessively pay for sex, the costs can be staggering. The income of participants doesn't seem to matter; all spend beyond their means. The guy with a $500,000 annual salary will spend $5,000 for a night with a high-priced prostitute, while the guy making $40,000 a year will continue to do $25 to $40 deals in the backseat of his car with street prostitutes. There are records of people who've spent $500,000 on prostitutes in just two months. All who pay for sex are focused, however, on the touching, foreplay, and intercourse dimensions while ignoring the work (and ultimately, the benefits) of a relationship.

Anonymous Sex

Perhaps no other medium serves the need for anonymous sex better than the Internet. It provides the ultimate in anonymity. Frequently, part of the attraction for people is the risk of unknown persons and situations. People go online for the sole purpose of finding someone they do not know to be a sex partner. By definition, anonymous sex is not about being in a relationship. With anonymous sex, you do not have to attract, seduce, trick, or even pay. It is simply sex. Frequently, part of the high for sex addicts is the risk encountered with unknown persons and situations. This stems in part from early sexual relationships that were fearful. Having to experience fear in order for arousal or sexual initiation to occur fundamentally distorts the courtship process. The safety of enduring bonds that allow deeper, profound risks of being known by another is never present.

Pain Exchange Sex

There are many fetish and S and M sites available on the Internet for people who have an interest in this kind of sex and who find it difficult to play it out in the real world. There is an important distinction to be made between people who are merely playing with roles, and engaging in mutually consensual S and M activities that cause no damage to either person, versus people for whom S and M is the only way they know to be sexual. When arousal is predicated on pain, degradation, or humiliation, it simply does not add to a person's health and well-being.

Unfortunately, such activities can and do escalate quickly once these behaviors become compulsive, and this is when people can be seriously hurt. People who take part compulsively in painful, degrading, or dangerous sexual practices, such as "blood sports" (creating wounds that bleed as part of sex) or asphyxiation, often have significant distortions of courtship. Specifically, touching, foreplay, and intercourse become subordinated to a dramatic story line that is usually a reenactment of a childhood abuse experience. Arousal that is based primarily on the experience of pain is a distortion of sexual and relationship health. People whose arousal scenarios are embedded in high-risk sex find enduring relationships to be difficult. They may be downloading S and M images and video clips, and because the only way they know how to act sexually involves degradation and humiliation, their behavior becomes damaging to themselves and others.

EXPLOITIVE SEX

To exploit the vulnerable is clearly distorted courtship. Sex offenders who rape have deep problems with intimacy and anger. Less obvious are nonviolent predators who seduce children or professionals who sexually misbehave with clients. In the workplace, where there is a differential of power, employees can be exploited. When arousal and attraction are dependent on the vulnerability of another, there is a significant courtship problem all along the courtship continuum. Sex addicts in this category will use "grooming" behavior that is carefully designed to build the trust of the unsuspecting victim. Attraction, flirtation, demonstration, romance, and intimacy are all used to gain the confidence of another for sexual exploitation. These people will go to the extent of professing an enduring bond with a much more malevolent intent. Online, exploitive behavior includes sex offenders who target teens and younger children via the Internet or men meeting women online with the intent of arranging an offline meeting so they can force them to be sexual.

PROCEEDING WITH CAUTION ON THE INTERNET

Our human relationships have evolved over millennia in the physical presence of other humans. Today's sudden development of the Internet offers a new and different way to meet others. Can the Internet serve as a healthy and valuable tool to facilitate meeting others? Certainly. Many people use it to meet people whom they may not otherwise have been able to meet. Visiting chat rooms and special interest sites, for example, can be a good way to find others with similar interests and to make valuable connections.

Our experience tells us, however, that the Internet provides only the starting point for friendship or romantic relationships. Too many people try to progress through courtship online only to find soon that it's not working out as they'd hoped. This is because it's simply not possible to progress through the steps of courtship online. All the Internet can provide is a kind of pre-noticing—a step zero, if you will. Real courtship can progress only if it includes physical connection and all that it brings. People who have had a long online relationship—for a year or two, for example—do learn quite a bit about one another (assuming that they are both being honest), but no matter how much they know, many relationship elements remain missing. The successful long-term online relationships we have witnessed progressed at some point to the phone, and finally (and carefully!) to an actual meeting. That's when courtship really began.

We all have friendships in which we have become physically separated. Despite being geographically apart, we can still maintain those very close relationships via the phone and Internet. When we see our friend, it can seem as though we've never been apart. This happens, however, because we had already completed many of the courtship dimensions before we were separated.

If many years pass without physical contact, however, even the strongest relationships will wane and some of the closeness diminish in the absence of physical companionship. Again, we need face-to-face contact to reinforce our connection; that is, to reinforce the courtship dimensions. Relationships require being in geographic proximity and actual physical contact.

IS IT REALLY CHEATING?

If you are struggling with online relationships and sexuality, you might be saying to yourself, "Well, if cyber-relationships aren't *really* relationships after all, then what's the problem having them? Cybersex isn't infidelity, so why not do it?"

The answer is that every moment you spend in an online relationship or activity is time you could be spending with the people in your life who matter to you. The more time you spend in cyberspace, the more you neglect those relationships. Regardless of whether cyber-relationships are true relationships, the repercussions of them on you, your partner, family, and friends are exactly the same as an offline illicit relationship. By not addressing this issue, you are also putting off the work you need to do to help yourself have richer and more fulfilling offline relationships.

In the next chapter, we will talk about how you can start to make positive changes in your life and begin the healing process.

6

Boundaries

WE'VE NOW TALKED ABOUT courtship and the relationships we have with others. In this chapter, we will look at another relationship, the one you have with yourself. We will introduce the idea of boundaries—what we define as a relationship with yourself—and look at how the computer and the Internet can foster boundary problems and magnify courtship problems and disorders.

We would like you to begin by imagining that you've cloned yourself. Now you must care for this baby, this miniature version of yourself. How would you raise this child? Exactly the way you were raised? Probably not. It's likely that you would raise this child differently—and better—than you were raised. In reality, you would care for this baby as though you were caring for yourself.

In this exercise of caring for your imaginary cloned child, you would regularly ask what would be the most loving thing you could do for him or her in every situation. And that's exactly how you should care for yourself. Treat yourself with the utmost compassion and never be afraid to ask what is best for you at any given time. Having parental feelings toward yourself is healthy. It is your chance to "reparent" yourself. It presents the opportunity to give yourself some of the love, affection, and guidance you missed when you were growing up. It is learning to love and respect and care for *you* that forms the foundation for building appropriate boundaries in your life. Learning to set appropriate boundaries is also the first step in creating a healthy zone in which to live—a Recovery Zone—an idea we will return to in chapter 8.

SAYING NO

Perhaps the most primitive of boundaries is abstinence itself—saying no to something. Let's look at a couple of examples of non-Internet and nonsexual boundaries. Perhaps you want to lose weight, and to do so you've decided to eat more healthy foods and get some exercise every day. For a few weeks, you maintain your new regimen. Then work and family life get busy, and you skip exercising for a few days and stop by some fast-food restaurants for quick lunches. How do you feel about yourself? Probably disappointed and maybe even somewhat disgusted. Perhaps you even want to say, "OK, to heck with it," and you pull into the nearest fast-food joint again on your lunch break and dive right into a couple of fat-laden burgers and a super-size order of fries. In so doing, you've broken a boundary you'd set for yourself.

Another example of boundaries might involve a promise made to better handle your finances. You've set a goal to try to save money and to pay off your credit card debt. You become depressed and go on a little spending spree to cheer yourself up. How do you feel about yourself after doing this? You probably thought that shopping would make you feel better, but instead you ended up feeling worse about yourself than before. The items you bought are a daily reminder that you couldn't afford them, so you don't enjoy them either. You've broken a boundary you set for yourself and now you feel bad.

If you were taking care of yourself, your greater goal would be to get to a point at which you have happiness, enjoyment, *and* relief from living paycheck to paycheck. You must ask yourself this: Is taking care of myself important enough to me that I will do what it takes to make that happen? Author Robert Bly expressed this concept well when he said, "The making of a man is making your body do what it doesn't want to do."[1] You may not *want* to create boundaries in your life, but doing so is absolutely necessary to achieve what you really want in life.

BOUNDARIES MUST BE TAUGHT AND LEARNED

Very young children have no boundaries.[2] Parents need to protect their children from being abused by others and to respectfully help children learn to put limits on their own behavior. It is through the protection and guidance of parents and other caregivers that we eventually learn to have healthy, firm, and flexible boundaries by the time we reach adulthood.

You can also think of boundaries as a kind of "force field," or safety barrier, that surrounds us. Emotional and psychological health requires that we know how to set individual boundaries in times of emotional pressure. It also means that we know how to let them down when we want love and nurturing. We also need to know how to set reasonable limits—boundaries—in our relationship with a partner.

The way boundaries are set varies from family to family. People who have grown up in dysfunctional homes with less-than-nurturing parenting usually have inadequately developed boundaries. They may have no boundaries at all or damaged boundaries. They may also use "walls" instead of boundaries, or they may move back and forth between putting up walls and having no boundaries whatsoever.

WHEN BOUNDARIES ARE TOO LOOSE

When boundaries are too loose, children are exposed to invasive abuse—physical, emotional, sexual, or religious—and experiences from which they should be protected.

Physical invasion takes place when one or both parents physically abuse their children. These children may be physically harmed, locked in their rooms, deprived of food, yelled at, or threatened.

Emotional invasion takes place when a parent or other caregiver expects and teaches the child to attend to that adult's own emotional needs. For example, a father who loves tennis relentlessly pushes his boys into playing tennis more than they want to because it makes him happy and he enjoys it. Emotional invasion also occurs when an adult expects from a child a level of understanding and support beyond a child's capabilities. For example, Dad's primary love is his work, so he is seldom home. Mom regularly says to her son, "I don't know what I'd do without you, Paul; I rely on you so much." Paul's mother has unfairly turned to her nine-year-old son for the understanding and emotional support that should be given by her husband, not her child.

Sexual invasion can occur in a variety of ways. It not only includes various forms of inappropriate touch, but it may also occur when children are teased regularly about their bodies, when they're told inappropriate sexual jokes, or when they're otherwise sexually harassed. Actually having sex with a child is the most obvious example of this category. It is important to note that if a child is living in an emotionally invasive relationship with a parent, then virtually any form of physical touching—kissing, hugging, lap sitting—can become erotically charged and is a form of sexual abuse.

Religious invasion occurs when, for example, children get messages from their parents that convince them that they are a mistake in the eyes of God. (This discussion about religious abuse is not intended to make a theo-logical statement; it merely recognizes that these behaviors exist.) For ex-ample, Lisa, a three-year-old, slid down a banister and fell off and bumped her head. Her mother responded by saying, "I wonder if Jesus wanted you sliding down that banister. If he did, I don't think he would have let you bump your head."

A BOUNDARY SYSTEM WITH "HOLES" IN IT

People with nonexistent boundaries have no sense of being abused or of being abusive to others. They allow others to take advantage of them physi-cally, sexually, emotionally, or spiritually without clear knowledge that they have the right to say, "Stop." Nor do they recognize other people's right to have boundaries, moving through the boundaries of others unaware that they are acting inappropriately.

A damaged boundary system has "holes" in it. People with damaged boundaries can set limits at certain times or with certain people. A person may, for example, be able to set boundaries with everyone but authority fig-ures, his or her partner, or his or her children. These people also have only a partial awareness that others have boundaries. Thus, they may step into certain people's lives to try to control or manipulate them. Damaged bound-aries can lead people to take responsibility for someone else's feelings, think-ing, or behavior. People may feel shame and guilt because their partners insulted someone at a party.

Some people substitute a system of walls made up of anger or fear for boundaries. These walls give off either verbal or nonverbal messages that say, "If you come near me or if you say anything about such-and-such, I'll explode! I might hit you or yell at you, so watch out." Others are then afraid to approach them for fear of triggering that anger. There are also walls created with silence or with words. People using a "wall of silence" become quiet and just seem to "fade into the woodwork." They prefer to observe others rather than interact with them. On the other hand, people using a "wall of words" talk and talk and talk, even when someone politely tries to contribute to the conversation by making a comment or attempting to change the subject.

WHEN BOUNDARIES ARE TOO RIGID

When parents set boundaries too rigidly, they create a "shell" around their children that overly insulates them from the surrounding world. Little can touch these children, including what ought to—love, care, nurturing, and touch itself in the form of physical affection. Such children feel lost, abandoned, and "on their own."

Physical abandonment occurs when a child doesn't have a sense of physical safety (this may happen to latchkey children, for example) or when the parents leave their children for long periods of time. It also occurs when children receive little or no instructions on how to take care of themselves, such as when to go to bed, how to brush their teeth, or how to eat well. Abandonment also occurs in situations where parents are physically present but pay little or no attention to their children.

Emotional abandonment occurs when children are regularly talked out of their feelings. When children come to their parents to talk about something upsetting and are told, "No, you're not upset; that was no big deal" or "Don't be sad," that is emotional abandonment. Though the child experiences feelings, the parents deny the existence or validity of these feelings.

Sexual abandonment occurs when the child does not receive appropriate modeling or instruction about healthy sexuality. Examples include parents who tell their daughter nothing about menstruation until she actually has her first period; parents who offer no support for their children for events that may be embarrassing (for example, the first time they have to take a shower with other kids after gym class); and parents who do not teach their children about safe sex.

Spiritual abandonment occurs when a child does not receive modeling or instruction in healthy spirituality. Parents may not, for example, give the child any opportunity for religious or spiritual instruction. Religious views may be actively or passively denounced. Children receive no teaching about their responsibilities as humans for the welfare of others and the importance of contributing to the greater good of society.

INCONSISTENT BOUNDARIES

It's not unusual for the same child to experience both loose and rigid boundaries. One parent may generally create loose boundaries, while the other parent is setting rigid ones. Here's an example: a father regularly shouts at and puts down his children (a loose boundary), while their mother ignores this situation even when the kids go to her for help. The children are not being heard, protected, and nurtured as they should be (a rigid boundary).

Children may experience abuse in subtle and indirect ways: "Well, we just don't expect you to be as good as your brother, because your brother is just good at everything he does. He's just naturally smarter than you are."

Many adults who are struggling in their relationships grew up in families in which boundaries were either regularly violated or inconsistently set. It is hard for adults to set boundaries and build healthy relationships when an appropriate model was never provided. Attempt to recall incidents of invasion or abandonment from your past. Your mind will allow you to remember incidents as you are able to deal with them.

THE INNER VOICE

Boundaries are a relationship with ourselves, one in which we seek to hear and follow our inner voice. Have your ever had the experience of being about to do something when you hear a voice inside that says, "No, don't do that," but then you do it anyway—even though you were pretty certain that the outcome wouldn't be good? You didn't listen to yourself and you felt bad about it afterward. When we hear, acknowledge, and follow that voice, we are holding to our boundaries. We are honoring our relationship with ourselves. But don't mistake what we are talking about for narcissism or arrogance. We mean making a real commitment to care for yourself in the way that a good parent would by nurturing, supporting, and protecting yourself. Respecting good boundaries means being able to say, "No, I'm not going to do that even though I want to, because if I do, I'm going to mess up my life."

Keeping boundaries means more than just paying attention to your conscience. Your conscience simply tells you what's right and wrong. We are referring to a level of discernment that grows out of a caring for self rather than from a worry about what the impact of your behavior might be on another. It means honoring your internal sense of what is the best for you. If you act in a way that always honors yourself, your actions will not harm others.

We all have an inner voice that can positively guide our actions. At times, however, we choose to ignore that voice. The ancient Greeks understood this very well, describing it in the myth of the Sirens. The Sirens were maidens who called out with irresistibly lovely voices to sailors, luring them landward toward shipwreck on rocky, dangerous shores. Because their call could distort all sense of time and weather and danger, countless ships followed the "Siren call" to destruction and death.

The Internet and cybersex provide an easy way to mute our inner voice. They are like the Siren call, a seemingly innocent and harmless beckoning to enter a portal that distorts time, perceptions, and values. Cybersex can override your inner voice and begin to collapse your boundaries, just as the reefs crushed the sailors' ships as they followed the Siren call. Cybersex is capable of casting a spell under which you no longer think about what you are doing, and distractions fall away as you slip deeper and deeper into the cyber-world.

SETH'S DESTRUCTIVE STORY

Seth, a married fifty-five-year-old man, father of two adult children, tells this story:

> I stopped drinking twenty-three years ago. During my thirteenth year of sobriety, I began treatment for serious problems with my sexual behaviors, which included going to prostitutes, pornography use, and extramarital affairs. After much struggle, I got my life back together and became an insurance claims adjuster. Eventually, I became one of my

company's best, often traveling throughout the country to handle the biggest and most complicated claims. I was doing quite well for more than a decade—so well that I even stopped attending Twelve Step meetings. I felt that the support they had provided for so long simply wasn't necessary anymore. And my life was going well—until I discovered cybersex. I became interested in pornography on the Net. Then I started looking around to see what else the Net had to offer in the sexual arena. Soon I discovered I could book prostitutes via the Net. It was quickly downhill from there. When I started using prostitutes and going to strip bars again, I became so despondent that I started drinking on the sly. Because I was on the road, my wife was not aware what was happening. Eventually, I made a pass at two women, both of whom were involved with claims I was investigating. They reported my inappropriate actions to the company and I was promptly fired. In only three short months of destructive behavior, all that I had worked for and built over many years was gone. My wife was devastated by this turn of events. It came as a complete shock to her. She had no idea that I'd been drinking again, let alone been unfaithful to her. She threatened to walk out on the spot. I was able to talk her out of it at the time, but I don't know what will happen to our relationship in the long term.

Seth had worked diligently for many years to create strong boundaries for his behavior. Here was a man who had a solid and long-term recovery with firm boundaries. After all, he was aware of the situations that could trigger his drinking and sexual compulsions. He knew how to stay away from their antecedents, the actions and situations that could become a slippery slope leading him closer to his triggers. Seth at first thought it was safe to dabble in cybersex. "It's not real sex," he told himself. What's more, it didn't seem like any trigger he'd ever encountered or like any of his trigger antecedents. Internet sex turned out to be very powerful, and by stumbling into the world of cybersex, Seth indeed set off many of his old triggers.

Again we see the power of cybersex. Passing through this portal creates an essential distortion in which there is the loss of self as you enter a trance-like state, mesmerized by the Siren call of the Net. Nothing seems real, which is precisely why the Internet makes it so easy to distort your relationship with yourself—your boundaries. It's so easy to tell yourself you're not really doing anything wrong or destructive to yourself or others. There are no impediments or constraints to going online—you need only a computer and a modem. You don't have to lie. You don't need money. You can be anonymous. You don't have to get into a car. You don't have to do anything more than boot up your computer. Boundaries become distorted and collapse easily and silently, almost without thought. "None of this is real," we tell ourselves. The Internet becomes a kind of sensory deprivation tank in which we float mentally, undistracted and untroubled by a suddenly muted inner voice.

INTERNAL AND EXTERNAL BOUNDARIES

There are two sets of boundaries—internal and external (concrete). External boundaries are marked by motivation that comes from outside of ourselves. Often we set external boundaries because we know there will be consequences if we don't set them. People who acknowledge their problems with cybersex may, for example, set an external boundary by:

- keeping their computer on the main floor of the house rather than in a more private home office
- choosing a nonsexual screen name
- using the computer only when at work
- not logging on to sexual sites
- giving the password to an accountability person (not a spouse or partner) so he or she can check computer usage or history files

External boundaries are very concrete steps that help you contain or control your behavior. They are often steps that a spouse or partner or counselor wants you to set, and they are usually easily measurable or verifiable. Going on a diet involves setting and maintaining external boundaries. Let's say that your doctor has told you that you need to lose weight because of heart problems. At her suggestion, you decide to limit your calorie intake to a thousand per day. You decide to cut back on fatty foods, eat more fruits and vegetables, and so forth. These are concrete and measurable steps, and they're also externally motivated.

Setting external boundaries is often a good place to start when making changes in your behavior, but it is only a first step. (In the next chapter, we will show you exactly how to set appropriate and concrete external boundaries that are the first step in recovering from cybersex behaviors.) Too often, people believe that this is the only step they need to take to get control of a problem. Establishing concrete boundaries, however, is not enough. You also need to establish internal boundaries, which is essentially the process of learning to care for your inner self. Without internal boundaries, you will, in the long run, always find ways around your external boundaries. Having appropriate internal boundaries means taking actions because you inherently know that by doing so, you are caring for yourself and doing what is good for you. This is, as you might recognize, a more difficult and longer-term project.

The good news is that keeping your internal and external boundaries becomes easier over time. A new system emerges. You will begin to build momentum and strength as the weeks, months, and years pass, in much the same way that your problematic behaviors became stronger and more difficult to control over time. As you set and keep boundaries, you'll find yourself feeling good about having met your goals. As time passes, you'll continue to feel better about yourself and your life.

As you know, boundaries are about the relationship that you have with yourself. Relationships with others also require us to establish boundaries. Before you can set any boundaries with others, though, you must have clear and firm boundaries with yourself. You have to be able to hear that voice that says yes or no, right or wrong. You have to understand your own limits and boundaries.

If you have a history of problematic or addictive sexual behavior, it's likely that you have trouble recognizing and trusting your inner voice and that you have weak or even nonexistent boundaries. The Internet has merely provided you with another way to act out.

If, on the other hand, you have become involved with cybersex but have never fallen into anything sexual like this before, it's likely that you can hear and pay attention to your inner voice and that you still have fairly intact internal and external boundaries. The power of the Internet and the lure of cybersex may weaken or bypass your boundaries.

CULTURAL CYBERSEX BOUNDARIES

The struggle so many people are having with cybersex is exacerbated by the fact that our culture has yet to establish clear boundaries with regard to the Internet. We have barely begun to discuss what is appropriate Internet content and behavior, with the exception of acknowledging the illegality of trafficking in child pornography and advertising for or booking prostitutes online. Even those boundaries, however, are blurred. Software currently exists that will "morph" sexual images of people, including children. Morphing is the process of taking various body parts (the face of one child and the torso of another child, for example) and combining them to create an entirely new image of someone who technically does not exist. Other software allows the creation of computer-generated images (CGI) completely from scratch. Similar to an artist's canvas, the final product may be of any type of image (including pornographic), the difference being that CGIs can be near photographic quality. The legal system continues to debate whether morphed images and CGIs cross the legal boundaries of child pornography. In some cases people have been found guilty of possessing and distributing child pornography even when the images were found to be morphed or computer generated. Regardless of the legal definitions, from a psychological perspective, such images continue to fuel a risky behavior that should be addressed.

In some of the personal stories we've detailed in this book, you've seen other examples of this cultural struggle. Is an affair on the Internet really an affair? If you're not actually having physical contact with another person, can we say that one has been unfaithful or adulterous? What about exposing one's genitals: it's illegal to do this in public, but is it illegal to do so on the Net from the privacy of your own home?

Because our culture is still struggling to develop boundaries for the Internet, people don't really have much support as they try to develop personal boundaries regarding cybersex. With the Internet, we have created an entirely new way to connect with one another. Thus far, at least, it is one without guidelines and without history. It's uninhibited. It's different from television and radio because of its interactivity. What's more, the technology developed, emerged, and has been embraced by so many people so quickly that we've been unable as a culture to keep up with the many different ways that people can use the Internet for sexual purposes (such as creating CGIs). Without culturewide consensus, the inner voice that helps keep us safe in other areas is compromised.

In 2000, the Catholic Church defined virtual sexual relationships as infidelity. That statement is an example of our culture beginning to sort out and define what is morally acceptable Internet behavior. Although the original edition of this book speculated that more institutions would follow the Catholic Church in establishing norms and boundaries for online sexual behavior, we were wrong. Nearly seven years later, few, if any, other influential institutions have stepped up to the plate to take a position on online sexual behavior. Until the time when other norms and guidelines are created, we will each need to set our own boundaries.

You might be thinking, "OK, since there aren't really any rules, how can I be breaking any? There's nothing wrong with my behavior." Just because few cultural boundaries exist doesn't mean that there shouldn't be boundaries, nor does it mean that we should feel free to do whatever we want. There are internal anchors available to help us determine whether our behavior is right or wrong: our own moral/value system. If you believe it's wrong, for example, to have an affair, then you can infer that it's wrong to have a cyber-affair. In addition, you can pay attention to your inner voice. How would it feel to you, for example, to carry out an online affair unbeknownst to your spouse or partner? How would that person feel if he or she discovered your "affair"? What would be the effect of your online behavior on others? Would it be any different from a physical-world affair? No. Both have similar effects on all involved and both cause a breach of trust. You can also look at the effect of your online behavior on other aspects of your life. Is it positive or negative? Is it making your life happier and more fulfilling or is it making things worse?

When people compromise their boundaries, even if they don't realize that they've done so, they still feel a sense of shame. That feeling of shame is a signal that you've broken a boundary. It's an indicator that you've done something that, on some level, you do not feel good about doing. It means that at some level, you wish that you had not done that behavior. And this brings you back to not caring for yourself, not knowing what you need to do to care for yourself, or not listening to what your inner voice is telling you is best for you. In most people, this feeling arises immediately after they've broken a boundary. They may say to themselves, "How could I do that again? I promised myself I wouldn't do that. I don't like myself when I do that." At a deep level, even if you didn't consciously recognize it, you have an internal boundary that tells you it is not OK for you to perform certain actions because you know they will hurt you and perhaps another person too.

We want you to ask yourself—to pay attention to—how you feel after participating in cybersex. Do you feel guilty? Do you feel ashamed? Disgusted? If you're thinking about this now, you might initially say to yourself, "No, this isn't me. I don't have any problem. I feel fine when I've been on the Internet. I'm just sexually liberated." If you scored high on the screening tests in chapters 1 and 2, and if you take some time to really think about this and to pay attention to your feelings, you may discover a different response. And you may realize that what you are doing is causing pain or shame in your life and sorrow in the lives of the people you love.

CHANGING BOUNDARIES

You may have the impression now that boundaries must be rigid, even absolute, in order to be effective. In fact, boundaries can, and in some cases should, change. To illustrate this idea, let's look at families and the ways they organize themselves into what are called family systems.

A healthy family has the capacity to organize and reorganize itself as it grows and changes—in other words, to develop, set, and change boundaries. Family system models generally recognize four levels of adaptability within families. Each of the four levels represents a range of behavior options.

- Rigid: Rigid families use extremely autocratic decision-making styles in which there is limited negotiation, with strictly defined roles and rules.
- Structured: Structured families mix authoritarian with some egalitarian leadership, resulting in stable roles and rules.
- Flexible: Flexible families use egalitarian leadership, seeking negotiated agreements and making for easily changed rules and roles.
- Chaotic: Chaotic families have erratic and ineffective leadership that results in impulsive decisions, inconsistent rules, and role reversals.

Structured and flexible systems are regarded as the best for optimum family and individual growth. Healthy families move between these two systems depending on various factors. For example, a family with two children under the age of five would thrive in a structured format, given the need for consistency and direction of small children. When the children are older, the same family will shift to a more flexible mode, given the need for and ability of the children to handle more autonomy and decision making.

Of course, every family has its moments of chaos and rigidity, but families that remain in the extremes damage their members. For example, children who live in rigid families end up with lifelong struggles with rules and authority—whether it is in excessive rebelliousness or excessive passivity—because of the unreachable expectations of their parents. Chaotic families produce children who have difficulty incorporating a consistent set of boundaries into their own consciences because no one ever showed them how to set boundaries or had any expectation of them to do so. An intriguing aspect of systems is that opposite extremes have similar consequences. Both rigidity and chaos affect conscience formation and boundary-setting ability.

A family's inability to adapt to children's needs becomes extremely important because of the close connection between a child's need to depend on others and compulsive/addictive behaviors. To illustrate, in rigid families, children who ask for help may receive assistance, but with a heavy price in the form of lectures, high expectations, and moralizing about failure. Under those conditions, children quickly learn not to ask for help. In chaotic families, when children ask for help, the assistance is incomplete, inconsistent, or doesn't come at all. Rather than embarrass their parents again and subject themselves to further confusion and disapproval, the children simply stop asking.

Children need to be able to count on—to depend on—their families for survival, nurturing, love, and approval. If the family doesn't provide it, they will look for what they can depend upon, and they find it. Drugs, alcohol, food, and sex always produce a predictable, albeit an ultimately self-destructive, high. If a child develops a reliance on these external sources, pleasurable experiences become the primary relationship upon which he or she relies.

Healthy adults have a range of boundaries covering all areas of their lives, including relationships with family members, work colleagues, legal issues, and so on. And at times, we change our boundaries. If, for example, a man is struggling with online sexual behaviors, we might suggest that masturbation is not an acceptable behavior for a time because that was what he did whenever he felt lonely, angry, or sad. In six months or a year, when he better understands himself and is feeling better about himself and his marital relationship, we might say that it's OK to masturbate. Boundaries can have a fluidity and flexibility to them, depending on what's going on in your life.

The danger, of course, is that we can all be good at coming up with reasons for changing our boundaries. Each of the examples of problematic online sexual behavior in this book shows how somebody rationalized boundary changes. You might, for example, have set a boundary that says you won't use your computer at work for sexual purposes. But during a particularly stressful day, you might find yourself thinking that just for today, just for five or ten minutes, you will log on to a sexually explicit Web site at work to feel a little better.

THERE IS HELP OUT THERE: NO NEED TO GO IT ALONE

We encourage people who are working to change their sexual behaviors to develop and rely on a strong support group. If you are thinking about changing a boundary in your life, it's important to talk it over with someone in your support group before you change it. And that means talking to a live person, not leaving a message on his or her answering machine, such as, "OK, today I'm changing my boundary about pornography at work. I'm sure this will be OK with you. Good-bye." You need to actually talk it over with another person who will help you look at why you're thinking about this change and determine whether this is a healthy change.

Again, we come back to asking what is really best for you—whether an action will support your relationship with yourself. If you cross that boundary at work, how will you feel about yourself when you get home or when you talk with those in your support group and tell them what you did? All the smaller boundaries are tied to this basic one.

Some people have a tendency to react to their problematic or addictive sexual behavior by saying something like this: "OK, so I have this problem.

Sex is a problem, so forget it. I just won't have anything to do with sex at all. I'll just stop."

Complete abstinence is not a solution, and this kind of thinking is just a move to an opposite extreme. It's similar to members of a chaotic family deciding to become rigid. As we've pointed out, we should seek the middle ground, which is a healthy sexuality.

Setting appropriate boundaries is critical to building and maintaining healthy relationships, successful recovery, and relapse prevention. It requires a critical restructuring of your relationship with yourself. Intimacy problems start with you and your boundaries. People who struggle with compulsive or addictive behaviors have not experienced or learned normal, healthy ways of nurturing themselves and respecting their own limits. What makes such a person vulnerable to the Net and to cybersex must be repaired in order to develop a healthy sexuality.

In previous chapters, you have explored the components that contribute to compulsive online sexual behavior. You have taken screening tests and you've learned about arousal templates, the components of courtship, and courtship disorders. In this chapter, we have talked about boundaries and how to set and maintain them. We have looked at ways to determine whether or not you are a person who can and does listen to your inner voice. You've seen how appropriate boundaries are a critical component of healthy relationships and that they play an important role in successful recovery from problematic and addictive online sexual behavior.

As you look at these areas of your life, can you recognize the role boundaries play in your life? Can you recognize a pattern in your sexual behavior? Can you see particular areas that are not going well? If so, you may be experiencing a number of feelings: guilt, sadness, shame, remorse, despair, and hopelessness. If you are, this is a good sign. It means that you are able to look more honestly at yourself and your behaviors. This is the first and critical step in making a positive change in your life.

Be assured that there is hope for successful change. In the next and subsequent chapters, we will help you leave problematic online sexual behaviors behind. We will show you how to develop healthier relationships and a more fulfilling sex life. We will help you set appropriate boundaries and determine which people in your life can help you through this transition and help you maintain this new, positive direction in your life.

7
Taking That First Step

AT THIS POINT, as you begin to look more closely at the situation you are in, you may be experiencing a range of feelings, such as confusion, concern, frustration, and anger, as well as loss and hopelessness. Such feelings are very common. The good news, although it may be hard to believe right now, is that understanding the significance of your problem is really the beginning of the recovery process. In this chapter, we will help you understand the extent of your problem and how, by doing so, you're taking a big step forward in attaining recovery. You've probably had many moments when you resolved to change, control, or stop your cybersex behaviors, but you didn't. That's because you didn't really understand that you had a serious problem. What we're talking about now is how you can get to the point of accepting your situation and, as a result, make positive changes.

NO MORE CYBERSEX

In the language of Twelve Step recovery, you are beginning to take a First Step. A First Step has two critical components, the first being to acknowledge your limitations. This means acknowledging that perhaps you aren't the same as most other people when it comes to cybersex. When you participate in it, you, unlike many others, can't control your usage. The second component of a First Step is to accept that you need help with this problem and that support may come in various forms such as therapy, medication, spiritual growth, behavioral changes, and personal exploration and growth.

In addition, it's time to recognize and acknowledge that your cybersex behavior is damaging you and others in your life and it can't continue.

We certainly don't advocate that people with compulsive addiction become celibate for the rest of their lives. We instead want to help them find a way to develop a healthy sex life, which is much different from a life immersed in cybersex. Just as an alcoholic must stop drinking completely, so, too, must you stop your cybersex activities. Cybersex is a behavior that some people simply cannot control. There's no middle ground. Cybersex is an activity you can't take part in any longer. "Controlled" use doesn't work because it's just too easy to fall back into compulsive behaviors. There's no room for negotiation.

THE GRIEVING PROCESS

Once you accept the fact that cybersex is an activity you can't take part in because you can't control it, you will begin a grieving process. Initially, this process involves some denial—denial that the problem exists and that there is any need to change. Eventually, we all go through a grieving process when we finally accept that there are limitations in our lives. There's a feeling of loss when you have to accept that there's an activity—drinking, gambling, or cybersex, for example—that other people can take part in that you cannot. Grief is part of addiction, and Twelve Step recovery programs are really a grieving process. We will return to this idea at the end of the chapter.

Your feelings of grief will likely center around the following four areas: (1) realizing that you can't engage in cybersex any longer; (2) the "death" of your sexual fantasy life; (3) the impact of past losses as a result of your cybersex behaviors; and (4) a fear of not knowing who you will be or what you will do without cybersex because it has been like a "friend" who provides you comfort.

REALIZING THAT YOU CAN'T ENGAGE IN CYBERSEX ANY LONGER
All recovering alcoholics, for example, eventually come to the realization that when they consume alcohol, they just aren't like most other people they know. Try as they might have, often over many years, they simply can't control their alcohol use. Cybersex presents a similar problem for you, and

you have to acknowledge that even though other people you know may be able to dabble in cybersex, you cannot. Occasional or moderate use quickly becomes an obsession.

THE DEATH OF YOUR SEXUAL FANTASY LIFE

You, like many people, probably had and still have numerous sexual fantasies, some of them "forbidden." At some point, you discovered sex on the Internet and soon realized that you could access any fantasy you ever had, not to mention new ones. You discovered a whole new world where you could have sex with hundreds of partners. Cybersex became the answer to your dreams. But eventually you became so wrapped up in those fantasies that you lost touch with life in the real world. You've discovered that you have to let go of your cybersex life and that there are sexual limitations. In reality, creating a rich, fulfilling relationship with one person is where the real challenge lies. Your fantasy life is nothing more than an imaginary trip beyond your limits, beyond what is really possible. By living in that fantasy world, you are actually preventing yourself from having a relationship that will be truly meaningful. With the realization that you can't have it all, however, comes a profound sense of loss.

THE IMPACT OF PAST LOSSES AS A RESULT OF YOUR CYBERSEX BEHAVIORS

At this point in the recovery process, when people begin to acknowledge what's been happening to them, they suddenly look back on their lives only to finally see the fallout that they've left behind—all the relationships that they've destroyed, the botched jobs, and the lost educational opportunities. The damage assessment begins, and they examine the consequences of their behavior.

You might think of the months or years you were participating in cybersex as riding the crest of a wave that became larger as it accumulated the consequences of your cybersex behavior. But now, time has run out. The wave is coming up against the shoreline of reality, and you can't pull off and paddle back out for another ride because it has simply grown too big. As the wave begins breaking, what you're feeling is all those consequences crashing down around you, tossing you like a pebble in the undertow. You see, feel, and are surrounded all at once by all of it.

Suddenly, you feel the pain of all the unacknowledged losses of family, friends, job opportunities, and relationships. The embarrassment of having been discovered by a spouse, partner, or employer comes crashing through. And perhaps you are realizing just how much time you've lost doing cybersex. There may have been countless hours that could have been spent enjoying friends and family, reading, taking classes, exercising, playing sports, achieving greater success and financial rewards at work, and much more.

These are the origins of your grief. It can feel overwhelming when it is with you all the time. Since you were unaware of or denied your losses along the way, you couldn't grieve them at the time they occurred. Now they appear in front of you all at once because you've finally been able to let yourself see them.

As you become more aware of your losses, you may also feel ashamed, so much so that you may be tempted to put a barrier between yourself and others. While these feelings are natural and common, you should not further isolate yourself. This is, in fact, what you have been doing all along with cybersex. It's only through reconnecting with others that you will begin to heal and recover from your struggle with compulsive sexual behavior on the Internet. Recovery comes only with the support of others. Later in this chapter, we will show you how to build a strong support group.

A Fear of Not Knowing Who You'll Be without Cybersex
Over time, your whole identity became wrapped up in your cybersex use as it became your life focus. Even though you knew at some level that this was unhealthy, your identity became firmly linked with your cybersex use. In a sense, it has defined who you are as a person. You grew comfortable in this identity. Cybersex became your best friend. Now, when you're anxious or upset, it is still your source of comfort. Without it, you feel lost. Shame also became part of your identity. You feel bad about what you're doing, you're incapable of stopping, and you're worried about what will take the place of cybersex and how you'll handle life without it.

GRIEVING THE LOSS OF CYBERSEX

For a person with problematic cybersex behavior, sex has been the primary relationship—the main source of nurturing in life. The end of that relationship is like a death.[1] The person who stops the compulsive cybersex cycle, which gave meaning and direction to life, suffers a very real loss. For example, the following signs of grief are typical in the beginning stages of recovery:

- confusion about how to act and what to do
- feelings of alienation
- fantasies about how things could have been different
- sadness over unfulfilled expectations and a wasted life
- desire for a quick fix
- feelings of exposure and vulnerability
- failure to take care of self
- uncontrollable emotions
- dark thoughts about death, including suicide
- sudden accident-prone behavior
- fear that the pain will not go away

Severe grief reactions are caused by many types of losses or major changes such as the death of a spouse or child, divorce, loss of job, or change of residence. In all of these situations, the signs of grief are predictable. This same process occurs for the addict in recovery.

One resource for people struggling with out-of-control cybersex behaviors is the Twelve Step program, which helps them through their grieving process. It disrupts preoccupation and obsession with sex and supports grieving over the loss of the pathological relationship. To make the connections explicit, let's explore each stage of the grieving process as it affects the recovering person, focusing on the help Twelve Step programs offer.

With all losses, most bereaved people initially deny reality and isolate themselves. They resent people who urge them to accept their loss, who would rob them of their denial. While living in denial and isolation, those with compulsive cybersex behaviors in particular deny the impact cybersex has had on their lives. Concerned friends, relatives, and professionals make an effort to confront that denial and often encounter extremely defensive behavior.

THE IMPORTANCE OF THE TWELVE STEPS

The First Step of the Twelve Steps adapted for sexual addicts helps with denial and isolation in several ways. It states: We admitted we were powerless over our sexual addiction—that our lives had become unmanageable. Usually, addicts do a methodical inventory of all the ways their addiction proved to be powerful, including all those events they would have done anything to avoid but were powerless to stop. Throughout the inventory, addicts note how life has become unmanageable and intolerable with the addiction. The process helps them own their loss. They admit (to acknowledge powerlessness) and surrender (to acknowledge unmanageability) to the illness and accept their need for help. This is the process you have begun in this chapter.

Once they have acknowledged a loss, most grieving persons become very angry. For addicts, the anger is similar to what people feel when a loved one has died. Often bereaved people feel angry with God, the deceased, and themselves for not having done more. Sometimes the anger is punctuated with moments when the bereaved bargains with God ("If only you change it, Lord, I will . . .") or continues to deny ("Maybe a terrible mistake has been made . . ."). Usually the person experiences alarm or panic that reflects the terror of facing life without the loved one.

You will also become angry. You may feel angry at God for letting this happen, anger at the compulsion and addiction, anger for loss of it, and anger at yourself for not having done something sooner. Bargaining and denial ("Maybe I'm only a partial or weekend addict . . .") provide relief for the pain. By taking the Second Step (Came to believe that a Power greater than ourselves could restore us to sanity) and Third Step (Made a decision to turn our will and our lives over to the care of God as we understood Him), you perform a significant act of trust, acknowledging a Higher Power who can help you regain sanity. You then turn your life over to your Higher Power. This leap of trust requires acceptance of the fundamental dependency of the human condition. You can then create meaning out of the experience, as did author Viktor Frankl during his time in a Nazi concentration camp during World War II. Like Frankl, you may discover that suffering has meaning in a spiritual context.

Those who suffer losses and pass through the stages of denial and anger come to accept themselves through letting go of the loved one. For those with compulsive or addictive behaviors, however, letting go does not repair all the damage the addiction has done to them. The enormity of the addictive patterns and the years of self-degradation overwhelm them. Steps Four and Five will help you bypass shame and gain self-acceptance. Step Four (Made a searching and fearless moral inventory of ourselves) asks you to make a thorough inventory of personal strengths and weaknesses, including all the ways you have not lived up to personal values. This careful look at yourself may cause sadness and remorse.

Step Five (Admitted to God, to ourselves, and to another human being the exact nature of our wrongs) invites you to share your inventory with another person. In sexual or cybersex recovery programs, this is usually a chaplain or pastor, although it may be another member of the fellowship. The experience of relating all that history to someone else exposes you to an extreme level of vulnerability. Being so exposed, and yet being affirmed and accepted, creates healing of the highest order. The spiritual skills of the clergy may play a key role in self-forgiveness and self-acceptance. In effect, you can feel restored to the human community. Often, great joy and relief occur after the Fifth Step has been taken.

As in all grief, the struggle does not subside with self-acceptance. Bereaved people have moments during which they intensely search for the lost relationship. You will experience pangs of loss when your sadness and desire for the old way return. This is a time for "slips," loss of courage, euphoric recall, and testing limits. Once again, the program provides a framework to help with this hanging on to grief. Steps Six and Seven ask you to be ready to let go of the defects of character that could bring back the active compulsive/addictive life. Again, part of letting go requires trust in a Higher Power and trust in the existence of a healing process. With Steps Six (Were entirely ready to have God remove all these defects of character) and Seven (Humbly asked Him to remove our shortcomings), you identify your compulsive "friends"—those beliefs, defenses, attitudes, behaviors, and other issues that supported your behavior when it flourished. For example, you may see how self-pity serves as a gateway back into the addiction. Since self-pity was very much part of it, in recovery it simply adds to the grief reactions. Now you must learn to stop giving in to these so-called former friends of the addict.

As the grieving process evolves, a new sense of identity emerges. With restored confidence, the bereaved seek reconciliation with people they had pushed away. For you, the renewal of identity takes concrete form in terms of celebrating your progress. Marking anniversaries (for example, at one, three, and six months; one year; two years; and so on) becomes extremely important.

When you build on this renewed sense of self, your shame will no longer prevent reconciliation with friends and family. With Step Eight (Made a list of all persons we had harmed, and became willing to make amends to them all) and Step Nine (Made direct amends to such people wherever possible, except when to do so would injure them or others), you list those people you have harmed and make amends to them in hopes of healing the breach in the relationship. Making these direct efforts brings comfort through further restoration of self and, in some cases, forgiveness.

All who suffer great losses reach a point where they must establish their renewed identity and recognize that life goes on. It is not true, however, that when grief subsides, pain goes away entirely. In effect, although the sadness never leaves, it is transformed, becoming incorporated into our beings as part of that suffering that brings wisdom and depth of feeling to all of us. One simply learns to adjust to life in order to carry the suffering.

Step Ten (Continued to take personal inventory and when we were wrong promptly admitted it) encourages a daily effort to take stock of your life using the principles of the first nine Steps. Step Eleven (Sought through prayer and meditation to improve our conscious contact with God as we understood Him, praying only for knowledge of His will for us and the power to carry that out) suggests that spiritual progress results from a daily effort to improve conscious contact with a Higher Power. Step Twelve (Having had a spiritual awakening as the result of these steps, we tried to carry this message to others and to practice these principles in all our affairs) asks you to tell other addicts about the power of the program. They, in turn, pass on what they have received.

These last three Steps help addicts integrate the program principles into daily life, and the program thus becomes an intervening system that disrupts the addictive system and provides ongoing support for the lifelong process of surviving the loss. In effect, you will join a community based on healing principles validated over time. The Twelve Steps consolidate these common principles into a discipline for living daily with suffering and loss. Although their simplicity can mislead the unknowing, these Steps require great courage and can result in profound experiences.

The table on page 122 summarizes the impact of the Twelve Steps on the loss of the cybersex relationship.

Those with compulsive or addictive sexual behaviors are particularly vulnerable to using preoccupation with these behaviors as a way to cope with the sorrow of loss and the sadness of life. Unlike alcoholics or compulsive gamblers, they cannot avoid the object of their addiction—their sexuality—so the compelling forces that were a part of their compulsion or

The Loss of the Cybersex Relationship

Typical Grief Reactions to Loss of a Loved One	Typical Grief Reactions to Loss of Cybersex Relationship	Steps	Therapeutic Tasks
Denial and isolation. Blame for those who press for acceptance.	Denial and isolation. Defensive around behavior.	1	Admission (powerlessness) and surrender (unmanageability)—acknowledge need for program.
Anger. Bargaining. Alarm reactions.	Anger and rage about loss of compulsion/addiction. Slips into denial about being addict to prevent loss. Efforts to bargain—the "partial" addict. Terror at life without compulsion/addiction—"Will I die?"	2, 3	Trust and mistrust issues worked through, including accepting Higher Power.
Acceptance of self.	Struggle to get past enormity of compulsive/addictive patterns and self-degradation.	4, 5	Bypass shame; self-acceptance.
Search for the lost relationships. Pangs of loss.	Time for slips, loss of courage, euphoric recall, testing limits.	6, 7	Identify the "friends of the addict."
Emerging new identity. Reconciliation.	Pride in progress; anniversaries and straight time important.	8, 9	Comfort with new sense of self. Reconciliation with old/new friends. Restoration and forgiveness.
Establish and maintain continuity.	Integration into lifestyle and behavior.	10, 11, 12	Establish network for new identity.

Figure 7.1

addiction will always be an integral part of their lives. Consequently, the tendency toward grief remains immediate, and the Twelve Step program becomes even more vital as a path to return to sanity.

Codependents use the Twelve Steps as well. (We will talk much more about the role of spouses and partners in chapter 10.) They have experienced the loss of a loved one to the compulsion or addiction. They, too, have a need to cut through their denial, replace anger with trust, alleviate their shame, and renew their sense of identity. The processes are the same, since the compulsive/addictive and codependent systems parallel each other so closely.

This "simple" Twelve Step program reaches far and touches many. Based on the commonality of human experience, the Twelve Steps can work for everyone.

Taking a First Step means admitting that you have a problem, that you can't use cybersex like other people can, that you admit your powerlessness to control your cybersex use, that your life has become unmanageable as a result, and that you examine the consequences of your cybersex behavior. As you move through this process, you will begin to grieve all that you've lost as a result of your uncontrolled cybersex use. You will also feel grief because you can no longer use cybersex. We have introduced you to the Twelve Steps as one way to work through this process of self-discovery and grief, and we strongly encourage you to attend a Twelve Step group or work with a therapist as you move further into recovery. In addition, as you read on in this book, you will find additional help for dealing with your grief and for strengthing your recovery.

THE CRITICAL IMPORTANCE OF A FIRST STEP

The First Step is not an easy one. It involves admitting that you have a problem with cybersex and that you cannot solve the problem alone. This is difficult because it brings many emotions to the surface, one of which is fear of the unknown. You may wonder how you can live without cybersex, since it has been your identity and life focus. Being worried about this admission is natural. Many other people have felt exactly the same way. Courageously, they took that First Step and eventually recovered from their compulsive or addictive behaviors to live happy and fulfilling lives.

Taking the First Step is absolutely necessary. It's a prerequisite for everything that follows. Without it, your chances of learning to manage your behavior are slim. Step One is the foundation for future work, and until you create this foundation, none of the other Steps will work.

Earlier in the book, we used food and eating as an analogy. In that same vein, when we are cooking, we follow a recipe, either from a cookbook or from one we keep in our memories. In most recipes, there are certain ingredients that can be manipulated or even left out altogether without substantially compromising the result. But there are other ingredients that are essential to each recipe. Step One fits in the latter category. Without Step One, the recipe for recovery will be a flop.

Yes, Step One is difficult and painful. But we want to emphasize again that it is really the beginning of recovery. It is true that life will seem worse before it feels better. But that's because you're eliminating your "medication"—the behavior you've been using to anesthetize the pain of all your losses during the time you've been doing cybersex. It has become an emotional anesthetic, hiding the pain.

If you look back, you can probably find points in your life when you started to feel some of the losses and consequences of your behavior. What did you do then? Did you turn away and flee back into cybersex behaviors? If so, what was the result? Probably nothing changed and your life just kept getting worse.

When you stop these behaviors, you experience your losses and pain. Remember, part of the goal of a First Step is to provide a safe place to begin experiencing this pain. It's OK—even necessary—to let yourself experience all the feelings that have been pent up inside you. In the end, you will feel better. This process is akin to going into a house that's been shuttered and closed for a long time and throwing open the doors and windows to let in the fresh air and sun. You are throwing open the windows on being fully human.

RATIONALIZATIONS THAT INTERFERE WITH THE FIRST STEP

We all have a natural tendency to develop rationalizations to protect ourselves from things that are frightening and painful. When we begin the grieving process, for whatever reason, it's likewise quite natural to develop certain rationalizations to protect ourselves from it.

As you begin your First Step, you will soon begin to see just how misleading and false the following eight rationalizations truly are. In Step One, you will look more closely at the three key tasks of a First Step: recognizing your powerlessness over cybersex behaviors, determining ways your life has become unmanageable because of these behaviors, and examining the consequences of these behaviors. People recovering from problematic cybersex behaviors typically experience some of the following eight rationalizations.

Rationalization 1: *It's not real.*
Cyberspace isn't real. There are no people. There are no rules. There are no consequences (that are immediately apparent, at least!). I can indulge in cybersex without worrying about it.

Rationalization 2: *Cybersex doesn't hurt others.*
I'm not having skin-to-skin contact, so it's not sex, and it's not affecting anyone. No one can get a disease. It can't hurt anyone if it's not a problem. I'm not unfaithful because I haven't really done anything with anybody. Even when I'm in a chat room, for example, it's all still make-believe. In reality, most of the time, I'm not even who I say I am. There is no direct harm to anybody and there isn't anything I need to be accountable for.

Rationalization 3: *Cybersex doesn't hurt me.*
I'm just on the computer, so what's the big deal? It's no different from surfing other kinds of Web sites on the Internet. There aren't any consequences. As long as I don't have skin-to-skin contact, I'm not hurting myself at all.

Rationalization 4: *I can stop anytime I want; I just need to turn off the computer.*
None of this is real, anyway. I'm not actually going to a strip club, seeing a prostitute, or exposing myself to a real person. Besides, all I need to do is shut down the computer and everything goes away.

Rationalization 5: *I've already done a First Step.*
People who are already in a Twelve Step recovery program might think, "I've already done a First Step for sex addiction (or for alcohol use, gambling, or another addiction), so why would I need to do another one? Besides, I haven't (fill in the blank) for years."

Rationalization 6: *Cybersex doesn't have any consequences.*
I can't get a sexually transmitted disease. It's not going to destroy my marriage if others don't have my mailing address or know where I live. Using the computer is so private. No one knows my access codes. When I'm online at work, well, that's no different from taking a short coffee break in the cafeteria.

Rationalization 7: It's just a game—it's virtual *reality.*
This isn't serious because it's not real. That's why it's called *virtual* reality.
It's fun, it's my entertainment, it really doesn't hurt anybody, and it doesn't
bother anybody. Who would ever take this seriously? I don't really mean
anything by any of this. It's really not any different from a video game.

Rationalization 8: I just use it occasionally. Cybersex doesn't interfere
with or jeopardize things in my life.
I'm not on the computer all the time or anything like that. I just go on when
I feel like it. It's just something to do. I'm still in a good relationship with
my partner, have a good job, and spend time with my kids. It's no big deal!

It is important to remember that these "rationalizations" may appear
to be true in the moment, but the cybersex compulsive's thinking is often
clouded and unable to ascertain the truth. Take for example the belief that
cybersex is a safe form of sex that does not lead to sexually transmitted
diseases. While this may seem true on the surface, researchers have learned
that those who engage in cybersex behaviors are more likely to engage in
sexually risky behaviors offline as well, leading to a higher incidence of
STDs among cybersex users.

The following four explanations show how reality could be substituted
for rationalizations.

Rationalization 1: They're just electrons; they're not real. They're only
virtual.
Regardless of the "unreality" of the Internet, real people *are* involved. You're
real. The other people online *are* real, even if you can't really see or touch
them. Your family is real. Your colleagues are real. Your children are real.
Your behavior affects real human beings.

Rationalization 2: Cybersex doesn't hurt others, it doesn't hurt me, and
there are no consequences.
There are few behaviors we engage in that have no consequences. Sometimes
the consequences are not apparent to us, or sometimes they do not appear
for weeks, months, or even years, but rest assured, there are consequences—
to you and others—for out-of-control cybersex behaviors. Consequences
come in all forms. Some are directly tangible (such as spending thousands of

dollars on pornography) while others are less tangible (such as the spiritual/ emotional drain it has on your life). Be honest with yourself and examine both the directly tangible and the indirect and intangible consequences to you and to others as a result of your online sexual behavior.

Rationalization 3: Occasional use isn't a problem for me. Besides, I can stop anytime I want. I just need to turn off the computer.
You probably often told yourself this, but did you stop? Did you turn off the computer? Did "occasional" use become "using whenever I had the opportunity"? Were you able to stop? And even when you did, did the fantasies stop spinning in your head? How about the desire to go back online? If you could have stopped whenever you wanted, you would have. But you didn't because you couldn't stop.

Rationalization 4: I've already done a First Step; why do another for this?
Regardless of other First Steps you may have done, it is imperative that you do a First Step that focuses on cybersex so that you can recognize powerlessness, unmanageability, and consequences in terms of this particular behavior.

POWERLESSNESS

"Powerlessness" means being unable to stop your cybersex behaviors no matter how hard you try and despite negative consequences. Have you tried to stop, cut back, set limits on, or change the patterns of your use?

You may, for example, have promised yourself you wouldn't use your computer at work for cybersex, especially after your information services department began monitoring Internet use, yet you continued to do so despite the danger. You might have promised yourself you'd never go to a particular sexual Web site again, but you ended up at a similar one. You may have promised yourself that you'd never stay online past 11:00 P.M. to engage in cybersex activities, but you found yourself online in the middle of the night at least three nights in the last week.

Consider how much you have been preoccupied with cybersex and how much you have been using it as a way to reduce anxiety in your life. How have your thinking and activities revolved around your cybersex use? Planning your day around your use, daydreaming about when you'll be free to participate in cybersex, and becoming anxious and angry when situations arise that prevent you from using are examples of preoccupation and powerlessness.

It's also important to note that any attempt to control your cybersex behavior is an indication that it is already out of control.

POWERLESSNESS INVENTORY

In the space below or on a separate sheet of paper, begin your own powerlessness inventory. List examples that show how powerless you have been to stop your Internet sexual behavior. Be explicit about types of behavior and frequency. Start with your earliest example of being powerless and conclude with your most recent. Write down as many examples as you can think of. By doing so, you will see the pattern of broken promises emerge and add significantly to the depth of your understanding of your powerlessness over these behaviors.

1.

2.

3.

4.

5.

6.

UNMANAGEABILITY

Unmanageability and powerlessness are closely intertwined. Unmanageability is, in fact, the manifestation of powerlessness. When you lose the ability to control your cybersex behavior, it affects all aspects of your life and soon becomes unmanageable. "Unmanageability" means that your cybersex use has created chaos and damage in your life. These are the consequences of powerlessness.

How do you see your life as unmanageable as a result of your cybersex behaviors?

1.

2.

3.

4.

5.

6.

CONSEQUENCES

When you stop and really look at the results of your cybersex behavior, you will see for the first time just how you and many others have been affected in a variety of different ways. Read and answer each of the following questions honestly. Spend as much time as you need to complete this exercise. Later, you may want to share your answers with others who are helping you in recovery, such as your sponsor or therapist.

SOCIAL LIFE
Have your cybersex behaviors affected your social life? If so, how?

Have you become more isolated from friends? If so, in what ways?

Do you spend so much time online that you're too tired to go out?

List three specific examples of how your cybersex behaviors have affected your social life.

1.

2.

3.

Physical Condition
What impact have your cybersex behaviors had on you physically?

Do you have difficulty sleeping?

Do you find yourself without energy?

Do you find it difficult to exercise as regularly as you once did?

List three examples of how your cybersex behaviors have affected your physical condition.

1.

2.

3.

ECONOMIC SITUATION

What impact have your cybersex behaviors had on your financial condition?

- Overspending?
- Loss of job or job promotions?
- Mismanagement of household funds?

List three examples of how your cybersex behaviors have affected your economic situation.

1.

2.

3.

JOB OR PROFESSION

What impact have cybersex behaviors had on your work and career? Problems can surface such as:

- lowered productivity
- frequent absenteeism
- deteriorating quality of product or decision making
- frequent tardiness

List three examples of how your cybersex behaviors have affected your job or profession.

1.

2.

3.

School

If you are a student, problems like these may surface as a result of your cybersex behaviors:

- not keeping up with homework assignments
- frequent absenteeism
- lower grades
- social isolation

If applicable, list three examples of how your cybersex behaviors have affected your education or school-related social activities.

1.

2.

3.

Emotional Problems

How has your cybersex use affected you emotionally? Emotional problems can include:

- depression
- feelings of low self-esteem
- difficulty in getting close to others or in expressing feelings
- extreme feelings of loneliness
- unexplained fears

List three examples of how your cybersex behaviors have affected you emotionally.

1.

2.

3.

FAMILY PROBLEMS

How have your cybersex behaviors interfered with relationships that mean the most to you?

- Loss of closeness?
- A feeling that other family members have lost respect for you?
- Using family members emotionally or financially?
- Extreme feelings of remorse or guilt?
- Withdrawing from family activities?
- Being unfaithful to your partner or spouse?

List three examples of how your cybersex behaviors have affected your closest relationships.

1.

2.

3.

ACCEPTING YOURSELF

Your admission of powerlessness and unmanageability marks the beginning of your recovery. But you must go beyond admission to acceptance—acceptance that your behavior has been compulsive—and come to the realization that you need ongoing help to achieve freedom from its power.

When you finally take time to really look at your behaviors, the result can be shocking. You're probably saying to yourself, "So I have this problem and it's out of control. What can I do? How can I get my life back together?" Regardless of your worries, take heart, because you are now on the road to recovery from these behaviors.

MAKING CHANGES

Before we look at specific changes you can make in your behavior, we want to introduce you to two levels of change: first-order changes and second-order changes.[2] These two levels parallel respectively the setting of external and internal boundaries, which we explored in chapter 6. First-order changes are very concrete actions that are taken to quickly stop a problem and to address specific consequences. First-order changes can also be well described by the French aphorism "The more things change, the more they remain the same." For example, think of Marie, a woman who's been married three times, each time to an alcoholic. She changed husbands but still found herself in the same situation. She did not change her life with each marriage. Instead, she continued to marry and live with alcoholics. First-order changes won't help anyone solve compulsive or addictive behaviors *on a permanent basis*. They are literally about trying harder at things that won't work in the long run.

It is important to understand that compulsion or addiction of any kind is a first-order phenomenon. The harder addicts try to stop their behavior alone and in secret, the more their failure is guaranteed. Only when they break the rules of compulsion or addiction by seeking help for their addiction will they be able to begin making the second-order changes needed to free themselves of these behaviors.

Second-order changes are those steps that you take to actually change the dynamics of your life and the way you live. Second-order changes for Marie, for example, include going to therapy and stopping dating. During therapy, she learns that she comes from an alcoholic family and that this background has been the basis for her selection of men.

Both first-order and second-order changes address the issue of unmanageability. In this chapter, we will offer suggestions for first-order changes, and in chapter 8 we will look at second-order changes.

To further illustrate the difference between the two types, let's imagine that you were hurt in an auto accident. When the paramedics arrive, the first action they take is to determine if you're breathing. Then they look for and control any severe bleeding that could bring immediate death. They would also immobilize any broken bones at this time. First-order changes are the splints, airways, and pressure bandages used to begin healing compulsive or addictive behaviors. They will stabilize your life in the short run by immediately controlling behavior and consequences.

Let's return again to that "accident." If you have internal injuries, your life will still be in danger. Dealing with such injuries takes more time and care, as well as professional staff in a hospital setting. Treating only the superficial wounds won't save your life. Likewise, you need second-order changes to recover in the long run from your compulsive or addictive behaviors. Second-order changes take more time, but eventually the whole person is healed, inside and out.

You may be tempted to skip over the first-order changes and go straight to the second-order changes. Carrying our analogy further illustrates why this is a bad idea. Focusing only on the internal injuries—with "second-order" care—would not be effective because you'd die of hemorrhage or shock before treatment for the internal injuries could be given. Thus, both first-order and second-order changes are necessary because both play a crucial role in healing.

EXAMPLES OF FIRST-ORDER CHANGES

The boundaries you'll start with may seem rather restrictive. That's because, for the time being, you need external limits and controls that will give you very little room to maneuver. Then, as you get more control over your behaviors and your life, you'll be able to loosen the restrictions and see how well you can cope with more flexibility. The first-order changes you need to put into effect fit into five categories. These categories suggest that you reduce access, reduce anonymity, reduce objectification, make yourself accountable, and develop healthy online habits.

REDUCE ACCESS

- Set a period of abstinence from all Internet use to see what issues arise for you and whether or not you are able to maintain the abstinence period.
- If your computer is in a relatively private setting in your home, move it into a higher-traffic area that is more regularly frequented by family members. Don't, for example, keep it in a home office, in your bedroom, or in an area where you can close a door for privacy. Instead, move it into your family room.
- Don't go online except when others are at home.
- Set limits for when and how long you're allowed to use your

computer. In addition, set a curfew for evening use, such as an
11:00 P.M. deadline.

- Use electronic limits to reduce your access. With an accountability
partner, use blocking or filtering software to help filter access to
sexual areas of the Internet (Web sites, chat rooms, newsgroups,
and so on).
- Switch to a "safe" Internet service provider. A number of family-
oriented Internet service providers, for example, carefully screen
out sexual sites. To find one in your area, type "family-oriented
service providers" into an Internet search engine such as Google
or Yahoo.
- If you were using your computer at work for cybersex, leave your
office door open whenever you're using the computer and place
your monitor so that others can see it as they walk by.
- Avoid any areas of the Internet that are sexual in nature.

Reduce Anonymity

- Be sure that your e-mail addresses and screen names actually identify you, even if it's only your real first name. No more hiding behind fictitious identities.
- Confide in at least two other people (in addition to your spouse
or partner) about your problem. (We'll talk more about finding a
sponsor shortly.)
- Minimize your electronic communications (e-mail, chat room conversation, instant messaging) to only those you already know in the
real world.

Reduce Objectification

- Regularly remind yourself that those with whom you communicate
on the Net *are* real human beings with feelings, hopes, worries, and
loved ones, just as you are, and they can be affected by your interactions with them. The Internet is *not* a video game.
- Place reminders of people you value in your life on or near your

computer (photographs of family members, a computer background of your partner, for example).

Make Yourself Accountable

- Allow a trusted friend, sponsor, or therapist to monitor your behavior and access. Give this person access to your computer history files. Make yourself accountable to this person for the time you spend online and what you did online.

Develop Healthy Online Habits

It is very important to understand that we are not saying you can't use your computer or the Internet. While that might actually be the best option, the Internet has become such an integral part of many of our personal and work lives that we simply have to have access for many reasons. You can learn to use the Internet for only healthy purposes by developing healthy online habits and accessing supportive online recovery resources. For example:

- Get an online sponsor.
- Develop e-mail buddies who are also recovering from problematic online sexual behavior.
- Find and use Web sites that can support your recovery rather than undermine it.
- Find and visit online support groups. For example, "Thought for the Day" at www.hazelden.org will provide you with an encouraging thought each day.

FINDING OTHERS TO SUPPORT YOUR RECOVERY EFFORTS

A word of caution: often the people who are involved in cybersex can't be objective enough to decide what they can and can't handle online. For this reason, it becomes increasingly important to seek therapy, join a Twelve Step group or other support group that focuses on this problem, or both. It is also important to find a sponsor (a trusted person with whom you can talk about sex and recovery).

We also encourage you to get an online sponsor, because such a person can truly understand the pitfalls of the Internet. This is another way a therapist and a support group can help—by steering you toward appropriate sponsors who understand the Internet and who will be able to effectively help you monitor your Internet behavior.

Therapists can help you in other ways too. If you're having a problem with online sexual behaviors, it's likely that they are a symptom of deeper, longer-term problems such as depression or issues growing out of your childhood and family of origin. Dealing with depression or anxiety requires help from a professional. Some people also find that medications help them with these problems. For all these reasons, we strongly recommend that you get a comprehensive psychiatric evaluation by a psychiatrist.

You may question whether you really need so much help in dealing with these behaviors. It's important to again acknowledge that you have a problem and that if you'd been able to handle it on your own, you wouldn't be in the spot you're in right now and reading this book for help. Depression and anxiety, for example, have nothing to do with your willpower or how strong a person you are. They often have roots in brain chemistry, and once it is in balance, you will be better able to work through these problems.

We also want to stress the importance of combined therapies. Too often, people seeking help for compulsive or addictive online sexual behavior will select only one source of help, such as a Twelve Step group, group therapy, or seeing a therapist. This strategy can work successfully, but using a combination of therapies increases the likelihood of your success. A comprehensive treatment approach is best. We believe that using individual and group therapy along with recovery groups and medication, if appropriate, is the most effective recovery strategy.

8

Changing the Way You Live

YOUR INVOLVEMENT WITH CYBERSEX and its effect on your life and the lives of those close to you may now be bringing up overwhelming feelings of fear, worry, confusion, sadness, anger, and guilt. The road to healing may seem difficult, even impossible, but don't give in to despair. There is hope. Perhaps you have reached that quiet moment of surrender, realizing that you have a problem with cybersex and that you really do need to do something about it. Or maybe you're not yet sure about your commitment to changing your cybersex behaviors. You may be wondering whether it's really worth the trouble and the effort. Whatever stage you are at, it is important to acknowledge your feelings and move on.

Our work with thousands of people who are recovering from compulsive or addictive behavior has shown us that there are predictable stages people pass through as they descend into more and more problematic compulsive and addictive behaviors and as they recover from these behaviors. These stages include the developing stage, crisis and decision, shock, grief, repair, and growth. While we can't say for certain what you will experience in recovery, if you follow the steps we lay out, you will be able to relate to these commonly shared experiences.

THE DEVELOPING STAGE

Jeremy was an executive responsible for some of the largest and most important accounts for his high-profile ad agency. He had it all—money, prestige, authority, responsibility—*and* a secret cybersex life. Jeremy initially began using the Internet for sex when he discovered online strip clubs. Jeremy tells his story:

> I'd often gone to real strip clubs in the past, but as my responsibilities in the agency increased, I just didn't have time to go anymore. The online clubs turned out to be a great substitute. In some ways, I enjoyed them even more than the real thing. I could "visit" whenever I wanted, right from my office, and I could actually request specific women and activities. Eventually, I also discovered that I could find and book prostitutes online too, which I did from both my work and home computers. My life was one of extremes. On the one hand, I managed ad campaigns for women's health care products, and on the other, I abused women through my use of prostitutes.

One doesn't have to be a high-powered executive to have the addictive pride that says you can manage the unmanageable, that you can do things others can't. It is this arrogance that pushes aside realities like AIDS, family commitments, and work priorities.

Things come apart, however, no matter who you are. For Jeremy, life began unraveling when his wife stumbled across one of the prostitution booking sites in his computer's history file. Confronted by this undeniable evidence, Jeremy confessed but minimized the problem, saying that he'd gone to the site only to see if one could really hire a prostitute online. He swore to his wife that he'd been faithful and to himself that he'd change his ways. Jeremy even talked about seeing a counselor, but he had not accepted that he had a problem—or at least one he couldn't handle.

Jeremy was, at this point, in the developing stage. Unmanageability and powerlessness forced him to acknowledge his problem, but he continued his problematic online sexual behaviors nonetheless. True recovery begins only after this stage, which can sometimes last two or more years. For Jeremy, it took over a year, and like many others, he made efforts to curtail his activities but his compulsive cybersex behavior continued.

Key characteristics of the developing stage include:

- seeking help but discontinuing it or deciding it isn't useful
- a growing appreciation of the reality of the problem but a tendency to counter this realization by minimizing the problem or thinking you can handle it by yourself

- temporarily curtailing or stopping the compulsive behavior or substituting other behaviors (Jeremy delved into sexualized online chat rooms)
- having the fear that stopping cybersex activities would mean stopping sex altogether

For most people struggling with compulsive or addictive sexual behaviors, these behaviors are seen as closely connected to survival. The behavior has until now been a "trusted friend," relied upon for some time. This "friend" has always delivered what it promised, but at a price. As the price grows intolerable, addicts prepare to face the fact that something in their lives has to change.

CRISIS AND DECISION

After three months of making some effort to curtail his online sexual behavior to please his wife, Jeremy felt his life was once again under control.

> One afternoon at work after everyone had left the office for the day, I went online to hire a prostitute. When my colleague's phone rang, I decided to answer it. I left my computer with the "order" information and a photo on my screen. While I was away, my boss returned unexpectedly for some papers he'd forgotten for a meeting. Noticing that the light in my office was still on, he stepped into my office to say hello, but was greeted instead by my computer screen with the prostitution booking service on it—in full view. Caught a second time, and confronted by both my wife and my boss, I agreed to seek counseling. Since neither could be conned or forced to budge, I finally had to be honest with myself.

Jeremy had entered the crisis and decision stage, the stage at which a commitment to change is made. This stage can occur within a single day or it can take some months; in any case, it marks the real beginning of recovery. Reaching this stage can happen in many ways. For some, there is a growing consciousness that something needs to be done. Others are frightened into action by the escalation of their behavior. Still others are so overwhelmed by their behavior that they will do anything to fix it.

Most people struggling with compulsive or addictive online sexual behaviors are forced to do something by events or by people—family members, partners, friends, therapists or the legal system. Because of their denial, the pressure may have to build up over a long period of time.

SHOCK

This stage is a time of emotional numbness, extraordinary disorientation, and efforts to control the damage. It's not unusual to spend some months in shock. It's OK to move ahead slowly. Maybe nothing major will happen for some time, even for as long as a year. Simply entering recovery and dealing with the implications of the problem can be so stressful that undertaking significant change would overload you. Time-honored sayings like "One day at a time" and "Keep it simple" are appropriate prescriptions for this stage of recovery.

The following experiences can characterize this stage:

- disorientation, confusion, numbness, and an inability to focus or concentrate
- periodic bouts with despair and feelings of hopelessness that can become more intense as the sense of reality grows
- angry feelings about limits set by therapists, sponsors, or family members
- in recovery or support groups, experiencing a sense of belonging along with the realization that recovery was the right decision
- feelings of relief and acceptance once the double life has ended

Perhaps the biggest struggle during this period is for people to be honest with themselves about the extent and nature of their problem. Jeremy says:

> In the beginning I was able to see how upset my wife was about the online prostitutes, but I didn't see how the lying, deception, chat room conversations, and other online behaviors really mattered. Then one day it struck me that I had been damaging my relationship with my wife for years and dishonoring my commitment to our marriage through my online behaviors. I became angry with myself, my wife, my boss, even my computer. I can honestly say I've never been so confused and flooded with so many emotions all at once.

With time and support, however, clarity about the problematic behavior will emerge. When you can see and accept reality, you will enter a stage of profound grieving.

GRIEF

Grieving involves denial or bargaining, anger over the losses, acceptance of the reality of your situation, and sadness. Actually, some aspects of grieving, particularly bargaining and anger, first emerge in earlier stages and simply continue in the grief stage. What really distinguishes this stage is the sadness and pain felt when losses are finally acknowledged.

Given the difficulty of this stage, it shouldn't come as any surprise that this is the point when people most often give up and revert to their old behaviors. Those behaviors had long been used to avoid pain, so when the pain becomes overwhelming, those problematic behaviors seem to bring relief, just as an old friend brings comfort and aid. This is a time when you will surely need outside support. You may be tempted to avoid this pain, but in order to heal and to begin a new life without the problematic behaviors, you simply have to pass through it. It is this pain that sets the stage for the next step; without it, you simply can't take that step.

Feelings may include:

- continued anger and defiance
- sadness and pain punctuated with periodic bouts of despair
- deep sadness over the losses incurred because of your behaviors
- a sense of profound loss as your problematic behaviors cease to serve as friend, comforter, and high

At this point, Jeremy finally began to see what he'd been doing:

I realized that my getting caught wasn't just bad luck; I realized that I had set these lessons up. The universe kept putting these lessons in front of me, and I'd been unwilling to pay attention to them. So the lessons had to get even more dramatic in order for me to finally say, "OK, I give up. I see the lesson. I'm ready to learn."

When that final acceptance occurs and you allow yourself to be vulnerable—to be human, ordinary, not unique—then significant change can begin. Awareness of your behavior will expand and deepen over the years.

Right now, however, it's important that you recognize its broad outlines and understand that your problem was more than just your behavior. It's important to recognize that these behaviors grew out of your beliefs, attitudes, and distorted thinking and were preserved with denial and delusion. With acceptance, you then enter the repair stage.

REPAIR

For Jeremy, the real watershed between grief and repair came when he finally told his wife and his sponsor the true extent of his behaviors and asked from his heart for forgiveness and the opportunity to begin anew.

That is when the chaos stopped and the rebuilding began. Jeremy began to build recovery.

> By this time, I was connected. I was part of a good support group, and I really used the help that they offered daily. We did things socially and I involved myself in meetings—and eventually as a sponsor for another guy who needed help. I immersed myself in therapy, including a weekly men's group. The result was that I was able to set aside my old behavior. I found that my relationship with my wife entered a new and deeply connected level and that I felt for the first time in my life a sense of spiritual connectedness.

For many, the repair stage is generally marked by a cessation or decrease in the amount of problematic online sexual behavior. Individuals report that they may occasionally have an online lapse. The lapses usually occur less frequently and individuals tend not to cross lines or take risks as much as they did during previous behaviors. For example, an individual's previous behavior may have included frequently logging on to a chat room and arranging for an offline meeting for sex with someone he or she just met. A lapse for this type of behavior may be logging on to the chat room one time and engaging in a conversation but then logging off before arranging for an offline meeting. Although this is still not healthy behavior for the individual, it is less risky and occurs only occasionally as compared to previous behaviors. Jeremy likened the steps he'd been taking to building the foundation for a new home:

It's brick, sunk in the ground, nothing fancy, just gray, cement blocks. And there's the beginning of a house on top that is in three dimensions and color. I'm not exactly sure what the house will look like, but I can tell already that I'm going to like it.

A number of crucial changes characterize this stage:

- a sense of productivity and renewal
- a new capacity for joy
- deepening of new bonds with others
- taking responsibility for yourself in all areas of life, including career, finances, and health
- learning to express your needs, accepting that you have them, and working to meet them
- a focus on completing tasks (degrees, projects, work, and so on) and being dependable (being punctual, following through, and responding to requests)
- living less "on the edge and at the extremes"

A common goal at this point is to achieve balance, to learn to live in the Recovery Zone, a concept we will explore in greater detail later. Since life has been out of control for so long, you must now focus on the basics. Working toward completion and staying low-key will feel good after all the unmanageability you've experienced. But the repair stage also requires developing new skills and forging new bonds. You will likely be forced to face fundamental issues that made you vulnerable to the draw of cybersex in the first place. Those behaviors can be stopped, but the deeply personal problems of distrust, victimization, and shame will remain. Few people are successful in dealing with them on their own, and it's for this reason that we strongly urge you to seek therapy and group support.

During this period of repair and personal growth, a greater understanding of your problematic behaviors will continue to grow. Essentially, you will be restructuring your relationship with yourself. You will begin to develop a much better understanding of your behavior and will come to realize what made you vulnerable to cybersex. You will be able to identify the governing themes and scenarios that connect all your problematic behaviors. Once you have a better relationship with yourself, you will be able to trust other people. You may also find yourself beginning to trust in a power greater than yourself—a Higher Power—and at that point a spiritual opening occurs. You will no longer be living in fear. You will acquire a vital perspective on your powerlessness, become more forgiving of yourself, and learn to care for yourself more deeply. And at this level of self-care, you will begin to nurture yourself into the growth stage.

GROWTH

Empowered by recovery, you will enter a stage in which you explore new options and restructure relationships. The changes that have occurred will enable you to open up what has been a closed system. Your problematic or addictive behaviors offered only decreasing options. Recovery creates an open personal system that allows for the expansion of countless options. Even better, once a system is open, it has the capacity to renew itself. Many people experience periods of dramatic personal growth years after their initial recovery.

Relationships with children, parents, and partners can all become richer and more sustaining. Many recovering people talk about being more emotionally present on the job, as well. They talk of more balance and greater intimacy, of an improved capacity to resolve conflict, and of being less judgmental and more compassionate. With the evolution of this new style of relationships, satisfaction with life dramatically improves.

Jeremy experienced these changes too: "The whole addiction was about me, me, me, me, me. In recovery, I turned to the opposite extreme of really taking care of 'me' in a healthy sense. Then I learned to be a conduit to allow this love that I'm receiving to flow through to others." Jeremy was very clear about the importance of creating a solid personal base. Of his relationship with his wife, he says, "It is now two wholes sharing a life together."

Characteristics of the growth stage include:

- profound empathy and compassion for oneself and for others
- developing trust for one's own boundaries and integrity in relationships
- feelings of achievement over new milestones in love and sex
- a new ability to take care of and nurture relationships
- transforming or ending old relationships

Another characteristic of this growth stage is a deep abhorrence of one's old behavior. Once people in recovery have enough distance from their old problematic behaviors, they often have extremely visceral reactions when they think about them. Many say they look back almost in disbelief at some of the things they've done.

The growth stage provides a special perspective on the course of recovery in general. It's clear that many people with problematic or addictive sexual behaviors were not always able to stop all their behaviors at once. Most people tend to focus initially on what got them into trouble. Then, as their awareness grows, they see the variations on the theme. Recovery moves them from crisis management to an expanded awareness and a more evolved consciousness. And this evolution takes time.

By the time recovery reaches the growth stage, it no longer involves false starts. Consciousness of sobriety and of richer relationships has brought the person to a new level of being. And it's at this stage that people in recovery often talk about the compulsive or addictive behavior as a gift. They have experienced a depth of humanity that many people never achieve. Their compulsive or addictive behaviors and subsequent recovery have given them a greater perception, compassion, and presence. Not only do they serve as models for other recovering people who follow them, but they also are literally helping our whole society heal.

It is important to keep in mind that in life, nothing happens in neat stages. The eleven-year-old child, for example, often has some adolescent traits along with traits typical of elementary-school children. Similarly in recovery, you can experience shock, grief, and repair in significant ways at the same time. Slips and relapses may slow development or even throw you back to the first stage of recovery. Other factors can impede development and recovery too, and lack of support from family, friends, and colleagues is perhaps the most devastating of all.

HERMES AND HERMES' WEB

A special tool that we find effective in helping people understand the complex nature of compulsive and addictive behaviors—as well as the process of recovery from them—is called Hermes' Web.[1]

Who or what is Hermes? One of the Greek pantheon, Hermes is the connector, the god of the crossroads. All things meet on Hermes' ground—

sexuality, business, ethics, medicine, and criminality. Hermes weaves them together. Hermes has the ability to move in and out of all other worlds freely and is never held captive. He is known for connecting high and low, living and dead, dark and light, and all manner of things. Hermes is an imaginal center in his own right.

Hermes is nonauthoritarian, an equalizer, creating symmetry and equality in relationships and politics. His aim is not power, but imagination and connection. Hermes is the friendliest of gods and works to connect the human and the divine, however estranged they may become. As the Greek god of thieves, borders, and commerce, Hermes is not afraid to combine elements, to take from here or there to put together what works rather than play by the rules and be ineffective.

Hermes seeks to keep life alive, mercurial, and vibrant. Hermes is also the desire for life, the yearning and urge to be alive, to explore, mix, and tangle. His fleetness is his excitement. He brings diversity and friendliness to the world, connecting all its elements.

Hermes' Web is a diagram that shows the interconnectedness of life, both internal and external, and honors the One whose role it is to bring awareness and soulfulness to life. Hermes' Web allows people to visualize their internal landscape and thus facilitate Hermes' work. It is a tool that demonstrates how everything in a person is interconnected, whether conscious or unconscious. Hermes' Web also demonstrates the negative consequences of various degrees of disconnection.

You can also view Hermes' Web as a representation of the human personality. As you look at the illustration on page 149, the top point represents the part of you that you like best, the part that best represents who you are. It's the part you "buff up" and show to the world; it's what we call the "ego." The opposite end of the piece represents the part of you that you keep hidden from the world. It's the "shadow" side, the part of you that you don't want others to see, the part of yourself you don't like so well, that you are even ashamed of and seldom acknowledge. The other pieces in Hermes' Web can represent opposites, or extremes, in your personality. The point on one might represent anger and on its opposite end represent passivity. Another might represent sexual compulsivity and its opposite end sexual abstinence. For a moment, think about your behaviors and their opposites. Can you see how you tend to live or act at one extreme and then another?

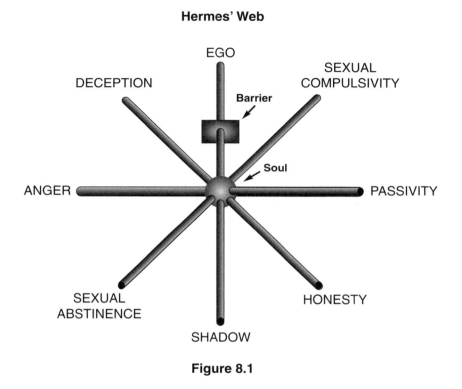

Figure 8.1

Now notice the section where all the pieces merge and cross paths. This section represents your core, and it contains your passion, your spirituality, the very best parts of who you are. The place where all these points come together we call the "convergence of soul." In each of us, ideally, there would be a strong connection between our ego and our soul. In other words, the parts of ourselves that we show the world and how we live in the world (the morals and values that we've learned in life) would reflect the soul, wherein lie our innate goodness, passion, and spirituality.

For some people, however, this is not the case. Instead, they begin, often at a very young age, to build a barrier between the parts of themselves they show to others and the convergence point. This happens for a number of reasons, all having to do with information from others—parents, relatives, teachers, siblings, and peers—that is negative. They may be told that they aren't good or worthy of love or wanted. These messages can be conveyed verbally, but often they are given through actions. In the extreme, they are given through physical, emotional, or sexual abuse or neglect.

We take in all messages that we receive about ourselves, be they positive or negative. And when they are negative, we all have to "do something" with them—and that "something" is usually to create an internal barrier between those negative messages and ourselves. It's a barrier between our ego and our core, the soul. As these messages continue to pour in over the years, they begin to accumulate. The "pile" grows larger and larger; the barrier between our outer self and our core grows more and more dense, making it more and more difficult for us to connect to our soul. Over time, we begin to lose touch with our passion, our spirituality, our soul.

When children living in chaotic or abusive settings create such a barrier, it is, ironically, a healthy process. They need to protect themselves. To stay sane, literally, requires that they create a thick barrier between their ego and their inner self as a way to avoid dealing with a difficult environment. Children who don't have the ability to erect such barriers actually can and do go insane. While this coping mechanism is useful and effective for self-protection in childhood, this is not the case once we are adults. These strategies become counterproductive and interfere with having relationships and with living a rich and fulfilling life.

COPING AND COMPARTMENTALIZATION

When you have been keeping secrets, you become like a volcano: the part of yourself that is visible above ground is serene, calm, and beautiful, even majestic and unthreatening, like the cone of the volcano. Underneath the surface, invisible to others *and* to yourself, are all the experiences and feelings you have kept hidden for many years, just as deep below ground under the volcano lies a mass of molten lava, heating and building pressure, month by month, year by year. By stuffing experiences into that barrier and out of sight—by keeping secrets—you've learned how to live a double life.

This "skill" is known as compartmentalization. You have seen examples of compartmentalization in the lives of public figures, but perhaps have never put a name to these actions. Presidents, ministers, politicians, and others create a public persona, a "self" that they show to the world. But too often there is another side, a shadow side, and occasionally, that shadow side is revealed to the world when news of sexual misconduct or financial misdealings, for example, splashes across the media and into our lives. These people have used compartmentalization to deal with the duality of their lives. Can you begin to see how secrecy, compartmentalization, and the private, hidden world of cybersex are all connected?

Over time, all the thoughts, experiences, and feelings that you put into the core begin to build up, and the older you are, of course, the more stuff you have buried. Deep under that volcanic peak, enormous pressure has been building for many years. Eventually, enough pressure builds up that an explosion, or a "flip," occurs and some of that hidden stuff is thrown out into the world. It may take the form of a violent crime, using alcohol or other drugs, or the compulsive use of cybersex. This acting out is a way to relieve the pressure that's built up in your core.

At the moment when the flip occurs, you also reveal your true self—your soul. That soul, however, is completely encrusted by all the "garbage" that you've piled on it for so long, while the person you consider yourself to be, that buffed, kind, moral person, is not there on the other side.

But the flip doesn't last long. Soon you flip back, denying to yourself and others what you've done. We call this a "truthful lie."[2] A person may deny having been drunk at the office party or having molested a child or having had sex with someone he or she met via the Internet. Because the part of us that we identify with—the ego on top—*couldn't* have done those acts, we deny them. Unconsciously, we tell ourselves that it was the part of us we *don't* identify with that did them. And that is the truthful lie.

Compulsive and addictive behaviors are a sure sign that there is a major barrier between the ego and the inner self and that we are feeling a great deal of pressure and stress. We are desperate for a way to relieve some of that pressure, and the three quickest ways to get some relief are sex, alcohol, and other drugs. We are trying to find a way to open ourselves up, and for a brief moment, these seem to do the trick. Other compulsive behaviors, such as gambling and overeating, may also seem to serve this purpose. But the relief is only temporary—very temporary. We feel alive and free, but before we know it, we crash. Eventually, the pressure builds up and again we act out. Soon we are in the midst of a cycle of compulsive/addictive behavior, one we return to over and over because we don't see any other option.

LIVING IN THE EXTREMES

In this state, we are living in the extremes, not in the convergence zone of the soul. Research has shown that people who have lived with a great deal of anxiety or fear—stemming from dysfunctional families, child abuse, sexual assault, trauma, or other causes—can actually experience an alteration of the brain that causes them to process information in the extremes. They tend to see life in terms of "all or nothing," "black or white," "all one way or all the other way." And when they turn to alcohol, other drugs, food, or sex, for example, to relieve the pressure and to fill the void they feel, they go to the extreme. They do not know that a middle way exists, that it's possible to have appropriate boundaries or to control their impulses. They stay in the extreme—extreme sex, extreme drinking, overeating, and so on. Perhaps, for example, they've been sexually abused as a child, and one of two things happens when they grow up: they either act out sexually or shut down sexually. Likewise, individuals who have experienced violence when they were children will, without help, either become victims or perpetrators of violence. Other people find themselves caught up in binge-purge cycles. They will binge on something such as alcohol or food and then go to the opposite extreme by trying to purge this behavior from their lives. They'll act out sexually and then decide to become celibate. In either case, these people don't know how to live a balanced life.

The answer to this predicament isn't just to go to the opposite extreme; abstinence, for example, is not the answer to problematic sexual behavior. Likewise, the answer is not, as too many people initially assume, to make the barrier even stronger. Doing so may seem to work, but if you take this course, you're actually just creating a very large "pressure cooker" that will eventually explode. Your next flip—and there *will* be a next one—will be even more dramatic with even greater negative consequences. All the stuff you've been trying to hide will come out despite your best efforts to hide it.

The task of recovery is essentially to dismantle the barrier you've created over the years and to reconnect with your shadow side—*and* with your soul. Once you start to take down that barrier, you will have to address all the issues, experiences, and consequences that you stuffed inside it. With this opening comes pain and grief. This is also the most likely point at which you'll relapse and turn back to your old behaviors. It's for exactly this reason that we have urged you to put your first-order changes in place. Having a support group, a therapist, boundaries for your computer use, and so forth will also help you get through this difficult time with less chance of a major relapse.

RELAPSING AND THE RECOVERY ZONE

If you do relapse, it's not the end of the world. Others, too, have relapsed. This doesn't mean you can't recover or that you should give up. It's just part of the process. In the next section of this chapter, you'll find more help for your journey into recovery.

At this point in recovery, it's easy to focus on the ability to become abstinent and to control your sexual behaviors. The real challenge, however, is to learn how to approach and work with deeper personal issues. It's about learning to deal with what Carl Jung called the "shadow self." It's not really the Internet or cybersex that has been casting a shadow over you; rather it's that you've been in the shadow of yourself. Once the barrier is down, you will start on a journey that will help you expose your shadow self and see who you really are. People who have been in recovery for a long time will tell you that one of the simplest tasks in recovery is abstaining from the problematic or addictive behavior. The more difficult task is to look at your relationships with other people and your relationship with yourself and to explore your life—past and present.

You will begin to move toward the center, what we call the Recovery Zone. When the barrier between the different parts of yourself is acknowledged and addressed, it becomes more permeable and allows the ego to develop a healthier relationship with the soul. The goal of recovery is not to remove the barrier completely—this would be far too frightening for any person. The goal is to see it for what it is and to be able to communicate with all parts of the self. Your life can become a reflection of the beauty of your inner self. You experience continual growth and expansion. You are living in the zone of the convergence of the soul.

SECOND-ORDER CHANGES—ON A PATH TO LONG-TERM CHANGE

In the previous chapter, we discussed first-order changes—the concrete actions taken to quickly stop a problem and to address specific consequences.

We will now introduce you to second-order changes—those steps that you take to actually change the dynamics of your life and the way you live. The following chart shows the difference in attitudes that exist during the change process.

Nonrecovery-Based Change Attitudes	Recovery-Based Change Attitudes
I don't have to tell others.	There are no secrets.
I can change behavior by myself.	I am powerless to change without the help of others.
I can always figure out or force a way to handle problems.	Sometimes there are events that I can't seem to control.
I work best alone.	I need contact with and the help of others.
No one is hurt by what I do.	Damage has rippled through the lives of people I know.
I have not been hurt by what I have done.	My behavior has disconnected me from myself.
I must operate in secrecy.	I must make a full disclosure.
I must isolate from others.	I must create support networks.
I cannot give anyone the whole story.	Trustworthy people get the whole story.
A double life is the only way to get my needs met.	Integrity must become the way I get my needs met.
Chaos is the norm.	I have a plan to reduce chaos and seek the help of others.

When working to make long-term behavioral changes in your life, the success of these changes is often dependent on the attitudes that underlie them. The above chart contains common nonrecovery attitudes that can block the recovery-based attitudes necessary for lasting and healthy change.

While your situation may feel quite hopeless or even desperate—and the struggle quite unwanted—those who have traveled this path before you have found that over time, a completely new way of living can emerge. This new life, you will discover, will be well worth the pain and effort of the work you're in the midst of right now. Though it may be nearly impossible to imagine, you may eventually come to see this struggle as a treasured gift, one that has given you a new life that is more rich and fulfilling than you ever imagined possible.

In making second-order changes, you will find that deeper tasks will emerge. The first-order changes of the previous chapter have enabled you to get a temporary handle on your problematic behavior, but now you need to look at the deeper issues that a lifelong solution will require of you. Surely more work and pain will be part of this journey, but if you commit to this process, you will not be disappointed with the result.

Second-order changes are the actions that will help you find the path to the deepest parts of yourself. They are the steps that will enable you to develop a new life in recovery. As you have seen, this is a difficult journey, one that often requires a number of interventions, including therapy, support groups, and spiritual guidance. It also takes time. It may help you to have more patience if you remember that it took you some time to get into the situation you're in and it will likewise take some time and work for a change to take place.

Second-order changes involve a lot of work and can be extremely difficult to face and move through. The resources listed on the following pages are not fail-safe, but they provide guidance from others who have been successful at coming into and moving through the second-order change process.

Finding and Working with a Good Therapist

There is a difference between going to therapy and actually being in therapy. "Going to therapy" means minimal involvement. It's basically showing up, sitting down, and waiting for the therapist to take charge. You don't voluntarily open up, share problems, or take any initiative. "Being in therapy," however, means that you come to each session with concerns and issues to work on. You have a commitment to being there mentally and emotionally, not just physically. You're there to take charge and to take responsibility for what happens. Therapy is not something your therapist "does" to you. Rather than resisting therapy, acknowledge your need for help. Open yourself up to the struggle and pain involved in recovery rather than trying to do everything you can to avoid it.

Once your therapist has helped you contain your behaviors, he or she can help you begin to look at the deeper issues that lie behind your compulsive and addictive behaviors, such as family-of-origin experiences, past trauma, and your relationship with your partner. Since working in therapy is a second-order process, this task will take time.

Finding and Using a Sponsor

Again, there is a difference between getting a sponsor and using a sponsor. "Getting a sponsor" is merely the act of finding someone who will agree to sponsor you. Your connections are brief and somewhat perfunctory; you don't really ask for help and you don't take advantage of all that a sponsor can do for you. "Using a sponsor" means connecting with a person who is willing to know everything about you—the whole dark side, the below-the-surface part of the volcano. A sponsor should be a person with whom you can discuss anything you want, someone who will support you without necessarily colluding with you, and someone who will be honest with you and who can confront you on any issue. Your sponsor may be someone who has already walked this road before. Or you may want to choose a close friend or colleague. We strongly urge you not to choose your partner as a sponsor, however, since partners are not only too close to the problem but often have their own individual struggles which they need to address. It is unfair to expect your partner to become your accountability person given all that he or she has to do for himself or herself. Once you have a sponsor, allow this person to help you. Having and using a sponsor is fundamentally about letting yourself be known. You must be willing to surrender to feedback regarding what it will take to get your life under control. And that means you have to let this person know how bad things really are right now, so he or she can see how best to help you.

Finding and Using a Support Group

As with therapy and sponsorship, there's a difference between going to group and using a group. If you are forcing the group members to work to get through to you, if you're trying to keep as much of your life as hidden as possible, then you're just "going to group." "Using your group" requires that you let down the barriers and allow others to know who you really are. This includes sharing when you're in trouble, taking chances, trusting the group, and asking for help.

PARTICIPATING IN TWELVE STEP MEETINGS

Many people have found tremendous support for recovery from a variety of compulsive and addictive behaviors—problems with alcohol, other drugs, bulimia, gambling, sex, and more—through attending Twelve Step meetings. As with support groups, you can go to meetings and just sit in a corner and people will pretty much leave you alone. Or you can go to meetings, listen, introduce yourself, socialize with people afterward, tell your story—your *whole* story—and talk and contribute at each meeting you attend. It may take some trial and error to find a meeting that feels right for you, but when you do, make a commitment to it. Remember, you're trying to build a support network, and meetings are a great way to begin this process. These people will understand you because they have been where you are now. And they know how to help and support you because they were helped and supported by those who came before them. Since intimacy seems to be at the core of many of the issues for cybersex compulsives, any type of group situation where you can develop and test new skills in relationship formation is going to be healthy. Developing healthy, intimate, nonromantic relationships with individuals of both sexes is critical in the recovery from cybersex compulsivity.

WORKING A PROGRAM

The phrase "working a program" grew out of the Twelve Step tradition. It means to actively participate in a Twelve Step program. While Twelve Step programs can be very effective, we are using the term "program" more broadly here. By "working a program" we mean that you need to make a firm commitment to participate in whatever recovery program or process you choose. That program may differ from a Twelve Step program in that it has different assignments and goals or is behaviorally oriented. Each therapy and recovery program looks a little different, but that's really not important. You could go to any number of different programs and still find help through each, as long as you are committed to the process of working that program. Conversely, you could go to the best program in the world and not be helped at all if you aren't committed. It's not so much the content of the program you attend that's critical as it is your willingness to open up and be known. Commitment to the process is the key to success. You truly need to "work" the program.

Watching Out for the Bounce Effect

Be aware of what we call the bounce effect. This happens when people begin working a program and attending support groups. They initially make big disclosures as they tell their stories, and having done that, they feel better—and then they stop. Often individuals feel better because the guilt they have held on to from their past behaviors is relieved. However, simply because one feels less guilty does not mean he or she is healthier. If guilt is "dumped" on others just to feel better, it can create an entirely new dynamic of emotionally victimizing other people just to get relief.

Individuals experiencing the bounce effect often don't take further steps beyond their disclosure. They rarely call their sponsor. They merely attend meetings; they don't participate in them. They have failed to understand that change, growth, and healing are *ongoing* processes and that they need to share continually what is happening in their recovery and lives. Opening up to others is not a onetime event or simply an end in itself. It is the first step in sharing who you are and who you are becoming. This kind of openness needs to become a way of life if you are to succeed in recovery. Our work with recovering people who have participated in Twelve Step programs has shown that those who committed to and followed the program through Step Nine are less likely to incur significant relapse.

The goal of treatment and recovery is not to immediately jump all the way to the other extreme—to make an enormous and dramatic splash at a meeting and to your sponsor and then be done with everything else. Instead, seek the middle ground. Begin the process and then continue it. Participate in your therapy groups, work the steps of your program, and begin to do service to others. You won't, at this point, know where this will all end, but have faith in the process and continue. Go on sharing your life and your problems and your challenges and your failures with others in your therapy program or recovery group and with your sponsor—and keep coming back week after week, month after month, and year after year. Recovery is not an event; it is an ongoing process, a process that will, over time, become far less focused on recovery from problematic sexual behaviors and more focused on personal and spiritual growth.

Making Social Connections

Reestablishing social connections is one of the most important steps you can take in recovery, particularly if you have problems with sexual behavior on the Internet. If you've been involved in cybersex, your social relationships have atrophied to the point where you have only one, and that's between you and your computer. Although there are some useful ways to develop and refine recovery with the Internet and to find support on the Internet, if that's as far as you take recovery, it means that your primary relationship is *still* between you and a computer. It is simply imperative that you begin to develop face-to-face contacts with other human beings, and the only way to do so is through actual social activities. Enroll in a photography or foreign-language class, join a church group or bike club, volunteer at a community organization, or take advantage of one or more of the countless other opportunities to meet people. One of the keys to breaking your link with the Internet is simply being with people in person. You need to have real, as opposed to virtual, interactions and relationships. You need to be out in the world interacting with people rather than sitting at home, isolated and alone with your computer. Through these social experiences, you'll meet people with whom you can become a companion and friend, and you'll find the opportunity for deeper relationships in your life. Developing good social support can, in fact, be just as important and effective for your recovery as finding a good therapist.

Involving Family and Friends

It's important to seek support from as many places as possible. Some people are comfortable talking with others in their lives, such as appropriate colleagues, good friends, and family members, while others find it enormously difficult to tell even one person. Those in the former group, however, have the best chance of achieving successful recovery.

A word of caution, however. When you begin to talk about your life, you may find that there are some people who don't really need to know what you have been through and for whom hearing your story would be painful and difficult. Hence, you need to respect the needs of others and to think about the consequences of revealing your story before doing so. It may not be appropriate, for example, to tell all your co-workers or your boss, if for no other reason than that you may be fired. It may also not be appropriate to tell your parents or other extended family members. This is really an example of working to develop good boundaries.

So start slowly. Find one or two people you can truly trust, get a sponsor, contact a good therapist, and then, with the help of this support system, slowly decide whom else you should include. Over time, you will find that the more people you can include in your support system, the stronger your recovery will be.

We can't overemphasize the importance of involving your partner early in the recovery process, because his or her involvement will dramatically increase your chances of success. It's also important that your partner have a therapist too, and that you, your partner, and both your therapists be involved in this process, especially for help in determining how much detail you reveal to others. You should reveal only information that will not be abusive to your partner. Disclosing every detail of everything you've ever done may simply be hurtful and unnecessary.

DEVELOPING AN INTERNET HEALTH PLAN

During recovery, many people are tempted to say, "Forget it! I'll just never use the Internet again." There are two problems with this. First, it isn't plausible for most people to give up the Internet in its entirety for the rest of their lives. The Internet is everywhere and has almost become a necessary part of our daily living. Second, deprivation of something that can be good, healthy, enjoyable, and entertaining sets up a dynamic of wanting it more and causing an eventual relapse. The goal is not to forgo the Internet completely, but, if possible, to develop a healthy relationship with it.

One way to explore developing a healthy relationship with the Internet is through an exercise called the Internet Health Plan. This exercise is designed to assist you in determining which of your Internet behaviors are unhealthy and which ones are healthy. You should review your Internet Health Plan at least every six months, or more often if necessary. This plan is designed to change and evolve over time as you learn more about yourself and effective Internet management skills.

Take a piece of paper and draw three circles similar to figure 8.2. In the inner circle, or the "red zone," list all Internet behaviors which are never healthy for you. This may include items such as going online after 10:00 P.M. or looking at certain sexual images on the Internet.

The middle circle is the "yellow zone." In the yellow zone you should list Internet behaviors about which you are uncertain whether they are healthy or unhealthy for you. This circle may also include Internet behaviors that

Internet Health Plan

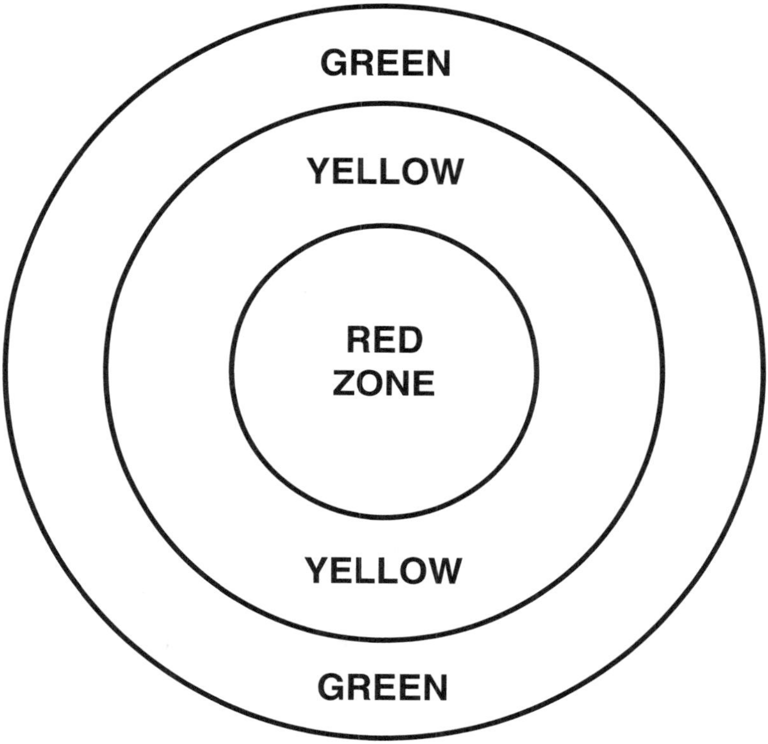

Figure 8.2

are sometimes healthy for you and are sometimes unhealthy. Examples include using the computer when you are alone, or going online when you are angry, tired, or lonely.

The outer circle is your "green zone." In this circle list Internet behaviors that you know are always okay for you. The green zone illustrates those behaviors that indicate healthy use of the Internet for you. Examples might be using the Internet in a high-traffic area, or finding recovery resources and support while online.

Enhancing Spirituality

Spiritual growth and development is an individual matter. How you pursue the spiritual aspects of your life can involve a variety of means, including meditation, membership in a religious organization, exploring Eastern spirituality, or practicing yoga, to name just a few. Involving someone else as a spiritual coach or mentor can be useful, as can joining a spiritual community with which you can readily identify. Your spiritual growth can become a tremendous source of support for your recovery.

Changing the Way You Live

To optimize your recovery, we strongly suggest that you embrace both the first-order changes laid out in the previous chapter and the second-order changes addressed in this chapter. First-order changes are meant to be stop-gap measures. If you stop with them, you will experience some healing, but the likelihood of falling back into your old behaviors will remain high. Keep in mind that first-order changes are only surface measures; they will not enable you to address the causes of the problem, which are deeper and take more time to work through. They will, however, help you quickly get your life under control and set the stage for the deeper work to be done with the second-order changes. As you can see, second-order changes help you build a strong support system. It's also likely that you'll be surprised to discover that this isn't a journey you have to take by yourself. In fact, it is a journey that you really *can't* take alone.

This brings us to the topic of the next chapter: relapse prevention. There you will find information based on the experiences of many others who have struggled with problematic sexual behaviors.

9
Preventing Relapse: Maintaining the Changes You've Made

FOR ALL OF US, making changes in our lives can be difficult. Each year in late January or early February, for example, we hear stories from friends about New Year's resolutions that have fallen by the wayside. Stories about failed diets or exercise plans are ubiquitous. You, too, have likely made promises to yourself about changing your cybersex behavior, only to find you've been unable to keep them.

Making life changes happen takes more than a promise to yourself. Yes, it is often difficult, but the lives of countless people who have done so is proof that it's possible. That's what this chapter is about: learning how to maintain the changes you've decided to make in your life.

It will help you to look more closely at the process of change. In the book *Changing for Good*, authors James Prochaska, John Norcross, and Carlo DiClemente state that there are six steps, or stages, that everyone goes through when making changes in their lives, regardless of what their goal is.[1] For example, if you think about a specific problem that you have resolved, chances are you will recognize immediately that its resolution didn't happen all at once. Perhaps for a while you ignored the problem; then you considered tackling it; after that, you may have made definite plans to change. Then, once you had garnered your forces—mental, physical, and social—you acted and began to struggle with the problem. If you succeeded, you worked at maintaining this change. If you failed, you probably gave up for a time, went back to the drawing board, and then tried once more.

Each of these steps is a predictable, well-defined stage: it takes place over a period of time and includes a series of tasks that must be completed before moving on to the next stage. Each stage doesn't inevitably lead to the next; it is possible to become stuck at one stage or another. However, by understanding these stages, you can gain control over the cycle of change and move through it more quickly and efficiently and with less pain.

As you read through these stages, we suggest that you keep in mind some changes that you've made, or tried to make, in your life and try to see how these stages apply to them.

STAGE 1: PRECONTEMPLATION

In this stage, it's not that you can't see the solution; it's that you can't see the problem! People at this stage usually have no intention of changing their behavior and typically deny having a problem. Although their families, friends, neighbors, doctors, or co-workers can see the problem quite clearly, the typical person in this stage can't.

Most people in this stage don't want to change themselves, just the people around them. Often they come to therapy because of pressure from others—a partner who threatens to leave them, an employer who threatens to fire them, or judges who threaten to punish them. Their first response in therapy is often, "How can I get others to quit nagging me?" When all else fails, they may change, but only as long as there is constant outside pressure. When that's gone, they quickly return to their old ways.

Precontemplators resist change. When their problem comes up in conversation, they shift the subject. They lack information about it and they intend to maintain ignorant bliss at all costs. Denial is characteristic of precontemplators, who place the responsibility for their problems on factors such as genetic makeup, family, society, or whatever, all of which they see as being out of their control. Precontemplators tend to be demoralized as well. They don't want to think, talk, or read about their problems because they feel the situation is hopeless.

So how can you change if you don't want to? The answer is in the approach; even precontemplators will progress toward change if they have the proper tools at the proper time.

STAGE 2: CONTEMPLATION

"I want to stop feeling stuck." These words are typical of contemplators. In the contemplation stage, people acknowledge that they have a problem and begin to think seriously about solving it. Contemplators struggle to understand their problem and to see its causes, and they wonder about possible solutions. Many have indefinite plans to take action within the next six months or so.

In this stage, you have become aware that something is amiss in your life. You've begun noticing that some difficulties have arisen. Your work supervisor recently had a meeting with you specifically to talk about those missed deadlines and the fact that you've been late getting to work more and more often. You know that both situations are due to your increasing cybersex involvement. The thought occurs to you that perhaps cybersex is a "bit of a problem." You contemplate making some changes, putting some controls on your use, and cutting down a bit.

The nature of contemplation can seem puzzling: you know your destination, and even how to get there, but you are not quite ready to go yet. Many people remain in this stage for a long time. Many spend years telling themselves that someday they'll change. When contemplators begin the transition to the preparation stage, their thinking is clearly marked by two changes. First, they begin to focus on the solution rather than the problem. Then they begin to think more about the future than the past. The end of the contemplation stage is a time of anticipation, activity, anxiety, and excitement.

STAGE 3: PREPARATION

Most people in the preparation stage are planning to take action soon, often within the very next month, and are making the final adjustments before they begin to change their behavior. An important step now is to make public the intended change. But although people in this stage are committed to acting and may appear ready to do so, they have not necessarily resolved their ambivalence. They may still need to convince themselves that this is what is best for them. People in the preparation stage may already have instituted a number of small behavioral changes, such as cutting their cigarette intake or counting calories. Awareness is high, and anticipation is palpable. People who cut short this stage—for example, waking up one morning and deciding to quit smoking cold turkey—actually lower their chances of success. It's better to make use of this time by planning carefully, developing a firm, detailed scheme for action, and making sure that you have learned the change processes you need to carry you through the process.

You might be asking yourself questions: "Do I need to get rid of the computer altogether?" "Do I need to put limits on how much time I spend on the computer or where I use it?" "What do I need to be cautious of?" "What is it exactly that I need to change?" In other words, what preparations do you need to make to effect the change?

Often anxiety is the impetus for finally taking action. While anxiety is often seen as a negative state, in this case, it has a positive effect in that it can impel us to finally move out of contemplation and into preparation and action. Without anxiety, there is often no change. If life is comfortable, why rock the boat? Concern and discomfort push us to take action to relieve anxiety.

STAGE 4: TAKING ACTION

The action stage is the one in which people most obviously change their behavior and their surroundings. They stop smoking cigarettes, remove all tempting desserts from the house, pour the last beer down the drain, send all the pornography to the dump, or confront their fears. In short, they make the move they've been planning.

The danger in this stage is that many people, including professional therapists, often mistakenly equate action with change, overlooking not only the critical work that prepares people for successful action but also the equally important (and often more challenging) efforts to maintain the changes following action.

It's important to recognize that the action stage is not the only time you can make progress toward overcoming your problem. Although modifying your behavior is the most visible form of change, it is far from the only one: you can also change your level of awareness, emotions, self-image, thinking, and so on. And many of those changes take place in the stages that precede action.

Furthermore, any movement from one stage of change to the next represents considerable progress. If, after years of avoiding a problem, you consciously begin to acknowledge that it exists and think seriously about changing it, the transition from precontemplation to contemplation is no less significant than from preparation to action.

STAGE 5: MAINTENANCE

There are great challenges at every stage, and the maintenance stage is no exception. It is here that people must work to consolidate the gains that they have made during the previous stages and struggle to prevent lapses and relapse. Change never ends with action. Although traditional therapy sees maintenance as a static stage, in fact it is a critically important continuation that can last from as little as six months to the rest of one's life. Without a strong commitment to maintenance, there will surely be relapse, usually to the precontemplation or contemplation stage. Programs that promise easy change—crash diets, one-day smoking-cessation sessions, or whatever— usually fail to acknowledge that maintenance is a long, ongoing process.

STAGE 6: RELAPSE

While Prochaska and his associates described this change process in a linear sequence—precontemplation, contemplation, preparation, action, maintenance—life is not so clear-cut and simple. Most people do slip up at some point, returning to earlier stages before renewing their efforts.

Relapse means slipping back into the behaviors you've decided to leave behind. Prochaska and many others who help people make changes in their lives strongly emphasize several points about relapse. First, relapse is a normal part of the change process. Making changes is not like flipping a light switch—as in "yesterday I did such and such" and then "click, and now today I do it differently and that's that." The average successful self-changer relapses several times.

Needless to say, the feelings relapse evokes are not pleasant. You may feel like a complete failure, embarrassed, ashamed, and guilty and may believe that all of your hard efforts at change have been wasted. Demoralization sets in, and you may want to give up entirely on changing. You may slide all the way back to the precontemplation stage.

After several setbacks, you may feel as though you are going in circles. But you're not. Think of the change cycle not as a circle, but as an upward spiral. You may be in the contemplation or preparation stage again, but this time you can draw on the lessons you've learned from your previous efforts. Relapse, or recycling, gives you the opportunity to learn. Viewed in this way, relapsing into old behaviors is not seen as a failure, but rather as a learning experience. You've prepared and taken action. Then, when you slip up, you simply move back to stages 2 and 3 to reevaluate what you're doing, how you slipped, and what you can do to minimize the chances of future relapse. Your goal is to learn from your slip. Prochaska and his associates say we can always expect some level of relapse to occur, particularly if the change is a difficult one like dealing with cybersex. Taking action and slipping is much better than taking no action at all.

You may find that you will cycle through these stages in various areas of your life at different levels for many years. Let's say, for example, that you've come to grips with your cybersex behavior. It's no longer a problem. Then, however, you notice that the relationship between you and your partner isn't all that you want it to be . . . so you apply the change process to this issue.

In its broadest sense, this change and recovery process is really a way of living life more fully and consciously. It's not something that you do for a few days, weeks, or months and then say, "Great! That's done. Time to move on."

Again, although we are applying these stages to the problem of cybersex, people move through these stages whenever they make changes in their lives. They are not just applicable to dysfunctional behaviors.

We have found that, when people are recovering from problematic sexual behaviors or cybersex addiction, there is a particular point when they are most likely to relapse. In the previous chapter, we explored the six stages that people with problematic or addictive behaviors go through as they move on in their recovery, and it is in the third and fourth stages, shock and grief, that relapse is most likely. Why then? Relapse normally occurs when people are most emotionally vulnerable. It is in these stages that people finally begin to be honest with themselves and to truly look at their behaviors and consequences for the first time. This is a wonderful point in recovery, but it is also a time when strong emotions surface. In the face of this emotional tempest, it's easy to revert to old dysfunctional behaviors for "comfort." This does not, however, mean failure. On the contrary, it means that we've taken another major step forward in recovery because we've been more honest and open with ourselves.

With the connection between shock, grief, and relapse made, it is important to remember that relapse can occur in any stage. In fact, throughout this book we have highlighted some things about the Internet that make it a unique and powerful force. Because of the nature of the Internet, its accessibility, and the factors in the CyberHex (page 14), we have found that cybersex compulsives are more likely to relapse than other addicts. Although hearing this may sound discouraging, it is actually good for you to know this in advance because you can work it into your change plan and be more vigilant for the signs of relapse. As with all problematic behavior, it is important not to become overconfident about the changes you have made, but this is even more critical in cybersex behavior. We have witnessed people with years of solid recovery in Alcoholics Anonymous or a sexual addiction recovery program quickly go back to square one when cybersex enters the picture.

To help you better understand the place of relapse in recovery, let's look at the experiences of two people, Rudy and Linda.

Rudy is a thirty-five-year-old, male, blue-collar worker who engaged in cybersex online. He used pornography chat rooms and other cybersex while masturbating. He felt tremendous guilt over this behavior because of his religious beliefs. As a result, Rudy entered treatment for problematic (offline) sexual behavior, in particular, for exhibitionism. Eventually during treatment, Rudy did admit that cybersex was a serious problem in his life too. Rudy participated in treatment by engaging in the minimum requirements of the program. There wasn't any reason to dismiss him from the group, but it was clear that Rudy never truly engaged in the therapy process. His counselor realized that Rudy was on a path toward relapse when he began to attend their sessions only infrequently while experiencing a series of stressful situations at work and within his family. Rudy clearly had applied first-order changes with regard to his cybersex behaviors by selling his computer and engaging in the minimum requirements of recovery. But Rudy had never made any second-order changes. Consequently, when stress in his life increased, he had no strategies or support in place to help him cope. His relapse included carrying out sexual activities online by using his brother's computer during the day, when his brother was at work. The only reason Rudy stopped his relapse behaviors was that he was caught.

Linda is thirty-eight years old, married, and the mother of two young children. Once her children were both in school, Linda began to log on to chat rooms to relieve her loneliness. Soon she developed several romantic online relationships with men there. On several occasions, she agreed to meet partners offline for sexual escapades. After one year, her husband discovered her online and offline affairs and demanded that they stop.

Linda entered treatment and began a solid recovery program by acknowledging that both her online and offline sexual behaviors were out of control. After two years of treatment and attendance in a Twelve Step group, Linda felt her life was back on track. She continued her counseling sessions and began to tap into painful childhood memories and childhood trauma that she had never dealt with. Her parents had been alcoholics and Linda had suffered neglect and emotional abuse. She began to realize for the first time that her family was not all that she had thought it was and that she really didn't have much support.

Not long after this, Linda's relationship with her husband became strained, finances grew tight, and she began to feel entitled to a better life. Feeling very vulnerable, Linda once again turned to the Internet. She logged on to one of her old chat rooms and found some of her old "friends" still there, ready to once again hook up sexually. Acting out brought on a great deal of guilt and shame, but Linda continued in her relapse for several weeks. She then realized that she was in trouble and needed to return to treatment.

The experiences of Rudy and Linda are examples of relapse handled in two very different fashions. Some individuals are impelled to enter treatment because of external factors in their lives. Perhaps it was a spouse or partner that insisted they enter treatment, or some other authority figure, such as the legal system. As such people "contemplate" their situation, they do not consider the deeper issues that have created the situation in which they find themselves. Instead, they are only thinking about what will happen to them if they don't accept treatment. They often see treatment participation as a way to "get the heat off" for a time while they figure out how to carry on in the future without getting caught. Their contemplation, preparation, and action steps don't grow out of an admission that they have a serious problem. Their focus is instead on developing tactics that will enable them to continue their cybersex behaviors without once again suffering the consequences that landed them in treatment. Theirs is a reaction to outside forces rather than action taken as a result of self-examination and inner growth. Still narcissistic, they are worried only about what will happen to them. They go through the treatment process but remain disengaged. They never really decide to give up their cybersex behaviors.

In Rudy's case, it's apparent from his relapse that he never really became engaged in the recovery process. He hadn't really moved beyond the contemplation stage, nor did he ever truly resolve to give up his cybersex activities.

Linda made both first- and second-order changes and was working a program. Linda reached a point in recovery at which she was emotionally vulnerable. She had finally begun to experience all the feelings that come with more self-awareness, including fear, remorse, anger, and pain. Though she relapsed, Linda recognized the problem on her own and decided, also on her own, to return to treatment. The impetus for this decision was not the result of outside forces. Had Linda planned for this time in her recovery, however, she may have been able to avoid her relapse.

SUDS: SEEMINGLY UNIMPORTANT DECISIONS

Relapses tend to be seen as a matter of impulse—as a moment of weakness when someone lets down his or her guard. Research has shown us, however, that this is not the case. Stress, coping strategies (or lack thereof), and decision-making skills all play a role, as do SUDs—seemingly unimportant decisions.[2] Relapse is really the culmination of a chain of events that starts days, weeks, or even months in advance of its actual occurrence. Often, the actual relapse act can't be carried out immediately because of situational constraints such as, in the case of cybersex, unavailability of computer and Internet access or the lack of privacy. The desire for immediate gratification may be temporarily put off and instead be redirected to secret planning or fantasies about cybersex. Because of the potential for conflict and guilt associated with these secret schemes and plans, people are likely to engage in rationalization or denial, or both. These two distorted ways of thinking can then combine to influence certain choices or decisions as part of a chain of events leading ultimately to a relapse.

We believe that people who are headed for a relapse make a number of mini-decisions over time, each of which brings them a bit closer to the brink of the triggering high-risk situation. An example is the abstinent drinker who buys a bottle of sherry to take home, "just in case guests drop by." Or the ex-smoker who decides it would be fine to choose a seat in the smoking section of a restaurant. Or the recovering gambler who expands a vacation driving trip to California to include a visit to Lake Tahoe, which is near the gambling mecca of Reno, Nevada.

The term "SUDs" describes these decisions. It is as though people slowly begin to set the stage for a possible relapse by making a series of SUDs, each of which moves them one step closer to relapse. A final advantage in "setting up" a relapse in this way is that people may be able to avoid assuming responsibility for the relapse episode itself. By putting themselves in an extremely tempting, high-risk situation, they can claim that they were "overwhelmed" by external circumstances that made it "impossible" to resist the relapse.

Stress can be a powerful relapse trigger too, one that should not be underestimated. Consider this scenario: over the past few weeks, one of your children has been having problems at school. This has taken extra time from you and your spouse. In addition, your spouse has been worrying about an impending visit from her parents. The result: There's a lot more tension around your house than normal, and it's been building up for a few weeks, wearing you down. You've been thinking more and more about how good it would be to jump online for a little dose of cybersex, just like old times. You've resisted this temptation with the help of your sponsor. But now it's Friday evening, and you're home by yourself . . . with your computer.

One of your primary relapse prevention goals is to become aware of the behavior chains that can lead you to relapse. If you can recognize them, then you can take action long before you get to the point of relapse. In the example above, talking with your wife about the stress you're feeling and your concerns about the end result would be a positive step in breaking the chain. Once you recognize your behavior chain, you can begin planning for ways to substitute new, positive, and supportive behaviors to prevent relapse. You realize that when life gets stressful at home, you need to spend time with a friend, for example, or talk with your wife about it, or get some exercise. Essentially, you need to do whatever seems to help relieve the stress before you feel the need to turn to cybersex for relief.

The concept of behavior chains and our power to change them points out another important difference between a first-order and a second-order relapse. People who have only made first-order changes always think that the cause of the relapse is something outside of themselves. The cause is external, something over which they have no control. They might say, for example, that it was their spouse's nagging that caused the relapse, or an argument with a relative, or a boss who is pressuring them. On the other hand, people who have made second-order changes would talk about this relapse in terms of their own responsibility: "I have been fighting with my wife a lot lately" or "I haven't really been responsible at work lately." These people realize that *they* are responsible for their behavior.

The concept of behavior chains and our power to change them also shows the importance of identifying your relapse triggers and determining ways to avoid them. We already have numerous procedures in our society that require us to prepare for the possibility (no matter how remote) that various problematic and dangerous situations may arise. For example, fire drills help us be prepared in case a fire breaks out in public buildings or schools. Anyone who has been on a cruise ship is familiar with lifeboat drills to teach the passengers what to do in the event that the ship encounters trouble at sea. Certainly no one believes that requiring people to participate in fire drills increases the probability of future fires; on the contrary, the aim is actually to minimize the extent of personal loss and damage should a fire happen. The same logic applies in the case of relapse prevention.

Include a "relapse drill" as part of your prevention strategy. Learning precise prevention skills and related strategies is more helpful than relying on vague suggestions to "work your program." Think of situations that you know could trigger a relapse for you. Begin with the scenarios that would be less likely to do so, and then move on to ones that would place you at higher risk until, finally, you list the situation that would be the most dangerous for you. For each of these situations, then, think of ways you could react that would enable you to escape the "fire" without being burned. As the intensity and risk of relapse increase with each situation, your escape plan will need to be better planned. List at least six to ten relapse-threatening situations. Finally, choose three—one that is quite low risk, one that presents a more moderate risk, and a high-risk situation—and write down your escape plan for each on an index card. Keep those three cards with you at all times. You may also find that referring to them occasionally will help remind you of your goals in recovery. Several popular slogans emphasize these ideas: "Forewarned is forearmed," "An ounce of prevention is worth a pound of cure," and "Be prepared!"

TEN RELAPSE PITFALLS

Even though you're gaining more insight and understanding about yourself and your behavior, the recovery road is not a smooth superhighway. There are potholes ahead, but you can avoid them, especially if you know what to watch out for. Here are ten pitfalls to beware of—and suggestions for bypassing them "unharmed."

Pitfall 1: Now that the crisis is over, there's no longer a problem.
This is a common pitfall because it's tempting to think this way after your initial crisis has passed. After that chaos, the first-order changes you put in place make your life feel almost carefree. It will seem as though the problem is solved.

Well, it isn't. You've only dealt with crisis management; you still need to deal with all the factors that led you into compulsive or addictive cybersex in the first place. This takes time. And effort. And the help of others. This is a lifelong issue that you will always need to be aware of and to manage. As time passes and your recovery strengthens, less vigilance will be needed, of course, but the potential for relapse will always remain.

Pitfall 2: Chaos helps me remember I'm alive.
It is not unusual for people who are involved in addictive or compulsive behavior to like the drama of crisis. And because they like it, "calm" isn't comfortable. It doesn't feel "right" because they are accustomed to crises and the adrenaline rush that crises bring on. If you're not familiar with life feeling calm, you may be tempted to create a situation in which a crisis will occur.

At times like this, you would do well to tell yourself the following: "Crisis isn't common; calm is OK." Yes, calm is OK. Life in recovery will feel different than life overwhelmed by cybersex, but just because it feels different or makes you uncomfortable doesn't mean it's bad. In fact, calm indicates that you have begun to create balance in your life. Life in crisis is life out of balance.

It's also common for people who are involved in an addictive or compulsive behavior to think that a life without the behavior will be boring—that they won't have any fun or excitement anymore. First, we suggest that thinking about your cybersex-obsessed life as being fun and exciting is not accurate—just review your consequences list for a reality check. As time passes, you will find much in your life that's interesting, exciting, and fun. You may even see your ability to manage and control your life as fun.

Pitfall 3: I'll start feeling better immediately.
As you begin recovery, you may expect to feel better immediately. Yes, once you've gotten first-order changes in place, you should feel some immediate relief. Once you begin the transition and especially the second-order changes, life may seem more difficult again—although in a different way than when you were involved in cybersex behavior. Strong feelings such as sadness, grief, anger, shame, regret, and failure may surface and cause great discomfort. You will likely feel worse again before turning the corner toward truly brighter days. Our culture teaches us to expect quick fixes for our problems: pop a pill to take care of pain—either physical or emotional—and it will be gone. Recovery—which means making fundamental changes in ourselves and our lives—is neither easy, quick, nor pain-free. But when you persevere, the rewards can be remarkable, even unimaginable.

Pitfall 4: I'll be able to handle or manage sex on the Internet.
Once people have progressed in recovery, they may reach a point at which it is tempting to say, "I can handle this," while dabbling in the problematic behavior. An alcoholic may say, "I've been sober for quite some time. I've finally got this drinking issue under control. It's now safe for me to have a drink once in a while." A person who's been involved in cybersex behavior may say the same thing.

"I had been in recovery from cybersex for nearly two years," said Terrence, a prominent lawyer. "One of the steps I'd taken was to not know the password to my computer. After a certain amount of time, I really felt

I didn't need this safeguard any longer and convinced my wife to reveal it to me. Sad to say, within six months I was back in trouble with cybersex again."

Don't fall into this pit. This kind of thinking is really no more than bargaining with your compulsion—"I'll give up *nearly all* these behaviors, but not all"—in an attempt to avoid the feelings of grief and loss over truly letting go of your problematic behaviors. This pitfall is an attempt to find ways that you can actually do the cybersex behavior without losing your sobriety totally. When you truly admit that you can't handle cybersex, then you will have to deal with painful feelings about losing that activity in your life.

This kind of self-talk is very seductive and it's likely that, at some point, you will go back to cybersex and soon find yourself in full relapse. If you do, try not to despair. Look at it as a lesson that you needed to learn, and then move on.

Pitfall 5: It wasn't *that bad when I was doing it.*
This pitfall is similar to the previous one. It's the result of a condition we call "addiction amnesia." After you have been in recovery for some time, a voice in your head will make statements such as "Doing what I did really wasn't that bad," or "I really didn't have too many consequences," or "I didn't have consequences that I couldn't handle."

When such thoughts surface, you need to do a reality check. Again, you might review the consequences list in chapter 7, and when you do, you'll quickly see just how bad the consequences of your cybersex behaviors were. You might also ask your spouse, partner, or someone else whose life was affected by your behaviors just how great the problem was. Ask that person how he or she was affected.

Pitfall 6: This problem is different for me than for others.
This kind of thinking is likely to arise once you begin attending a support group or Twelve Step group. After hearing many people's stories, you may find yourself thinking that your situation is unique, that your problem is either worse or less serious than everyone else's. If you think that you're better than the others and that your situation is not very serious, you aren't accepting the true extent of your problem—and you're more likely to relapse. On the other hand, if you begin to believe that you're worse off than

everyone else, you are likely to trigger your feelings of shame. You may then tell yourself that you'll never be able to control your cybersex behaviors anyway, so why even bother trying to stop?

The pitfall here is "unique thinking"—believing you're different from other people. Comparing your situation with that of others is pointless. Severity is irrelevant. You all have the same problem and you all need to stay in recovery.

Pitfall 7: A slip (or relapse) equals a failure, so why continue recovery?

Let's say you're on a diet. You've lost twelve pounds already, but you are still a bit less than halfway to your weight goal. One evening, you're visiting a friend's home and she offers you some Oreo cookies. You know you should decline, but you eat three anyway. Later, you're in the kitchen by yourself when you discover a cookie jar filled with more Oreos. You think, "What the heck, I've slipped already so I might as well eat all of these that I can." Is eating three (a small slip) a good reason to go back and eat the rest of the bag?

Slips and relapse are often part of recovery. Think about the stages of change that we discussed at the beginning of this chapter. Do you remember how the process sometimes means taking a few steps backward before permanently moving ahead. Having a slip is not reason for despair, nor is it a justification for surrendering to your compulsive and addictive behaviors again. You've made progress in your recovery. Much good has happened. You slipped; so get up, brush yourself off, and get back on the path. Then talk with your sponsor or therapist about what happened and develop a plan for avoiding such a slip or relapse in the future.

Pitfall 8: I can't do recovery for the rest of my life; therefore there's no hope for me.

Particularly during early recovery, after that first rush of good feelings has passed and suddenly things look much more difficult again, you may say something like this to yourself: "Oh, my God, I've been struggling with this for six weeks. It's so hard. I can't even *imagine* going through this for the rest of my life! There's really just no hope."

Many, many people in recovery have had such thoughts. They are typical of early recovery. What you need to do is to turn your focus away from the future and stay in the present. Right now, you are not involved in cyber-sex behaviors. Take life one minute, one hour, one day at a time. Recovery does become easier with time—and not just because you're "stronger," but because it feels better and better to be in recovery. Your life begins to have more joy. Recovery is something you want because it's making your life better. And sooner than you think, all those "one day at a times" turn into weeks and months and even years. Pay attention to today; the future will take care of itself.

Pitfall 9: I can do this on my own.

"I don't need other people to help me." "I don't need God or a spiritual connection that people talk about." "I'm strong; I can do this on my own."

This kind of thinking indicates that you have not moved beyond first-order change. You were isolated in your cybersex behaviors, and now you are still isolated in your recovery. Isolation will draw you back into your compulsive or addictive behaviors.

As we have emphasized throughout this book, you cannot recover on your own. You need others to help you take this path successfully. People are ready to help you. You need only ask. In fact, by not allowing other people to help, you are actually denying them an opportunity to give you a gift.

Pitfall 10: My partner didn't leave me, so what I did couldn't have been so bad for him/her.

Just because your partner or spouse—or friends and colleagues—didn't completely abandon you does not mean that your behaviors didn't hurt them. Forgiveness does not mean permission to return to your compulsive behaviors. Forgiveness is based on the hope and the promise you've made to work on your behavior and not repeat your mistakes.

When you find yourself thinking like this, we suggest that you talk with the people in your life who were affected by your cybersex behaviors and ask them to tell you how they were affected. As time passes, you may forget what happened (again, this is addiction amnesia). While there's no need to revisit the past regularly, it is useful to occasionally re-member when you were out of control, when people were upset with you, and when you were creating havoc in your life and the lives of others.

Bringing that time to light serves as an effective remedy for this kind of thinking.

Twelve Step groups and support groups are effective in part because they serve as a means of reminding members what a life of compulsion and addiction is like. When newcomers join and tell their stories, all are reminded of the place they once lived and how far they've come.

RELAPSE ATTITUDE TRAPS

We are now going to introduce you to four relapse attitudes: entitlement, resentment, deprivation, and stress. Getting them out in the open helps you avoid relapse.

ENTITLEMENT

People who fail at some task, who are struggling with problems, or who feel put upon often feel so much self-pity that they believe they are entitled to some kind of reward for their struggles. Conversely, people who are very accomplished and overreach themselves can likewise feel that they deserve some reward for all their hard work. Many people who struggle with compulsive and addictive behaviors stretch their lives to the extreme. Often they have a difficult time saying no to others' requests and find themselves overcommitted. Ministry and medicine, for example, are two professions that reinforce overcommitted behaviors. The people who are drawn to these professions are often very good at them and committed to helping others, repeatedly giving in positive ways, but often they also do a poor job of taking care of their own needs. It then becomes easy for them to think that, because they work so hard for others, they are entitled to some reward. And some rewards, such as cybersex or affairs, can be very self-destructive. Their feelings of entitlement don't derive from a sense of narcissism; instead they grow out of an inability to say no to the needs of others. Sadly, their attempts at self-care are counterproductive. The struggles and hard work of recovery can also lead people into feelings of entitlement.

RESENTMENT

During the recovery process, it's common for feelings of anger and resentment to surface. These feelings may come from many sources: resentment about difficult predicaments, losses suffered, past and future consequences of out-of-bounds behavior, family-of-origin issues, and so on. It is important to acknowledge and address these feelings with a therapist or sponsor. If they remain unaddressed, they can lead to ever stronger feelings of self-pity and entitlement—and eventually to relapse.

Deprivation: Abstaining from All Things Sexual

In recovery from any problematic sexual behavior, it is tempting to say to yourself, "That's it, I'm just going off sex. It has caused me so much trouble, and I don't seem to know how to handle it in a healthy way. I'm just going to quit." The problem is that you can't quit being sexual, and more important, you don't have to. Trying to abstain will only set you up for a relapse. Many people who are on food diets experience similar problems. They diet carefully, denying in the process all the foods they really like. The result? Inevitably they leave their diet behind, only to fall into eating binges and regaining the lost weight. Entitlement thinking plays a key role here too. It's easy to tell yourself that you've been good for so long and you've deprived yourself of the foods you love for so long that you're now entitled to engage in the "forbidden" loves. That's relapse. If you live in a state of deprivation, you will be more vulnerable to feelings of entitlement.

People who successfully lose weight instead learn how to eat healthfully. They also take time and effort to look inside themselves to see what emotional needs or family issues lie behind their habit of overeating, and they make plans to deal with the cravings that will inevitably arise.

Successful recovery from your dysfunctional cybersex behaviors won't happen through sexual abstinence, but instead through following the steps we have laid out, in particular the second-order changes you make. These steps lead to personal awareness and growth, to an ability to nurture yourself, to intimacy with those you love, and to a healthy sexuality in which you will no longer need your old behaviors to feel good.

Simply stopping problematic or addictive behaviors does not equate with recovery. Again, we are talking about making only first-order changes. Without the introspection and inner growth that come with second-order changes, you are merely setting yourself up for relapse. Feelings of deprivation and entitlement will surely arise. And you may find yourself engaging in compulsive behaviors of another kind, such as drinking or gambling.

Until the issues underlying your problematic or addictive sexual behaviors are addressed, there will be no recovery.

STRESS

Higher-than-normal stress levels can quickly increase your risk of relapse. Remember, too, that stress is not always created by negative situations or events. Receiving a long-sought work promotion, moving to a new city, the birth of a child, or a new relationship can all create stress too. If you are un-sure about ways to handle the stress in your life, seek out a course on stress management skills, relaxation training, or meditation—and then put these skills to use.

TRANSFORMING RELAPSE

As previously discussed, relapse is a normal part of the change process. Cybersex compulsives tend to be more prone to relapse than those with other forms of addiction because of the accessibility and anonymity associ-ated with the Internet. The key to making relapse part of change is your responses and actions following a relapse: a relapse followed by thinking errors, distortions, and false beliefs ("This wasn't that bad." "I can handle this alone.") versus deciding how to learn from the experience ("How can I learn from this experience?" "What might I do differently in the future?").

Below is a list of questions that will help you transform relapse into healthy change. Write out your answers to the following questions as hon-estly as possible following a relapse. Pay attention to whether you are dis-torting the truth in your responses. Then find an accountability partner such as a therapist, sponsor, or friend to share your responses with. The accountability partner will serve as a sounding board to help keep you hon-est in your answers.

1. What behaviors (looking at pornography, chatting online with a teenager, for example) were involved in your online relapse? Be sure to list *all* the behaviors involved.

2. Describe the chain of online events immediately preceding the actual online behaviors that accounted for your relapse. (For example, were you surfing the Internet and stumbled on a Web site accidentally? Did you intentionally sit down to look for sex chat?) Did this chain of events trigger an old ritual for you?

3. What thoughts, feelings, and behaviors were occurring in your offline world immediately before you sat down at the computer? (Were you fighting with your partner? Yelling at your kids? Thinking about work? Feeling lonely? Feeling angry?) Are these thoughts, feelings, or behaviors a recurring theme that has led to past problems?

4. What thoughts, feelings, and behaviors occurred within the first thirty minutes after your relapse was over? How about within the next six hours? The next twenty-four hours? (For example, "I need to keep this a secret," "I am never going to recover," or "My stress is relieved.") Are these thoughts, feelings, or behaviors a recurring theme that has led to past problems?

5. Is it possible to trace the chain of events that led to your relapse into the weeks before it actually occurred? (For example, did you feel an increase in stress at work? Did you notice a lack of self-care? Were you tempting yourself online?) Did you encounter common triggers that have led you to relapse or near-relapse in the past?

6. What are your plans to transform this relapse into a healthy change process? (For example, what will you do differently in the future? What did you learn from this relapse?) Who can you process this relapse with?

STAY ALERT FOR SIGNS OF TROUBLE

Social pressures, internal challenges, and special situations are common threats to maintenance and recovery. Social pressures come from those around you who either engage in cybersex themselves or don't recognize its impact on your life. Internal challenges usually result from overconfidence and other forms of defective thinking, such as those mentioned on pages 179–81 as the tried-and-true relapse traps. While many of the more common temptations will occur for you during the action stage, most people learn to deal with them before moving out of that stage. During maintenance, however, the relatively rarer temptations come into play. They are difficult to anticipate and pose serious threats to your confidence, convictions, and commitment.

ADDITIONAL SUGGESTIONS FOR MAINTAINING COMMITMENT
AND RECOVERY

- Write down the difficulties you encountered in your early efforts
  to change your cybersex behaviors. Next, review the lists you made
  in chapter 7 in which you described the negative aspects of your
  cybersex behaviors. Keep both of these lists, look at them periodically, and refer to them at the first sign of slipping.
- Take credit for your accomplishment. This is not the time to criti-
  cize yourself for having had problems; instead take both credit and
  responsibility for change. Use the new year, your birthday, or the
  anniversary of your change (it doesn't have to be a year; celebrate
  month by month at first) to reflect on the success you have had and
  to renew your commitment.
- As you progress in your recovery, you will gradually become more
  and more comfortable in the presence of certain temptations or
  situations. But you may not become completely immune to them.
  Especially during the early months of maintenance, it's best to continue to avoid people, places, or things that could compromise your
  recovery. Pay attention to the behaviors you need to avoid (found
  in your Internet Health Plan).
- Make a crisis card for your wallet or purse. On it, write a list of the
  negative consequences of your problem, as well as a set of instructions to follow when you are seriously tempted to slip. The instructions could read as follows: (1) review the negative consequences of
  the behavior, (2) substitute a positive alternative for the cybersex
  behavior, (3) remember the benefits of changing, (4) engage in distracting or positive behavior, and (5) call someone (write down a
  support person's name and phone number).
- Last, but by no means least, seek help and support from your support group, therapist, partner or spouse, and friends. Having someone to call on who has been where you are, who can understand,
  and who can help is simply invaluable.

Though recovery may seem to be a daunting and endless task, we encourage you to begin thinking in a new way about these changes. If you
think of recovery as a burden akin to a diet, it just won't work. Try to view

the path on which you've set out as a truly remarkable opportunity, because that is exactly what it is. Once you begin to change, to accept the support others are offering to you, and to live in your Recovery Zone, you will find that you love your new life so much that you don't want to give it up. Gradually, staying in your Recovery Zone will no longer seem like something you have to do (because otherwise your partner will leave you or you'll be incarcerated), but something you *want* to do. You will begin to truly cherish what you've found. This newfound caring for yourself and the pride it creates will build a new feeling of being capable—of self-confidence and self-esteem. This is a hope-filled process.

Even if you are not yet at the point where you have started to experience these feelings, it's important that you know that this place exists. If you've read the book to this point without having done the work we suggested, you're unlikely to understand or believe that this is possible. But by doing the work, you can get there. This is not a fantasy or an illusion. You *can* reach a point where you *want* to be in recovery—a point where your passion for recovery is as strong as your passion for cybersex once was.

10

Family Dynamics and Cybersex

KATHLEEN IS AN attractive, thirty-five-year-old professional woman married to Tom, her second husband.

Our marriage had been somewhat problematic, and I was frustrated because it felt like I was carrying most of the weight in the business that we were in together. For some time, my husband had talked of a fantasy of a sexual threesome with another woman. I didn't really like the idea, but he brought it up so often that I finally agreed. So Tom booked a prostitute via the Internet. She came to our home and we all had sex together. This was a very painful experience for me, but I felt that somehow maybe there was something wrong with me because I didn't like it.

After some months and a number of threesomes with different women, things were just getting worse for me so I sought help from a therapist. The therapist handed me a copy of a book on sex addiction in the first session, and said, "You have a problem, and there's more going on here than you know." I continued therapy for eighteen months but felt that I just wasn't really making progress. And we still were having threesome-sex occasionally too. During this time, I began to have migraine headaches that kept increasing in severity as the months passed. Eventually, I had to be hospitalized. I just couldn't function anymore. In the hospital, I was medicated constantly with few positive results.

One day, however, I woke up and realized that I was slowly dying.

I was just wasting away in the hospital. And I realized that the migraines were due to the terrible unhappiness in my life because of my sexual relationship with my husband. I finally called my sister, who came and took me out of the hospital and brought me to her home. While living with her, I slowly began to recover. I continued therapy, and after some months, the migraines disappeared. The sexual demands and activities to which I had acquiesced had been so emotionally painful that they had actually caused a physical illness.

Adam and Gordon are professionals in their mid-thirties. Says Gordon:

Adam and I had been partners for four years when I discovered that he had been using the Internet to meet and have sex with other men. I was devastated at this revelation, as you can imagine. But more than that, I was plagued by the feeling that this happened because I wasn't attractive enough to hold his attention—to keep him interested just in me. Now I'm so angry. I don't know how I can trust him anymore. I'm afraid that our relationship will disintegrate. And most of all, I'm furious with him because he got infected with syphilis, and now I have it too.

Cindy and Steve, a Caucasian couple, had been married fifteen years when Steve discovered Cindy had been having an affair with an African American:

When I confronted her about this, Cindy admitted that during the last five years of our marriage, she'd had four affairs, each time with black guys she'd met through the Internet. Needless to say, I was very hurt and angry. Even worse, this situation began eating at me. It wasn't long before I began to pester Cindy for details about these affairs. Then we'd have very aggressive, violent sex. This situation continued for some time, with me wanting more and more details of her exploits with these men. Eventually, Cindy's revelations weren't enough for me, so I turned to the Internet myself and began searching for interracial sex sites. Upon discovering them, I literally spent endless hours at a time on the Net. Cindy didn't like this situation at all, but she didn't feel she had any right to complain because she felt bad about the affairs she'd had. Besides, she told herself, I wasn't having affairs with people; I was just on the Internet. Yet I was spending so much time with it. I just couldn't stop. It was like a drug to me. Next, I began buying "black-and-white" pornography. At that point, Cindy felt so awful that she sought help from a therapist who told her that I was clearly addicted to Internet sex. When she told me this, I told her she was nuts. But soon Cindy's therapist helped her intervene on me and both of us entered treatment. Looking back, it seems so ironic that initially I was responding to Cindy's sexual behavior, but then I ended up ensnared myself by cybersex.

THE CYBERSEX IMPACT

The experiences of these people typify the powerful and adverse consequences to those whose spouse or partner has become compulsively involved in cybersex. The results of a 2000 survey examining the effects of cybersex addiction on the family further describe the serious consequences of cybersex addiction for the partner and children of cybersex addicts.[1] They include feelings of hurt, betrayal, rejection, abandonment, devastation, loneliness, shame, isolation, humiliation, jealousy, and anger, as well as loss of self-esteem. Being lied to repeatedly was a major cause of distress. Cybersex was also a major contributing factor to separation and divorce in couples who took part in the survey.

Among 68 percent of the couples in this study, one or both partners had lost interest in relational sex. Some couples had had no relational sex in months or years.

Partners of cybersex addicts compared themselves unfavorably with the online women (or men) and pornographic pictures, and they felt hopeless about being able to compete with them. These partners overwhelmingly felt that online affairs were as emotionally painful to them as live, or offline, affairs, and many subsequently believed that virtual affairs were just as much adultery, or "cheating," as live affairs.

The impact of cybersex on children was equally distressing. Adverse consequences included:

- exposure to computer-based pornography
- involvement in parental conflicts
- lack of attention because of one parent's involvement with the computer, the other parent's preoccupation with the cybersex addict, and breakups of the marriage or partnership

Negative consequences on marriages and partnerships included:

- depression and other emotional problems
- social isolation
- worsening of sexual relationship with spouse or partner
- harm done to marriage or primary relationship
- exposure of children to online pornography or masturbation
- career loss or decreased job performance
- other financial problems
- legal problems

A companion online study conducted in late 2000 surveyed forty-five men and ten women, age eighteen to sixty-four, who identified themselves as cybersex participants who had experienced adverse consequences from their online sexual activities.[2] When asked about the nature of their online sexual activities, 77 percent of the men mentioned pornography, 46 percent mentioned chat rooms, and 26 percent reported participating in online real-time sexual activities with another person. Among the women, only 10 percent mentioned pornography, while 80 percent reported chatting and 30 percent engaged in online real-time sexual activities. When asked whether their online sexual activities had led to actual sexual encounters, 33 percent of the men said yes, as did 80 percent of the women. In addition, 92 percent of the men and 90 percent of the women stated that they considered themselves sex addicts.

THE DISCOVERY

Discovering that a partner or another family member has engaged in compulsive or problematic use of sex on the Internet can be shocking. A person's first inclination may be to gather all the details he or she can with the hope of somehow understanding how this happened and what to do next; however, the disclosure of secrets should be a process, not a onetime event.

Authors M. Deborah Corley and Jennifer Schneider have written numerous articles and an entire book outlining the healthy ways for disclosure to occur in a family.[3] Although space doesn't permit us to repeat all of their research and suggestions, it is important to keep in mind that there are healthy and unhealthy ways to discover and disclose information within a family—whether it is between partners or with children.

One point made repeatedly is that disclosure should be helpful, not harmful to the receiver. In order to ensure that this is the case, most experts on this issue suggest that disclosure occur in a safe therapeutic environment so it can be somewhat controlled and directed. Each person in the room can receive the support he or she needs, and the process can be stopped or altered if necessary to reduce the harm caused by the disclosure as much as possible.

The most common disclosure occurs between partners or spouses. Each partner or spouse should spend some time preparing individually with his or her therapist before coming together for the actual disclosure session. Following are some questions to consider and discuss with a therapist *before* the disclosure meeting:

- What do you hope to hear during the disclosure process?
- What do you hope to gain?
- What do you think you will feel upon hearing/giving the disclosure?
- How do you think the disclosure will be helpful to you?
- How much detail is enough? How can you maintain this boundary?
- What support do you have in place following the disclosure?
- How will you deal with feelings that may emerge later?
- What do you anticipate saying to your partner after the disclosure?

Keep in mind that even in this controlled setting, disclosure is extremely difficult for everyone. No person responds the same, and people should be given adequate time to both disclose and hear disclosures. It may take several weeks or even months before a full, healthy disclosure can be made.

PARTNERS AND CODEPENDENCY

Partners of people who are compulsively engaging in cybersex find themselves in a very difficult position, and most have no idea how to react to the situation. They respond in a variety of ways, including:

- trying to take responsibility for people, tasks, and situations they're not responsible for.
- trying to "be good enough" to earn the love of their partners and others.

- reacting to their partners' behavior instead of responding to their own motives.
- becoming consumed with their partners to the point of putting their own needs on hold.
- becoming so emotionally tied to their partners that they can't admit their partners' illness.
- losing all sense of themselves, of how they feel and what they need. They become so obsessed with their partners and their problems that they no longer deal with their own lives—their pain, needs, shortcomings, joys, and growth.

THE LOSS OF SELF

In other words, partners often become codependent on their addicted mates. Codependency, or coaddiction, is an illness too, in which reaction to compulsivity and addiction causes the loss of self. Like the addicts, codependent partners lose an essential sense of self. They may put up a front for the world that says everything's fine, but the reality of what is happening proves this to be a lie. The front has little to do with the codependent's true self. It is only an image that shields the reality of what both partners have become. The codependent becomes part of his or her partner's double life.

The preserving of appearances doesn't prevent the erosion of self. Terri, whose husband used the Internet to view pornography and live sex, and eventually to book prostitutes whom he met at home during his lunch hour, was caught in the web of codependency. Upon learning of her husband's activities, Terri obsessed about her husband—about where he was, what he was doing, and whom he was with. She did all the "detective" work, spying on him, checking his computer, and installing Internet-tracking software. She became paranoid about other women, saw them through his eyes, and compared herself with them. She rationalized that he was more liberal and open-minded about sex than she was. She risked disease because of his sexual habits. She felt embarrassed to go out with him because other people knew about his exploits. For a long time, she never questioned whether she loved him, only whether he loved her. "I never thought about being happy, only whether I could keep him with me," she said.

I never thought about my needs, only whether I could meet his. Feeling less and less, because nothing I did was enough. Thinking there was something wrong with me that I could not meet his sexual needs. Hating myself for being "weak." Having no pride. Putting up with abusive treatment. Having no interests outside of the relationship. It was a disaster for me, but for a long time, I didn't know how to escape the cycle we were in together.

All codependents experience such feelings. These attempts at accommodation lead to powerlessness and unmanageability. While codependents are powerless to control their partners' behaviors, they continue to try to do so, and as a result, their own lives become unmanageable and they become coaddicts.

THE SIGNS AND CHARACTERISTICS OF COADDICTION

COLLUSION

Most codependents actively support their partners' compulsive sexual behavior by covering up for them in some way. Powerful childhood rules about family image and secrecy have helped make them unwitting partners in the addictive process. Many codependents keep secrets about their partners. Many lie to cover up for their partners' behavior or actively work to present a united front to the world. Another form of collusion is to become "hypersexual" in an effort to join with the partner. In the example on pages 186–87, Kathleen's husband presented the threesome idea in such a way that she felt something was wrong with her if she didn't participate. So she colluded, joining her husband in activities that gave her no pleasure, because she believed that if she didn't, she might lose the relationship altogether. Partners can also feel pressure to go along because the images presented on the Net are always those of smiling partners cooperating. Codependent partners may also feel that their mate's behavior isn't so bad if he or she is only doing cybersex, as opposed to going to strip clubs or using prostitutes. If the partner has a history of using strip clubs, for example, the codependent may actually see cybersex as a sign of improvement in the partner's compulsive sexual behavior. To summarize, the characteristics of collusion include:

- joining your partner to present a united front
- keeping secrets to protect your partner

- lying to cover up for your partner
- becoming hypersexual for your partner
- feeling cybersex isn't so bad because it's not "real"

OBSESSIVE PREOCCUPATION

Codependents obsess about their partners and their lives. They think constantly about their partners' sexual behavior and motives. Many actually play detective by checking mail, computer history files, Internet bookmarks, credit card and telephone bills, and briefcases. They may also become obsessed with the Internet themselves, working so hard to find out what the partner is up to on the Net that they spend countless hours online too, entering chat rooms or checking out porn sites. This is a trap many partners who install surveillance software fall into. To summarize, the characteristics of obsessive preoccupation include:

- focusing totally on your partner to avoid feelings
- constantly thinking about your partner's behaviors and motives
- checking your partner's mail, purse, briefcase, computer history files, and so on
- forgetfulness
- spending time on the Net investigating sites your partner uses

DENIAL

When not obsessing, codependents lapse into ignoring what is really happening in their lives. Many speak of setting aside their intuitive feelings or totally denying their problem. Many try to stay very busy and overextended to avoid the problem. Despite failures, most codependents believe, at least for a time, that they can eventually change their partners. When cybersex is involved, often codependents tell themselves that it's virtual, not real; that if there's no physical contact, nothing's really happening; that at least the partner is going to work and staying at home at night. Characteristics of denial include:

- denying your own intuition
- keeping overly busy and overextended
- believing you can eventually change your partner
- totally denying the problem
- telling yourself that it's virtual sex, not real sex

EMOTIONAL TURMOIL

Life for codependents is an emotional roller coaster. They go on emotional binges, sometimes to the extent that their emotions are simply out of control and they experience free-floating anxiety and shame. Many say that they are always facing a crisis or problem. Cybersex involvement can also dramatically accelerate the codependent's emotional turmoil because of how quickly and deeply a partner can be overwhelmed by cybersex and by the range of sexual activities available with so little effort. Everything can be done at home. Codependent male partners are often rapidly overwhelmed emotionally because they just don't know how to handle such a situation. A physician, for example, was filled with self-righteous rage when he discovered that his wife had been having Internet-arranged affairs with ten of his colleagues and friends. To him, everything was her problem, not his. He couldn't see his role in the relationship's troubles. Characteristics of emotional turmoil include:

- out-of-control emotions
- going on emotional binges
- experiencing free-floating shame and anxiety
- always having a crisis or problem

MANIPULATION

Codependents become manipulative in their drive to control their partners. They try and fail over and over again to control their partners' sexual acting out. They may use sex to manipulate their partners or to patch up disagreements. Many threaten to leave but never follow through. Almost all codependents see themselves as having played martyr, hero, or victim roles. Before cybersex, spouses and partners tried to keep tabs on their sexually compulsive partner's schedule. With cybersex, codependent partners may actually control computer access. They may become the keeper of the computer's password, or they may install automatic surveillance software to keep tabs on their partners. Manipulation enters even more areas of life. Since there are additional opportunities for acting out, there's more behavior to try to control over more parts of the day (and night). Characteristics of manipulation include:

- playing martyr, hero, or victim roles
- using sex to manipulate or patch up disagreements
- failing at efforts to control your partner's sexual acting out

- making threats to leave but never following through
- taking control of the computer via a password in an effort to control your partner's behavior
- installing automatic surveillance software to keep tabs on your partner

EXCESSIVE RESPONSIBILITY

In their obsession, codependents can be extremely hard on themselves. They blame themselves for the problem. They believe that if *they* change in some way, their partners will stop. Codependents now find themselves having to contend with and compare themselves with all the beautiful people on the Net—and with endless sexual variations and opportunities available on the Net. They may also try to take responsibility for their partners' behavior. Many actually seek extra responsibility by trying to create dependency situations where they will be indispensable. Characteristics of excessive responsibility include:

- blaming yourself
- believing that if you changed, your partner would stop
- taking responsibility for your partner's behavior
- creating dependency situations to make yourself indispensable

COMPROMISE OR LOSS OF SELF

Codependency involves a constant series of compromises that erode one's sense of self. Codependents can act against their own morals, values, and beliefs. They give up life goals, hobbies, and interests. Many change their dress or appearance to accommodate their partners and even accept their partners' sexual norms as their own. When Kathleen began participating in threesomes, she compromised her own values and betrayed herself, since she did not want to take part in these activities. Characteristics of compromise or loss of self include:

- giving up life goals, hobbies, and interests
- acting against your own morals, values, and beliefs
- changing dress or appearance to accommodate your partner
- accepting your partner's sexual norms as your own

BLAME AND PUNISHMENT

Codependents become blaming and punishing in their obsession. They perceive themselves as having become progressively more self-righteous and punitive. Some have affairs to punish their partners and to prove that they are worthwhile and attractive. For example, a woman who has discovered her husband's online affairs may become involved in one herself just to spite and punish him. Other women post nude pictures of themselves after ending a marriage, sending a message to their former husbands that says, "See what you're missing. See how desirable I am!" as an act of revenge. Many see their behavior as destructive to others. Some even admit to homicidal thoughts or feelings. Meredith discovered her husband's online affairs. To strike back at him, she initiated an online affair with him while posing as someone else. At home, she pretended that nothing was happening. She had become so obsessed with his betrayal that she actually became part of that betrayal.

Both partners may also binge on sex outside of the marriage or partnership while staying compulsively nonsexual with each other, as was the case with Stan and Cheryl.

"I had been having sex with people in an adult video bookstore, among other things," said Stan.

> Cheryl was absolutely infuriated with me because of what I'd been doing and that I'd had unprotected sex. She was worried that both of us may have been exposed to AIDS. Cheryl, I later realized, felt very lonely and ignored, since we'd rarely had sex for some time. Eventually, Cheryl started going into chat rooms, where she arranged meetings with men and had unprotected sex with them. I guess she was trying to punish me. So here we were, having lots of sex with others and none with each other.

Characteristics of blame and punishment include:

- becoming increasingly more self-righteous and punitive
- being destructive to others
- having homicidal thoughts or feelings
- having affairs (online or offline) to punish the partner or prove worth
- withholding all sex from partner as punishment

SEXUAL REACTIVITY

Codependents go to various extremes in reacting sexually to their partners' behavior. When one partner gets out of control sexually, it's not unusual for the other partner to close down sexually. Many numb their own sexual needs and wants. Codependents may change their clothes out of sight of their partners. They may make excuses not to be sexual. And many rarely feel intimate during sex. Characteristics of sexual reactivity include:

- numbing your own sexual needs and wants
- rarely feeling intimate during sex
- making excuses not to be sexual
- changing clothes out of sight of your partner

CYBERSEX CODEPENDENCY INVENTORY

How do you know if you have become part of your partner's compulsive or addictive behaviors? The following inventory can help you determine that. If you agree with eighteen or more of the thirty-five items in the following exercise, you may have a problem with codependency and need to address your own issues with a professional counselor. While you may or may not be codependent, a score of eighteen or more indicates that you might be at risk for codependency problems.

1. I constantly think or obsess about my partner's cybersex behaviors and motives. Yes   No
2. I engage in self-destructive behaviors (physically, sexually, or emotionally). Yes   No
3. I check my partner's e-mail accounts, computer files, and the like for evidence of sexual material. Yes   No
4. I blame myself for all the problems related to my partner's sexual use of the Internet. Yes   No
5. I believe that if I changed, my partner would stop acting out sexually on the Internet. Yes   No
6. I feel shame as a result of my behavior or my partner's behavior related to cybersex. Yes   No
7. I feel anxiety as a result of my behavior or my partner's behavior related to cybersex. Yes   No

8. I use my own sexuality as a way to manipulate my partner.
Yes   No

9. I feel numb to my own sexual needs and wants. Yes   No

10. I accept my partner's norms as my own. Yes   No

11. I find myself doing sexual things I don't want to do. Yes   No

12. I am overly sexual to satisfy my partner. Yes   No

13. I take responsibility for my partner's cybersex behaviors and their consequences. Yes   No

14. I keep secrets to protect my partner. Yes   No

15. I rarely feel intimate during sexual encounters with my partner.
Yes   No

16. I lie to cover up for my partner. Yes   No

17. I totally deny that there are any problems with cybersex. Yes   No

18. I always seem to be in the midst of a crisis or problem. Yes   No

19. I threaten to leave my partner, but never follow through. Yes   No

20. I am giving up my own life goals, hobbies, and interests as a result of my partner's cybersex. Yes   No

21. I have changed my dress or appearance to accommodate my partner's wishes. Yes   No

22. I believe I can eventually change my partner. Yes   No

23. I play martyr, hero, or victim roles. Yes   No

24. My life seems increasingly unmanageable. Yes   No

25. I go against my own morals, values, and beliefs. Yes   No

26. I deny my intuitions. Yes   No

27. I am feeling more and more unworthy as a person. Yes   No

28. I shut down sexually from my partner as a result of his or her use of cybersex. Yes   No

29. I am obsessed with learning more about cybersex through the media, the Internet, and so on. Yes   No

30. I am considering engaging in cybersex as a way to make my partner understand my feelings. Yes   No

31. I have fantasies about getting revenge on my partner and his or her online "friends." Yes   No

32. I am in competition with the computer for my partner's time and attention. Yes   No

33. I am irritable with others when I think about my partner's cybersex use. Yes   No

34. I neglect important areas of my life because of my partner's cybersex use. Yes   No
35. I am a cybersex codependent. Yes   No

THE EFFECT OF CYBERSEX ON FAMILY LIFE

When a parent is caught in the web of cybersex, one of the primary effects on the rest of the family is the loss of time with that person. In the beginning stages of the cybersex compulsion, codependents often begin to feel that their partners are slowly drifting away and becoming more distant, but they don't know why.

LOST FAMILY TIME

There are only so many hours in each day, and hours spent on cybersex are hours that cannot be spent with your partner or children. In some ways, cybersex is more time-devouring than other forms of compulsive sexual behavior, such as going to strip clubs or using prostitutes. The Internet gives you access to your sexual activities at any time of the day or night for as long as you want—and from your own home. Many couples use the time after children are in bed to reconnect and talk about their day. But when a partner is using cybersex, this opportunity often disappears. Cybersex addiction is easy to hide, so the partner may not have any clue about what's happening but does know that something isn't right. Communication decreases. The sexually compulsive partner becomes more and more unavailable. This can be confusing for children too, because the sexually compulsive parent may be home but not available to the children, who can't understand why Mom or Dad can't spend time with them.

Al's story is a poignant example of this situation:

One night I finally realized what I'd been doing to my kids. I was in my home office on the computer when my two children came in and wanted to play. I screamed at them to shut up and go find something else to do and to leave me alone. When I turned back to the screen, it finally hit me. I was screaming at my own children to leave me for cybersex. I finally saw the impact of my addiction and how it was affecting my relationship with them. I wasn't asking them to leave me alone so I could work or to prepare for a meeting or a community activity. No, I was saying, in effect, "Leave me alone because I'm having sex on the Internet."

Arlene, too, was seduced by cybersex to the detriment of her children.

I was married to a wealthy man. We had four children and a live-in nanny. When my husband died, I became very morose. I didn't know what to do, so I just began living in my bedroom. We'd had a computer and Internet access, though I'd never used it much. But one day, I went online. Somehow I discovered a very curious and interesting chat room. All the participants were philosophical and intellectual. They were always talking about philosophers like Nietzsche, Heidegger, and Sartre. There was also a kind of hierarchy among the forty or so participants. The top guys called themselves silverbacks. It was like a group of philosophizing primates. There was also verbal sparring going on continuously while they were talking. What's more, the whole scene was underlaid with very sexual talk. Very quickly I got hooked. I was pretty depressed at the time, feeling very alone, and it just drew me in. It was intellectually and erotically very stimulating. It was like an online, real-life soap opera. I spent hours and hours there, day after day, hunkered down in my room. I wouldn't get up until 10:00 or 11:00 A.M. I'd get something to eat and then go online and stay online until two or three in the morning. What about the kids? The nanny assumed complete care for them. For a long time, I totally ignored them. I might as well have been dead too, for all the care, love, or time they got from me.

CHILDREN EXPOSED TO CYBERSEX

Aside from the loss of time with their parents, children living in homes where a parent is participating in cybersex are much more likely to be exposed to sexual images or activities. The problem here is the ease of access children have to sexual information and activities. What's more, such exposures can happen inadvertently because of the way the Internet works. For example, a client told of her ten-year-old doing an astronomy research project on black holes. She typed in the term "black hole" and was greeted by a Web site dedicated to the genitalia of women and a screen full of women's vulvas. Another client spoke of how his son wanted to learn more about the president of our country and the White House. He made a mistake when typing "www.whitehouse.gov" into the search engine and ended up in a porn site. Even accidental discovery gives kids access.

If a parent is using the Net for sex, however, the possibility for access and exposure to sexual sites increases. Even a child with limited computer knowledge can stumble into, or deliberately access, the parent's history files and visit any of those sites, not to mention any bookmarks that have been set up. Furthermore, if a parent is regularly using the Internet for sex, at some point a child *will* happen upon him or her in the middle of sexual activity.

Having a sexually compulsive or out-of-control person living in the house also creates a sexualized energy that permeates the entire home. Children may not understand what is happening, but they do sense this sexualized atmosphere, and when they get older, they recognize in retrospect what had really been happening, even though they were never directly exposed to it.

As the age of children who access the Internet continues to decrease, we are also noticing an increase in problematic online sexual behavior for children themselves. The average age of first exposure to pornography is eleven years old. Given that children are being exposed to sex online at earlier ages, we can expect that compulsive online sexual behaviors may also begin earlier. We mention this so that parents and caregivers can pay attention to children's online Internet use and, we hope, prevent some cases of lifelong compulsivity due to Internet sexuality.

Focus on Yourself as a Partner

Recovery from cybersex compulsion or addiction includes three separate, yet interrelated, components: your partner's recovery, your recovery, and your relationship's recovery. We can't emphasize strongly enough that you must let your partner take responsibility for his or her own recovery.

A word of caution: If life with your partner has become truly out of control and he or she is not willing to get help, you may need to consider having an intervention. For recommendations on additional resources for help, please refer to the appendix.

Most codependents beginning recovery feel as if they are running inches ahead of an avalanche of hopelessness and despair. The possibility of a peaceful life and a nurturing relationship seems terribly remote. One codependent told us, "I simply couldn't envision it at the start." Most cannot.

The burning question for codependents as they face their relationship with a sexually compulsive partner is "Should I leave the relationship?" Although for some that question will have to be confronted in the course of recovery, it is usually best not to do so at this point. In the first place, it's not in your best interest. You need to work through your codependency issues in order to recover yourself, and that often happens best with your partner's support. The question at this point is not "Should I divorce my partner?" Rather it is "How do I start my recovery?"

As a codependent, you have a right to receive help. A good analogy is to think of marriage as a "reincarnation" event. The things you do not work out in your current relationship will simply have to be dealt with in the next. Consider this a kind of marital karma. Without help, the probability of ending up in another dysfunctional relationship is almost certain. You must stop running and face the avalanche. Many people will be there to help you.

Recovery requires that you take certain steps. It's not your job to monitor your partner's sexual behavior. It's not your job to keep your partner "sober." It's not your job to ensure your partner's sexual satisfaction. You simply can't guarantee your partner's recovery, and the more you try to help, the more you'll get in the way. Finally, you must take responsibility for your own recovery.

STEPS FOR CODEPENDENCY RECOVERY

Your most immediate task concerns detachment. You need to refocus your life and recovery on yourself—the person who has been lost in the codependency. The following four guidelines will help you to do so.

1. LEARN TO LOVE WITHOUT INTERFERING WITH CONSEQUENCES
By this we mean caring for another person without intervening in his or her life. Disaster at work, financial chaos, arrests—whatever happens because of your partner's addictive behavior is your partner's problem and responsibility, not yours. As part of recovery, sexually compulsive or addicted partners must feel the full brunt of their powerlessness. Any effort to protect your partner diverts energy from your recovery. Extend support, but not help.

2. Acknowledge Your Own Powerlessness over Obsession

In a Twelve Step support group or therapy—or both—you need to acknowledge that you don't have control over your partner's behaviors. You must survey all the ways you obsess about or attempt to control your partner. This includes all the ways you try to influence your partner's recovery. You must reach a point of surrender, which means committing to stop.

3. Acknowledge the Consequences of Codependent Behavior

Part of surrender is to fully comprehend the costs of your codependent behavior. Accepting powerlessness is admitting what did not work. Acknowledging chaotic unmanageability due to consequences is admitting what did happen. Recognizing the costs deepens the commitment to stop.

4. Define a Codependent's Sobriety

Becoming more clear about personal codependent patterns will tell you which of your behaviors are self-destructive and need to be stopped. Sexually compulsive partners aren't the only ones who need to achieve "sobriety." You must also abstain from your obsessional and dysfunctional behaviors. And you must be clear about what constitutes a slip for you.

DETACHMENT AND ITS ROLE IN RECOVERY

As detachment proceeds, you will discover much. You will learn how you can better handle anxiety. You'll see the ways you tried to control your partner's behaviors. You'll work on being able to say what's acceptable and what's not in a way that's not angry or accusatory. You may have felt responsible for your partner's sexuality. Now you'll see that there's no way you can do that.

Recovery requires that you change your expectations of yourself. You'll learn that you're not the one who needs to supply your partner's boundaries, monitor choices, or set priorities. It's not unusual for a codependent to have entered a relationship with someone who has a lot of problems. Typically when that happens, the partner's needs absorb all the codependent's time and energy, preventing the person from looking at his or her own problems.

Working on your recovery is extremely important. An invaluable part of this process is to seek help from a good therapist. Unfortunately, many codependents are reluctant to enter therapy because they feel that they are not the ones with the problem. That's correct, but only to a point. No, you don't have your partner's problem, per se, but you do have problems of your own, and they are related to the behavior of your partner. Therapy will help you look at the role you've played in your partner's addictive behavior; doing so can dramatically improve your recovery.

Our research shows that the first six months of recovery will include times of intense emotional turmoil and pain.[4] It is at this point that you may experience health problems. In the next six months, you will likely see significant change and gain. Career, finances, and self-image improve dramatically and continue to improve in the coming years. Significant improvement in communication with your partner and in the overall quality of the relationship is common. And in the second and third years, codependents find themselves much more able to cope with stress and to develop spirituality and friendships. In addition, codependents can expect progress in sexual health and overall life satisfaction.

Our findings also indicate that the stages of progress you and your partner experience will often be mismatched. As a result, you may become impatient with your partner, even though he or she is proceeding at a rate similar to other recovering addicts. You may also prematurely conclude that the relationship cannot be saved. To prevent premature or bad choices, we urge you to commit to your own recovery.

WHAT YOU CAN EXPECT DURING YOUR RECOVERY PROCESS

- Things will get worse before they get better.
- You will need to monitor your expectations.
- There is no magical solution.
- There will be relapses.
- A year of hard work will be needed before you'll feel that recovery has begun to take hold.
- Recovery will be on track when you and your partner are working independently in therapy.
- For your recovery to progress, you will need to
  —develop a plan so you know what to do when a relapse occurs

—make decisions with the support of others (a support group, your therapist, or a Twelve Step group)

—avoid, if possible, making major decisions (divorce, moving, or changing jobs, for example) during the first year

—fulfill the tasks asked of you by your therapist

—focus during the first year on your individual recovery, not on the recovery of your relationship

—do couples work while your independent therapy progresses

—seek help from Recovering Couples Anonymous (RCA) when you decide to work on your relationship.

Recovering Couples Anonymous stresses the idea that recovery is a three-pronged process that includes your recovery, your partner's recovery, and your recovery as a couple.[5] Your recovery as a couple cannot take place without the individual recovery of each partner. Conversely, while it is possible for two partners to achieve a solid recovery independent of one another, that alone will not guarantee the creation of a healthy relationship. You must learn how to integrate your recovery together with your partner's. Three ideas lie at the root of this issue:

- People who haven't completed certain developmental tasks look to their partners to solve them.
- Two shame-filled people make a shame-based couple for whom there is no possibility of a healthy relationship.
- The harsh reality is that making individual changes is not enough to give you the skills needed to create a fulfilling relationship.

UNDERSTANDING FAMILY DYNAMICS

Each partner in the relationship brings along his or her unique family history. We don't seek to judge or blame our families for the difficulties we're having in our current relationships. Instead, we seek to understand our family roots and dynamics. Then we can gain a better understanding of the family models each of us brings to the relationship. In addition, we can better understand the dynamics involved as we try to combine our own family histories into a new family. This is called the "blending of the epics." Each of us is on a life journey. When we join with another person to create a couple, these individual journeys take on even greater importance. Two people are now trying to merge their individual journeys. They are at different stages in their journeys, each coming from a different background.

Those individual journeys make up each partner's family epic, adding to the complexity and difficulty of this merger. Every family is really a great, transgenerational story—of all the many people involved, their personal struggles, and their ways of interacting, expressing emotion, loving, arguing, and communicating.

Our families help determine the kind of person we look for in a partner. We look for a partner who can help us resolve the problems we experienced when we were growing up. If we become more aware of our family histories, we can become more aware of the reasons we are attracted to particular types of people.

TELLING YOUR STORY

In our culture today, many people have lost or forgotten parts of their stories. Recovery groups such as Alcoholics Anonymous, Overeaters Anonymous, and others encourage people to discover and tell their stories. Partners need to go through this same process together as a couple. They need to tell their stories to each other to begin forming a joint story. When partners share this process, a new truth begins to emerge that is critical to the relationship's success.

First we must discover what happened to us in our families, the ways we learned to deal with feelings, conflict, and anger. Next we need to share that knowledge with each other. Then we can understand why we react to one another and others the way we do. Until we can do this, real communication and intimacy are not possible.

If two people are at varied points in their journeys, they can be mismatched. As mentioned, individuals who haven't completed certain developmental tasks look to their partners to solve them. When people try to solve these developmental issues through their partners, they are doomed not only to fail but also to create further problems.

COUPLESHAME

Living in the midst of the destructive cycle created with intimacy problems, partners find that they aren't honest with each other, they don't communicate, and they either withdraw or fight. Any problem with money, the children, or their social life only serves as further evidence that they and their relationship are a terrible failure.

Because these couples haven't had a source of support, they are operating with family-of-origin problems, and they struggle with intimacy and codependency—all of which lead to feelings of "coupleshame": shame as a couple.

Coupleshame closely parallels individual feelings of shame. Coupleshame appears when two people with core feelings of shame join in a relationship. As in mathematics, adding two negatives together makes an even greater negative. Two shame-filled people make a shame-based couple for whom there is no possibility of a healthy relationship. Sam and Paula's story illustrates this situation clearly.

Sam and Paula had been going to Alcoholics Anonymous meetings for years. Both divorced from extremely dysfunctional marriages right after they began their recovery from alcohol addiction. They had avoided relationships for years, basically because they were afraid.

Sam and Paula met at their AA meetings and began dating. Soon they had fallen in love with each other and decided to marry. Then they discovered that many of the same issues that had been part of their first relationships were surfacing again in this marriage.

Miserable in the marriage, they began to feel as if the marriage had been a mistake and they'd chosen the wrong partner. Both were also saddened and disillusioned because they couldn't understand how, after all the work they'd done individually in their years of recovery and fellowship meetings, they could so quickly fall right back into the negative and destructive patterns of their first marriages.

Sam and Paula's story exposes the reality that merely making individual changes is not enough to give you the skills needed to create a fulfilling relationship. These skills can be developed only in a relationship. When faced with a situation similar to Sam and Paula's, many couples reach the conclusion that they shouldn't be together and that they deserve to divorce.

It is important to know that you will not solve coupleshame through separation. Nor will relationship difficulties and problems be solved by working separately outside of a relationship. If you do not work on your relationship issues in this relationship, you are doomed to repeat them in the next . . . and the next and the next. Although they parallel individual skills, couple recovery skills develop only in a relationship.

If and when you and your partner reach a point at which it seems right to begin working on the recovery of your relationship, Recovering Couples Anonymous can be an enormous help. RCA uses the following questions to help couples better understand themselves and their relationship to each other. If you believe that exploring such issues could help your relationship, we encourage you to contact your local RCA group (see appendix for more information). They will be happy to help.

QUESTIONS TO ASK FOR BETTER MUTUAL UNDERSTANDING

GIVING AND PARENTING
- In what ways have we given so much outside the relationship that it was harmful to ourselves or others—for example, spending so much time on community activities, work, or our children that we had nothing left to give each other?
- In what ways has our giving to others been meaningful and satisfying, while maintaining a balance in our time and energy?

ISOLATION/COMMUNITY
- In what ways have we become isolated from other couples and friends, cutting ourselves off from their support and community?
- In what ways have we sought community for our relationship by seeking out other couples and friends?

CRISIS
- In what ways have we handled crises poorly—in our family, relationship, and friendships?
- In what ways have we created a crisis by blowing a situation out of proportion?
- In what ways have we dealt with crises well?

CONFLICT

- How have we dealt with conflict? Have we repeated fights over the same issue? Have we deliberately created conflict over relatively superficial issues to avoid a deeper issue?
- How have we dealt with conflicts so that they were resolved and both of us were generally satisfied with the process and the result?

STRESS

- In what ways have we allowed ourselves to become so mutually depleted of spiritual, physical, and emotional energy that we have nothing left to give anyone?
- What steps have we taken to manage stress so that we could maintain balance in our lives and ensure a continuous reservoir of energy with which to nurture both ourselves and others?

DENIAL/ACCEPTANCE

- What are the issues in our relationship that we pretend don't exist and have avoided dealing with?
- What are the issues we have acknowledged, faced, and talked about?

Though it may seem impossible right now, thousands of couples have reinvigorated and enriched damaged and foundering relationships. Don't give up hope. Seek help from others—they are waiting for your call. Healthy and fulfilling intimacy is possible. For additional reading and resources, please turn to the appendix.

II

The Web Frontier

THROUGH THE INTERNET, cybersex has begun affecting our society in subtle and profound ways. It is changing relationships and forcing us to examine and reevaluate our ideas about sexuality. More significant, the impact of cybersex has only begun, and its influence will grow for years to come. What its ultimate impact will be, we can only guess. Clues, however, can be found in the experiences of the people who are struggling with problematic and compulsive cybersex behaviors. We have learned from them that while cybersex has positive aspects, its effects can be overwhelming and damaging, both to the people who engage in it and to their partners, friends, family members, and colleagues. People struggling with and recovering from this problem will encourage us, and perhaps force us, as individuals and as societies, to be more open and honest about our sexuality and to more closely examine our relationships and the role our sexuality plays in our lives. Their experiences and their recovery will also create a path for others with similar struggles to follow—one that also offers the hope that healing is possible.

People recovering from problematic and compulsive cybersex behaviors are basically trying to define what healthy sexuality means for them. With the easy access to sexual information and activities that the Internet provides, each of us will also need to determine how we will use this technology as well as how much and in what ways we will allow it to affect our sexuality and our relationships.

This process of pursuing and taking on greater personal responsibility can be seen on a much broader scale as we look out across our planet to see the amazing drive for self-determination and self-government among so many cultures and nations. More and more cultures are reaching a point at which they can no longer tolerate domination by authoritarian leaders. In their landmark book *The Paradigm Conspiracy,* authors Denise Breton and Christopher Largent describe this worldwide shift in power from autocratic and authoritarian models to new modes that incorporate shared power, interaction, and interdependence.[1]

The science of ecology is also revealing just how intricately all parts of our planet and its ecosystems are intertwined. Ecologists are showing us that we must be responsible for our actions and that there are limits to what we as a species can do without destroying all that we depend on for our survival.

And what if one's actions are irresponsible? We have long had laws governing our behavior, as well as penalties for misbehavior. What went on within the family, including spousal and child abuse, however, was long considered outside of society's purview. This is no longer true, as we have now begun to take a stand regarding domestic abuse. Such steps are also being taken with countries at the international level. The multicountry intervention in the Yugoslav state of Kosovo in 1999, in response to the mass killing and deportation of Kosovars by the Serbian government, was an example of nations intervening within another sovereign state not primarily out of self-interest, but to come to the aid of a persecuted and vulnerable group of people.

As individuals, members of cultures, and citizens of countries, humans struggle with issues of appropriate limits, self-determination, and interdependence. Not as individuals, citizens, nor as a species can we do whatever we like. We are all interdependent, and all of us must live within limits.

THE HUMAN CONNECTION

If you are using sex compulsively, you know that it can be very isolating. Sex can become your most important need, to the exclusion of the rest of your life. This flies in the face, however, of our human need for connection. Humans live and actually thrive in community.

Heart researcher and internist Dean Ornish, for example, developed a regimen that can not only halt hardening of the coronary arteries but also actually reverse it without surgery. This regimen includes meditation, a low-fat vegetarian diet, yoga, and support-group participation. Subsequent research by Ornish revealed that the key factor in the success of his program was support-group participation.[2] Mounting evidence suggests that people without close, durable ties to family and friends are at high risk for everything from cancer and heart disease to ulcers and infections. "Love and intimacy are at the root of what makes us sick and what makes us well," says Ornish. "I am not aware of any other factor in medicine—not diet, smoking, or exercise—that has a greater impact."

Similar studies of men and women throughout the world have revealed a similar pattern. Women who say they feel isolated go on to develop and die of breast and ovarian cancer at several times the expected rate. College students who report "strained and cold" relationships with their parents suffer extraordinary rates of hypertension and heart disease decades later. Heart attack survivors who happen to live by themselves die at twice the rate of those who live with others.

What's going on here? How can something as mushy as "social support" affect the growth of a tumor or the function of a coronary artery? For starters, such support helps regulate our behavior. People with commitments to honor are less likely to abuse themselves. They drink less, eat better, and avoid needless risks. Companionship also lets us share feelings that would otherwise fester and modulate our body's response to stress. Again, people, societies, and nations cannot survive, let alone thrive, in isolation.

Seventy percent of all cybersex traffic occurs Monday through Friday between 9:00 A.M. and 5:00 P.M. Millions of Americans are engaging in cybersex activities every day, and much of that activity is happening in the workplace. It might be a key executive or a technology guru or an invaluable scientist who couldn't possibly be fired but whose cybersex compulsion is simply out of control. Or it could be an employee or a colleague who clearly needs help. Business bottom lines are being dramatically affected by losses in time and productivity due to cybersex. As more employers are forced to confront the reality of compulsive or addictive cybersex, more people will begin to understand and accept the reality of sex addiction. Employers will search for ways to help these people. The power of cybersex addiction will put to rest the doubts of skeptics that sex addiction isn't just weird and perverted anomalous behavior taken up by a few mentally ill people. It is a disease with clear roots, an illness that can strike close to home.

Cybersex addiction is already being recognized in popular culture. In his book *The Bear and the Dragon,* one of author Tom Clancy's characters speaks of this problem: "He had considered prowling some Internet pornography sites. For one reason or another the Asian culture made for an ample collection of such things. He wasn't exactly proud of this addiction, but his sexual drive needed some outlet."[3] Here is a best-selling author whose books are read by millions of people throughout the world acknowledging the power and addictive nature of cybersex and the struggle people have trying to control their addiction.

THE POWER OF THE SEX DRIVE

For much, if not all, of human history, societies have placed strict controls on sexual activity. These controls were easily enforceable, since people lived in tight-knit communities where violation of sexual mores could mean ostracism, a terrible and sometimes even fatal consequence.

Today, however, even before the advent of the Internet and cybersex, attitudes toward sexual activity have become much more relaxed. At this point, we must not underestimate the power of sex to influence behavior. A noted laboratory experiment with rats shows this immense power. First, rats were habituated to heroin. Next, an electrode was placed in their brains that, when activated, stimulated the sexual pleasure centers of the animals. The rats were then given two choices: touch a button that would give them heroin or one that would sexually stimulate them. They consistently chose sexual stimulation over heroin, one of the most addictive drugs known, with extremely uncomfortable withdrawal symptoms. In another experiment, rats were deprived of food for a week. They were then put into a cage with their mates and food. Every rat chose to mate rather than eat the food.

Sex is an enormously powerful drive. In a sense, cybersex is enabling people to "mainline" sex whenever they want it. The many vignettes we've related in this book have shown people choosing to put sex above all other life activities. They ignored their families, work, partners, friends, food, and sleep for lengthy periods of time. Sex became their most important need.

They became lonely, hungry, and tired. They knew they needed other people in their lives, yet they found that they couldn't stop their cybersex activities.

TECHNOLOGICALLY ENHANCED SEX:
CYBERSEX IS ONLY THE BEGINNING

We fear, too, that cybersex is only the beginning of what is coming in the way of increased and enhanced sexual activities and opportunities. For many years now, people have used drugs like cocaine, marijuana, and "poppers" to enhance sexual experiences. Ecstasy, known as the "love drug," is now commonly used by high school and college students for this same purpose. Given the incredible advances in molecular biology, it is not at all difficult to imagine a new designer drug that will incredibly alter and expand the sexual experience—one that will be extremely addictive too.

WHY A WAR ON CYBERSEX WON'T WORK

Science fiction writers have for years written of fantastically enhanced sexual experiences and their addictive qualities. Frank Herbert, in his remarkable classic science fiction Dune series, wrote of an order of women who had perfected the art of enhancing the male sexual and orgasmic experience.[4] The feelings and sensations they could elicit in men were so profound as to be instantly addictive—and enslaving. Men would do *anything* for the promise of another experience. In Aldous Huxley's classic *Brave New World,* a group of characters spends an evening at the "feelies," a movie theater in which, by holding special handles on their seats, viewers could feel all the physical sensations the actors felt as they made love on screen.[5] And finally, there's the holodeck in *Star Trek: The Next Generation,* a virtual-reality room that the user can program to produce any kind of experience he or she wants. While the use of the holodeck for sex was only implied in the series, it's not hard to imagine the potential of such a device. Any kind of sexual experience you could ever imagine with real people could be accomplished with no fear of disease or need for a relationship.

In all probability, inventions like these will be developed in the future because there is so much money to be made. Today's video streaming and Webcam technology were developed predominately by the pornography industry because it recognized the enormous potential for profit. That profit potential is always there, waiting for the next innovation. This is why we believe we are seeing only the leading edge of the cybersex and sex addiction problem. It is imperative for society to acknowledge this situation. It would be fruitless, though certainly tempting, to simply stick our collective head in the sand and pretend that nothing like this will happen or to roll our eyes and write off the issue as a fringe problem among a few "perverts."

A more likely and extremely tempting step in dealing with cybersex would be for the state or federal government to set controls on Internet sex. Logically, this would never work. No matter how clever a blocking software might become, people would be able to bypass it. Previous failed attempts at governing people's behaviors include Prohibition and the "war on drugs." Though begun with the best of intentions, Prohibition failed miserably in its goal to stop alcohol use in the United States. In addition, it spawned a sophisticated and powerful network of organized crime that plagues our society to this day.

Our more recent war on drugs has turned out to be equally futile. The United States imprisons a higher percentage of its citizens than any other country in the world except South Africa, and the vast majority are nonviolent substance abusers who can be rehabilitated. Most crimes in this country are either the direct or indirect result of the criminal's drug or alcohol abuse. Current correctional trends toward longer sentences, fewer prison programs, and limited access to drug and alcohol treatment have only served to guarantee a continuation of the massive recidivism rates we currently experience. Billions of dollars have been spent to stop the flow of illicit drugs into the United States (including $1.2 billion given to Colombia in 2000 for drug interdiction) and to stop domestic production. Yet demand and use is higher than ever for many drugs.

Other countries—Switzerland and the Netherlands, for example—have taken a much different approach to the drug problem by decriminalizing its use. In addition, they provide extensive counseling and medical and treatment services at little or no cost to those who have problems with drugs to help them recover from their addictions and live more meaningful and productive lives. These countries have extremely low rates of drug abuse.

What's more, criminal activity associated with drug trafficking and use in these countries is nearly nonexistent.

So often when our society determines that some behavior is wrong or a problem, we enact a law in an attempt to control that behavior. In some cases, this is the wrong approach. Clearly, some people are having problems with the easy access to sex provided by the Internet and are exhibiting behavior that is regarded as wrong, even criminal, in the offline world. Arranging for prostitutes, for example, generally goes unmonitored and uncontrolled on the Net. What's more, minors have easy access to sexual sites and information too. We have already seen attempts to use the legal system, with the threat of incarceration, to regulate behavior or content on the Internet. It will be very hard, if not impossible, however, to enforce such laws. We will not be able to control cybersex, and a war on cybersex that parallels the war on drugs would be similarly ineffective.

Trying to control the Internet by legal means is really an attempt to solve the problem with first-order changes. Just as that is merely a temporary fix on the personal level, it will not work at the societal level either. The Internet is not inherently good or bad. It enables us to stay in touch with one another from nearly anywhere on Earth. It can be used to help people create new and rewarding relationships. It's not the enemy. As a society, we have to view this cybersex problem in terms of second-order changes. We need to ask ourselves what our goals are. What kind of behaviors do we want vis-à-vis the Internet and cybersex? What will make us better human beings? What will contribute to the growth of healthy sexuality and loving relationships?

At issue is how we will learn to control our own sexual behavior given the reality of this new technology and how we will teach others to do the same. Once again, we return to the theme of self-determination. We must look within as a culture to decide what behaviors will be best for society.

When a new technology emerges, its impact on society often forces us to change how we interact with one another. The Internet is doing just that. The impact of instant access to so much information on sex and the opportunities for cybersex are exacerbating the tremendous changes in our gender-related and sexual mores that have been under way for most of the past century. Fifty years ago, for example, only a small percentage of women worked outside the home and the majority of those who did were concentrated in just a few professions, such as teaching, nursing, and secretarial work. Today, men and women work alongside one another in virtually all workplaces and professions. As this change occurred, new rules for interaction between men and women in the workplace had to develop. "Sexual harassment" is not only a relatively new expression, it's a new concept too—one that grew out of the need to more clearly define the behavior of men and women in the workplace.

DISCUSSING SEX OPENLY

The Internet is enabling us to relate to one another in new ways. But as yet we don't really have any rules about how to use this technology. As a society, we are only beginning to develop these rules. What should they be? Who should develop them? And how? Who will have input? And what should the rules be about sexuality? As a society, we tend not to talk about sex openly. Studies continue to show that few American parents talk with their children about sex. We push the topic under the table. The Internet and access to cybersex force us to bring sexuality out in the open in a way we have never done before. The Internet has amplified this process enormously. The media, which use sexual images to sell just about everything, have been pushing this issue for some years, but now we are at a point where we simply must be out in the open with it. As a culture—and as a species—we will have to decide how we are going to deal with this new technology and its relationship to our sexuality.

This is an inevitable struggle that will bring the human race to a higher level. It is a struggle that is affecting societies across the globe because the Internet knows no borders. In many countries in which the population is predominantly Muslim, for example, women are struggling to have the rights that they now know many other women have. Television and the Internet have played a powerful role in exposing them to information about how other women in the world live. Throughout the world, the media are forcing us to look at how we relate to one another during this time of extraordinary change.

The problem we face is not cybersex, per se. It is learning new ways to relate to one another and to our sexuality. There is much to be sorted out, and this process will take some time. In another hundred years, historians will likely look back and see that the technology of the Internet created a cultural earthquake and that part of that change was directly related to a vastly more open discussion about sexuality and the relationships between men and women.

THE INTERNET: CREATING A NEW TYPE OF RELATIONSHIP

The Internet created the possibility for a new type of relationship, one for which we had no guidelines. For example, is a cyber-affair really an affair if the two people were never in physical contact with one another? These technology-based relationships are uninhibited and interactive. The technology has developed so quickly that we're unable to keep up with the many different ways that people can use—and abuse—the Internet. We simply lack the cultural anchors needed to deal with this technology.

Without cultural anchors, what do we do? On the one hand, it's easy to think that since there are relatively few rules or laws about the Internet and cybersex, anything goes. Besides, existing laws, such as those against soliciting sex on the Net and exchanging child pornography, are difficult to enforce. Because there are few cultural norms in this area doesn't mean that doing whatever one pleases is a good idea. This book has been devoted to helping people see the devastating results of cybersex addiction in people's lives. Just because there are few societal norms for cybersex doesn't mean there won't be individual consequences for such behavior. We have to do as a society what you are doing as an individual. Without cultural anchors, you have no choice but to turn to your own value system and make some inferences about what is appropriate behavior. You're trying to determine how to live with this new technology without destroying all that is dear to you. You're creating new first- and second-order changes and developing appropriate boundaries in your life. You're learning to live in your Recovery Zone. You as an individual—and we as a society—will make some mistakes along the way. We'll have some slips, but the glimpse of a better life will help us persevere.

We have become a culture that believes not only that "we can have it all," but also that we deserve it. We are constantly inundated by social and media messages telling us that we are entitled to whatever we want: a well-paying, fulfilling job; a great marriage or partnership; two or three cars; closets packed with fine clothes; a large and well-appointed house; perfectly mannered, talented children; time for golf, tennis, skiing, and the health club; vacations in exotic locales; personal fulfillment; and great sex. The U.S. Army's ad slogan "Be All You Can Be" might actually reflect society's message to us, but perhaps with this addition: "And Buy All You Can See."

LIVING IN THE RECOVERY ZONE: MAKING CHOICES

More than thirty years ago, Alvin Toffler, in his prophetic book *Future Shock,* had already foreseen and named this phenomenon; he called it "overchoice."[6] Engulfed by far more possibilities than we can handle, we are discovering that, in fact, we can't have everything we want. Each of us is faced with the task of determining the limits we have to put on our lives. We simply can't experience all that is potentially available to us. Some families, for example, decide to limit the after-school activities of their children in order to preserve family time together. Partners may each decide to forgo promotions—and the new "toys" that could come from higher income—because they want more personal time.

At its most basic level, we are talking about self-determination. We must decide how and where to focus our attention in a way that will let us live the life we want. We must learn what works for us and what doesn't.

Cybersex, called by some "the biggest porn shop in the world," presents this same problem of overchoice. While the good news is that there's more easily accessible information about sex available to more people than ever before—and more and different opportunities to engage in it—we still cannot do it all. Each of us must determine appropriate boundaries for our sexual activities that allow us to balance all our life goals and needs—those involving work, family, friends, hobbies, and so forth. In other words, we must learn to live within our Recovery Zone.

The limits we set on our lives—the boundaries we create—are based on a relationship with ourselves, one in which we seek to hear and follow our inner voice. These limits enable us to nurture, support, and protect ourselves. As we said earlier, setting appropriate limits also means being able to say, "No, I'm not going to do that, even though I want to, because if I do, I'm going to mess up my life." We take a particular stand because it reflects a belief we have about who we are.

As sex becomes more accessible, less regulated, and more public, it may also become more casual, even to the point of actually being trivial. Given its availability, sex could come to be seen as just another recreational activity, one that, as we know, can become addictive. Sex—an action that can hold tremendous personal and interpersonal significance—may soon no longer be seen as connected to Self, but rather little more than a biological expression having nothing to do with Self. At some point, we have to ask ourselves what sex is and what it means in our lives. If we want to maintain sex as an integral and meaningful part of our relationships, we may find that we simply cannot experience all the sexual choices available to us. We may have to say that sex isn't just another pleasurable diversion. We stand to lose much if an act that can create such profound feelings of connectedness becomes trivialized.

A SPIRITUAL JOURNEY OF DISCOVERY

This is, in the end, a spiritual quest, a spiritual journey to discover who we really are and what we can be as human beings. One of the most important ways we discover who we are is through interactions with other human beings. The Internet and cybersex are leading us to develop a greater awareness of our sexual selves and to discover how our sexuality fits into our lives and our interactions and relationships with others.

Too often in our culture, the relationship of sexuality and spirituality is seen as a war in which one must defeat and destroy the other. This view is futile and counterproductive. The desire to unite through the sexual act can metaphorically be seen as a drive to once again be united with the Divine. This is a yearning for our lost wholeness, a search for our other half, so that we might, if even for only a moment through sexual union, reexperience the lost bliss of our godlike totality. Our sexuality arises out of a sense of incompleteness that is manifested by an urge toward wholeness and a yearning for the One. But what, then, is spirituality? Is it not this same desire, a yearning for the Divine? While spirituality and sexuality are not exactly the same, they are cut from the same cloth. They are, as noted author M. Scott Peck says, "kissing cousins." The sexual and spiritual parts of our being lie so close together that it is hardly possible to arouse one without arousing the other. They are like two snare drums sitting side by side. If you strike one, the other vibrates too.

This is not myth; it's human experience. In Peck's *The Road Less Traveled,* he writes:

> When my beloved first stands before me naked, all open to my sight, there is a feeling throughout the whole of me. Awe! Why awe? If sex is no more than an instinct, why don't I simply feel horny or hungry? Such simple hunger would be quite sufficient to ensure the propagation of the species. Why should sex be complicated with reverence?[7]

Sex is "complicated with reverence" because it is, in fact, the closest many people ever come to a mystical experience. Indeed, this is why so many people chase after sex with such desperate abandon. Whether or not they know it, they are searching for God. The Internet and cybersex enable people to chase all the more frantically and intensely.

SEX AND SPIRIT UNITE

Abraham Maslow, in his studies of self-actualizing people, discovered that they often experience orgasm as a religious, even mystical, event. Maslow made it clear that these people were not speaking metaphorically. With another human in a deeply loving relationship, we can touch the Divine through sex.

Ironically, however, though we need the other to reach these heights, we briefly lose that other at the climactic moment, forgetting who and where we are. Mystics and spiritual teachers through the ages have spoken of an "ego death" as a necessary part of the spiritual journey, even its goal, and the French actually refer to orgasm as the "little death." We have entered the realm of spirit. Sex and spirit become one as we become one with All.

Sex does, however, complicate relationships. It is the search for God in human romantic relationships that lies at the root of the problem, says Peck. We look to our spouse or to romantic love to meet all our needs and fulfill us. This never works, or at least not for long. We can live in the bliss of new love perhaps for a few months, a year, or several years if we are lucky. But after a while, we change or our partner changes or everything changes—and suddenly it's all up for grabs. Throughout this long journey, however, we learn a lot about vulnerability, intimacy, love, and our own narcissism. It is natural for us humans to want a tangible God, but the Divine is not ours to possess. Instead, we must learn to accept that we live within the Divine or, as some describe it, within "the one in whom we live and move and have our being."

The common denominator of sex and spirituality is the search for meaning. Sexuality and spirituality connect through meaning. As we deepen our understanding of ourselves, of others, and of our planet and all its myriad life, we heighten both our spirituality *and* our sexuality. As M. Scott Peck is fond of saying, "I distrust any religious conversion which does not also involve an intensification of one's sexuality." The deeper and more meaningful our sexuality, the more we touch the mystical.

We need to recognize that we are part of a much larger whole. When people are unable to make this connection, they turn to relationships with objects—the false gods, in the biblical sense, of alcohol, money, sex (including cybersex), food, whatever seems to fill the void inside. While still searching for meaning, this path leads to addiction and an unmanageable life.

Despite its novelty, allure, and power, and no matter how intense and momentarily wonderful and fulfilling the experience, cybersex is no different. For all the reasons we've mentioned, it is ultimately an emotionally and spiritually empty and isolating experience.

CHOOSING HOW TO LIVE LIFE

Here is a critically important point. The choice is not to be in control or out of control; the choice is *how* we will live without control. We can "lose" control by admitting that there are larger forces at work in our lives and that we are part of a Divine plan. This will, in fact, bring us closer to our true selves and the Divine. Our other choice is to lose control via compulsive and addictive behaviors. This brings pain, misery, and ultimately self-destruction.

Through prayer and meditation, we seek conscious contact with a Higher Power, a connection that we strengthen as we learn to accept nurturing, to be open to our senses, to trust ourselves and others, and to become more centered within ourselves. As we do this, we are better able to enter into healthy relationships with a partner. Our search for meaning weaves the strands of relationship, self, spirit, and sensuality and sexuality together.

The information, suggestions, and guidelines we've provided can help you start on the road to recovery. Yes, you *can* change. You *can* create better relationships and live a richer, more fulfilling life. Remember that you *can't* do this alone. And you don't have to. Reach out to others for strength, support, and encouragement. All that you need will be given to you.

$\mathcal{A}$ppendix

The Twelve Steps of Alcoholics Anonymous*

1. We admitted we were powerless over alcohol—that our lives had become unmanageable.
2. Came to believe that a Power greater than ourselves could restore us to sanity.
3. Made a decision to turn our will and our lives over to the care of God *as we understood Him.*
4. Made a searching and fearless moral inventory of ourselves.
5. Admitted to God, to ourselves, and to another human being the exact nature of our wrongs.
6. Were entirely ready to have God remove all these defects of character.
7. Humbly asked Him to remove our shortcomings.
8. Made a list of all persons we had harmed, and became willing to make amends to them all.
9. Made direct amends to such people wherever possible, except when to do so would injure them or others.
10. Continued to take personal inventory and when we were wrong promptly admitted it.
11. Sought through prayer and meditation to improve our conscious contact with God *as we understood Him,* praying only for knowledge of His will for us and the power to carry that out.

* The Twelve Steps of AA are taken from *Alcoholics Anonymous,* 3d ed., published by AA World Services, Inc., New York, N.Y., 59–60. Reprinted with permission of AA World Services, Inc. (See editor's note on copyright page.)

12. Having had a spiritual awakening as the result of these steps, we tried to carry this message to alcoholics, and to practice these principles in all our affairs.

The Twelve Steps of Alcoholics Anonymous Adapted for Sexual Addicts*

1. We admitted we were powerless over our sexual addiction—that our lives had become unmanageable.
2. Came to believe that a Power greater than ourselves could restore us to sanity.
3. Made a decision to turn our will and our lives over to the care of God *as we understood Him.*
4. Made a searching and fearless moral inventory of ourselves.
5. Admitted to God, to ourselves, and to another human being the exact nature of our wrongs.
6. Were entirely ready to have God remove all these defects of character.
7. Humbly asked Him to remove our shortcomings.
8. Made a list of all persons we had harmed, and became willing to make amends to them all.
9. Made direct amends to such people wherever possible, except when to do so would injure them or others.
10. Continued to take personal inventory and when we were wrong promptly admitted it.
11. Sought through prayer and meditation to improve our conscious contact with God *as we understood Him,* praying only for knowledge of His will for us and the power to carry that out.
12. Having had a spiritual awakening as the result of these steps, we tried to carry this message to others and to practice these principles in all our affairs.

Contact List for More Information

For more information about Dr. Patrick Carnes and his speaking engagements, access his Web site at www.sexhelp.com or call him at 800-708-1796.

For information about Dr. David Delmonico and his speaking engagements, contact him at Duquesne University at 412-396-4032.

For information about Elizabeth Griffin and her speaking engagements, contact her at Internet Behavior Consulting at 952-210-5778.

For information on training for counselors and other helping professionals, call the Society for the Advancement of Sexual Health at 770-541-9912 or access its Web site at www.sash.net.

Resource Guide

The following is a list of recovery fellowships that may be helpful to you in your particular situation.

Al-Anon
888-425-2666
www.al-anon.alateen.org

Alcoholics Anonymous
212-870-3400
www.alcoholics-anonymous.org

Co-Anon
800-898-9985
www.co-anon.org

Co-Dependents Anonymous
602-277-7991
www.codependents.org

COSA
763-537-6904
www.cosa-recovery.org

Internet Behavior Consulting
952-210-5778
www.internetbehavior.com

Society for the Advancement of Sexual Health
770-541-9912
www.sash.net

Recovering Couples Anonymous
510-663-2312
www.recovering-couples.org

S-Anon
800-210-8141
www.sanon.org

Sex Addicts Anonymous
800-477-8191
www.sexaa.org

Sex and Love Addicts Anonymous
210-828-7900
www.slaafws.org

Sexual Addiction Resources/Dr. Patrick Carnes
www.sexhelp.com

Sexual Compulsives Anonymous
800-977-4325
www.sca-recovery.org

U.S. Drug Rehab Centers
866-449-1490
www.usdrugrehabcenters.com

Books of Related Interest Authored by Dr. Patrick Carnes

The Betrayal Bond: Breaking Free of Exploitive Relationships (Deerfield Beach, Fla.: Health Communications, 1998).
In a savage psychic twist, victims of abuse and violence often bond with their perpetrators to the stunning point that they will die rather than escape. Carnes's breakthrough book focuses on how betrayal intensifies trauma and illuminates the keys to escaping destructive relationships.

Contrary to Love: Helping the Sexual Addict (Center City, Minn.: Hazelden, 1989).
This sequel to *Out of the Shadows* traces the origins and consequences of the addict's faulty core beliefs. Building upon his earlier work, Carnes describes the stages of the illness and lays the groundwork for potential recovery.

Don't Call It Love: Recovery from Sexual Addiction (New York: Bantam, 1991).
This landmark study of one thousand recovering sex addicts and their families explores how people become sex addicts and the role of culture, family, neurochemistry, and child abuse in creating addiction.

A Gentle Path through the Twelve Steps: The Classic Guide for All People in the Process of Recovery (Center City, Minn.: Hazelden, 1994).
A guidebook for people in recovery that helps them understand their own stories and begin planning a new life of recovery. With more than 250,000 copies sold, it holds invaluable insights for beginners and old-timers alike in any Twelve Step program.

Out of the Shadows: Understanding Sexual Addiction, 3d ed. (Center City, Minn.: Hazelden, 2001).
The groundbreaking book that first identified and defined sexual addiction. A must for anyone looking to understand the illness, it's an expert and in-depth look at the origins of sexual addiction and the addictive cycle.

Sexual Anorexia: Overcoming Sexual Self-Hatred (with Joseph M. Moriarity) (Center City, Minn.: Hazelden, 1997).
The devastating mix of fear, pain, and betrayal can lead to obsessive sexual aversion. Tracing the dysfunction's roots in childhood sexual trauma, neglect, and abuse, Carnes explores dimensions of sexual health, targeting key issues that let recovery proceed.

Videos by Gentle Path Press

For more information or to order videos from Gentle Path Press, call 800-708-1796.

Addiction Interaction Disorder: Understanding Multiple Addictions
Few addicts—about 17 percent—have only one addiction. More commonly, assorted compulsions combine in a complex systemic problem called addiction interaction disorder. This video outlines how to screen for the disorder (a major factor in relapse) and explores the role of addiction as a "solution" to trauma.

Contrary to Love: Helping the Sexual Addict
A twelve-part PBS video series in which noted addiction psychologist Dr. Patrick Carnes discusses the spectrum of compulsive-addictive behavior and its treatment. The titles of the twelve parts are
   "Our Addictive Society"
   "Cultural Denial of Addiction"
   "Am I an Addict?"
   "Interview with Three Addicts"
   "The Addictive Family"
   "Interview with Melody Beattie"
   "Child Abuse"
   "The Twelve-Step Recovery Process"
   "Healthy Sexuality and Spirituality"
   "Finding a Balance in Recovery"
   "Coping in a World of Shame"
   "The Ten Risks of Recovery"

Trauma Bonds: When Humans Bond with Those Who Hurt Them
Victims often cling to destructive relationships with baffling desperation. In this riveting video, Dr. Patrick Carnes analyzes how trauma bonding develops and outlines strategies for breaking free from its compulsive torment.

Audiocassettes by Gentle Path Press

For more information or to order audiocassettes from Gentle Path Press, call 800-708-1796.

Addiction Interaction Disorder: Understanding Multiple Addictions
Sexual Abuse in the Church
Sexual Dependency, Compulsion and Obsession
Towards a New Freedom: Discovering Healthy Sexuality
Trauma Bonds: When We Bond with Those Who Hurt Us

For Further Reading

The following list contains books referenced in this book, in addition to further readings that may be helpful.

Co-Sex Addiction Recovery

Beattie, Melody. *Codependent No More: How to Stop Controlling Others and Start Caring for Yourself.* 2d ed. Center City, Minn.: Hazelden, 1992.

Calof, David L., and Robin Simons. *The Couple Who Became Each Other and Other Tales of Healing of a Master Hypnotherapist.* New York: Bantam Books, 1996.

Carnes, Patrick J. *The Betrayal Bond: Breaking Free of Exploitive Relationships.* Deerfield Beach, Fla.: Health Communications, 1998.

Fossum, Merle A., and Marilyn J. Mason. *Facing Shame: Families in Recovery.* New York: Norton, 1989.

Friel, John, and Linda Friel. *Adult Children: The Secrets of Dysfunctional Families.* Deerfield Beach, Fla.: Health Communications, 1988.

Schaeffer, Brenda. *Is It Love or Is It Addiction?* 2d ed. Center City, Minn.: Hazelden, 1997.

Schneider, Jennifer. *Back from Betrayal: Recovering from His Affairs.* New York: Ballantine Books, 1990.

Schneider, Jennifer P., and Burt Schneider. *Sex, Lies, and Forgiveness: Couples Speaking Out on Healing from Sex Addiction.* Center City, Minn.: Hazelden, 1991.

Family

Bradshaw, John. *Bradshaw on the Family: A Revolutionary Way of Self-Discovery.* Deerfield Beach, Fla.: Health Communications, 1988.

———. *Family Secrets: What You Don't Know Can Hurt You.* New York: Bantam Books, 1996.

Evans, Patricia. *The Verbally Abusive Relationship: How to Recognize It and How to Respond.* Holbrook, Mass.: Adams Media Corporation, 1996.

Love, Patricia. *Emotional Incest Syndrome: What to Do When a Parent's Love Rules Your Life.* New York: Bantam Books, 1991.

Mellody, Pia, with Andrea Well Miller and J. Keith Miller. *Facing Codependence.* San Francisco: Harper San Francisco, 1989.

Key Recovery Works

Beattie, Melody. *Journey to the Heart: Daily Meditations on the Path to Freeing Your Soul.* San Francisco: Harper San Francisco, 1996.

Bradshaw, John. *Healing the Shame That Binds You.* Deerfield Beach, Fla.: Health Communications, 1988.

Breton, Denise, and Christopher Largent. *The Paradigm Conspiracy: Why Our Social Systems Violate Human Potential—and How We Can Change Them.* Center City, Minn.: Hazelden, 1996.

Bryan, Mark, and Julia Cameron. *The Money Drunk: Ninety Days to Financial Sobriety.* New York: Ballantine Books, 1993.

Cameron, Julia. *The Artist's Way: A Spiritual Path to Higher Creativity.* New York: Putnam, 1995.

Covey, Stephen R. *First Things First.* New York: Fireside, 1996.

———. *The Seven Habits of Highly Effective People: Powerful Lessons in Personal Change.* New York: Simon & Schuster, 1989.

Hope and Recovery: A Twelve Step Guide for Healing from Compulsive Sexual Behavior. Center City, Minn.: Hazelden, 1987.

Milkman, Harvey B., and Stanley Sunderwirth. *Craving for Ecstasy: The Chemistry and Consciousness of Escape.* New York: Free Press, 1987.

Millman, Dan. *Way of the Peaceful Warrior: A Book That Changes Lives.* Tiburon, Calif.: Kramer, 1984.

Mundis, Jerrold. *How to Get Out of Debt, Stay Out of Debt & Live Prosperously.* New York: Bantam Books, 1990.

Nouwen, Henri J. *Reaching Out: The Three Movements of the Spiritual Life.* Garden City, N.Y.: Doubleday, 1986.

Peck, M. Scott. *People of the Lie: The Hope for Healing Human Evil.* New York: Simon & Schuster, 1985.

———. *The Road Less Traveled.* New York: Simon & Schuster, 1997.

Sex Addiction and Cybersex

Carnes, Patrick. *Contrary to Love: Helping the Sexual Addict.* Center City, Minn.: Hazelden, 1989.

———. *Don't Call It Love: Recovery from Sexual Addiction.* New York: Bantam, 1991.

———. *Out of the Shadows: Understanding Sexual Addiction*. 3d ed. Center City, Minn.: Hazelden, 2001.

Cooper, Al, ed. "Cybersex: The Dark Side of the Force." Special issue, *Sexual Addiction and Compulsivity: The Journal of Treatment and Prevention* 7 (2000): 1–2.

———. *Sex and the Internet: A Guidebook for Clinicians*. New York: Brunner-Routledge, 2002.

———. "Sexuality and the Internet: Surfing into the New Millennium." *Cyber-Psychology and Behavior* 1, no. 2 (1998): 181–87.

Cooper, A., C. Scherer, S. Boies, and B. Gordon. "Sexuality and the Internet: From Sexual Exploration to Pathological Expression." *Professional Psychology* 30, no. 2 (1999): 154–64.

Cooper, Al, and L. Sportolari. "Romance in Cyberspace: Understanding Online Attraction." *Journal of Sex Education and Therapy* 22, no. 1 (1997): 7–14.

Delmonico, David L. "Cybersex: High Tech Sex Addiction." *Sexual Addiction and Compulsivity: Journal of Treatment and Prevention* 4, no. 2 (1997): 159–67.

———, ed. "Cybersex." Special issue, *Sexual and Relationship Therapy* 18, no. 3 (2003).

Delmonico, David L., Elizabeth J. Griffin, and Joseph Moriarity. *Cybersex Unhooked: A Workbook for Breaking Free of Compulsive Online Sexual Behavior*. Phoenix, Ariz.: Gentle Path Press, 2001.

Diamond, D. "The Sleaze Squeeze." *Business2.0,* (February 1999): 35–45.

Goodman, Aviel. *Sexual Addiction: An Integrated Approach*. Madison, Conn.: International Universities Press, 1999.

Milkman, Harvey, and Stanley Sunderwirth. *Craving for Ecstasy: How Our Passions Become Addictions and What We Can Do About Them*. San Francisco: Jossey-Bass, 1987.

Schneider, Jennifer. "Sex Addiction: Controversy within Mainstream Addiction Medicine, Diagnosis Based on the DSM-III-R and Physician Case Histories." *Sexual Addiction and Compulsivity: Journal of Treatment and Prevention* 1, no. 1 (1994): 19–44.

Schneider, Jennifer, and Robert Weiss. *Cybersex Exposed*. Center City, Minn.: Hazelden, 2001.

Weiss, Robert, and Jennifer Schneider. *Untangling the Web: Sex, Porn, and Fantasy Obsession in the Internet Age*. Los Angeles: Alyson Books, 2006.

Young, Kimberly S. *Caught in the Net: How to Recognize the Signs of Internet Addiction—and a Winning Strategy for Recovery*. New York: John Wiley & Sons, 1998.

———. *Tangled in the Web: Understanding Cybersex from Fantasy to Addiction*. Bloomington, Ind.: 1st Books Library Publications, 2001.

Young, Kimberly S., and R. C. Rogers. "The Relationship between Depression and Internet Addiction." *CyberPsychology and Behavior* 1, no. 1 (1998): 25–28.

Sexual Health

Bechtal, Stephen. *The Practical Encyclopedia of Sex and Health.* Emmaus, Pa.: Rodale Press, 1993.

Berzon, Betty, ed. *Positively Gay.* Berkeley, Calif.: Celestial Arts, 1995.

Covington, Stephanie. *Awakening Your Sexuality: A Guide for Recovering Women.* Center City, Minn.: Hazelden, 1991.

Diamond, Jed. *Male Menopause: Sex and Survival in the Second Half of Life.* Naperville, Ill.: Sourcebooks, 1997.

Eisler, Riane. *The Chalice and the Blade: Our History, Our Future.* San Francisco: Harper & Row, 1987.

Hastings, Anne S. *Discovering Sexuality That Will Satisfy You Both: When Couples Want Differing Amounts and Different Kinds of Sex.* Tiburon, Calif.: Printed Voice, 1993.

Klausner, Mary A., and Bobbie Hasselbring. *Aching for Love: The Sexual Drama of the Adult Child.* San Francisco: Harper San Francisco, 1990.

Maltz, Wendy, ed. *Intimate Kisses: The Poetry of Sexual Pleasure.* Novato, Calif.: New World Library, 2001.

———, ed. *Passionate Hearts: The Poetry of Sexual Love.* Novato, Calif.: New World Library, 1997.

Maltz, Wendy, and Suzie Boss. *Private Thoughts: Exploring the Power of Women's Sexual Fantasies.* Novato, Calif.: New World Library, 2001.

Renshaw, Domeena. *Seven Weeks to Better Sex.* New York: Random House, 1995.

Sex and Religion

Burkett, Elinor, and Frank Bruni. *A Gospel of Shame: Children, Sexual Abuse, and the Catholic Church.* New York: Viking Penguin, 1993.

Laaser, Mark. *Faithful and True: Sexual Integrity in a Fallen World.* Grand Rapids, Mich.: Zondervan, 1996.

———, ed. *Restoring the Soul of a Church: Reconciling Congregations Wounded by Clergy Sexual Misconduct.* Collegeville, Minn.: Liturgical Press, 1995.

Rossetti, Stephen J. *A Tragic Grace: The Catholic Church and Child Sexual Abuse.* Collegeville, Minn.: Liturgical Press, 1996.

Sipe, A. W. Richard. *Sex, Priests, and Power: Anatomy of a Crisis.* New York: Brunner/Mazel, 1995.

Trauma Resolution

Bass, Ellen, and Laura Davis. *The Courage to Heal: A Guide for Women Survivors of Child Sexual Abuse.* New York: HarperCollins, 1994.

Courtois, Christine A. *Healing the Incest Wound: Adult Survivors in Therapy*. New York: Norton, 1996.

Crowder, Adrienne. *Opening the Door: A Treatment Model for Therapy with Male Survivors of Sexual Abuse*. Philadelphia: Brunner/Mazel, 1995.

Davis, Laura. *Allies in Healing: When the Person You Love Was Sexually Abused as a Child*. New York: HarperCollins, 1991.

Dolan, Yvonne. *Resolving Sexual Abuse: Solution-Focused Therapy and Ericksonian Hypnosis for Adult Survivors*. New York: Norton, 1991.

Fossum, Merle A., and Marilyn J. Mason. *Facing Shame: Families in Recovery*. New York: Norton, 1989.

Hunter, Mic. *Abused Boys: The Neglected Victims of Sexual Abuse*. New York: Fawcett, 1991.

Maltz, Wendy. *The Sexual Healing Journey: A Guide for Survivors of Sexual Abuse*. New York: HarperCollins, 1991.

Maltz, Wendy, and Beverly Holman. *Incest and Sexuality: A Guide to Understanding and Healing*. Lexington, Ky.: Lexington Books, 1987.

Miller, Alice. *For Your Own Good: Hidden Cruelty in Child-Rearing and the Roots of Violence*. New York: Farrar, Straus, Giroux, 1990.

White, William L. *The Incestuous Workplace: Stress and Distress in the Organizational Family*. Center City, Minn.: Hazelden, 1997.

Hermes' Web and the Web Sight Program

Hermes' Web

- is an innovative new tool for working with difficult clients
- helps communicate essential psychological concepts
- demonstrates treatment dynamics
- compensates for learning and comprehension difficulties
- helps build the connection between intention and behavior
- meets clients where they are—dubbed "the equalizer"
- works on multichannels: visual, tactile, abstract, spiritual
- can be used with many treatment models and modalities

Hermes' Web, Ltd., also offers the Web Sight Program, which incorporates the use of the Web. The Web Sight Program is unique—it combines ten essential and difficult components that, when brought together, have the capacity to reach, work with, and affect the most difficult clients.

The following are the components of the Web Sight Program:

1. Presenting problems and disorders
2. The Web
   - Ego/core
   - The flip
   - Black box
   - Mirroring
   - De-repression
   - Dismantling the victim identity
   - Tracking the perpetration
   - Incorporating the Web into your program
3. Interactive drama
   - Principles of drama therapy
   - The interactive strategy
   - The repertoire of characters
4. Process psychology
   - Group process skills
   - Conflict work
   - World work
   - Racism and privilege
5. Violence prevention
   - The roots of violence
   - The criminal mind
   - The holocaust self
6. Real sexuality
7. Guild philosophy
   - The new ethic
   - Democracy
   - Spirituality
8. Rights of passage
   - Moving from adolescence to adult—the essential lessons
9. Reading contemporary culture
10. Firebelly work
    - Movement
    - Rhythm
    - Team movement/working in unison on body level

For more information about Hermes' Web or the Web Sight Program, contact
Jerry Fjerkenstad
Hermes' Web, Ltd.
235 Bedford Street SE
Minneapolis, MN 55414
Phone: 612-623-3982
Fax: 612-362-9310
E-mail: jrfnh@aol.com
www.hermesweb.com

Jerry Fjerkenstad, M.A., L.P., is the creator of Hermes' Web and its Violence Prevention Curricula as well as TNT: Toys n' Tools for Core-Level Change. He has extensive national and international teaching, conference, and workshop presentation experience. He served as executive director of MASC (Minnesotans Actively Seeking Community), a nonprofit corporation providing violence prevention programming to public schools, and worked for sixteen years in Project Pathfinder, Inc.'s adult outpatient sex offender treatment program, including four years as clinical director. He is currently in private practice in the Minneapolis area, and works as a consulting psychologist for a maximum security prison. He also provides training and consultation for juvenile detention centers, addiction programs, and federal prisons.

$\mathcal{N}otes$

Chapter 1: The Shadow Side of the Net

1. Nielsen//NetRatings Resources: Data and Rankings (August 2006). Available online at www.nielsen-netratings.com.

2. Family Safe Media: Pornography Statistics (2006). Available online at www.familysafemedia.com/pornography_statistics.html.

3. Nielsen//NetRatings Resources: Data and Rankings (August 2006). Available online at www.nielsen-netratings.com.

4. Lynn Townsend White, *Medieval Technology and Social Change* (Oxford: Clarendon Press, 1966); Alvin Toffler, *Future Shock* (New York: Bantam, [1970] 1991).

5. Ibid.

6. David L. Delmonico, Elizabeth J. Griffin, and Joseph Moriarity, *Cybersex Unhooked: A Workbook for Breaking Free of Compulsive Online Sexual Behavior* (Phoenix, Ariz.: Gentle Path Press, 2001). Available online at www.internetbehavior.com/services/cyber_unhooked.htm.

7. Al Cooper, David L. Delmonico, and Ron Burg, "Cybersex Users, Abusers, and Compulsives: New Findings and Implications," *Sexual Addiction and Compulsivity* 7, nos. 1 and 2 (2000).

Chapter 2: Do I Have a Problem with Cybersex?

1. J. P. Schneider, "Sexual Addiction: Controversy within Mainstream Addiction Medicine, Diagnosis Based on the DSM-III-R and Physician Case Histories," *Sexual Addiction and Compulsivity* 1, no. 1 (1994): 19–44.

2. David Delmonico, published on the Internet at www.sexhelp.com (1999).

Chapter 4: What Turns You On? The Arousal Template

1. John Gage, "Old Brains, New Tricks," *Time* 7 (August 2000): 70.

2. Helen Fisher, "Lust, Attraction, Attachment: Biology and Evolution of the Three Primary Emotion Systems for Mating, Reproduction, and Parenting," *Journal of Sex Education and Therapy* 25, no. 1:96–105.

3. John Money, *Love Maps: Clinical Concepts of Sexual/Erotic Health and Pathology, Paraphilia, and Gender Transposition in Childhood, Adolescence, and Maturity* (Amherst, N.Y.: Prometheus Books, 1989).

Chapter 5: Courtship Gone Awry

1. Havelock Ellis, *Psychology of Sex* (New York: Harcourt Brace Jovanovich, [1933] 1978).

2. K. Freund and R. Watson, "Mapping the Boundaries of Courtship Disorder," *Journal of Sex Research* 27, no. 4 (November 1990): 589–606.

3. Patrick J. Carnes, *Don't Call It Love: Recovery from Sexual Addiction* (Phoenix, Ariz.: Gentle Path Press, 1991).

Chapter 6: Boundaries

1. Robert Bly, *Iron John: A Book about Men* (New York: Vintage Books, 1992).

2. Pia Mellody, *Facing Codependence* (San Francisco: Harper San Francisco, 1989).

Chapter 7: Taking That First Step

1. Patrick Carnes, *Contrary to Love: Helping the Sexual Addict* (Center City, Minn.: Hazelden, 1989).

2. Paul Watzlawick, John H. Weakland, and Richard Fisch, *Change: Principles of Problem Formation and Problem Resolution* (New York: Norton, 1988).

Chapter 8: Changing the Way You Live

1. The use of Hermes' Web as a tool for addiction recovery was developed by Jerry Fjerkenstad. (See appendix for more information.)

2. The phrase "truthful lie" was first used by Jerry Fjerkenstad, Hermes' Web, Ltd.

Chapter 9: Preventing Relapse: Maintaining the Changes You've Made

1. James O. Prochaska, John C. Norcross, and Carlo C. DiClemente, *Changing for Good* (New York: Avon Books, 1995).

2. G. Alan Marlatt and Judith R. Gordon, eds., *Relapse Prevention: Maintenance Strategies in the Treatment of Addictive Behaviors* (New York: Guilford Press, 1985).

Chapter 10: *Family Dynamics and Cybersex*

1. J. P. Schneider, "Effects of Cybersex Addiction on the Family: Results of a Survey," *Sexual Addiction and Compulsivity* 7, no. 1 (2000): 31–58.

2. J. P. Schneider, "A Qualitative Study of Cybersex Participants: Gender Differences, Recovery Issues, and Implications for Therapists," *Sexual Addiction and Compulsivity* 7, no. 4 (2000): 249–78.

3. M. Deborah Corley and Jennifer Schneider, *Disclosing Secrets: When, to Whom, and How Much to Reveal* (Center City, Minn.: Hazelden, 2002).

4. Patrick Carnes, *Don't Call It Love: Recovery from Sexual Addiction* (Phoenix, Ariz.: Gentle Path Press, 1991).

5. Patrick Carnes, Debra Laaser, and Mark Laaser, *Open Hearts: Renewing Relationships with Recovery, Romance, and Reality* (Phoenix, Ariz.: Gentle Path Press, 2000).

Chapter 11: *The Web Frontier*

1. Denise Breton and Christopher Largent, *The Paradigm Conspiracy: Why Our Social Systems Violate Human Potential—and How We Can Change Them* (Center City, Minn.: Hazelden, 1996).

2. Dean Ornish, *Love and Survival* (New York: Harper Collins, 1999).

3. Tom Clancy, *The Bear and the Dragon* (New York: Putnam, 2000).

4. Frank Herbert, *Dune* (New York: Ace Books, 1999).

5. Aldous Huxley, *Brave New World* (New York: HarperPerennial, 1998).

6. Alvin Toffler, *Future Shock* (New York: Bantam, [1970] 1991).

7. M. Scott Peck, *The Road Less Traveled* (New York: Simon & Schuster, 1997).

Index

About the Authors

PATRICK CARNES, PH.D., is an internationally known speaker and authority on addiction and recovery issues. He is the bestselling author of fifteen books, including landmark classics such as *Out of the Shadows, A Gentle Path through the Twelve Steps,* and *Don't Call It Love.* He pioneered inpatient treatment for sex addiction, and currently serves as the executive director of the Gentle Path Program at Pine Grove Behavioral Health Center in Hattiesburg, Mississippi. Dr. Carnes founded the medical journal *Sexual Addiction and Compulsivity: The Journal of Treatment and Prevention.* He received a lifetime achievement award from the Society for the Advancement of Sexual Health (SASH). As the primary architect of the "task-centered" approach to therapy, his research is the core of the Certified Sex Addiction Therapist program of the International Institute for Trauma and Addiction Professionals (IITAP). More information about Dr. Carnes can be found at www.sexhelp.com. For more information about the Gentle Path Program please go to www.pinegrovetreatment.com, and for information about the Certified Sex Addiction Therapist program go to www.iitap.com.

DAVID L. DELMONICO, PH.D., is an associate professor at Duquesne University in Pittsburgh, Pennsylvania. He conducts research, consultation, and training on topics such as cybersex, cyberoffense, and cybersafety. He also lectures on topics such as general Internet psychology and sexually addictive and compulsive behaviors. Dr. Delmonico is co-author of *Cybersex Unhooked: A Workbook for Breaking Free of Compulsive Online Sexual Behavior* and has published numerous scholarly articles on a variety of addiction and sexuality topics. He is director of the Online Behavior Research and Education Center (OBREC) at Duquesne University and editor-in-chief of the *Sexual Addiction and Compulsivity* journal. Dr. Delmonico is the co-director of the Internet Behavior Consulting group, which provides research, training, education, and direct care service for problematic online sexual behavior. More information can be found at www.internetbehavior.com.

ELIZABETH GRIFFIN, M.A., is a licensed marriage and family therapist with more than twenty-five years of experience treating individuals with problematic sexual behavior. She lectures and consults internationally on the assessment and treatment of individuals, couples, and families struggling with problematic online behaviors, sexually compulsive behaviors, and sexual offense behaviors. Ms. Griffin has lectured and consulted in legal/forensic settings, religious communities, HR/EAP settings, and educational settings. She co-authored *Cybersex Unhooked: A Workbook for Breaking Free of Compulsive Online Sexual Behavior* and has published numerous academic articles on issues related to problematic sexual behavior. Ms. Griffin is the co-director of the Internet Behavior Consulting group, which provides research, training, education, and direct care service for problematic online sexual behavior. More information can be found at www.internetbehavior.com.

JOSEPH M. MORIARITY, B.S., B.A., has worked for twenty years as a freelance writer with a primary focus in the fields of health care, addiction and treatment, science, and education. He has previously written two other books for Hazelden, *Winning a Day at a Time* with John Lucas and *Sexual Anorexia* with Dr. Patrick Carnes.

OTHER TITLES THAT MAY INTEREST YOU:

Out of the Shadows
Understanding Sexual Addiction
Patrick Carnes, Ph.D.
The definitive resource for understanding sexual addiction. This book, in its third edition, identifies the danger signs, explains the dynamics, and describes the consequences of sexual addiction and dependency.
Softcover, 240 pp.   Order No. 1853

Contrary to Love
Helping the Sexual Addict
Patrick Carnes, Ph.D.
The long-awaited sequel to *Out of the Shadows*. *Contrary to Love* builds on the original descriptive framework while adding new insights and findings.
Softcover, 304 pp.   Order No. 7611

A Gentle Path through the Twelve Steps
The Classic Guide for All People in the Process of Recovery
Patrick Carnes, Ph.D.
This revised edition of *A Gentle Path through the Twelve Steps* offers exercises, inventories, and guided reflections for those facing the challenge of attaining or maintaining an addiction-free lifestyle.
Softcover, 328 pp.   Order No. 7625

Confusing Love with Obsession
When Being in Love Means Being in Control
John D. Moore
A must-read book for anyone involved in a dangerously obsessive intimate relationship. Drawing from dozens of real-life stories, Moore calls attention to this largely hushed, but intensely harmful problem.
Softcover, 208 pp.   Order No. 2630

Hazelden books are available at fine bookstores everywhere. To order directly from Hazelden, call 1-800-328-9000 or visit www.hazelden.org/bookstore.

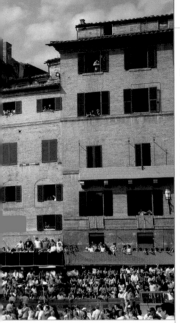

LEFT: crowd at the Palio, Siena.

updated throughout by **Lisa Gerard-Sharp**, an experienced travel writer who is knowledgeable about all things Tuscan. Lisa has contributed to many Insight Guides for Italian destinations, after living in several places in the country. It was commissioned and edited by **Rebecca Lovell** at Insight Guides.

This edition builds on the work of previous contributors. These include **Angela Vannucci**, **Adele Evans**, **Sarah Birke** and **Robert John**, who all gave their expertise to the Places chapters and Travel Tips sections.

Christopher Catling wrote the original history chapters, and the Renaissance art chapters were penned by **Russell Chamberlin**.

The routes on the accompanying touring map were planned and written by travel writer **Rebecca Ford**.

The majority of stunning pictures were taken by **Steve McDonald**, winner of the 2011 Insight Guides/The Independent on Sunday annual photography competition. He has captured the timeless beauty of the Tuscan landscape and its historic towns.

The book was proofread by **Hildegarde Serle** and indexed by **Helen Peters**.

CONTACTING THE EDITORS

We would appreciate it if readers would alert us to errors or outdated information by writing to:

Insight Guides, P.O. Box 7910, London SE1 1WE, England. email: insight@apaguide.co.uk

NO part of this book may be reproduced, stored in a retrieval system or transmitted in any form or means electronic, mechanical, photocopying, recording or otherwise, without prior written permission of *Apa Publications*. Brief text quotations with use of photographs are exempted for book review purposes only. Information has been obtained from sources believed to be reliable, but its accuracy and completeness, and the opinions based thereon, are not guaranteed.

www.insightguides.com

◆ A special section of photographic features highlights Florentine museums and other aspects of Tuscan culture, such as Chianti and its wine.

◆ Photographs are chosen not only to illustrate the landscape and buildings but also to convey the moods of the region and the life of its people.

◆ The Travel Tips listings section provides a point of reference for information on travel, hotels, shops and festivals. Information may be located quickly by using the index printed on the back cover flap – and the flaps are designed to serve as bookmarks.

The contributors

This edition of *Insight Regional Guide: Tuscany* was thoroughly

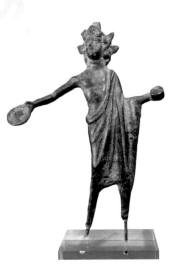

Contents

LEFT: classic Tuscan countryside.

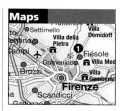

Maps

Travel Tips

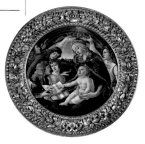

THE BEST OF TUSCANY: TOP ATTRACTIONS

The enigmatic Etruscans, the wine-loving Tuscans, Italy's loveliest hill towns, the world's finest museum of Renaissance art, the iconic Leaning Tower, countryside that inspired Leonardo da Vinci – Tuscany has it all

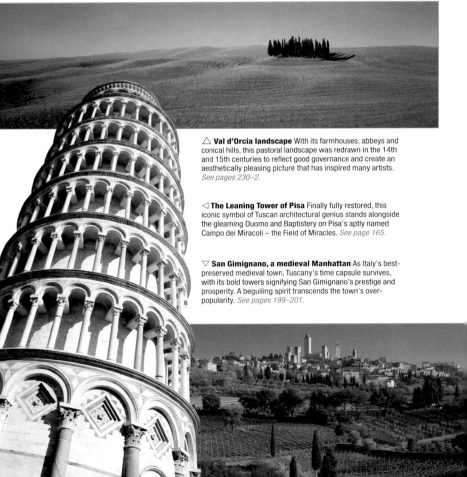

△ **Val d'Orcia landscape** With its farmhouses, abbeys and conical hills, this pastoral landscape was redrawn in the 14th and 15th centuries to reflect good governance and create an aesthetically pleasing picture that has inspired many artists. *See pages 230–2.*

◁ **The Leaning Tower of Pisa** Finally fully restored, this iconic symbol of Tuscan architectural genius stands alongside the gleaming Duomo and Baptistery on Pisa's aptly named Campo dei Miracoli – the Field of Miracles. *See page 165.*

▽ **San Gimignano, a medieval Manhattan** As Italy's best-preserved medieval town, Tuscany's time capsule survives, with its bold towers signifying San Gimignano's prestige and prosperity. A beguiling spirit transcends the town's over-popularity. *See pages 199–201.*

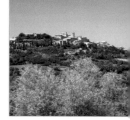

▷ **Hill towns of Montepulciano and Montalcino** Montepulciano and Montalcino draw you in with their palaces, seductive lifestyle and cellars of famed wines. Sip Vino Nobile in Cantine Contucci or sample Brunello di Montalcino in the Fortezza. See pages 227–29 and 237–8.

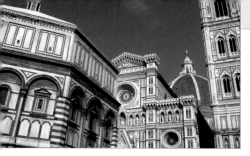

△ **Florentine churches** From Brunelleschi's dazzling Duomo to Romanesque San Miniato, Gothic Santa Croce and Michelangelo's Medici tombs in San Lorenzo, Florentine churches are mesmerising repositories of art and history. See pages 96–105.

▷ **Wine-tasting in the Chianti** Ignore the "Chiantishire" tag and visit a chequered landscape of vineyards, villages and fortified-wine estates that include the Castello di Brolio, birthplace of the modern Chianti industry. See page 202.

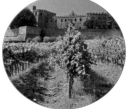

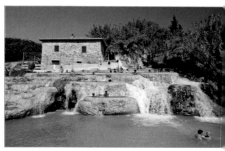

△ **Tuscan spas** Despite dating back to Etruscan times, Tuscany's new breed of thermal spas combine sophisticated pampering with authentic water cures in incomparable natural settings – as in Fonteverde Terme or Terme di Saturnia. See page 138.

▽ **Siena, the quintessential medieval city** Siena, the feminine foil to Florentine masculinity, is the city that most lives enfolded in its own private world, from the compelling medieval mood to the pageantry of the Palio horse race. See pages 211–23.

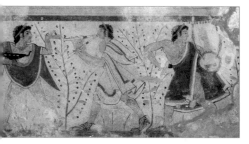

△ **Etruscan Tuscany** Whether in Volterra's intriguing Etruscan museum or Chiusi's painted tombs, the colour and life of Etruscan art contrasts with the cold perfectionism of the Greeks and Romans. See pages 27–31, 191 and 233.

◁ **The Uffizi Gallery in Florence** The world's greatest collection of Renaissance art includes masterpieces such as Botticelli's *Birth of Venus*, and works by Leonardo da Vinci, Michelangelo, Raphael, Titian and other masters of the High Renaissance. See pages 110–3.

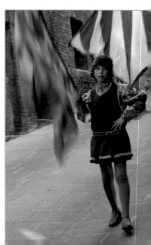

THE BEST OF TUSCANY: EDITOR'S CHOICE

Art, culture, food and history... Here, at a glance, are our recommendations for your visit

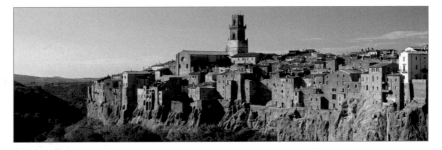

CHURCHES AND MONUMENTS

- **Brunelleschi's dome.** An incredible feat of engineering by the father of Renaissance architecture. *See page 98*
- **Monte Oliveto Maggiore.** A secluded 14th-century monastery set among groves of cypress trees. *See page 224*
- **Sant'Antimo.** An abbey church built of creamy travertine framed by tree-clad hills. *See page 238*
- **Siena cathedral.** A magnificent Gothic structure of banded black and white stone. *See page 215*
- **San Michele in Foro** in Lucca. A fine example of the exuberant Tuscan Romanesque style. *See page 135*
- **Santa Maria della Grazia.** The domed church just outside the Etruscan walls of Cortona is a hidden gem. *See page 259*
- **San Pellegrino in Alpe.** An ancient monastery deep in the Garfagnana mountains, with sweeping, glorious views. *See page 153*

THE BEST TUSCAN HILL TOWNS

- **Pienza.** The ideal Renaissance city is famous for its scenery and its production of tasty pecorino cheese. *See page 225*
- **Monteriggioni.** The Sienese hilltown encircled by walls and 14 towers is a truly spectacular sight. *See page 203*
- **Massa Marittima.** This town is perched on top of a high hill on the edge of the Colline Metallifere and is the loveliest springboard for exploring the Maremma. *See page 194*
- **Cortona.** An enchanting hill town in eastern Tuscany with attractions out of all proportion with its tiny size. *See page 261*
- **Vinci.** The genius of Leonardo is proudly celebrated in his birthplace, a tiny hill town situated between the cities of Florence and Pisa. *See page 129*
- **Pitigliano.** Once one of the most important settlements in southern Tuscany, this dramatic tufa haunt is found in a forgotten corner of Tuscany. *See page 248*
- **San Miniato.** An ancient town straddling three hills in the province of Florence. On a clear day, you can see Volterra and the Apuan Alps from this vantage point. *See page 129*

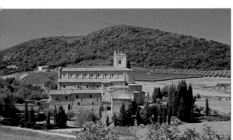

ABOVE: the Pitigliano skyline. **LEFT:** Abbazia di Sant'Antimo, southern Siena.

TUSCANY FOR FAMILIES

- **Florence or Lucca by bike.** Or, in the case of Florence, also by rickshaw, Segway, horse-drawn carriage or summer boat along the Arno. *See page 269*
- **Giardini di Boboli.** The gardens behind the Pitti Palace are fun for children to clamber around. There is an amphitheatre, strange statues and grottoes, and a handy café. *See page 115*
- **Trips to the Tuscan islands.** Explore the Tuscan archipelago with the ferries and hydrofoils that sail from Porto Santo Stefano to Giglio, and from Piombino to

Elba. *See pages 186 and 268*
- **Giardino dei Tarocchi.** A bizarre garden full of colourful fantasy figures. *See page 246*
- **Parco di Pinocchio.** Pinocchio's park at Collodi, near Pisa, has a certain old-fashioned charm. *See page 140*
- **Museo dei Ragazzi.** Dressing up, model-making and other fun activities for kids in the Palazzo Vecchio bring the Renaissance to life. *See page 93*
- **Ice cream.** When all else fails, an ice cream on a town square, most of which are traffic-free, rarely fails to win them over.

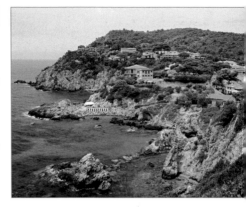

ABOVE: Talamone on the Maremma coast. **BELOW LEFT:** the Teatro Romano in Fiesole.

SEASIDE AND SPAS

- **Elba.** A beautiful island with dramatic scenery and a series of small beaches and coves. Perfect for families. *See page 181*
- **The Maremma.** Backed by a nature reserve, it is one of the most unspoilt stretches of beach on the coast. *See page 241–4*
- **Forte dei Marmi.** With its villas and chic cafés, this cycle-friendly summer resort is a magnet for the beautiful people.

See page 152
- **Monte Argentario.** A craggy peninsula with several chic fishing ports make it tempting to explore by yacht or by car. *See page 244*
- **Spas.** From the simple but charming (Bagni San Filippo) to the sophisticated and stylish (Grotta Giusti, in a villa) to a cool castle spa (Castello del Nero), Tuscany is Italy's most pampering spa destination. *See pages 138 and 301*

TOP ETRUSCAN SITES

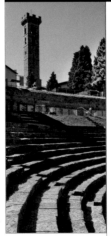

- **Volterra** has some of the best Etruscan funerary art to be found

outside Rome. *See page 189*
- **Chiusi.** Etruscan tombs and tunnels are the highlight of a visit to Chiusi. *See page 231*
- **Tufa towns.** Superb Etruscan sites and trails are found around Sovana, Sorano and Pitigliano. *See page 248*
- **Museo Archeologico** in Florence has a fine collection of Etruscan art. *See page 102*
- **Fiesole.** An Etruscan temple and a Roman theatre a 30-minute bus ride from Florence. *See page 123*

BELOW: sunbathing on one of the Tuscan coast's many pleasant beaches.

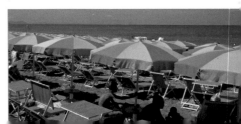

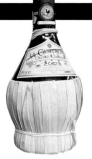

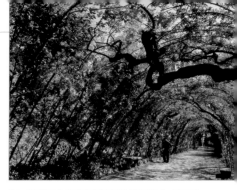

ABOVE: walking in the Boboli Gardens, Florence. **LEFT:** famed Chianti wine. **BELOW:** a detail of the magnificent bronze doors of the Baptistery, Florence.

A TASTE OF TUSCANY

- **Wine tasting.** As well as in the Chianti *(page 202)*, Montepulciano *(page 227)* and Montalcino *(page 237)*, visit Bolgheri for the Super-Tuscans and Maremma for Morellino di Scansano *(page 241)*.
- **Food festivals.** Tuscans are proud of their local produce, which they celebrate with festivals *(sagre)* – white truffles, chestnuts, Valdichiana beef, wild boar and pecorino cheese all have festivals dedicated to them.
- **Cookery courses.** The best include: Cucina Giuseppina in medieval Certaldo (www.cucina giuseppina.com); Camilla in Cucina in Florence (www.link firenze.it; tel: +39 055 461 381); and Badia a Coltibuono,

where you can eat, sleep and cook. *See page 290*
- **Mushrooms.** In autumn, mushroom-loving Tuscans forage for *funghi*. Wild mushrooms, especially the prized *porcini* and *tartufi* (truffles), are also on the menu. *See page 76*
- **Sweet treats** include candied fruit cake, *panforte*, sweet almond biscuits, *ricciarelli*, crunchy *cantucci* biscuits, and irresistible *gelati*. *See page 218*

VILLAS AND GARDENS

- **Giardini di Boboli.** The regal gardens of the Pitti Palace, now a vast museum. *See page 104*
- **Villa Medicea Poggio a Caiano.** The perfect frescoed Medici villa, with beautiful gardens. *See page 128*
- **Villa Demidoff and Parco di Pratolino.** The gardens contain extraordinary Mannerist sculpture and grottoes. *See page 126*
- **Lucchesi villas.** The area around Lucca is

rich in villas, all surrounded by beautiful parks. *See page 137*
- **Villa Medici (Fiesole).** A delightful villa and garden with superb views of Florence. *See page 126*
- **Villa Medicea della Petraia.** An elegant villa decorated with wonderful frescoes. *See page 126*
- **Villa Medicea di Castello.** This villa has beautiful Renaissance gardens. *See page 126*

RENAISSANCE ART

- **Masaccio's Florentine frescoes** in the Brancaccio chapel and Santa Maria Novella in Florence reflect a range of true Renaissance values: the importance of the human form, human emotion and the use of perspective. *See pages 101 and 104–5*
- **The Bargello.** A major collection of Renaissance and Mannerist sculpture is housed in this building – a former prison. *See page 120*
- **The Baptistery.** Ghiberti's bronze doors are so dazzling, Michelangelo called them the "Gates of Paradise". *See page 96*

- **Lorenzetti's frescoes.** Located in Siena's Palazzo Pubblico – a striking allegory of good and bad government, one of the earliest secular paintings. *See page 215*
- **The two Davids.** Michelangelo's *David* is Florence's icon, but Donatello's *David* was the first free-standing nude since antiquity. *See pages 119 and 121*
- **Giotto's frescoes** in Florence's Santa Croce displays a significant departure from the flat Byzantine style. *See pages 102–3*
- **Piero della Francesca's frescoes** in Arezzo are marvels of pastel shades awash with cool light. *See page 254*

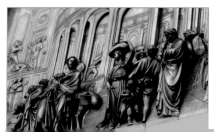

TUSCAN LANDSCAPE

- **The Crete Senesi.** The dramatic landscape of rounded hills, stately cypresses and isolated farms, this the Tuscany of postcards and posters. *See page 224*

- **Parco Regionale della Maremma.** Beautiful, unspoilt beaches backed by steep cliffs, parasol pines and wild Mediterranean scrubland. *See pages 71 and 243*

- **Chianti Country.** Gentle hills cloaked in vineyards and dotted with medieval castle estates where winetasting is on offer. *See pages 69 and 204–6*

- **Parco dell'Orecchiella.** A wild mountainous area, rich in wildlife, the region's most spectacular park. *See page 71*

- **Apuan Alps.** Behind the well-groomed beaches of the Versilia is a rugged hinterland of marble quarries, mountain ridges and narrow gorges. *See page 154*

- **The Casentino.** Ancient forests of the upper Arno valley. *See pages 68 and 255*

- **Monte Amiata.** The site of an extinct volcano with a profusion of thermal springs and quaint hamlets. *See pages 236 and 248*

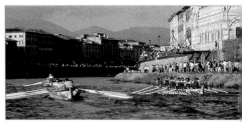

ABOVE: the boat race at the Luminaria di San Ranieri festival, Pisa. **BELOW LEFT:** a typical landscape in southern Siena.

FESTIVALS AND EVENTS

- **Il Palio.** Siena's traditional horse race is a heart-racing and passionate affair, involving all of the town's *contrada*. *See pages 222–3*

- **Lucca Summer Music Festival.** This takes place in July and attracts some big celebrity names. *See page 293*

- **Puccini Festival.** This celebration of Puccini's musical genius is held at the composer's villa on Lake Massaciuccoli. *See pages 151 and 291*

- **Luminaria di San Ranieri.** A lovely Pisan festival when thousands of candles light up the River Arno and celebrations are brought to a close with a boat race. *See pages 171 and 293*

- **Carnevale.** Viareggio's riotous carnival is a memorable experience and one of the best carnivals in all of Italy. *See page 294*

- **Estate Fiesolana.** This enjoyable music and arts festival held in Fiesole in the province of Florence is well worth catching. *See page 293*

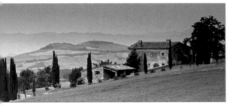

MONEY-SAVING TIPS

Travel by train: this is inexpensive and a lovely way of travelling between cities, but a car is essential for reaching most hill towns and exploring the countryside (www.trenitalia.com).

Bicycle hire: in city centres such as Florence (www.florencebybike.it, from €8 for 5 hours); Lucca (www.puntobici.lucca.it, from €7.50 for 3 hours); and Pisa (www.pisacruiserbiketours.com, bike or Segway in Pisa or Florence).

Museum cards: the new **Firenze Card** (www.firenzecard.it) costs €50 for 3 days and includes all Florence public transport (www.ataf.it) and 33 museums, including all booking reservations. It can be booked online or bought at six places in the city.

Friends of the Uffizi Card: it offers unlimited access for one calendar year to Florence's state museums (including the Uffizi and the Accademia) and costs only €100 for a family of four, or €60 for adults (www.amici degliuffizi.org).

Uffizi booking: avoid the queues by booking directly, cheapest through the Uffizi (www.uffizi.com), from €20 per person, but the ticket (not the booking slot) is free to EU citizens over 65 or under 18.

Designer outlets: save money at Tuscany's outlets, with free shuttle services from your Florence hotel to **The Mall** (www.themall.it) or a fare-paying service to **Barberino Designer Outlet** (30km/18.5 miles away) from the Fortezza da Basso in Florence.

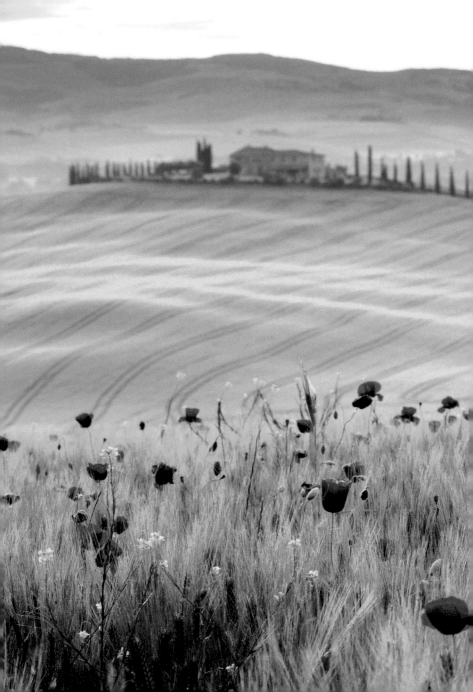

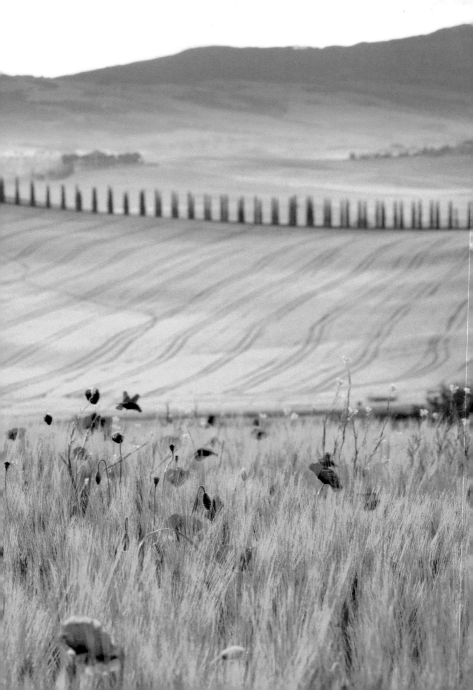

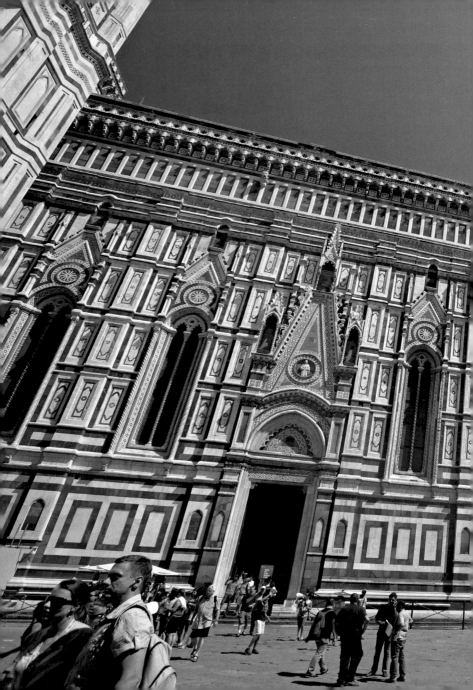

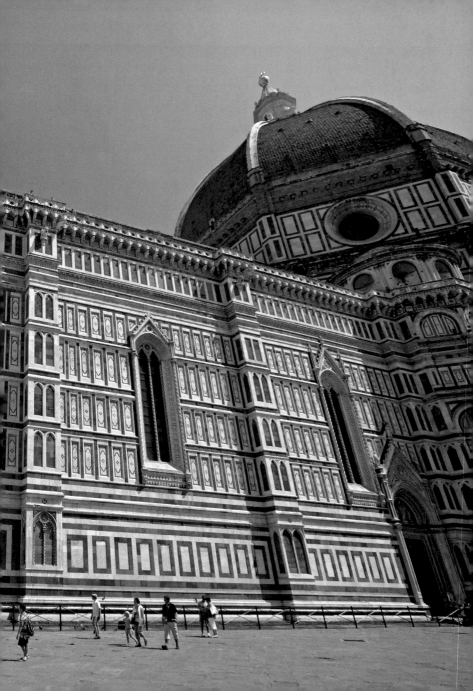

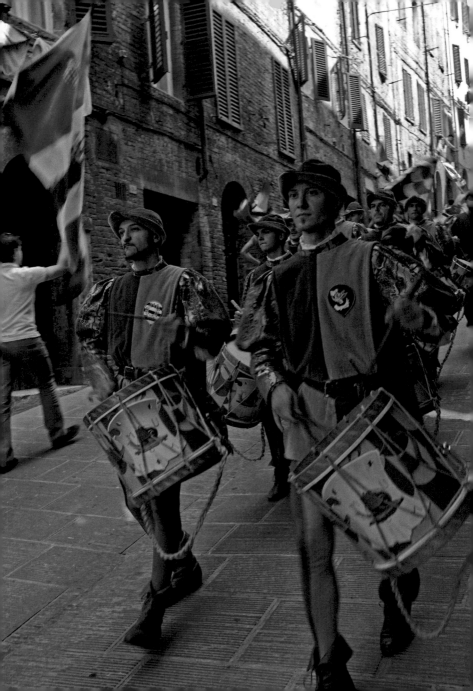

THE TUSCAN MIRACLE

**Birthplace of the Renaissance, a strong tradition of
village life, picturesque countryside: these factors
and more contribute to the enigma that is Tuscany**

From the top of a village tower, the Tuscan landscape lies below: the most civilised rural scene on Earth. Yet driving through southern Tuscany at night, there is little sense of civilisation, still less of domesticity – even farm animals are kept indoors. In the distance, a succession of small lights trails across the black countryside: tenuous links with separate inward-looking communities. The spaces in between are remote, uncivilised. The blackness and emptiness of the countryside go back to medieval times and beyond; the "Tuscan Miracle" only illuminates the cities, leaving the gaps unfilled.

In giving birth to the Renaissance, Tuscany designed the modern world. In his paintings, Giotto projected Tuscany into space. Brunelleschi crowned space with his Florentine dome, the greatest feat of Renaissance engineering. In the Carmine frescoes, Masaccio peopled space with recognisably human figures. His *Expulsion from Paradise* reveals Adam and Eve in all their naked beauty. Gone is the medieval coyness; present is the palpable suffering of a couple who have lost everything.

The Tuscan miracle, however, is not a frozen Renaissance portrait but a living procession of Tuscans completely at ease with their artistic setting and identity. Tuscans do possess an innate aesthetic sense but the Tuscan tapestry is a rich weave that has been created by many different threads. Literary Tuscany is a strand that can be clearly traced through Boccaccio, Petrarch and Dante. Republican Tuscany is best glimpsed through its fortified town halls, while humanist Tuscany is enshrined in poetry, sculpture and art, the fruits of patronage and craftsmanship. Aristocratic Tuscany still lingers in Medici palaces, villas and sculptured gardens, as well as the ancestral homes of the Rucellai, Corsini and Frescobaldi. Bourgeois Tuscany parades along Florence's Via Tornabuoni, patronises the arts and restores family farms. Peasant Tuscany traditionally takes a little of everything from the land: game, beans, chestnut flour, unsalted bread, olive oil and, of course, the grapes needed to make Chianti and Brunello. Tuscan cuisine combines proportion and variety to produce delicious, hearty fare. Like the Tuscans themselves, it is of good peasant stock. ❏

PRECEDING PAGES: the beautiful Val d'Orcia landscape; the Duomo in Florence, built with different-coloured marble and topped by Brunelleschi's famous dome. **LEFT:** a parade during the Palio in Siena.

TUSCANY TODAY

Despite the region's resounding popularity, Tuscany is not succumbing to "Disneyfication" – and a new environmental awareness means that the lifestyle is more seductive than ever

It's a travesty to equate Tuscany to "Chianti-shire", a parody of an English country-house party transposed to Italy. It is also misleading to reduce the region to Renaissance art, Florentine architecture and Chianti vineyards. The Tuscan landscape is as beautiful as the art. The soothing scenery, dotted with hill towns, inspired the Renaissance masters and nurtured a lifestyle with timeless appeal. This rose-tinted Tuscan lifestyle is arguably now the greatest lure, with villa-living or farm-stays the ideal way of living the dream. The Tuscans seem to have found a perfect balance between country and city living. And, as bedazzled fans, we come in search of the secret, as if it lay in the princely countryside, the pasta feasts and the pampering hot springs.

Pienza is perfect Tuscany. This tower-capped outpost overlooking sun-baked valleys is all an Italophile could wish for – so much so that this town of 2,300 has 100,000 visitors a year. In the rush to enjoy the rural idyll, we risk turning high-season Pienza into an elbow-to-elbow mêlée. And this is Tuscany's dilemma. Her beauty is in danger of becoming her beast. While Rome does government and Milan does commerce, La Toscana does cypress-lined rolling hills and the Renaissance. The region's wealth is her landscape and heritage, and the question for the future is how to preserve this while finding room for 10 million visitors a year.

The price of paradise

As Italy's most popular region, Tuscany's long-standing relationship with tourism is finely balanced. Pisa is grappling with the quick-fire habits of the tourist in search of little more than

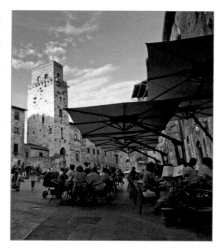

a snapshot of himself, arms askew, mimicking the Leaning Tower behind him. Florence is reeling. The city that caused Stendhal Syndrome – the dizzying disorientation some visitors experience when they overdose on Florentine Renaissance masterpieces – is in danger of sending tourists' heads spinning in front of the Uffizi Gallery.

While ostensibly true, this snapshot is still misleading and restricted to tourism "hotspots" such as the Leaning Tower, the great Florentine galleries and San Gimignano. Beyond these beautiful bottlenecks, Tuscany is as spacious yet enveloping as ever it was. Many evocative hamlets on Monte Amiata see far too few visitors, as do Maremma's Etruscan sites, wild Garfagnana and cities of the stature of Massa Marittima. But even just beyond San Gimignano's walls, you can still lose yourself on walks through epic countryside that has been cultivated since time immemorial.

Environmental factors and "Slow Travel"

Tuscany has also woken up to environmental issues, with classic hill towns, such as Montepulciano, closed to traffic, or partly pedestrianised, as is Siena. Florence is dabbling with trams to the suburbs and electric buses in the historic centre, with a futuristic Norman Foster-designed

the Val d'Orcia villages, Montepulciano, Pietrasanta, and the "tufa towns" (a type of local stone) around Pitigliano.

Such places embody the essence of "Slow Travel" – confident enough to be revitalised by tourism, careful not to be denatured by it. The secret of Tuscan identity lies in each town's sense of completeness. Tuscan towns go against the grain, shunning spurious modernity if it simply means homogeneity. Instead, without being fossilised, Florence is becoming more Florentine and Siena more Sienese. For a Tuscan, city life feels narrow but it is also invitingly deep. The watchwords are tradition, civility, good taste and a sense of ease with the past.

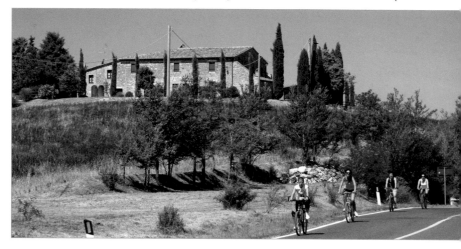

rail hub opening in 2014. And Tuscans, not just tourists, have taken to cycling, especially in Pisa, Lucca, the Chianti and the Versilia coast. Pisa currently boasts more pedestrians than cars, and more bicycles than motorcycles and mopeds. Despite traffic restrictions, cities such as Siena, Lucca and Massa Marittima are more liveable than ever, big enough to take tourism in their stride, but small enough for civic pride to define who they are. Equally harmonious are Volterra,

Left: dining alfresco in the Piazza Cisterna, in the popular medieval hilltop town of San Gimignano. **Above:** cycling through southern Siena – a fantastic way to see the stunning countryside.

The heritage scene

Temperamentally left-wing, Tuscans can be deeply conservative when it comes to heritage – and with good reason. Apart from being the cradle of the Renaissance, Tuscany boasts the most Unesco World Heritage Sites of any Italian region: from Florence, Siena, San Gimignano, Pisa and Pienza to the landscape and lifestyle of the Val d'Orcia. The Pisan Unesco site was expanded to embrace the cluster of sacred buildings on the Campo dei Miracoli beyond the legendary Leaning Tower.

Safe in its historical time capsule, Florence has often struggled to break free from its self-serving reputation as a museum-city, marooned in its glorious past. Recently, its sleepy attitude to culture post-Michelangelo has been shaken up by the success of the Palazzo Strozzi, which has put the city on the contemporary art map. The duality of the Tuscan temperament when it comes to heritage – conservatism with a dash of radicalism – is reflected in the Renaissance Palazzo Strozzi, and its contemporary-arts space, La Strozzina. The Establishment space can stage art blockbusters, leaving its cutting-edge sister to play with new trends and talents. As its director James Bradburne says: "Florence has a deep connection to its Renaissance past, but citizens have a right to have a place that feels like a city of today."

Reconciling the cultural past and present

Encouraged by a charismatic young mayor, Florence is experiencing a cultural revival. The Palazzo Vecchio stays open until midnight, and there is pressure on the more staid State-owned museums to follow suit. The greatest, the Uffizi Gallery, is being expanded and the city also has a new opera house and auditorium. In addition, former convents, a fortress, a station and even a prison have been converted into cultural centres, concert halls, libraries, galleries and venues for fashion shows, exhibitions and eclectic events. This new dynamism is not restricted to Florence. Prato's Pecci museum of contemporary

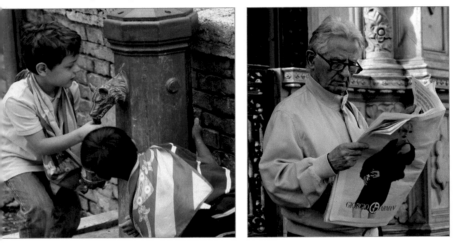

THE NEW MEDICI OF WINE

Many Tuscan wine estates are still the preserve of aristocrats who trace their lineage back to Medici Florence or beyond. The noble names include the Antinori (the largest family-run wine business in Italy), Frescobaldi and Ricasoli. But now the rock stars are moving in as the new Medici of wine.

In Tenuta degli Dei, flamboyant Florentine designer Roberto Cavalli creates Tuscan Merlots at his wine estate and stud farm in the heart of Chianti country (www.deglidei.it). Tuscan opera legend Andrea Bocelli also dabbles in wine-making, his greatest passion after music and horses. Sienese rock star Gianna Nannini crafts Sangiovese-style reds in a former monastery near Siena (www.certosadibelriguardo.

com). In gentleman-farmer mode, superstar Sting sells his wine, organic oil and honey on his Tenuta il Palagio retreat in Chiantishire. Bob Dylan quaffs his own Visions of J Montepulciano, named after an old Dylan hit. His wine maker, Antonio Terni, compares the Montepulciano grape to "a block of marble waiting to be turned into a statue".

Tuscan actors and artists are equally keen to till the soil. Actress Stefania Sandrelli produces genuine Chianti on her estate, and artist Sandro Chia makes award-winning Brunello. Castello Romitorio, Chia's 12th-century estate, is dotted with arresting artworks that would have caught the Medici eye. (www.castelloromitorio.com).

art is thriving, and an elite group of Tuscan arts festivals are gaining international recognition, from Florence's Maggio Fiorentino to Cortona's Tuscan Sun festival and Lucca's celebrity-studded summer music festival.

But there's no escaping the constraints of the 16th-century straitjacket. If the glory of Florence is that it contains the world's greatest concentration of Renaissance art and architecture, the price is responsibility to future generations, and perpetual restoration. Critic Mary McCarthy put the dilemma forcefully: "Historic Florence is an incubus on its present population. It is like a vast piece of family property whose upkeep is too much for the heirs, who nevertheless find themselves criticised by strangers for letting the old place go to rack and ruin."

Renovation and protection

Yet there is much to celebrate in the capital and in Tuscany as a whole. In Siena, the glorious pilgrims' hospital of Santa Maria della Scala has become a magnificent medieval museum. In Pisa, the (slightly straighter) Leaning Tower was finally unveiled in 2011. In the Maremma, Sovana's monumental Etruscan trails have recently been restored. A welcome trend in conservation is the return of artworks to the churches for which they were created. In Florence, Michelangelo's wooden Crucifix returned to Santo Spirito, as did Masaccio's fresco of the Trinity to Santa Maria Novella. More recently, a once-neglected Crucifix has been restored, declared a genuine Giotto, and returned in glory to its home in the Ognissanti church.

Even so, restoration is never-ending in Tuscany, with each project accompanied by public scrutiny from some of the most artistically aware citizens in Europe. In Piero della Francesca's superb fresco cycle in Arezzo, for instance, the restorers were accused of repainting rather than simply restoring. As for major sculpture, the threat of pollution means that "cloning" carries the day, with restored statues replaced by copies. In a sense, the pattern was set by the removal of Michelangelo's *David* to the Accademia. The cloning issue divides critics, with realists opting

for copies and romantics preferring the works to grow old gracefully, or disgracefully, in the place for which they were created. But given Florence's new environmental initiatives, more sculptures may well remain *in situ*.

Tuscans and their landscape

The counterpoint to the compact urban artistic heritage is the endless countryside. Etruscans cultivated it, Tuscans civilised it, and foreigners romanticised it. Tuscans still prefer living in large villages or small towns, echoing the Etruscan ideal, which was confirmed by the rural perils of medieval Europe. These deeply urban people cultivate a close relationship with the land, but

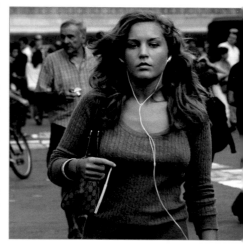

CHIANTISHIRE COMMUTERS

Peasant farmers could not believe their luck when crumbling, empty farmhouses began to be seen, in the 1960s, as an opportunity to create a rural idyll. A British presence in this revival gave birth to the nickname Chiantishire.

Tuscans often protest that the Chiantishire commuters have priced locals out of their native villages, but foreigners argue that they saved places such as Sovicille near Siena, or Bugnano near Lucca from total abandonment.

Agriturismo (farm-stays) helps to generate funds for further restoration. What's more, many foreign residents are now well integrated, as in the village of Barga, in Garfagnana, or in the marble-carving town of Pietrasanta.

FAR LEFT: young boys wearing the colours of their *contrade*, drinking from a fountain during the Palio, Siena. **LEFT:** reading a daily newspaper in Florence. **RIGHT:** young woman walking through Florence.

it is a wary bond that doesn't imply mastery. Even so, rural traditions have deep roots. Lucca's olive trees date back to Roman times, while the region's ancient vineyards are terraced on slopes that have been cultivated for centuries.

World War II shattered rural life in Tuscany – ending the feudal *mezzadria* system of land being governed by the wealthy nobility. With the ancient paternalistic social structure gone, thousands of farmers and villagers abandoned their homes and headed for the cities in search of jobs. Villages that had been the hub of rural life for thousands of years became ghost towns. Although the medieval *mezzadria* system of sharecropping (in which a landowner allows a tenant use of the land in return for a share of the crop produced) was banned in 1978, old traditions die hard. Apart from large wheat and cattle farms in the Val d'Arno and Val di Chiana, farming is mostly labour-intensive, under-mechanised and organic. Partly through poverty and tradition, Tuscany has gained a reputation as a leading region for small-scale sustainable farming.

The countryside revival

Even so, beyond the sought-after wine and oil estates, the countryside has been suffering from depopulation. The influx of the olive-nibbling classes has helped to reverse the trend, with tumbledown farmhouses being snapped up by

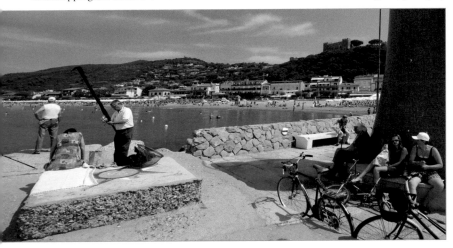

TUSCANY IN THE CINEMA

Tuscany is cinematic by nature, with its rolling hills and quaint villages perfect for expat dramas, from *Room with a View* (1985) to *Under the Tuscan Sun* (2003). Bernardo Bertolucci's *Stealing Beauty* (1996) plumped for Chiantishire, while Jane Campion's stylish *Portrait of a Lady* (1996) preferred the Lucca countryside. Franco Zeffirelli's semi-autobiographical *Tea with Mussolini* (1999) is set in wartime Florence, a period also perfectly evoked by Anthony Minghella's *The English Patient* (1996). In the last film, Piero della Francesca's frescoes in Arezzo's Basilica di San Francesco are revealed by flares to the enchanted Hanna (Juliette Binoche).

Tuscan film sets transcend period drama. Ridley Scott made his epic, *Gladiator* (2000), in lush Val d'Orcia, while *Hannibal* (2001) saw the charismatic psycopath lap up Florence, from the Ponte Vecchio to the Porcellino. More recently, Carrara's marble quarries saw action in *Quantum of Solace* (2008), with the film thundering to a climax during Siena's Palio horse race.

Artier films include Zeffirelli's Oscar-winning *Romeo and Juliet* (1968) and Tarkovsky's *Nostalgia* (1983), set in the mysterious spa pool at Bagno Vignone. And just when many feared that Tuscany had fallen out of favour with directors, along came *Twilight: New Moon* (2009) to seduce impressionable adolescents with vampires in Volterra.

the Chiantishire set *(see page 21)*. Villas, castles and fortified estates have been turned into sleek spa resorts *(see page 138)*. Semi-abandoned villages are being reborn as boutique retreats, as in the case of Il Borro, a resort restored by the Ferragamo family. Castelfalfi is the most ambitious rural resort, with a castle and cluster of hamlets developed by TUI, the huge German tour operator. When complete, the resort should house 3,000 guests in farmhouses, villas and apartments scattered throughout the estate. Critics mutter about "the German conquest", but the lovely village, with views towards Volterra, was previously abandoned. Other slumbering villages are being saved by novel local schemes.

mystery, its wild pine groves a reminder that Tuscany is blessed with more forest than any other region in Italy. These remote swathes are the riposte to those who decry Tuscan "Disneyfication". The same is true of the beaches, such as Marina di Pisa, Castiglione della Pescaia and the silver coast of Monte Argentario, which win Tuscany awards as one of the cleanest coastlines in Italy.

In Tuscany, quality of life is cultivated like an olive grove: few would jeopardise this heritage by turning to heavy industry. The industries Tuscans speak of with pride, such as Siena's *panforte*, Carrara's marble, Volterra's alabaster and Arezzo gold, date back to medieval times. In

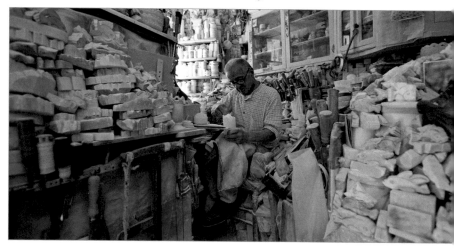

Pari, a depopulated village between Monte Amiata and Petriolo, is running a "reopen the shutters" project to win back young families, offering to pay their rent for three years. Proof, indeed, that tourism is not the only answer.

In fact, beyond the Florence–Siena axis, the effects of tourism fade away. Here another Tuscany emerges, in the Apuan Alps and Garfagnana, with their rugged mountains, plunging valleys and marble mines. And to the west, the Maremma is still imbued with a sense of

keeping with tradition, true Tuscans are provincial, conservative and independent; civic culture and rural pride are their touchstones. For all its Dantesque grandiloquence and Renaissance finery, Tuscany's heart is rural. Its largest city is home to less than half a million people, and the nickname for Tuscans is *"Mangiafagioli"* (bean eaters). So it is perhaps not surprising that the province's best-loved son comes from the Arezzo countryside. Italy's tragicomic clownprince – Oscar-winning actor Roberto Benigni – speaks lovingly of his homeland as "a region of hunters and hares, of large peasant women and wild and poetic beauty". And who would argue with Tuscany's *"grande Roberto"*? ❏

LEFT: enjoying the sun in Castiglione della Pescaia on the Maremma coast. **ABOVE:** alabaster craftsman working in Volterra.

DECISIVE DATES

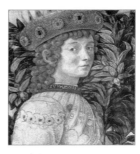

ETRUSCANS AND ROMANS

800–500 BC
Etruscan civilisation flourishes. Etruria Propria, a confederation of 12 states, includes Arezzo, Chiusi, Fiesole and Volterra.

480–290 BC
Romans annexe Etruria and found colonies at Ansedonia, Roselle, Volterra, Luni and Lucca.

80 BC
Faesulae (Fiesole) becomes a Roman military colony.

59 BC
Colony of Roman veterans founds Florentia (Florence) on the banks of the Arno.

AD 200–600
Region invaded by Lombards, Goths and Franks.

AD 306
Constantinople capital of Roman Empire; the Byzantine period follows.

AD 476
The Fall of Rome.

MEDIEVAL TUSCANY

1000–1300
Germans conquer Italy; warring between Guelfs (supporters of papacy) and Ghibellines (supporters of Holy Roman Empire).

1062
Pisa triumphs over Saracens in battle off Palermo.

1115
Florence becomes an independent city governed by a mercantile-class council.

1118
Pisa Cathedral consecrated.

1125
Florence begins expansion with takeover of Fiesole.

1173
Bonnano Pisano begins Pisa's Leaning Tower.

1246–50
Work on Florence's Santa Maria Novella begins and Bargello built.

1260
Sienese defeat the Florentines in battle of Montaperti.

1294
Arnolfo di Cambio begins Florence's Santa Croce.

1296
Di Cambio begins Florence's Duomo.

1310
Siena's Palazzo Pubblico is completed.

1314
Dante Alighieri begins *The Divine Comedy*.

1334
Giotto begins Florence's Campanile.

c.1345
Florence's Ponte Vecchio is erected by Taddeo Gaddi.

1348
Black Death hits Florence, killing a third of population.

1390
John Hawkwood becomes Captain General of Florence; inter-city wars.

THE RENAISSANCE

1406
Pisa is defeated, becoming part of Florentine state.

1420
Papacy returns to Rome.

1434–64
Cosimo de' Medici rules Florence.

1436
Brunelleschi completes dome for Florence's Duomo.

1452
Alberti's *Ten Books on Architecture* is published.

1469–92
Lorenzo de' Medici rules Florence.

1478
Sandro Botticelli paints *La Primavera*.

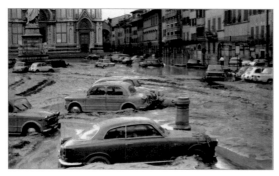

1498
"Mad monk" Savonarola hanged for heresy in Florence's Piazza della Signoria.

1504
Michelangelo completes *David*.

1513
Niccolò Machiavelli writes *The Prince*.

1527
The Sack of Rome.

1530
Republic of Florence ends as armies of Pope Clement VII and Emperor Charles V besiege the city.

1550
Giorgio Vasari's *Lives of the Artists* first published.

1554
Siena is defeated, becoming part of Florentine state.

1564–1642
Galileo Galilei discovers the principles of dynamics.

LEFT: Lorenzo de' Medici. ABOVE: debris from the 1966 flood outside Santa Croce, Florence.

GRAND DUCHY TUSCANY
1716
Grand Duke establishes Chianti wine laws.

1737
Gian Gastone, the last male Medici, dies.

1796
Napoleon's first Italian campaign.

1815
Grand Duchy absorbed into the Austrian Empire.

MODERN TUSCANY
1848
The War of Independence.

1861
Kingdom of Italy proclaimed.

1865–71
Florence capital of Italy.

1915
Italy enters World War I on the Allies' side.

1922
Benito Mussolini elected.

1940
Italy enters World War II against Allies.

1945
Mussolini executed.

1946
Italy becomes a republic.

1957
The Treaty of Rome; Italy a founder member of EEC (now EU).

1966
Massive flooding in Florence – artworks damaged.

1993
Mafia bomb kills five and damages Uffizi, Florence.

1994
Right-wing government ushers in Second Republic. Silvio Berlusconi elected premier.

2001
Silvio Berlusconi elected premier of coalition.

2004
Val d'Orcia declared Unesco World Heritage Site.

2005
Pope John Paul II dies, succeeded by Benedict XVI.

2008
Berlusconi elected prime minister for the third time.

2009
Left-leaning Matteo Renzi elected Mayor of Florence, Italy's youngest mayor.

2011
Restoration on Pisa's Leaning Tower ends after 20 years of work. Oldest-ever Etruscan necropolis found near Livorno.

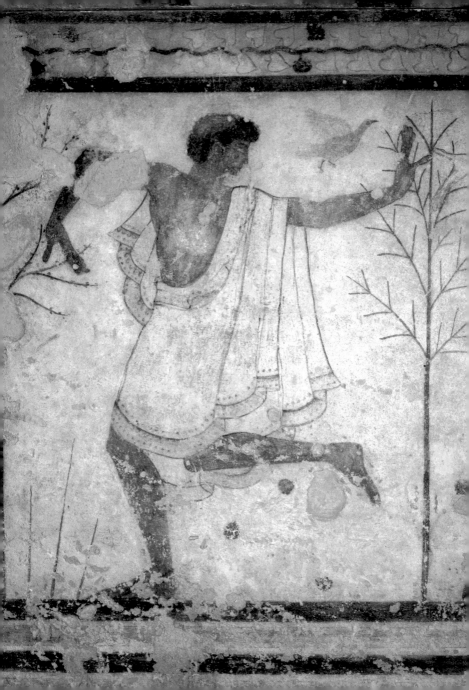

THE ETRUSCANS

Long before the Romans left their mark on the landscape, the Etruscan people established their own sense of regional identity, humanistic values and peaceful society in Tuscany

The story of Tuscany begins with the Etruscans, its earliest known inhabitants, whose origins are shrouded in myth and mystery. The Romantics and latter-day writers believed that the Etruscans sailed from Asia Minor. However, Dionysius, writing as the Etruscan civilisation neared its end, held that the Etruscans were natives with an indigenous culture too deeply ingrained to be oriental. Most modern scholars believe that the Etruscans migrated from Eastern Europe over the Alps and represent the flowering of the early Italic tribes. What is clear is that between the 8th and 4th centuries BC, "Etruria Propria" flourished as a confederation of 12 city-states in central Italy.

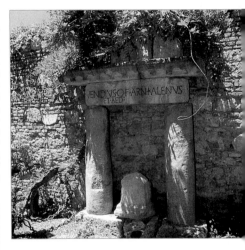

Northern Etruria, roughly equivalent to modern Tuscany, included Arezzo, Chiusi, Cortona, Populonia, Vetulonia and Volterra.

Etruscan seafarers and merchants first settled on the coast and began smelting iron ore from Elba and importing oriental ceramics, glass and silverware. Greek naval supremacy meant an opening to Hellenistic culture: ships sailed to Corinth with honey, gold and bronze figurines, and returned to Vetulonia and Populonia with perfume and painted wine jars. The inland cities such as Chiusi

LEFT: detail from Tomba del Triclinio, Monterezzi Necropolis, Tarquinia. **RIGHT:** part of the fortification wall at Chiusi, one of Tuscany's major Etruscan sites.

and Volterra thrived on hunting, farming and trade. Over the next two centuries, the Etruscans allied themselves to the developing Roman power, and by the 1st century BC, all Etruscan territory was annexed. Although Etruscan and Latin co-existed, Etruscan culture was crushed; its role degenerated into the provision of soothsayers, musicians, dancers and fighters for Rome.

Etruscan society

The original confederation had a complex urban and social structure: each city was originally run by a king, later by local aristocrats, and finally by a priestly oligarchy. The lords owned large land-holdings or navies and were served by serfs and slaves. Whereas the serfs were rewarded with agricultural plots, the slaves danced and sang for their supper. With urbanisation, an independent class of artisans and merchants began to emerge. The granting of the same Roman citizenship to the middle classes as to the aristocratic priests and magistrates was a severe blow to the Etruscan princely tradition.

The Etruscans were expert builders. Their cities followed the contours of the land and sited the necropolis below the city walls and the living city above. If cities of the dead predominate today, it is by accident and not by design. Public buildings, constructed of wood and clay, did not survive. From what remains of the cities, there was enough to impress Roman and Renaissance architects. Volterra's Porta all'Arco, a deep gateway inspired by Mesopotamian architecture; the huge drystone walls at Saturnia, rebuilt to defend the city against Roman incursions; the neat town plans of Pitigliano and Sovana – all these scattered remains are evidence of the vitality and ingenuity of Etruscan builders.

New discoveries of Etruscan artefacts continue to be made around the region. Recently, east of Livorno, archaeologists unearthed a 3,000-year-old necropolis, dating from the end

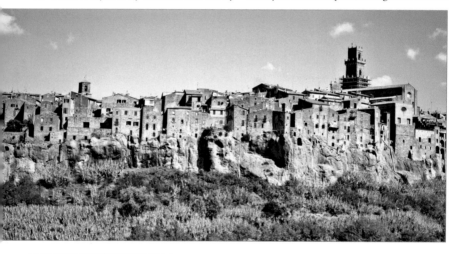

BEST ETRUSCAN SITES

Scrape the surface of the most enigmatic Tuscan towns and an Etruscan spirit lies beneath, with temple walls recycled into Roman buildings, or ancient epigraphs encrusted within Renaissance palaces.

In Volterra, the Porta all'Arco Etrusco reveals a Roman arched vault, incorporating three Etruscan basalt heads, on massive Etruscan bases. The superb Etruscan Museum displays *The Shadow of the Evening* sculpture. Although over 2,000 years old, this bronze figure seems modern in both message and design. Florence's Archaeological Museum boasts the reconstructed Inghirammi Tomb, a semicircular Etruscan tomb from Volterra. Finer still is the museum's

bronze *Chimera* from Arezzo.

Chiusi has one of the best museums, stuffed with *bucchero* ware and Canopic urns, cinerary urns with an idealised effigy of the deceased on the lid. The only painted tombs in Tuscany are here, along with underground galleries and a mysterious labyrinth that reputedly conceals the sarcophagus of Lars Porsenna, mythical king of the Etruscans.

In the Maremma area, Sovana is riddled with deep, ravine-like Etruscan roads and "pigeonhole" tombs, niches cut into the rock. In Vetulonia, the remote, rural setting contrasts with tangible proof that this was once one of the richest cities in Etruria.

of the Bronze Age, and the oldest Etruscan site ever found. To trump that, a Palaeolithic man, Tuscany's oldest *Homo sapiens*, was found in Monteriggioni in 2011. In Sesto Fiorentino, outside Florence, the Etruscan Tomb of La Montagnola has recently been opened, with its impressive secret vaulted corridor and noble burial chamber.

Etruscan art

Fascinating tombs, in every shape and form, can be seen in the Etruscan necropolises: "temple" tombs at Saturnia; melon-shaped tombs at Cortona; oriental "trench" tombs at Vetulonia. It is the tombs that remain as a cultural

Greek myths. The women were depicted as pale, while the men were uniformly reddish-brown, either suntanned or ritually painted. Friezes of serene married couples, tender lovers, absorbed wrestlers, erotic dancers or grieving warriors reflect the fullness and variety of Etruscan life.

Noblewomen had freedom, influence and social status. They are frequently depicted attending banquets without their husbands, riding covered wagons to their land-holdings and playing flutes or lyres at funerals. The men are rarely still: they charge through games, boar-hunts, processions, journeys, dances, banquets and diving competitions. The "ordinary"

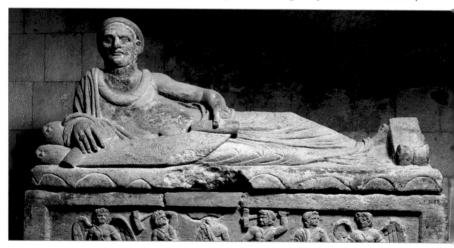

testimony to the power, wealth and beliefs of their owners. Death reflected life: the poor were often buried in shallow graves or their ashes put in small urns; the rich were buried in chamber tombs and stone sarcophagi decorated with pottery.

Since there is no extant Etruscan literature, our knowledge of the living Etruscans is oddly dependent on a reading of this funerary art for clues. We know them as they would like to be known, these idealised aristocrats elevated by

LEFT: the town of Pitigliano, inhabited during Etruscan times. **ABOVE:** sarcophagus dating from the 2nd century BC, Tarquinia.

Etruscan is only glimpsed in passing: a prized blonde courtesan flits past dancing slaves; a serf mourns his dead master.

The Roman legacy

Rome annexed Etruria in 351 BC, and, from the 3rd until the 2nd century BC, as part of the massive road-building programme that was to transform the entire country, four great Roman roads were built across the territory: the Via Aurelia, which ran up the western seaboard to Pisae and the naval base at Genua in Liguria; the Via Clodia, which stopped at Saturnia; the Via Cassia, built in 154 BC to connect Rome with Florentia; and the Via Flaminia, built in

Roman Tuscany

Apart from the roads, the Romans' greatest legacy is their template for the classic town plan, with the forum – evolving into the piazza – the focal point

It's hard to imagine the impact that Roman roads, giant engineering projects, must have had on the colonised Etruscans, as regimented teams spanned rivers with elegant stone bridges,

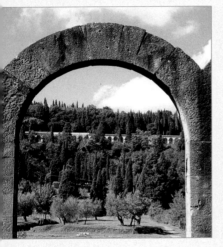

built drains to prevent their new roads from flooding, and at times even cut through the hills themselves.

Detective work is necessary to unearth Roman Florence, Florentia; the Roman gridiron street plan is clearly visible in maps, with the Piazza della Repubblica following the outline of the old *castrum*. Nearby, Fiesole, which possibly dates from the 8th century BC, was an Etruscan settlement but, as Faesulae, became a Roman military colony from 80 BC and later became the capital of Roman Etruria. The Piazza Mino da Fiesole occupies the site of the Roman forum. The archaeological site, set on a hillside near the Duomo, features a remarkably well-preserved Roman theatre, still used for performances. Beyond are Roman baths, and on the far side, the ruins of a Roman temple, both 1st century BC, as well as a 3rd century BC Etruscan temple, set against the Etruscan city walls.

In Lucca, the original street plan is also still evident. Lucca began as a military colony in 178 BC and featured a 10,000-seat amphitheatre, outside the walls. In time, it was largely dismantled, and most of its remains are below street level. During the Middle Ages, however, houses were built using the remaining walls of the amphitheatre, thus fossilising its outline and four main entrances. Fragments of it are still visible from the surrounding lanes, incorporated in the outer walls of the houses. Volterra, which became an important Roman municipality in the 4th century BC, also recycled its history, as well as retaining the ruins of the 1st century BC Roman theatre beyond the city walls.

Luni, called Luna by the Romans, was founded in 177 BC and was the springboard for the conquest of the Ligurian tribes. The Roman city, its forum, a number of houses and its amphitheatre have been excavated.

Another extensively excavated site is at Roselle, the Roman Rusellae. Originally an island, the Etruscan city was taken by Rome early in the 3rd century BC. The ruins are satisfyingly complete, with Romano-Etruscan walls, a Roman forum, paved streets, basilicas, villas, amphitheatre and baths.

Ansedonia, the Roman Cosa, was founded as a Roman colony in 273 BC. The ancient hilltop city has been excavated, and the site contains the ruins of a main street, forum, walled acropolis and the *capitolium* – a tripartite sanctuary for the triad of Jupiter, Juno and Minerva. The city's 1.5km (1-mile) wall is virtually intact, as are many of its 18 guard towers. The site is overgrown, and many of the ruins are covered in brambles, creating a beguilingly elegiac mood. ❑

LEFT: view from the Teatro Romano, Fiesole.

220 BC to connect Rome to Umbria and the Adriatic Sea.

Etruscan roads were all designed to connect the interior with the coast, whereas Roman roads all led to Rome, thus the axis was turned 90°, from east–west to north–south. The more impressive new Roman roads purposely avoided the great Etruscan cities, which slowly fell into decline, whereas the new Roman cities such as Pistoriae (Pistoia), now better connected, grew in importance.

New colonies were founded at Ansedonia, Fiesole, Roselle, Populonia, Volterra, Luni and Lucca. The cultural identity of the Etruscans was gradually absorbed into that of the

of gods and competent soothsayers, the Etruscans also added a set of religious, humanistic and regional values that far outlived the Roman Empire itself. But by creating the roads and major cities of Tuscany, the Romans also left a permanent imprint on this part of the Italian landscape.

A millennium later, the ruins of their great bridges, amphitheatres and city walls were the inspiration for the next great blossoming of Italian culture: Tuscany's coming of age, the Renaissance. The art critic John Ruskin even saw an unbroken line of tradition from the tomb paintings of the Etruscans to Giotto and Fra Angelico. ❏

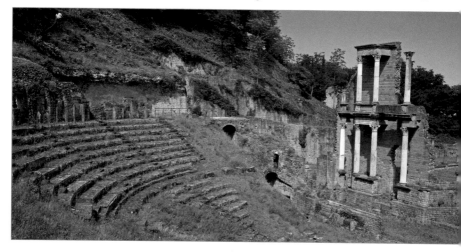

Romans, a process that was accelerated in 91 BC when Roman citizenship was extended to the Etruscans.

The Romans learnt many things from the Etruscans – principally, the Tuscan arch, which they developed as a key element in their extraordinary aqueducts, bridges and buildings, relegating the classical columns of Greece to a more decorative role in their architecture.

Certainly, the Etruscan influence on the Romans was considerable. Apart from introducing to Rome the purple toga, an abundance

ABOVE: the remains of the Roman theatre in Volterra.

MYSTERY LANGUAGE

The Etruscan language may be as mysterious as the people's origins, but its unintelligibility is still part of a glamorous myth. Although the alphabet is borrowed from Greek, the language, read from left to right, belongs to no known linguistic group. True, there are no external keys such as dictionaries or bilingual texts, but the core grammatical and phonetic structure is known, and, by deduction, most of the 10,000 shorter texts can be read accurately. These elusive texts are mostly funerary inscriptions and religious dedications as there is no extant literature. The one known book, a priest's manual discovered wrapped around an Egyptian mummy, has still only been partially deciphered.

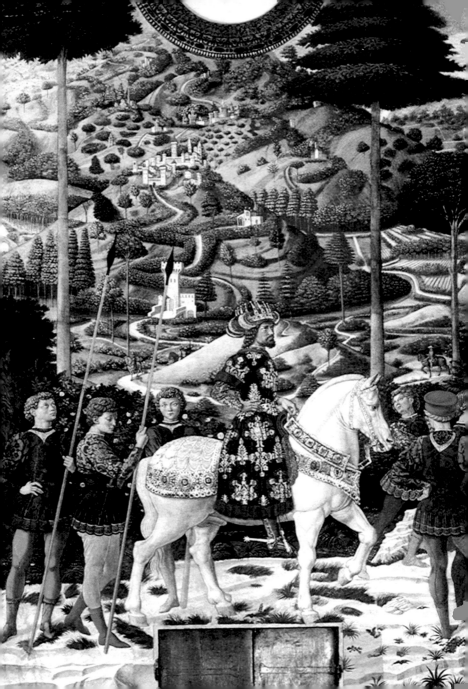

THE RENAISSANCE AND THE MEDICI

From feuding factionalism to the rise of the Medici, the aspirations of small city-states to remain independent were often dashed – but wealth, power and patronage still fostered an artistic flowering

Between the ending of the Roman Empire in the 5th century AD and the beginning of the foreign invasions in the 16th century, the story of Italy is a catalogue of conflict between its cities, each of which was a sovereign state. In Tuscany, a three-way battle was conducted between Florence, Pisa and Siena.

The *condottieri*

In the early stages, the battles between the city-states were conducted by the citizens themselves, but when Florence crushed Arezzo in 1289 at Campaldino, the bloodshed was so great that thereafter the cities began to fight out their differences with mercenaries, the *condottieri*.

Throughout the 14th century, the *condottieri* held the balance of power. Commanding companies numbering thousands of men, they sold their services to the highest bidder. The city that could afford them – and control them – dominated its neighbours. Few could control them, however, and that is why the *condottieri* system failed. The *condottieri* had a vested interest in conflict: from being paid to fight on behalf of a city, it was a short step to blackmailing that same city into paying you not to attack them.

Some *condottieri* were bought off – Sir John Hawkwood, the piratical leader of the much-feared White Company, was given a palatial villa and a substantial estate as his reward for retiring gracefully from the fray. Hawkwood craved

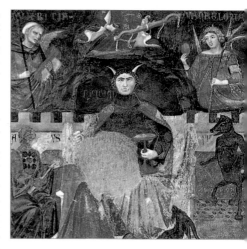

immortality and wanted an equestrian statue to be erected in Florence – instead, the miserly Florentines opted for the less expensive solution of an illusionistic fresco, painted by Paolo Uccello to look like a statue, in Florence Cathedral.

The burden of paying the *condottieri* fell to the merchant class. They were caught on the horns of a dilemma, desiring domination over their trade rivals, and yet aware of the high cost of war, in terms of both taxes and economic instability. When they waged war on neighbouring cities, they often did so in the name of "Guelf" or "Ghibelline" partisanship. The Guelfs were broadly made up of the rising merchant class, bankers and members of the trades

LEFT: *Procession of the Magus Balthasar* (fresco from the Magi Chapel of the Palazzo Medici Riccardi) by Benozzo Gozzoli (c. 1420–97). **RIGHT:** detail from Ambrogio Lorenzetti's *Effects of Good and Bad Government* (1338).

guilds, who nominally supported the papacy in its long battle against the Holy Roman Emperor, and who wanted a greater role in city government. Conversely, the Ghibellines, the old feudal aristocracy, supported the emperor, because he seemed the best guarantor of their virtual autocracy. Since the emperor was often German or Spanish and an absentee ruler, paying nominal allegiance to such a distant figurehead was far preferable to the threat of the pope exercising real and temporal power much closer to home.

Outside Tuscany, many city-states fell under the dominion of a single ruler – some of them former *condottieri* who ended up rulers of the cities they once protected, founding dynasties. The Tuscan city-states and republics maintained their independence far longer, but eventually even they fell to a dynastic power, as the Medici transformed themselves from private citizens to grand dukes.

The rise of the Medici

Ruefully reflecting on the mistakes that had led him to be imprisoned and tortured before being cast from office, Niccolò Machiavelli, former Chancellor of Florence, wrote his masterpiece *The Prince*, in which he admiringly recounted the ruthless methods used by the Medici to claw their way to absolute power in

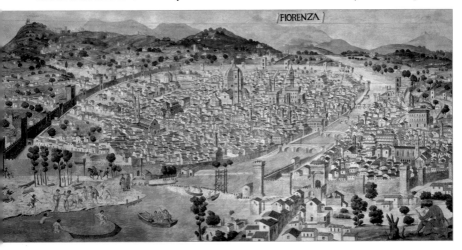

DANTE'S FLORENCE

In the medieval heart of Florence, an unassuming tower-house is reputedly the birthplace of Dante Alighieri (1265-1321), Italy's most revered poet. His epic poem, *The Divine Comedy*, set the Tuscan dialect as the model for Italian literature. The Casa di Dante is an evocation of Dante's Florence rather than an attempt to explore the poet's genius.

As a citizen of Florence, Dante's horizons embraced the Bargello, the Baptistry and the Badia Fiorentina. The museum presents the Guelf-Ghibelline political struggles, including family crests and battle maps. Unjustly cast into exile after disputes within the Guelf faction, Dante declared himself "a Florentine by birth but not by character". The poet died in exile in Ravenna, but his native city belatedly redeemed itself with a Dante memorial in Santa Croce.

On display in the poet's home is a copy of Henry Holliday's Pre-Raphaelite painting, *The Meeting of Dante and Beatrice*, alluding to the doomed infatuation that inspired much of the poet's work. The earliest-known portrait of Dante was recently discovered in the medieval meeting hall of the Magistrates Guild. Now both a moody museum and restaurant, Alle Murate reveals portraits of other Florentine legends, including Petrarch and Boccaccio. (Alle Murate: 6 Via del Proconsolo, Florence; www.allemurate.it. Casa di Dante: Via Santa Margherita, Florence; www.casadidante.it).

"Whoever desires to found a state and give it laws must start with assuming that all men are bad and ever ready to display their vicious nature whenever they may find occasion for it." (Niccolò Machiavelli)

Tuscany. Even more remarkable is the way that the dynasty threw up gifted individuals, generation after generation. The Medici were masters of realpolitik and military strategy but also patronised the arts, helping to make Florence and Tuscany the engine of cultural regeneration that we know as the Renaissance.

The man who laid the foundations for the family's meteoric rise was Giovanni de' Medici (1360–1429), founder of the Medici bank. This was just one of 100 or so financial institutions in 15th-century Florence, but Giovanni's masterstroke was to develop a special relationship with the Church, eventually securing a monopoly over the collection of the papal revenues.

Giovanni's son, Cosimo, developed this relationship still further: one of his great coups was to attract the prestigious General Council of the Greek Orthodox and the Roman Catholic churches to Florence. These two great Christian churches had been at loggerheads for six centuries. Their assemblies in Florence were intended to find ways of burying their differences and creating a unified Christian church. This they failed to do, but the meetings had a lasting impact on Florence. Not only did they create a stimulating climate of theological and intellectual debate, out of which the Renaissance was to grow, but also they fuelled artistic debate. The pomp and pageantry of the papal entourage, and the flamboyance of its Greek counterparts, provided artists with an array of exotica.

Cosimo himself eschewed such riches. He took pride in simplicity, ordering Brunelleschi, the temperamental genius behind the dome of Florence Cathedral, to modify his designs for the Medici palace, as they were too ostentatious. More to his taste was Michelozzo, who designed the marvellously airy library in San Marco, Flor-

ence, as a repository for the Medici book collection, the world's first-ever public library. Such generosity was typical of Cosimo, who spent a fortune endowing Florence with public buildings. Among his friends he counted humanists who shared his thirst for classical knowledge, for this was an era in which the lost classics of Greece and Rome, including works by Plato and Cicero, were being rediscovered.

Though a devout Christian who regularly retreated to his private cell at San Marco, Cosimo believed strongly that God's grace was best leavened by human reason. This made him an effective and humane ruler – even if, following his father's advice to "keep out of the public eye",

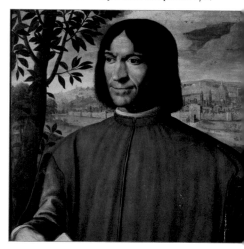

GOOD AND BAD GOVERNMENT

In Siena's Palazzo Pubblico, Lorenzetti's great frescoes, *The Effects of Good and Bad Government*, served as a lesson to the city's medieval rulers. *Bad Government* depicts a countryside ravaged by bandits, with fields left uncultivated, churches in ruin, and women raped in broad daylight. By contrast, *Good Government* depicts a city-state populated by peaceable citizens, attentive students and prosperous merchants. The message was not lost on the city rulers or the citizens. The adjoining room is dominated by a portrait of Guidoriccio da Fogliano in ceremonial battledress. As the city's *condottiero*, he was responsible for delivering the peace that underpinned the Sienese social order.

LEFT: the map known as the *Carta della Catena* showing Florence around 1470. RIGHT: a portrait of Lorenzo de' Medici.

Cosimo never sought public office. Instead, he wielded immense influence behind the scenes.

Lorenzo de' Medici inherited his father's love of the classical philosophers, and his gift for diplomacy. An outstanding poet in his own right, he promoted the study of Dante in Tuscan universities, elevating the Tuscan dialect to equal status with Latin. His greatest gift was peace. By using his diplomatic gifts to hold the great rival powers of the papacy and the Holy Roman Empire apart, Tuscany enjoyed a period of relative prosperity, in which merchants thrived and great fortunes were made. With the countryside no longer ravaged by war or held to ransom by lawless mercenaries, wealthy

Michelangelo had carved his *David*, the boy hero standing up to the bullying giant Goliath, as a symbol of the city's desire to rid itself of the Medici. He also fashioned new defences for the city, but when the combined forces of the Medici and the Holy Roman Emperor held the city to siege in 1530, he took himself off to hide – irony of ironies – in the Medici mortuary chapel, attached to San Lorenzo. Vasari attributes his cowardice to the artistic temperament, and while he was in hiding he worked the masterly reclining figures of *Dawn, Evening, Day* and *Night*, which now adorn the Medici tombs.

Alessandro de' Medici, who led the victorious siege, rubbed salt into the wounds of his

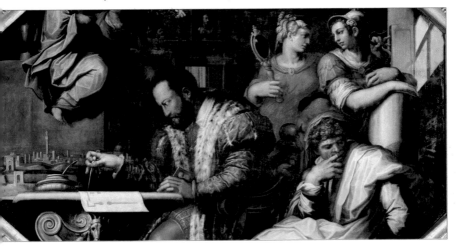

individuals began to build the villas that are still such a characteristic feature of the Tuscan countryside. Lorenzo himself led the way, staying regularly to his rural retreats at Fiesole and Poggio a Caiano.

The Medici lose support

Prophetically, Pope Innocent VIII declared that "the peace of Italy is at an end" on learning of Lorenzo's death in 1492. A period of turmoil ensued when Lorenzo's successors, who lacked the political acumen of their forebears, were expelled from the city and Savonarola, a firebrand preacher, took centre stage.

But the Medici swiftly returned in 1512.

Bonfire of the Vanities

From 1494, Girolamo Savonarola, a Dominican preacher, filled the Florentines with anti-Medici zeal. He argued that their fondness for pagan philosophers and the artistic depiction of heathen gods would bring God's wrath on the city. In 1497, erotic sculptures, fine clothes, secular poetry, mirrors and paintings were burnt in what Savonarola termed "the bonfire of the vanities". Even Botticelli supported the movement, renouncing his past attachment to humanist ideals, and turned to painting Christian allegories, such as *Nativity*. But the Florentines tired of their firebrand friar, and burnt him at the stake in Piazza della Signoria, on the very spot where his moral crusade had begun.

fellow citizens by having himself crowned Duke of Florence, claiming absolute power where his predecessors had been content with influence. When he was murdered in 1537 by his own cousin, with whom he had been having a homosexual affair, the city sought a successor. Cosimo, descended from Giovanni de' Medici via the female line, emerged victorious, partly by convincing his fellow citizens of his probity.

Once in power, Cosimo revealed his true colours, as he systematically set about destroying all opposition. Not only was he unrelenting in his pursuit of the republican leaders who had opposed his election, tracking them down in

security in the region, he also set up an effective civil service to administer the dukedom, based in the Uffizi (literally, the "Offices") in Florence. This proved effective right up to the point when Tuscany joined the United Kingdom of Italy in 1861. So effective was this civil service that Tuscany continued to be ruled effectively even when Cosimo's successors proved to be corrupt, incompetent, self-indulgent or mad. Few made a major mark on the city, though Cosimo II did the world a great favour by patronising Galileo, making him court mathematician to the Medici and providing him with a home after his trial and excommunication by the Inquisition.

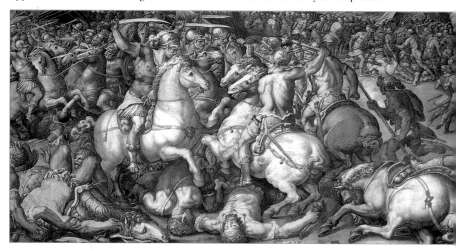

their exile and bringing them back to be tried and executed in Florence, he also set about conquering old enemies – Pisa, Siena, Massa Marittima, Montepulciano – with a ruthlessness and brutality that is still remembered and resented to this day. The whole story is told on the ceiling of the Palazzo Vecchio council chamber in a series of bloody frescoes painted by Vasari to honour Cosimo I in 1563–5.

To his credit, Cosimo not only forced Tuscany into political unity and established

The Medici art collection

The dynasty also amassed an astonishing art collection, which Princess Anna Maria Lodovica, the last of the Medici line, bequeathed to the city of Florence upon her death in 1743, along with all the Medici palaces and gardens, ensuring that many of the greatest works of the Renaissance were not sold off or dispersed, but would remain in the city that gave them birth. Today, these priceless works of art form the backbone of Florence's three main galleries: the Uffizi, the Pitti and the Bargello.

For more about Renaissance art and architecture, see pages 49–65. ❑

LEFT: painting depicting Cosimo I planning the conquest of Siena in 1555. ABOVE: detail from a painting by Vasari portraying Florence's victories over Pisa and Siena.

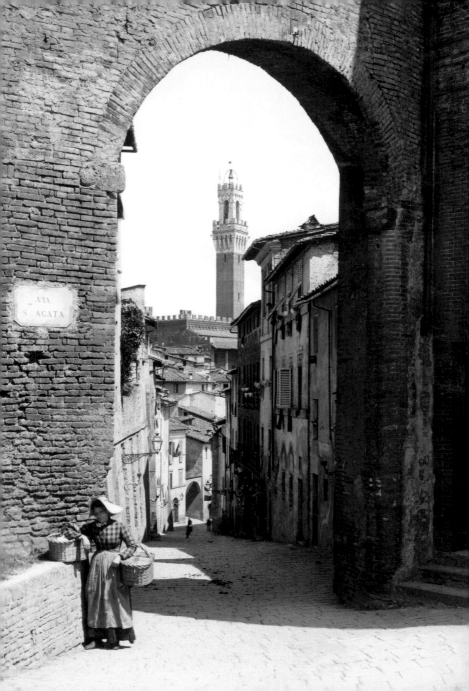

MODERN TUSCANY

After the Renaissance, Tuscany became an economic backwater. Italian Unification, international conflict and political corruption have all had an impact on modern Tuscany, and the "Tuscan model" is now often seen as a wise balance between prosperity and a peaceful pace of life

Since the glories of Rome and the Renaissance, Italy has written little history. The head of Italy's Bureau of Statistics likens modern Italian history to a muddle, "a happy antheap where everyone is running about and no one is in control". The alternative is the "strong man" view of recent history, as expressed in the Florentine saying, "Whose bread and cheese I eat, to his tune I dance". But, while Rome danced to martial music, Tuscany sometimes starved or burned.

Tuscany has been buffeted rather than enriched by its recent past. Well-kept war memorials in shabby towns attest to the loss of two generations, one abroad and one at home. Look at Asciano, a village dwarfed by its *carabinieri* stronghold, built by Benito Mussolini and still used to this day to maintain law and order. Visit Montisi where, for the price of a drink, locals will describe the German bombing of the village tower, a story complete with sound effects, gestures and genuine sorrow. Ask proud Florentines why the medieval houses on the south side of the Arno are lost for ever.

The effect of Italian Unification

In 1865, Florence briefly became the capital of the newly united Italy. Although its exalted role would only last five years before Rome was then made the permanent capital, Florence underwent profound and rapid change during this time. An ambitious plan of expansion

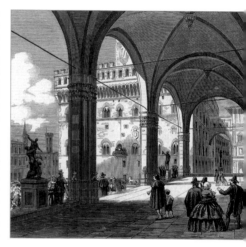

and modernisation sadly led to the demolition of, among other things, the old city walls, and their replacement with a wide ring of avenues punctuated with large piazzas in keeping with the French urban taste of the times. Quarters for the middle classes and the Piazzale Michelangelo were built. Later, old areas of the centre, including the Ghetto, were declared to be in dangerous condition and unwholesome, and were razed; the soulless Piazza della Repubblica was created partly in their place. The square remains a bold flourish of nationhood, but when the capital was transferred to Rome, Tuscan allegiance unquestionably remained in Tuscany. Unification, under the leadership of Count Camillo Benso Cavour,

LEFT: the Arch of Saint Joseph, Siena, in 1890. RIGHT: painting of 1860 depicting the event of Tuscany becoming part of a newly unified Italy.

a French-speaking Piedmontese, was seen as a foreign threat to the *de facto* sovereignty of Florence and the smaller city-states. Defenders of the Risorgimento, the movement for Italian unification, appealed to nascent patriotism. Critics of unification cited Dante's pleas to Tuscan liberty, before both sides settled down to start subverting the power of the new rulers. The merging of Tuscans into Italians started promisingly enough, but the end result is still only to be seen abroad or at international football matches.

World War I

Unification represented a missed chance for Italy. By failing to help shape a national identity,

Tuscans also fell victim to the clearer vision of a "strong man". Even before World War I, Mussolini was making inflammatory speeches while a weak parliament practised the art of "timely resignation", a ploy used ever since to stage-manage a new coalition.

Although the pre-war Tuscan economy thrived under weak government, it was no match for growing social pressures and a deepening gulf between society and state. With few real policies, one of the last liberal governments blundered into World War I. Italy's unpopular late entry into the conflict cost Tuscan lives and support. The pyrrhic victory was exacerbated by a power vacuum, economic problems and a revo-

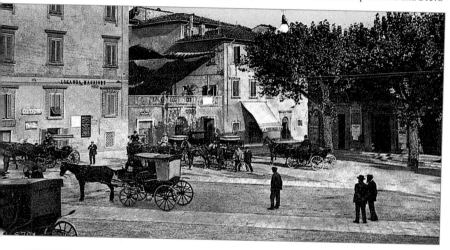

THE GROWTH OF THE GRAND TOUR

The most anglophone city in Italy, Florence has been a magnet for foreign visitors since the 17th century, when daring adventurers explored this strange land. By the 1700s, rich aristocrats were attracted to the region's alien psyche, perfect climate, low cost of living and undervalued art.

Florence became an essential stop on any European tour and, in the 18th century, the middle classes joined the aristocratic *dilettanti* and *literati* on the road to Tuscany. Art was on the agenda, with foreign visitors flocking to see the Uffizi sculptures and Botticelli's *Birth of Venus*. By the 1850s, visitors from Victorian England had made Florence *"une ville anglaise"*. "They toil not, neither do they spin"

was the cool judgement on his contemporaries by Irish novelist Charles Lever. Lever's biographer, William Fitzpatrick, damns the expatriate circle as "the society of diplomats and demireps, swells and snobs, princes and pretenders, wits and worthies, snarlers and social men".

By the 20th century, the Anglo-Florentine community was well established, though World War I chased many away. The Grand Tour resumed in the 1920s, mainly for society figures and intellectuals. The tradition continues today, with sons and daughters of the Establishment coming to learn Italian and attend art courses on the Renaissance – occasionally enjoying the designer labels rather than the artistic treasures.

lutionary working class. Benito Mussolini, from neighbouring Emilia, wasted no opportunity in claiming, "Governing Italy is not only impossible, it is useless", before proceeding to govern it impossibly but fairly usefully for 20 years.

By 1922, the corporate state was literally under construction. The economic benefits lasted until 1929, but the aesthetic effects linger on in functionally "improved" cities all over Tuscany. Florence railway station was the first Functionalist station in Italy.

World War II

At the outbreak of World War II, most Tuscans were cautiously neutral. Mussolini, despite hav-

the Resistance, it also harboured strong Fascist sympathisers. Even after the city was captured by the Allies, individual Fascists held out, firing from the rooftops. Surprising loyalties emerged: while the director of the British Institute was a known Fascist sympathiser, the German consul risked his life to protect Florentines who had been denounced. After the liberation he was granted the freedom of the city.

Florence was liberated in August 1943, but Mussolini and the German forces survived the winter behind the so-called "Gothic Line" in the Apennines. Apart from Florence, the partisans were very active in the Monte Amiata area, as well as in the Val d'Orcia, where the writer Iris

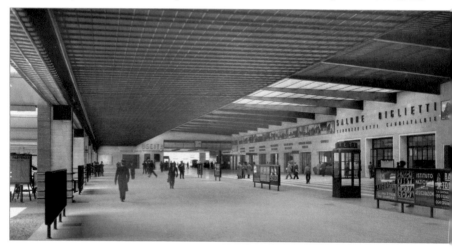

ing signed the Pact of Steel with Germany, only entered the war in 1940, after the fall of France. By 1943, the north was under German control, but the Allies were progressing northwards from Sicily. Allied bombing, German entrenchment and an emerging Tuscan Resistance transformed Tuscany into a battleground.

Anti-Fascist cells had been secretly set up by the Communists and Catholics in key towns under German and neo-Fascist control. Florence was split: while it was the intellectual centre of

LEFT: Montecatini in the early 1900s. **ABOVE:** Santa Maria Novella railway station in Florence, one of the key architectural works of Italian Modernism.

Origo, an Englishwoman married to an Italian *marchese*, sheltered many refugees and prisoners of war in her villa, La Foce.

Writing about it at the time, she observed: "In the last few days I have seen Radicofani and Cortignano destroyed, the countryside and farms studded with shell holes, girls raped, and human beings and cattle killed. Otherwise the events of the last week have had little effect upon either side; it is the civilians who have suffered."

Nor were the Allies completely blameless. The modernity of Grosseto, Livorno and Pisa today owes much to Allied bombing in 1943. The British War Office reports naturally exonerated the Allies: "No damage of any significance

Foreign Writers in Tuscany

Generations of enraptured writers have penned paeans to Tuscany, which often say more about themselves, and their romantic projections, than they do about Tuscany

Shelley pronounced Tuscany a "paradise of exiles" tempted by art, adventure and escape from persecution. But the exiles' motives were as varied as their prose styles. The Scottish

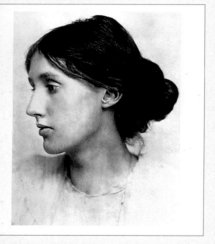

writer Tobias Smollett (1721–71) failed to appreciate the entrepreneurial nature of the Tuscan aristocracy, finding it undignified for "a noble to sell a pound of figs or to take money for a glass of sour wine". The Romantics were more enthusiastic. Lord Byron was "dazzled, drunk with Beauty" in Santa Croce. Shelley adored Pisan landscapes and Livornese seascapes, tragically drowning near La Spezia. Tuscany soon became a place of pilgrimage for the later Romantic poets, such as Tennyson and Wordsworth.

Although officially a diplomat in Florence, the French novelist Stendhal spent most of his time absorbing Renaissance frescoes and planning his novel, *Le Rouge et le noir* (1830). As with Byron, the Santa Croce Effect sent Stendhal reeling: "I walked in constant fear of falling to the ground." This aesthetic sickness is now known as Stendhal Syndrome.

Henry James was one of the few foreign writers able to see through Tuscany's literary and artistic veil, taking a more pragmatic approach. His *Portrait of Places* gives an opinionated but sensitive picture of the region in the 1870s.

The most romantic Victorian couple was undoubtedly the poets Elizabeth Barrett Browning and Robert Browning. Robert brought his wife to Florence because of her poor health. There he used Chianti to wean Elizabeth off her addiction to laudanum. Their 15th-century palazzo, redecorated in Victorian style, is now a museum.

The 20th century brought E.M. Forster, with his ironic analysis of the resident English community at play. Forster's *A Room with a View* portrays the heroine's encounter with an alien culture and alien passions. Virginia Woolf saw her own image reflected in the landscape, "infinite emptiness, loneliness, silence", while D.H. Lawrence, living in his "grave old Tuscan villa", imagined that he was communing with the original Etruscans.

World War II prevented further literary flowering, but in *War in Val d'Orcia*, Iris Origo, an Anglo-Florentine, painted a dramatic picture of the Tuscan battlefield. Soon after the war, the Welsh poet Dylan Thomas came to Tuscany and was entranced: "The pine hills are endless, the cypresses at the hilltop tell one all about the length of death, the woods are deep as love and full of goats." He apparently enjoyed a hedonistic lifestyle, vegetating in the sun and devouring strawberries and wine.

Tuscany still draws literary pilgrims. Frances Mayes' bestseller, *Under the Tuscan Sun*, brought a fresh wave of American tourists in search of the Tuscan dream. Her memoirs are only the latest in a long line of tributes penned by besotted foreigners. ❑

LEFT: Virginia Woolf saw "loneliness" in the landscape.

is attributable to Allied action [in Florence]." The Allies issued their troops with booklets listing various buildings to be protected, including the tricky prospect of safeguarding the "living museum" of Florence: "The whole city of Florence must rank as a work of art of the first importance." According to one report, "the great monuments, nearly all of which lie north of the river, escaped practically undamaged because, though the enemy held the northern bank against an advance, our troops deliberately refrained from firing upon them".

Despite Allied concern and care, Florence nevertheless lost innumerable bridges, streets, libraries, churches, palazzi, paintings and Tuscan

building exercise: "Without it [we] would surely have sunk into a morass of low politics and intrigues." That was still to come.

"Red belt" Tuscany

Tuscans may be conservative by nature, but they are also fiercely independent. Since World War II, they have tended to vote for right-wing governments nationally, but for left-wing councils locally. Until 1994, this meant Christian Democracy at national level and Communism at regional level. On the surface, this appeared a rather curious recipe for success.

Given the level of national opposition to Communists, the Communist Party evolved an

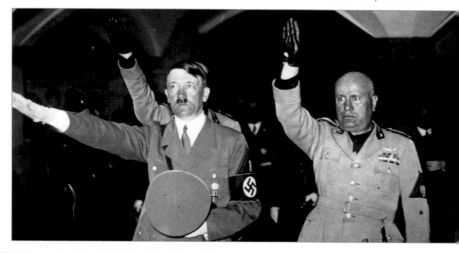

lives. But, in contrast to the "mutilated victory" of 1919, Italy lost the war but won the peace.

Massimo Salvatore, a supporter of the partisans in Florence, saw the war as a character-

Commendable feats of Allied bravery included the penetration of enemy lines via the Vasari Corridor, a secret route used by the Medici in similar crises.

ABOVE: Hitler and Mussolini salute at Florence's Tomb of the Fascist Martyrs.

aggressively pro-regionalist stance. The reward was the "red belt" across central Italy, run by left-wing coalitions since the first regional elections in 1970. Red Tuscany formed the central strand between Emilia Romagna's model economy and rural Umbria. Despite the transformations in the "new Italy", left-leaning Tuscany survives as one of the most efficient of regional governments.

The Tuscan left believes in a broad but increasingly secular Church. Civic culture, regional pride and fierce individualism form the real faith. The power of the left is as much a reflection of regional hostility to Roman centralisation as an espousal of social democratic principles. Even in "red belt" Tuscany, the region's most popular newspaper is the right-wing but regional *La Nazione*, not the left-wing but national *La Repubblica*. How could a Roman product possibly compete with a Florentine/Sienese masterpiece?

At a national level, however, by the early 1990s, more than 50 post-war "swing door" governments had come and gone. To many observers, the source of this crisis lay in Italy's administration and dubious morality. Senior party leaders tended to die in office, governments suffered from opportunism, not lack of opportunity. *Partitocrazia* (party influence) supplanted democracy, extending from government to public corporations, infiltrating banking, the judiciary and media, and the public tacitly condoned this "old boys' network".

Corruption and terror

The early 1990s saw a series of political scandals involving bribes, and the result was the *Mani Pulite* ("Clean Hands") campaign under the fiery leadership of Antonio di Pietro, a former magistrate who became Italy's most popular moral crusader. A vast network was uncovered, in which public contracts were awarded by politicians to businesses in return for bribes. Italian public life was convulsed by the scandal, dubbed *Tangentopoli* – literally, "Bribesville". Dozens of MPs and businessmen were arrested,

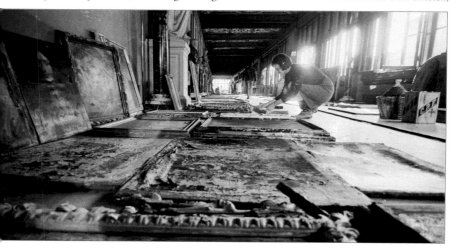

ECCENTRIC EXPATRIATE COLLECTORS

Anna Maria Gastone, the last of the Medici, left centuries of art treasures and palaces to Florence in perpetuity. In her wake came a succession of patrons who, despite their self-indulgence, left treasures that can still be seen *in situ* today. Among connoisseurs, the 19th-century race for progress produced an artistic backlash, a desire for escapism coupled with nostalgia for an idealised past. In response, the Florentine foreign collectors pursued a private Arcadia. Often the reaction took the form of a romanticisation of the Gothic era, a period perceived as a heady amalgam of medieval chivalry and costumed romp. Other collectors were inspired by the Florentine heyday, conjuring up a Renaissance stage set.

The art historian Herbert Percy Horne (1864–1916) left his idealised Florentine Renaissance palazzo to posterity. Frederick Stibbert (1838–1906) was the classic case of a collector who succumbed to *fin de siècle* aestheticism, leaving behind his museum of armour in a villa steeped in decadent Gothic gloom. Charles Loeser, heir to Macy's store, bequeathed his collection of Old Masters to the Palazzo Vecchio in 1928. The art historian Bernard Berenson (1865–1959) pioneered Renaissance studies so it is fitting that his villa, I Tatti, is now Harvard's Centre for Renaissance Studies. The Anglo-Florentine aesthete Sir Harold Acton (1904–94) left Villa La Pietra, his home and art collection, to New York University.

with others committing suicide. The Christian Democrat Party, which had dominated Italian politics since the war, collapsed under the weight of its own corruption. Two former prime ministers – the socialist Bettino Craxi and the Christian Democrat veteran and seven-times former prime minister Giulio Andreotti – were investigated.

Craxi died in self-imposed exile in Tunisia in 2000, while Andreotti, charged with Mafia ties, was eventually acquitted. The appeal judges found Andreotti to have enjoyed "friendly" and direct relations with the Mafia "up until 1980", but not later – so "Beelzebub" escaped prosecution thanks to the statute of limitations.

In the midst of the political upheaval, in May 1993, Florence suffered a devastating blow when a bomb planted by the Mafia behind the Uffizi gallery rocked the city. Five people were killed, priceless paintings and sculptures damaged and a handful destroyed. The Uffizi's buildings were damaged, and several medieval buildings around the corner were virtually destroyed.

The Mafia's aim was to use the attack, and others in Milan and Rome, to force the Italian state into submission, and to agree to a deal of mutual convenience with the Mob, as had been enjoyed with the Christian Democrats. The jailed Sicilian Godfather, Salvatore "Toto" Riina, was sentenced to life for the Uffizi bombing in 1998. Meanwhile, while no area of Italy appeared to have been left untouched by corruption, including Florence, in the end few, if any, *Tangentopoli* politicians served much real time in jail.

In a frank interview in July 2005, the film director Bernardo Bertolucci told the *Corriere della Sera*: "Italy lost a great opportunity after *Tangentopoli*. It should have had a real examination of conscience, in order to understand how on earth it could be that there were so many corrupt figures populating our landscape, accomplices of a system which goes from small tips in return for small favours, to large *tangenti* (bribes) for big contracts. And instead we have wound up with an illegal prime minister, who was elected amid conditions of almost complete control of the media." He was referring to Silvio Berlusconi, the media tycoon-turned-prime minister.

Silvio Berlusconi

Berlusconi, the populist, perma-tanned tycoon, was first elected premier in 1994, on an anti-corruption ticket, and has led two further administrations. Ironically, Berlusconi's career has been dogged by charges of everything from conflict of interests to embezzlement and false accounting. His classic response is that such allegations have been politically motivated by rivals and a biased judiciary.

Clowning, corruption and "bunga bunga" sex scandals aside, Berlusconi has dominated Italian life, as much by his oversize personality as by his vast wealth. Some see Berlusconi as a product of Italian culture, tapping into the traditions

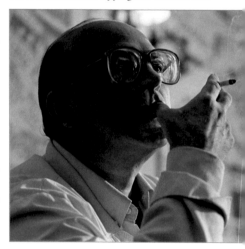

Left: paintings from the Uffizi laid out for restoration after the 1966 flood. **Right:** Bettino Craxi, former Prime Minister of Italy.

of patronage and family. The billionaire's business empire spans the media, entertainment, insurance, construction and sport (the tycoon owns AC Milan football club). Berlusconi's fans felt that only a successful businessman could transform a recalcitrant country into a model business. His critics cite conflict of interests, including the media mogul's ownership of three television channels, and undue influence over the public-broadcasting networks. They believe that Berlusconi entered politics to protect his empire and evade legal charges. The right may wear the trousers in Rome but, almost as a matter of regional pride, far fewer Tuscans voted for Berlusconi than in other regions.

Berlusconi's second term, from 2001-6, made him the only post-war prime minister to govern for a full five-year term. Despite bringing a semblance of stability, the empire-builder narrowly lost out to Romano Prodi in 2006, ceding to a fragile left-wing coalition whose eventual collapse prompted fresh elections. Disillusionment with a lack of leadership from the left led to the right regaining power in 2008, masterminded by Berlusconi's People of Freedom party. The flamboyant billionaire businessman was elected on a platform of reducing public spending, lowering taxes, reforming the judiciary, and modernising the infrastructure.

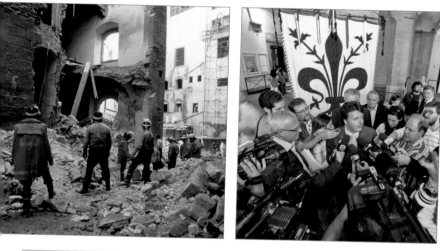

A TUSCAN HALL OF FAME

There's a saying that Tuscany is "equally blessed by the genius of man and nature". And history has proved the proverb, with the greatest Tuscans achieving worldwide fame. Unsurprisingly, many are from the world of art: Giotto, Leonardo da Vinci, Michelangelo, Donatello, Masaccio and Cellini were all born in or around Florence, as was the architect Brunelleschi. The painter and art historian Giorgio Vasari is famed for his *Lives of the Artists*, and was celebrated in Italian-wide events in 2011, the 500th anniversary of his birth.

Literary celebrities include the triumvirate of Dante, Petrarch and Boccaccio (born in Paris, but raised in Florence). In the music field, the composer Puccini hailed from Lucca,

and opera itself was born in Florence in the late 1500s. Tuscany was also home to the astronomer Galileo, mathematician Leonardo Fibonacci, political theorist Machiavelli, and merchant-turned-explorer Amerigo Vespucci. Alas, in the banking field, the great Florentines are anonymous, including the creators of the florin (*fiorino*) in 1189, and the inventors of double-entry book-keeping.

Many famous modern-day Tuscans are linked to the fashion world: the late Emilio Pucci, Guccio Gucci and Salvatore Ferragamo (a transplanted Neapolitan), plus Roberto Cavalli. Showbiz representatives include the singer Andrea Bocelli, film-maker Franco Zeffirelli, and comedian Roberto Benigni.

The consensus is that Berlusconi, bogged down by personal scandals and pursuing his own interests, failed to deliver on all fronts. By mid-2011, the country was in a perilous position amid fears that it would fall victim to the eurozone debt crisis. Despite being its third-largest economy, Italy had not embarked on reforms or tackled public debt. After faring badly in local elections in 2011, Berlusconi's chances of surviving until the general elections in 2013 looked slim. He was also involved in four trials, with charges ranging from illegal sex with an underage prostitute to corruption and perverting the course of justice.

After dominating the political scene for 17 years, Berlusconi, the country's longest-serving post-war prime minister stepped down in 2011. Overwhelmed by the scale of Italy's debt crisis, the consummate survivor finally made way for respected economist Mario Monti, who formed a government of technocrats to steer the country through uncharted waters.

Florentine revival

Fortunately, on the Tuscan stage, politics is being rejuvenated by the dynamic mayor of Florence, Matteo Renzi. When elected in 2009, the youngest mayor in Italy declared that Berlusconi's sleazy generation of politicians should stand aside. Apart from introducing merit as the main criterion for council jobs in Florence, Renzi appointed women to half of the posts. Meritocracy is a bold new concept in such a closed, clubby and recalcitrant political culture. Elected on a platform of making the city cleaner, more liveable and more accountable, the mayor's first public act was to pedestrianise Piazza del Duomo, since extended to other areas, notably Piazza Santa Maria Novella and chic Via de Tornabuoni. Returning visitors can now savour the Duomo without the din of traffic, apart from the clatter of hooves from the horse-drawn carriages. You can even take in the stripy Gothic facade of Santa Maria Novella without fear of being hit by careering cabs shooting out of the station. The Mayor has pledged to reduce the city's carbon footprint

dramatically. The rules governing access to the restricted traffic zone are also being simplified, and Green-friendly electric buses introduced in the Oltrarno.

Still, the changes go beyond pollution-cutting measures and spruced-up squares. Culturally, the revitalisation extends to revamped galleries and museums, more cosmopolitan nightlife, and a fresh perception of Florence as a creative, contemporary city, not mired in the past. To this end, the administration admits that Florence, and by extension Tuscany, had rested on its laurels as far as tourism was concerned. Bicycles will be more readily available, inspired by schemes in Paris and London, while Segway tours and rickshaw

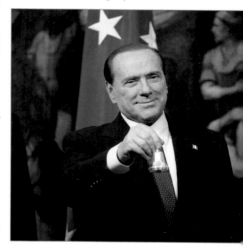

rides are also being encouraged. Museums are becoming more user-friendly, with longer opening hours and better ticketing. Major galleries are seeking to take invisible masterpieces out of the store-rooms and put them into the public domain. A "Firenze Card" has finally been introduced, a simple, convenient three-day pass that combines public transport and the top museums. As Mayor Renzi says: "Being radical and forward-thinking is in the genes of Florentines, this is the city of Savonarola and Machiavelli." Refreshing news, but perhaps not the wisest of parallels, with the latter a master of murky realpolitik and the former burnt at the stake. Tuscan politics is rarely dull. ❑

FAR LEFT: aftermath of the Uffizi bombing. **LEFT:** Mayor of Florence Matteo Renzi at the Palazzo Vecchio reopening. **RIGHT:** outgoing Prime Minister Berlusconi; the Ceremony of the Bell signals a change of Italian leadership.

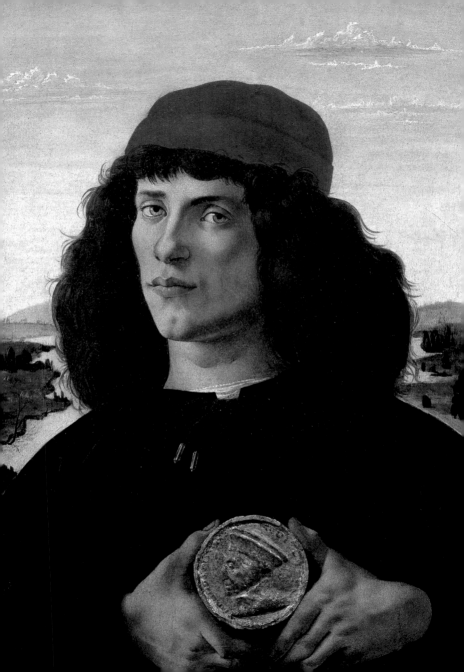

RENAISSANCE ART

Art historians divide the Renaissance into three waves: the trecento (1300s) was the era of the workshop and fresco; the quattrocento (1400s) welcomed a new realism featuring perspective and emotion; the cinquecento (1500s), or High Renaissance, was the apogee followed by a sharp decline, as political and economic decay eventually took its toll

One of the great myths of history provides a kind of Hollywood scenario for the "birth of the Renaissance", linking it to the fall of Constantinople in 1453, when scholars were supposed to have escaped, clutching their precious Greek manuscripts, to Italy. There, these manuscripts became a kind of magical seed, taking root, growing and bearing fruit almost immediately as "the Renaissance".

Of course, this is nonsense; like any other human phenomenon, the Renaissance had roots deep in history. It was the political fragmentation of Italy that created the Renaissance, each little city-state contributing something unique to the whole. But the process certainly started in Florence, and the city dominated the cultural scene until the early 16th century. Again and again over the centuries, attempts have been made to analyse the causes of the Florentine flowering, with reasons ranging from the poverty of the soil to the quality of the light. But it is no more possible to "explain" this than it is any other mystery of the human spirit.

Defining the Renaissance

The very word "renaissance" is a Florentine invention. In his book *Lives of the Most Excellent Architects, Painters and Sculptors,* first published in 1550, Vasari, first of the art historians,

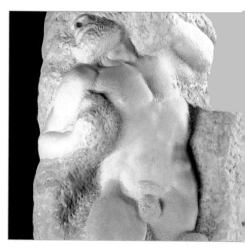

remarks that the reader "will now be able to recognise more easily the progress of [art's] rebirth *(il progresso della sua rinascita)*".

But what, exactly, did Vasari mean by *rinascita*? What was being "reborn"? Vasari was referring to a rebirth of the art and architecture of classical times, that is, before Emperor Constantine transferred the seat of empire to Constantinople at the beginning of the 4th century AD, causing it to become the centre of art and culture. A distinctive architecture, based on Roman models, using bricks and featuring domes and cupolas, was developed. Byzantine art was hierarchical in style, using flattened forms and no perspective.

LEFT: portrait of a young man (c.1475), probably a member of the Medici dynasty, by Botticelli (Uffizi). **RIGHT:** *The Awakening Slave* (1519–20), one of four "unfinished" *Slaves* by Michelangelo (Accademia), intended for the tomb of Pope Julius II in Rome.

Architects drew and measured the ruins of the Roman cities, rediscovering their building techniques and their rules of proportion, the "classical orders". Vitruvius's *Ten Books on Architecture*, the only surviving manual from classical times, was studied anew and became the basis, in the 15th century, for Alberti's treatise of the same name.

Painting, which of all the arts is preeminently *the* art of the Renaissance, owed little to antiquity, partly because no Roman examples survived to be used as models. Renaissance artists broke new ground, discovering perspective and observing the natural world that surrounded them. The 14th-century Florentine

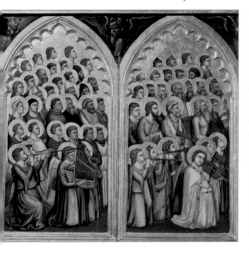

BYZANTINE ART

Byzantine artists covered interiors with mosaics, a Roman decorative device that became a sumptuous art form, with myriad glazed-stone fragments catching the light in a way no fresco ever could. Inspired by cupolas in Constantinople, the best Byzantine art in Italy is in Ravenna, dating from the 5th century. But the style prevailed in 11th-century Venice, and even influenced 13th-century Florence, in the magnificent Baptistery. But to its Florentine critics, notably Vasari, Byzantine art was static and stiffly formalised. It was this aspect that Vasari decried as "a certain residue of the Greeks" – and that was completely overthrown by the new naturalism of the Renaissance artists.

artist Cennino Cennini gave good advice to his fellow artists. "If you wish to draw mountains well, so that they appear natural," he wrote, "procure some large stones, rocky, not polished, and draw from these." The idea of a handful of stones standing in for the Alps or the Apennines might seem ludicrous, but it was a pointer to the new road the artist was taking, the road to reality in nature.

The classical world provided the inspiration for the artist to rise above the narrow medieval world, with its emphasis on theological studies. But, once he had started, he went his own way. What was reborn was an artistic sensibility but not a recycled past.

The trecento

Until the quattrocento (15th century), the term "artist" had no particular significance, being virtually interchangeable with "artisan" or "craftsman". All were members of guilds, or *arti:* there was an *arte* for the shoemaker, no more and no less valid than the *arte* for the goldsmith, itself a subdivision of the immensely powerful Silk Guild. Everything was linked to the power of the guilds and the emergence of artistic workshops.

The growing popularity of the process known as *buon fresco* also demanded a cooperative approach. The medium of fresco painting had been introduced about a century earlier, and time had shown that it was the most permanent of all forms of mural art to date, since the colouring became an intrinsic part of the plaster itself.

In addition to large commissions, the workshop (or *bottega*) would produce a variety of smaller articles for sale, ranging from painted scabbards to holy pictures and statues. There was widespread demand for religious art, which provided the bread and butter for hundreds of small *botteghe*. A peasant might have scraped together enough for a tiny picture; a parish priest might have a large sum at his disposal to commission a mural or even an altarpiece; or a wealthy merchant might be anxious to propitiate fate and show an appropriate level of piety.

The potential client had little interest in the identity of the craftsmen producing his order. But, if expensive colours were used (gold, silver, or blue made from the semi-precious lapis lazuli), then the fact was clearly stated in the contract, along with the date of delivery of the finished piece. Commissioned work was almost invariably recorded in a contract that, in addition, usually specified how many figures were to appear in the finished painting, as well as their activities and attributes. Sacred art touched on the delicate area of religious orthodoxy, and the wise craftsman ensured that his client stated exactly what he wanted.

The identity of most of the workers in the *botteghe* is unknown. They were conscientious and skilled, rather than brilliant, but they formed the subsoil from which the genius of the quattrocento could flourish. The actual working pattern of the *bottega*, whereby a group of lesser craftsmen would paint the main body of a picture, leaving it to the identified master to put the finishing touches to it, would continue into the High Renaissance, the cinquecento. This made it difficult, at times impossible, for the most skilled art critic to say that such a painting was, beyond a doubt, the work of a particular famous artist.

Early Renaissance art

Comparing trecento (or Gothic) paintings in any Tuscan art gallery with the work of quattrocento (or early Renaissance) artists reveals a compelling difference: whereas Gothic paintings are iconographic, revelling in the use of celestial gold and presenting a spiritual Madonna and Child for worship and contemplation, the same subject in the hands of Renaissance painters becomes a study in living flesh, the figures of mother and child endowed with attitudes, character, emotions and psychological motivation. Scholars argue endlessly about why this great change occurred, but there is near-universal agreement on who started it: Giotto di Bondone (1267–1337), who, according to Vasari, "restored art to the better path followed in modern times".

But Giotto was not entirely alone in injecting life, and naturalism, into art. Nicola (1223–84) and Giovanni (1245–1314) Pisano, the father-and-son team, were achieving similar advances

in sculpture at the same time as Giotto was breaking new ground in painting.

When the Pisani were living and working in Pisa, it was the fashion for Pisan merchants to ship home Roman sarcophagi from the Holy Land or North Africa for eventual reuse as their own tombs. Scores of them still line the cloister surrounding Pisa's Campo Santo cemetery. Inspired by the realistic battle scenes carved on these antique marble tombs, the Pisani created their own versions: great pulpits sculpted with dramatic scenes from the life of Christ, which can be seen in Pisa's cathedral, and in Sant'Andrea church in Pistoia.

In architecture, the classical inspiration

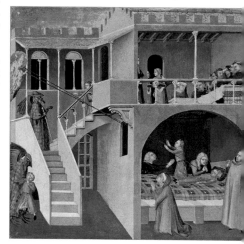

THE GUILDS

The guilds extended their control over the decorative as well as the practical arts. Sculptors and architects were enrolled with the masons, and painters formed a subdivision of the apothecaries, as they needed a grasp of chemistry to prepare their colours. Far from resenting the obligation to join associations, painters and sculptors formed their own groups, or *compagnie*, within larger guilds. This meant members could help one another, sharing profits and losses. Increased teamwork also meant that several men might be engaged at successive stages in the shaping of a pillar, from rough hewing to final carving, conveyor-belt style. The same was true of fresco painting.

LEFT: detail from the *Coronation of the Virgin* (c.1330) altarpiece by Giotto (Santa Croce, Florence). **RIGHT:** scene from the *Life of St Nicholas* (c.1327–30) by Lorenzetti (Uffizi).

that helped to define the Renaissance had never disappeared to quite the same degree as it had in art. The very term Romanesque – meaning derived from or in the Roman style – indicates the essential continuity between the architecture of Rome and that of Tuscany in the 1300s. Churches were still built to the same basilican plan as those of the late Roman period, and, though the facades of many Tuscan churches look quite unclassical, they are still based on the geometry of the Roman hemispherical arch, as distinct from the four-centred arches of Venice or the pointed arches of French Gothic. What distinguishes Tuscan Romanesque from Lombardic or Piedmontese

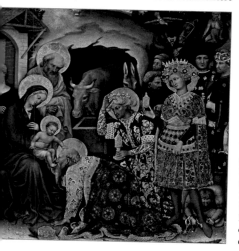

is the exuberant use of polychrome marble to create complex geometrical patterns. Pisa was the seminal influence here – trade links with Spain and North Africa led to the adoption of Arabic numerals in place of Roman, and to the fondness for surface patterning in architecture, copying Moorish tilework and textiles. From Pisa the oriental influence spread to Lucca, Prato, Pistoia, and even to Florence, where it was to pave the way for the great polychrome Campanile designed by Giotto.

The quattrocento

A great breakthrough took place in Florence at the beginning of the 15th century, a moment so important that it can be dated to within a few years, and a new philosophy of life flowed through the city. Until the 1470s, Florence was a dynamo, providing light and energy for the entire peninsula. The city retained its dominance in art for barely a lifespan, however, because it exported so much of its native talent – which ensured the spread of Renaissance values but, with them, ensured Florence's own relative eclipse.

The breakthrough began when the Florentine *Signoria*, or government, decided to refurbish the ceremonial centre of Florence: the group of buildings consisting of the cathedral, the Campanile – begun by Giotto in 1334 and finished after his death but to his design in 1359 – and the octagonal Baptistery. This little black-and-white building had a special place in Florentine affections, and when, in 1401, it was decided to offer a thanksgiving for the city's escape from plague, the Baptistery was chosen

---

GIOTTO DI BONDONE

Tradition has it that Giotto (1267–1337) was working as a shepherd boy until Cimabue, himself a pioneer of greater naturalism in art, discovered that Giotto could draw a perfect circle freehand, and offered to train him as an artist. Pupil soon surpassed master, and Giotto went on to create the great *St Francis* fresco cycle in the Upper Basilica in Assisi and the *Life of Christ* fresco series in the Scrovegni Chapel in Padua. In Florence, his main masterpiece adorns the Franciscan church of Santa Croce, where his work (and, of course, that of his *bottega* of assistants) covers the walls of the two chapels to the right of the choir. To measure the breadth of the Giotto revolution, it is enough to compare his

frescoes with the static 13th-century altarpiece nearby.

Despite Giotto's supposedly rural background, in his work nature is formalised and subservient to humanity. It is the figures who occupy the foreground, vibrantly *alive*. Giotto was ahead of his time in introducing character and individuality to his art. Straddling two ages, Giotto has been claimed both as a Gothic artist and as the pioneer of the Renaissance. Perhaps if war and the Black Death had not ravaged Europe from the 1340s, the Renaissance might well have blossomed sooner than it did. As it was, another 60 years were to pass before the naturalism pioneered by Giotto was to re-emerge, this time as a mass artistic movement.

to benefit. The wealthy Wool Guild announced that it would finance the design and casting of a second set of bronze doors that would be even grander than those of Pisano. The design for them was thrown open to competition.

Out of the many entrants, seven were chosen, each to execute a panel on the same subject: the sacrifice of Isaac. Two of the entrants, the 21-year-old Brunelleschi, later credited as the creator of the "Renaissance style" in architecture, and the 20-year-old Lorenzo Ghiberti, produced work that caused considerable difficulty to the judges. Both the panels exist today, one preserved in the Museo dell'Opera del Duomo, the other in the Bargello museum.

changing status of the artist. In the first contract he is treated essentially as an artisan, expected to put in a full day's work "like any journeyman".

In later contracts for his employment, he is treated far more as a free agent, permitted to undertake commissions for other work. Ghiberti, too, made explicit this change by boldly including his own self-portrait among the reliefs on the door.

Learning from the ancients

Meanwhile, in Rome with his friend Donatello, Brunelleschi was discovering how the ancients had built their enormous structures. In an entirely new approach to the past, he examined

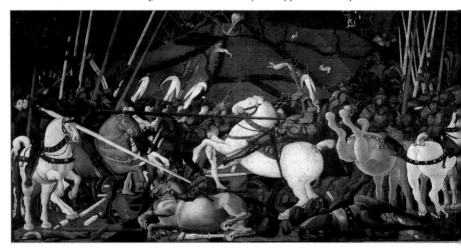

Comparing the two, posterity finds it impossible to say which is "better". The *Syndics*, at a loss to choose, came up with a compromise, suggesting that the artists should share the work. Brunelleschi declined and set out for Rome, while Ghiberti began work on the doors, completing them 22 years later.

He was offered the commission to produce a second pair: these took him 27 years. During the almost half-century that he worked on the project, it is possible to see in his contracts the

originals rather than copies of copies. One of his findings – or, possibly, inventions – was the *ulivella*. Intrigued and puzzled by the existence of regular-shaped holes in the huge stone blocks of the ancient buildings, he assumed that they had been made to allow the block to be gripped by some device, and designed a kind of grappling iron to fit. Whether or not the Romans had actually used such a device, it was very useful – and a demonstration of the benefits to be gained by studying the past.

Brunelleschi returned to Florence at about the time that the *Syndics* of the Wool Guild, who also had the responsibility for the cathedral, were puzzling over the problem of completing it.

LEFT: *Adoration of the Magi* (1423) by Gentile da Fabriano (Uffizi). **ABOVE:** *The Battle of San Romano* (1432) by Paolo Uccello (Uffizi).

Arnolfo di Cambio had begun it in 1296, and it had been completed, all except for the dome, by 1369. Nobody knew how to bridge this immense gap, which, for half a century, had been covered by a temporary roof.

In 1417, a special meeting was called to debate the problem and consider suggestions, and Brunelleschi put forward his solution. He was mocked for it because it dispensed with the wooden centring over which architects traditionally built their arches and vaults, supporting their weight until the keystone was in place. But, in desperation, the *Syndics* offered him the job. Brunelleschi solved the problem by building a dome that was pointed in sections,

supported by ribs with the lightest possible in-filling between them. He built two shells, an outer skin and an inner one: one way in which the crushing weight of the dome, the problem that had prevented its construction, was considerably reduced.

The work took 16 years, and was completed on 31 August 1436. This was the first Renaissance dome in Italy, the largest unsupported dome in Europe, bigger than the Pantheon in Rome, which Brunelleschi had studied, bigger even than the great dome that Michelangelo raised a century later over St Peter's in Rome.

It was Brunelleschi's successor, the scholar Alberti, who first applied the classical orders

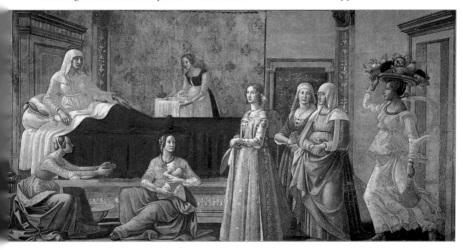

BOTTICELLI'S *SPRING*

La Primavera (1478) is Sandro Botticelli's most famous painting – and certainly the most mysterious of the Early Renaissance. Hung in the Uffizi, it depicts nine supernatural creatures placed in an exquisite natural setting. On the left, a young man is pointing at something. Next to him a group of grave-faced women are performing a solemn ritual dance. On the right is the only figure who seems to be aware of the observer: Botticelli's stunningly beautiful "mystery" woman with a provocative half-smile. Beside her what appears to be an act of violence adds a discordant note: a bluish figure is leaning out of the trees and clutching at a startled girl.

In the background, but dominating the whole, is the most

enigmatic figure: a pale woman whose expression has been variously described as frowning, smiling and melancholy; whose stance has also been described in conflicting ways, as dancing, as that of a consumptive, as pregnant and as offering a blessing. The figure is claimed to be both Venus and the Virgin Mary. Botticelli was trying to restate classical mythology in Christian terms while remaining true to the original – and to his own quirky self. However, he was later influenced by the gloomy, savage friar Savonarola – who turned Florence into a puritan reformatory in the 1490s – and, almost overnight, ceased his joyous mythological paintings, concentrating instead on orthodox religious subjects.

to domestic architecture and created what we now think of as the Renaissance palazzo. Whereas Brunelleschi introduced the columns, pediments and cornices he copied from Roman ruins into his churches, there were no surviving examples of Roman domestic architecture for the 15th-century Florentines to copy. When Rucellai, a wealthy Florentine merchant, asked Alberti to design a palace for him, Alberti took as a model the Colosseum in Rome and applied its tiers of arches to the facade of a three-storey palazzo. Although it was the only palazzo he built, and though Brunelleschi's design for the Medici Palace never got beyond the model stage, these two architects developed a new type of building, a system of proportion and an elegance of line that is still in use today.

Brunelleschi's other major breakthrough was his use of perspective. Alberti described its effect to a generation for whom it appeared almost a magical technique: "I describe a rectangle of whatever size I wish, which I imagine to be an open window through which I view whatever is to be depicted there." Donatello (1386–1466) eagerly used the technique in his bas-relief of *Salome Offering John's Head to Herod*. The observer is looking at a banquet where the diners are recoiling in horror from the offering. Beyond the banqueting rooms can be seen a succession of two more rooms, giving a remarkable and, for contemporaries, almost eerie sense of depth.

A new perspective

Like the difference between Giotto's mobile, dramatic figures and their static, formal predecessors, perspective gave a new vista to civilisation. Its most dramatic form was that employed by the young Masaccio. His great painting of the *Trinity*, in the church of Santa Maria Novella, is an intellectual exercise in the use of perspective that is also infused with religious awe. Beneath a trompe l'oeil classical arch stands the immense figure of God the Father, half-supporting a cross on which there is an equally immense figure of Christ; below them are various saints and donors and a memento mori of a skeleton in a sarcophagus revealing

an ancient warning: "I am what you are, and what I am, you shall be."

The huge figures stand out from the background and appear to loom over the observer. As a young man, Michelangelo used to stand before these, copying them again and again to fix the style in his mind. Eventually, therefore, some essence of this experimental period of the Renaissance found its way into the Sistine Chapel, that shrine of the High Renaissance dominated by Michelangelo's work.

The classical arch in Masaccio's painting is a pointer to a curious development that took place during the quattrocento – the clothing of biblical figures in a totally anachronistic way,

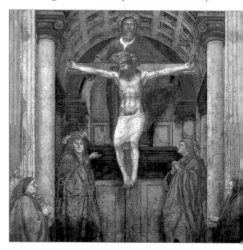

either in classical Roman attire or in contemporary Florentine dress. The frescoes that Ghirlandaio (1449–94) painted in the Sasseti Chapel within the church of Santa Trinità supposedly concern the prophecies of Christ's birth, and the location should be Augustan Rome. But it is a Rome that bears a remarkably close resemblance to 15th-century Florence, and the people waiting for the awesome news are all citizens of Florence in normal dress. Lorenzo de' Medici is there, as is his mother, his children, friends and various colleagues.

Early Renaissance painters were preoccupied with technique. Their subject matter remained largely unchanged: religion was still the most

LEFT: *Birth of John the Baptist* (1485) by Ghirlandaio.
RIGHT: *Trinity* (c.1425) by Masaccio, the pioneer of perspective (both in Santa Maria Novella, Florence).

important concern. But in the second half of the quattrocento a new, exciting and somewhat disturbing element began to appear: the mythological and the allegorical. The supreme practitioner in this field was Sandro Botticelli, who worked with Leonardo da Vinci in Verrocchio's workshop but developed in a totally different direction.

The High Renaissance

Even to the untutored eye, there is a profound difference between the work produced before and after the 1520s in Tuscany and elsewhere, most noticeably in Florence. Partly this was the result of an immense political crisis. Italy

had become a battleground, invaded again and again by warring foreigners. In 1527 a savage army, composed partly of mercenaries, sacked Rome and held the pope to ransom. Italy was never to recover from that experience, which was the curtain-raiser for a period of foreign domination that would not come to an end until the 1800s.

The apogee of the Renaissance – in Florence, at least – was ushered in with Leonardo da Vinci and Michelangelo. But the decline swiftly followed, particularly when Michelangelo and Raphael left for Rome, to work for Pope Julius II. Other artists followed suit: the major Florentine families – other than the Medici – could no

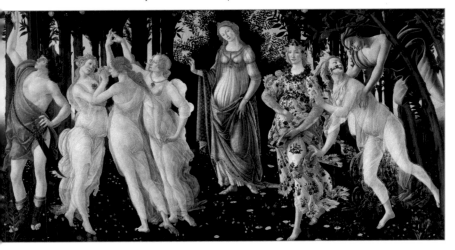

MICHELANGELO IN FLORENCE

A Vasari anecdote describes how a 13-year-old Michelangelo Buonarroti (1475–1564) made a drawing of the tools in the workshop. His master, Ghirlandaio, was so impressed that he told Lorenzo de' Medici, who invited Michelangelo to enter his princely household and study with his own children.

Michelangelo also worked for the next 40 years on a thankless task: the great tomb for his patron, Pope Julius II. The unfinished statues for this tomb, the famous *Slaves,* are now in Florence's Accademia gallery. Five centuries later, the sculptor's technique is still clearly visible; shallow depressions surrounding the figure, made by the rounded head of a chisel, seem to be "freeing" the figures.

Florence boasts many statues by Michelangelo; although often unfinished, they always reveal the chisel strokes of a master. They include the iconic *David,* and the statues of *Dawn, Evening, Day* and *Night* in the Medici Chapel. Florence's Casa Buonarroti (Via Ghibellina; www. casabuonarroti.it), once owned by Michelangelo, showcases the sculptor's working drawings and a few early works. The quintessential Renaissance man is not fully represented here, either in spirit or in sculpture. Still, thanks to his descendants, the palace conveys the atmosphere of a family home and remains a touching tribute to the great sculptor, painter, architect and poet.

longer afford to make commissions, so the art scene moved on.

Shortly after the sack of Rome, the Medici Pope Clement VII clamped down on his native city of Florence, ending republicanism and preparing the way for the first dukedom. Meanwhile, in the world of art, the glory was departing from Florence, as the impetus of the Renaissance shifted to Rome and Venice. From the middle of the 16th century, Florentine artists tended to be court artists, dancing attendance on the Medici dukes. Among them was the artist-turned-art historian Giorgio Vasari (1511–74).

Until recently, Vasari's work as an artist was dismissed almost as contemptuously as his work as an art historian was received enthusiastically. However, posterity owes him a debt of gratitude, both as an architect and as a painter. In 2011, worldwide celebrations to mark the fifth centenary of his birth provoked a re-evaluation of his artistry. Not only did he build the Uffizi for Duke Cosimo I, and the Vasari Corridor, but he frescoed the interior of Brunelleschi's dome. Vasari also remodelled the Palazzo Vecchio and decorated its parliamentary chamber, the great Salone dei Cinquecento, with outstanding contemporary representations of the city and its surrounding countryside.

Leonardo da Vinci

Although the glory was departing from Florence, the sunset was stupendous. It could scarcely be otherwise with two such giants as Michelangelo and Leonardo still on the scene. Leonardo, born in 1452, trained in Vérrocchio's *bottega*, thus carrying the medieval systems on into the new era. One of Vasari's anecdotes claims that Verrocchio, on seeing his young apprentice's work, laid down his brush and never painted again. Unlikely though the incident is, the anecdote shows that Leonardo was recognised as being almost a freakish genius in his own lifetime.

Leonardo left Florence for Milan at the age of 30. He returned in 1502 when commissioned by the *Signoria* to create the great mural, the *Battle of Anghiari* in the Council Chamber, and eventually crossed the Alps to

become court painter to François I of France. His contribution to the history of ideas is incalculable, but his legacy in Tuscany is restricted to several Madonnas and the unfinished paintings of the *Battle of Anghiari* and the *Adoration of the Kings*, all in the Uffizi. The two best-known masterpieces, the *Mona Lisa*, set against an exquisite Tuscan background, and the *Virgin of the Rocks*, are in Paris and London respectively. However, there is at least a museum of his fantastical creations in Florence, which displays working models of his flying machines, armoured tanks and swing bridges, all before his time *(see page 94)*.

Michelangelo is another story, however.

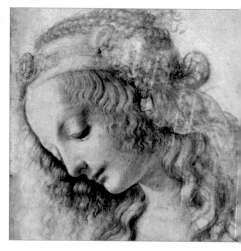

His greatest work, the Sistine Chapel, is also situated outside Florence, but he did leave an enduring imprint upon his home city, in the form of the walls that gird it and the sculptures that grace it.

Michelangelo

Michelangelo was nearly a generation younger than Leonardo, born in 1475 when the Renaissance was approaching its apogee. His father was a poor but proud country gentleman who disapproved of the idea of his son becoming an artisan or artist; in his mind, there was no clear distinction. Indeed, Michelangelo was apt to be touchy on the subject. Although he served

LEFT: *La Primavera* (1478) by Botticelli (Uffizi). RIGHT: a sketch in charcoal by Leonardo (Uffizi).

his apprenticeship in a *bottega*, he later rejected the idea that he touted for trade: "I was never a painter or a sculptor like those who set up shop for the purpose."

Michelangelo was just 18 when Lorenzo de' Medici died in 1492. Florence was plunged into chaos, because Lorenzo's son, Piero, was extravagant and unpopular, and the Florentines chased the tyrant out of the city. The artist's links with the Medici were no longer so advantageous, and so he took the road to Rome, where the Sistine Chapel awaited. Although Michelangelo is remembered as a painter and sculptor, he was also a gifted engineer and a poet of a good deal of sensitivity and insight.

della Signoria – a message to anyone in Florence who dared to resist the might of the Medici. But it is indicative both of Cellini and of the enveloping atmosphere of artistic decadence that his best-known work would be the elaborate golden salt cellar crafted for François I of France.

Raphael

Raphael (Raffaello) was a gentle, handsome young man who seemed to have no enemies. Born in Umbria in 1483, he received his basic training in the workshop of Perugino, working on frescoes in Perugia. In 1500, at the impressionable age of 17, he came to Florence, where he absorbed the works of Leonardo da Vinci and

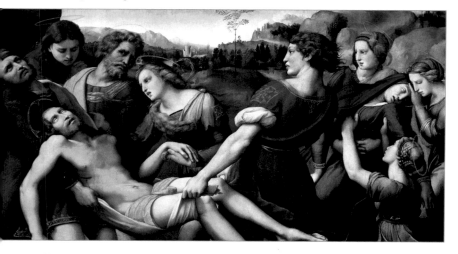

Cellini

Michelangelo was just 25 when Benvenuto Cellini was born in 1500. Like so many of the artists of his time, Cellini was a jack of all trades – including, improbably enough, a gunner. He played a role in the tragic sack of Rome which, in effect, brought the Renaissance to an end. Acting as gunner in defence of the Vatican, he assured his supporters that the pope promised him absolution "for all the murders that I should commit".

In Florence, his most famous work is that beautiful but curiously heartless statue of *Perseus Slaying Medusa*, commissioned by Cosimo I for the statue-filled Loggia dei Lanzi on the Piazza

Michelangelo. He left Florence in 1508, attracted to Rome by the fiery Pope Julius II, who was planning a series of architectural embellishments to the Vatican. There the young Raphael made a mark by painting the series of rooms known as the Stanze della Segnatura. Under the Medici Pope Leo X, he was placed in charge of archaeological excavations in Rome itself.

Thus, the last true artist of the Renaissance introduced into the mother city of Europe that passionate search for the past that had triggered the Renaissance in Florence nearly two centuries earlier. ❏

ABOVE: *Entombment* by Raphael.

Literary Classics

"Florentine firsts" are not restricted to the art world – Dante, Italy's finest poet, and Machiavelli, the first political theorist, are just two names to conjure with

In a crowded field, three towering figures provide some orientation to Tuscan literature. Dante, Petrarch and Machiavelli follow each other chronologically and, as each caused, as well as recorded, great changes, it is possible to plot the course of the region's history through them.

Born in 1265, Dante was an exact contemporary of Giotto, whose work he admired. But where Giotto kept out of politics, Dante involved himself wholeheartedly and was exiled for his pains. *The Divine Comedy*, which deals with the great mysteries of religion, had a profound effect on Italian thought.

Francesco Petrarch, though a Florentine, was born in Arezzo, where his parents had been exiled during the same feuds that caused Dante's expulsion. Petrarch was one of the first to retrieve the lost classical literature that helped to usher in the Renaissance. He travelled widely, had an enormous circle of friends and it was often through his letters that the "new learning" was disseminated. In poetry, he devised the sonnet form that took his name – Petrarchan – which was greatly to influence the poets of Elizabethan England.

Niccolò Machiavelli was born in 1469. Viewed from almost any angle, his life appears a failure. As a career diplomat, he never wielded real authority. As a republican, he was obliged to curry favour with the openly despotic Medici. In his political writings, the tone is ice-cold, logical, in total command. In real life, he was lecherous and adulterous. But he was, nonetheless, a realist who exposed the immorality of leaders. *The Prince* is still treated as a

political manual today. Classic advice includes: "When neither their property nor their honour is touched, the majority of men live content"; and "It is better to be feared than loved, if you cannot be both."

Although innovations in literature were less spectacular than in art and architecture, there are a number of outstanding "firsts". Francesco Guicciardini wrote the first true *History of Italy*, and Giovanni Boccaccio (1313–75) produced Europe's first novel, *The Decameron*, a collection of tales told by 10 young aristocrats who retreat from the plague that struck Florence in 1348. Staying in a country house,

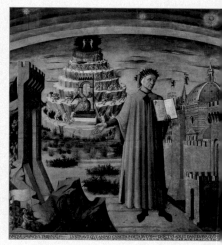

they spend the time telling erotic stories and reciting poems, and poking fun at the clergy. All the stories demonstrate Boccaccio's well-honed skills as a storyteller.

Finally, there were the true "Renaissance men" who mastered both art and literature – as exemplified by Michelangelo's poetry and Cellini's swashbuckling *Autobiography*. Cellini, a brilliant sculptor and soldier, was also a superb writer and wrote an account of the casting of the exquisite bronze sculpture *Perseus* for the Loggia dei Lanzi. At a crucial moment, he ran out of metal and had to throw in the family pewter in order to complete the statue. ❑

RIGHT: *Dante and the Divine Comedy* in Florence's Duomo.

Architectural Treasures

Tuscany combines a rich urban heritage
with a delightful rural legacy, to create
a unique architectural tableau

Curiously, Tuscan architecture is characterised as much by diversity as it is by harmony: harmony in its aesthetic sweetness;
diversity in its range of buildings, from Romanesque cathedrals to Renaissance palaces, town
halls to tower-houses.

Tuscan town halls

Civic architecture is particularly rich. The Tuscan town hall, with accompanying bell tower,
encapsulates a civic ideal. In the past, it promised a degree of democracy to the merchant
guilds, the nobility and the people. The Palazzo
del Comune, known by different names, has
been the seat of local government since medieval times. This imposing, fortified building
dominates the square today, as surely as it has
always dominated the lives of local citizens. The
best known is the fortress-like Palazzo Vecchio
in Florence, its austerity belying its palatial interior. However, even the smallest commune has a
grand town hall. In the Mugello, Palazzo Vicari
in Scarperia resembles Palazzo Vecchio, with its
impressive 14th-century merlons and corbels.
Such public palazzi are often studded with *stem-
mata*, stone-carved coats of arms belonging to
prominent citizens or noble clans.

In numerous cities, including San Gimignano, there is also an adjoining balcony known
as the *arengo*, from which politicians would
harangue the crowd. Nearby is usually a loggia, providing shelter from the sun or rain, as
well as a meeting place, today often used as a
small market. Thus, Tuscany's grandest buildings serve much the same purpose today as they
have always done.

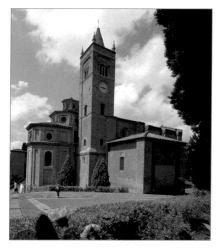

Urbanisation

Visually, urban Tuscany is the product of medieval and Renaissance builders, even if Roman
and Etruscan stones were recycled. Dismissing
the Middle Ages as a period of decadence and
decay does an injustice to the region's prosperity and architectural heritage. In Tuscany, the
period represented a marked social rebirth, with
the flowering of independent city-states in the
11th century. By 1200, most towns had become
burgeoning centres with distinctive identities
and a civic pride evident in the grandiose town
halls and tower-houses. The medieval cathedrals
and civic buildings were a testament to the citizens' refined taste, just as the ordered country

estates later became a Renaissance symbol of peace and prosperity.

The medieval "skyscrapers" of San Gimignano signified the civilising effect of urban living, with the *signori* (feudal lords) encouraged to relinquish their castles for city life. The *borgo*, or fortified city, was also home to landowners and merchants, particularly with the rise of the *popolo grasso*, the wealthy middle class in the 14th century. The medieval city became a symbol of safety during the city-state conflicts.

Tuscan Romanesque

This style is less solemn, less philosophical than French, English or German Romanesque.

Pisan Romanesque is more eclectic, as befits its cosmopolitan heritage. The maritime republic of Pisa was an 11th-century power, trading with northern Europe and the Muslim world. As a result, the severe colonnaded galleries owe much to Norman models, while Sicily inspires the seductive decoration, including exuberant arabesques. A hallmark of the style was its talent for selecting a theatrical space: in Pisa the main buildings present a unified whole, placed on the lawn like prisms on a baize cloth.

Medieval cityscape

Given the rich Roman heritage that was available to them, Tuscans did not take to Gothic

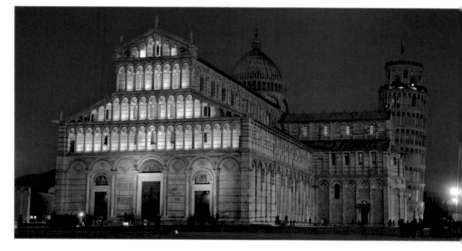

Its hallmarks are surface decoration and space rather than sobriety and solidity, with simple bricks transformed by a marble veneer. The style, centred on Florence, favours contrasting patterns of dark and light marble as well as striking geometric designs. The form was first realised in the city baptistery, with its round-headed arches, classical proportions and a striving for weightlessness. The Florentine model retains a certain simplicity of form, contrasting the austerity of Romanesque with the traditional Tuscan love of polychrome marble patterns.

LEFT: the Abbazia di Monte Oliveto Maggiore. **ABOVE:** Pisa's glorious "Square of Miracles" at night.

MARBLE CATHEDRALS

Inspired by Pisa, the cathedrals of Siena, Pistoia, Florence, Prato and Lucca use stripes and an interplay of light and shade. The geometry of multicoloured marble is quintessentially Tuscan, striking visitors as bold or brash, spellbinding or superfluous. The palette contrasts white marble from Carrara, rosy pink from Maremma and dark green from Prato. The predominant Pisan style combines a Tuscan taste for marble with an austere Norman Romanesque form, in turn inspired by a Moorish Sicilian aesthetic. The Pisan Duomo was the prototype, with its contrasting bands of colour, blind arcading, colonnaded gallery and, of course, the geometry of inlaid marble.

> *In medieval Tuscan architecture, a* castello *was a fortified village or a castle, a* rocca *was a defended garrison post, and a* fortezza *was a fortress of strategic importance.*

gables and sheer verticality, but preferred symmetry instead, balancing height with breadth. In great churches such as Santa Croce in Florence, naves and aisles are not vaulted, but use the open trusses favoured by Romanesque architecture.

as *borghi* and built on hilltops, so that advancing enemies would be easily spotted, are emblematic of the Tuscan cityscape. Anghiari, Buonconvento, Monteriggioni and Montepulciano all provide proof that walls help preserve a distinct identity. The region abounds in ruined or restored examples, including castles at Poppi and Prato, and the pair of fortresses in Florence. Siena province alone boasts San Gimignano's *rocca* and watchtowers, as well as the massive *fortezza* in Siena and Montalcino, both of which have now been converted into wine-tasting centres.

Tower-houses were castle residences serving as both warehouses and fortresses, self-sufficient

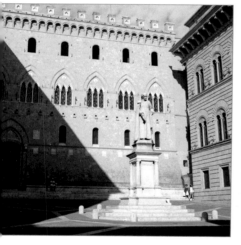

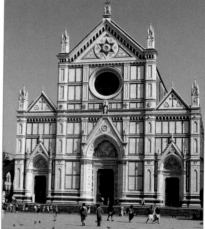

Not that Gothic gables are a guide to a medieval atmosphere, of course. Many Tuscan towns are authentically medieval, as is the case with Cortona, Lucca, San Gimignano and Volterra. As the largest medieval city in Europe, Siena is arguably the most authentic of them all, with strict building regulations in place since the 13th century. Certainly, its Gothic spirit is intact, from red-brick palaces to herringbone alleys, all moulded to a mystical Sienese sensibility.

Tuscan fortifications

Fortifications played an important role in medieval Tuscany. Walled towns, often known enclaves symbolising the wealth and influence of the feudal nobles or prosperous merchants and their scorn for civil authority. Key features of these grand buildings included a well for a constant water supply, an inner courtyard to provide light and ventilation, and an external staircase to the *piano nobile*, the grand residential first floor.

Medieval domestic architecture

As the great Tuscan families grew wealthy on banking and the cloth trade, their homes became more palatial and domesticated. In time, decorative details were added, notably graceful courtyards complete with sculpted

Renaissance palaces

The Florentine palazzo was a direct descendant of the tower-house, but without an outmoded defensive function. In keeping with the new humanist spirit, architects designed gracious private palaces as proof of their revivalist skills, not simply as symbols of patrician pride. Foremost amongst the trailblazers was Michelozzi (1396–1472), who pursued the architectural principles of Alberti and Brunelleschi. Michelozzo designed the Florentine Palazzo Medici-Riccardi, the Medici home and banking headquarters, a massive mansion with an arcaded inner courtyard. He also designed Palazzo Pitti (1444), the prototype of a patrician

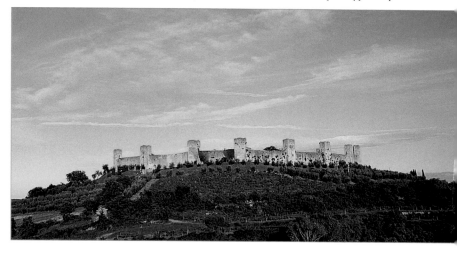

wells, coats of arms, ornate arches and a loggia above. The Florentine Palazzo Davanzati *(see page 95)* preserves much of its medieval atmosphere, from its iron-bolted doors and formidable facade to an internal courtyard boasting a well with a pulley system designed to supply water to each floor. The interior presents a charming portrait of domestic life, from 15th-century frescoes and tapestries to the *cassoni*, Tuscan wedding chests, and even a privileged child's bathroom.

palace, boasting strict classical proportions and a rusticated facade. Yet there are lingering traces of feudal times in the Gothic windows and heavy cornices. Built for Cosimo de' Medici, Palazzo Pitti clearly symbolises the power and prestige of the owner.

However, some nobles simply modernised their feudal seats. Palazzo Spini-Ferroni, a crenellated three-tiered fortress close to the Arno, was a 13th-century watchtower before becoming a palatial home. Just around the corner looms the grandiose Palazzo Strozzi, a rusticated stone cube of mammoth proportions built for the greatest banking dynasty. Rustication was intended to underline the Strozzi's

FAR LEFT: Piazza Salimbeni, Siena. **LEFT:** the Basilica of Santa Croce in Florence. **ABOVE:** the fortified town of Monteriggioni.

power. Whereas Palazzo Strozzi emphasises strength and stability, homes such as Palazzo Rucellai were more harmonious, embellished with elegant loggias, classical motifs and decorative friezes.

Renaissance architects

As the cradle of the Renaissance, Tuscany is where the profession of architect first came into its own. Imbued with a new humanist spirit, architects of the stature of Brunelleschi, Alberti, Michelozzo, Rossellino and Sangallo made their mark on churches, palaces and villas. Florence, which saw itself as the inheritor of Roman grandeur, is the Tuscan city with the greatest concentration of Renaissance monuments. Strongly influenced by Tuscan Romanesque, the buildings were models of visual restraint, dedicated to proportion, perspective and classical motifs. Brunelleschi (1377–1446), the father of Renaissance architecture, left his masterpiece on the Duomo in Florence. His spectacular dome was the fulfilment of the Renaissance ideal, an astounding feat of Florentine engineering *(see page 98)*.

Alberti (1404–72) rivalled Brunelleschi in his gift for geometry and desire to revive "the immutable laws of architecture", yet also respected the Tuscan taste for decoration. As an architectural historian, he revived Vitruvius's

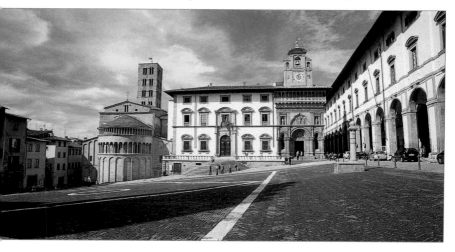

SACRED SIGHTS

Religious architecture represents one of the highlights of Tuscany. Any tour would certainly include the cathedrals of Florence, Lucca, Pisa and Siena. Lesser-known gems include Barga's Romanesque cathedral, Montepulciano's Renaissance San Biagio and the Romanesque San Miniato al Monte in the Florentine hills. Given city rivalries, Tuscan Romanesque delights in distinctive regional variations, as in the differentiated stripes and arcading in Lucca. In San Michele, a city masterpiece, the chiselled style of the delicate colonnades emphasises the height and exuberance of the facade. In many cases, architecture is inextricably bound up with artistic wealth on the walls, as in Santa Maria Novella in Florence or Arezzo's San Francesco. However, exteriors can be austere or unfinished, a sign that patrons argued or ran out of funds.

Setting is also significant, with cathedrals usually constructed on spots hallowed since Roman and Etruscan times. Mendicant churches were often built outside city walls, with surrounding squares becoming major city markets. Abbeys and monasteries, often as large as medieval towns, were built on new sites, and blended civic and Christian concerns. Some good examples are the Romanesque abbey of Sant'Antimo the Baroque Certosa di Pisa, the Carthusian foundation of Camaldoli; the hilltop monastery of La Verna; and the Benedictine Monte Oliveto Maggiore, in the woods south of Siena.

theories and put them into practice in Florence. The laws of proportion, perspective and the use of the classical orders all came into play in the Duomo and in the Florentine Palazzo Rucellai (1446). This landmark palace was inspired by the Colosseum and classical Rome. The Roman

> Alberti is considered the archetypal Renaissance man; a patrician playwright, humanist and philosopher, composer and lawyer, athlete and architect.

influence is present in the porches and panelled doors, as well as in the frieze. The magnificent Rucellai loggia was the last to be built in 15th-century Florence, such was the profligacy it engendered. Weddings and festivities in the loggia may be no more, but the family remains ensconced in the palace.

Rural retreats

Tuscany's rich urban heritage risks overshadowing the delightful rural legacy of sunny villas and picturesque hilltop farmhouses. In medieval Tuscany, the traditional battlemented manor or fortified seat evolved into the gracious villa residence of Renaissance times. In the 13th century, there were two forms of rural retreat, the feudal domain – the grand preserve of the landed nobility – and the *casa da signore*, the hub of a country estate. This was a crenellated property with a watchtower, surrounded by farm buildings and cottages, and owned by the gentry or bourgeoisie.

The villa as a country retreat was a Renaissance concept, reflecting the gracious rural lifestyle cultivated by the Tuscan nobility, even today. The villas were mostly elegant but unostentatious, reflecting the cultural conservatism of the Florentine nobility. However, the grandest Medici villas, such as Cafaggiolo, designed by Michelozzo, were sumptuous princely estates. Poggio a Caiano *(see page 128)* is the model Renaissance villa, with its harmonious design and colonnaded loggia harking back to the grandeur of classical times. The rural design

reflected a desire for symmetry and a rationalisation of form and function. Embellished by porticoes, the villa was built on a square plan around an inner courtyard, with a loggia on the first floor. Set in ornamental gardens and encircled by walls, the villa enjoyed superb views, often from a hilltop.

At a time when peace reigned in the Tuscan countryside, the gardens were regarded as a bucolic retreat, featuring a *giardino segreto*, a geometrical walled garden, with formal parterres and topiary, kitchen and herb gardens, lined by stately avenues of cypresses or lemon trees. The design, enlivened by water gardens, was set in the 16th century, when the Mannerist

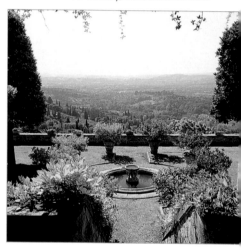

style acquired colonnades and statuary, grottoes and follies.

By the 17th century, the crisp geometry of the gardens was matched by formal terraces, virtuoso waterworks and sculptures of sea monsters cavorting with mythological figures. In their ease and openness, the gardens demonstrated a harmony with the house and with the patrician owner.

As the Renaissance architect Alberti declared, "Only the house of a tyrant can look like a fortress: an ideal home should be open to the world outside, beautifully adorned, delicate and finely proportioned rather than proud and stately". ❑

LEFT: Arezzo's stately main square. **RIGHT:** a garden of Villa Medici, a rural retreat built by Michelozzo.

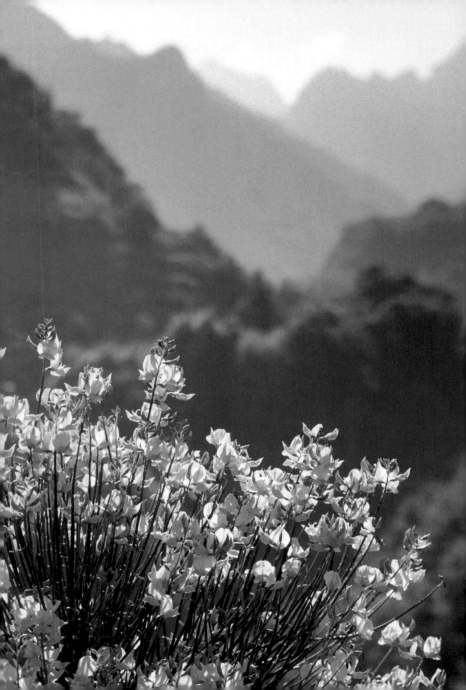

WILD TUSCANY

Nature-lovers sated with the art treasures of the
region will find plenty of wild refuges
in which to rest or roam

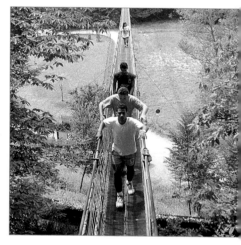

Classic Tuscany is a civilised scene of silvery olive groves, vine-cloaked hills, sunflowers shimmering in the heat and dark silhouettes of cypresses, arranged in double file along timeless avenues. The Welsh poet Dylan Thomas, who was no stranger to life on the wild side, praised the Florentine countryside – "The pine hills are endless, the cypresses at the hilltop tell one all about the length of death, the woods are deep as love and full of goats" – a seductive rural image that has attracted so many visitors to this lush region in search of their version of earthly paradise.

Given the civilisation of the landscape, "wild Tuscany" might seem a misnomer. Yet, beyond the classic chessboard of vineyards, a rugged wilderness awaits keen explorers. Tuscany is Italy's most thickly wooded region. Mountains soar, and in the northwest there are woods as thick as rainforests, while on the west coast the Maremma marshlands remain the emptiest and most ecologically pure stretch of coastline in the country. The south, meanwhile, has the unexpected primeval emptiness of the Sienese moonscape.

The Apuan Alps, Lunigiana and Garfagnana

This mountain chain, with its awe-inspiring landscape, runs parallel to the coastline and the Apennine ridge. Behind the well-groomed beaches of Versilia, on the western side of the chain, lurks a rugged hinterland of marble

LEFT: wild flowers in the Apuan Alps. **RIGHT:** negotiating a suspension bridge near Pistoia.

quarries and mountain ridges, narrow gorges, deep caves and thermal springs.

> The Apuan Alps are named after the Apuani Ligures tribe who lived in this region in ancient times.

Mountainous Lunigiana, north of Carrara (famous for its marble), is wedged between Emilia and Liguria. The region is crisscrossed by streams, with canoeing popular in the clear waters of the river Magra. From Aulla, a convenient base, there are organised tours of glacial moraines, karst gorges, caves and botanical gardens.

Garfagnana lies on the borders of Emilia Romagna and northern Tuscany, between the Apuan Alps and the Apennines. Parco dell'Orecchiella is the region's most spectacular park. While closely resembling the Apuan Alps, it is higher and wilder, with a mixture of woodland and pasture, picturesque clearings and mountain streams.

The Apennines

While the Apuan Alps are more varied, the Apennine range of mountains has not been ravaged by quarrying. They include the range on the Emilian border, the loftiest in the northern Apennines, as well as those in the Casentino and Mugello.

The Casentino, north of Arezzo, forms a series of razor-like crests and deep woods that straddle Emilia and northeast Tuscany. Centred on Bibbiena in the Upper Arno, these ancient forests are the region's finest. While the Emilian side is characterised by steep bluffs and stratified outcrops, the Tuscan side presents a softer atmosphere and range of scenery, with picturesque waterfalls and streams.

The Mugello, the hilly region north of Florence, resembles a landscape painted by Giotto, whose homeland this was. The Mugello can

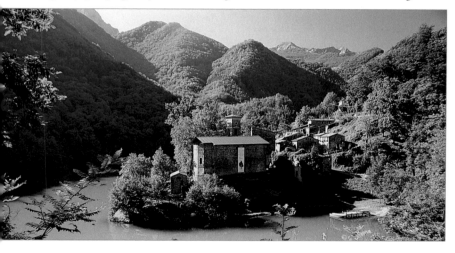

HIKING FOR TUSCANY

Tuscany is beguiling walking country, with a typical hike from Volterra to San Gimignano encompassing an old Etruscan trail and the Via Francigena, the route that led medieval pilgrims from Canterbury to Rome. The dusty trail, mostly along typical Tuscan *strade bianche,* follows these unpaved roads past vineyards, sunflowers and honey-coloured hamlets. Naturally, you wind into a sleepy hilltop hamlet, such as Casole d'Elsa, in time for lunch in an arty *trattoria*, with olive-oil coated *crostini* and *panzanella* salad washed down with a crisp Vernaccia di San Gimignano. After fording a few streams and passing abandoned farmhouses, you can fall into a farm-stay for a *Fiorentina* steak and bed. Tuscany at its most seductive.

But without the right planning, the reality can shock you out of any reverie. The region is often let down by poor maps, haphazard signposting and the lack of passing help. Contrary to popular belief, Tuscany is not Chiantishire: far from being assailed by linen-clad compatriots, you may not meet a soul *en route*, apart from languid-eyed Chianina cattle. For "soft hiking", opt for a walking holiday through a specialist operator *(see page 294)*. You can still do the trails independently, but following a wonderfully detailed route-map without nasty surprises – no getting lost in the forest, or arriving at the sole *trattoria* on closing day. The walking itinerary described is available through Headwater (www.headwater.com).

> The Apennines are divided into three sections: northern (Appennino setten-trionale), central (Appennino centrale) and southern (Appennino meridionale).

be explored on horseback, by following the old bridle paths between the cities of Bologna and Florence. The valleys along the Sieve, the main tributary of the Arno, are dotted with villages, olive groves and vineyards. The transition from valley to mountains means that olive groves give way to chestnut and oak forests before culminating in beech woods and waterfalls. Upper Mugello is a harsh, wild landscape of mountain peaks and passes, with ridges and ravines carved out by flowing rivers over the years.

Classic Chianti

While the Florentine Chianti is devoted to wine, the Sienese side is wilder, with vineyards gradually giving way to slopes covered in holm oaks, chestnuts and juniper. A 15km (9 mile) hilly hike from Greve in Chianti to Panzano covers the Via Chiantigiana and its offshoots, passing farms, cypresses and chestnut groves along the way.

In subtle Siena province, much of the landscape is classic Tuscany, with olive groves, gently rolling hills and dark cypresses standing sentinel. However, stretching from Siena to Montepulciano is a singular moonscape known as Le Crete Senesi, the strange hillocks marking the Sienese badlands. Barren or virtually treeless, this is beguiling territory nonetheless, with solitary farmhouses marooned on the crests of hills. This seemingly empty terrain is in fact home to a range of wildlife including foxes, badgers and wild boar.

Monte Amiata, the site of an extinct volcano further south, presents the province's wilder face, with a profusion of thermal springs bubbling amid the beech and chestnut groves. With its mossy banks and majestic grandeur, the mountainous setting is suitable for hiking, horse riding and skiing.

LEFT: a verdant scene in the Garfagnana. **RIGHT:** the wooded regions of Tuscany should not be overlooked.

Marshy Maremma

Maremma, the southern coastal strip, is a composite of natural Tuscany. The Parco della Maremma, with its soft whalebacked hills parallel to the coast, is dotted with Spanish watchtowers, parasol pines and coastal dunes.

On La Spergolaia ranch, the legendary *butteri*, the last of the Maremman cowboys, break in sturdy wild horses. The park can be explored on horseback or on foot from Alberese, where waymarked paths connect the shoreline and steep cliffs (*see overleaf and page 241*).

For more information on hiking in Tuscany, see pages 294–6, and consult the Italian parks website, www.parks.it. ❑

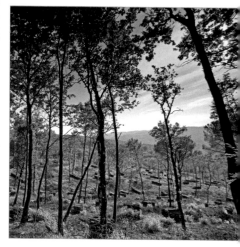

ANIMAL MAGIC

Italian hunters' fondness for the chase means that the wildlife has taken flight. The power of the hunting lobby has severely depleted numbers, with the exception of wild boar. Outside designated reserves, wildlife-spotters fare less well than botanists. Hawks and golden eagles still enjoy the majesty of the mountains, but life is no pastoral idyll for deer, ravaged by hunting. But, against the odds, Apennine wolves have made a comeback in the mountains, encouraged by the profusion of their favourite dish, short-fleeced mouflons (mountain sheep). Even so, sightings of the short-fleeced sheep, porcupine or wild boar are more frequent than glimpses of the eagle owl, weasel, wildcat or wolf.

A Walk in the Park

Tuscany's parks and wild places are increasingly becoming centres for rural pursuits, whether a stroll in the park with the family or a major mountain trek

A way from the cultural crowds, nature-lovers and adrenalin junkies can indulge in hiking, skiing, horse riding, mountain biking, climbing, caving, gliding, paragliding, sailing and surfing.

Riding is very popular in Tuscan parks, with more riding stables and well-trodden mule tracks than anywhere else in Italy.

This is also a rambler's paradise. The trails are marginally better mapped than in most Italian regions, and run from relaxed to rigorous. Serious hikers can follow the long-distance trails organised by the Italian Alpine Club (CAI) (see website www.cai.it for more details).

Parco Appennino Tosco-Emiliano

The Apennine ridges that span the border between northern Tuscany and Emilia Romagna offer diverse landscapes, from moorlands and lakes to craggy summits and waterfalls. The wildlife includes golden eagles, wolves and roe deer.

The new visitor centre is at Fivizzano (tel: 0585-947 200; www.appenninopark.it).

In the Parco dell'Alto Appennino, Abetone, commanding the mountain pass separating Tuscany and Emilia, is the region's most important winter-sports resort. Fortunately, the mountain air also makes Abetone invigorating during a stifling Tuscan summer, when the cable car takes walkers up to the leafy heights.

Despite the ravages of hunting, the forest is home to roe deer, mouflons and marmots, with golden eagles swooping over the crags. One of the most rewarding stretches of the rugged long-distance path (GEA) lies between here and Cisa.

Yet Abetone is also suitable for less energetic walkers – well-marked trails in the woods are available for those who prefer to stroll.

Parco delle Foreste Casentinesi

Home to the secluded monasteries of Camáldoli and La Verna, this corner of the Casentino lies along the ridge that divides eastern Tuscany and Emilia Romagna. Deer, golden eagles and wolves inhabit these ancient beech and chestnut woods.

The park headquarters are in Prato Vecchio (Via Brocchi 7; tel: 0575-50301; www.parcoforestecasentinesi.it), with information offices at Camáldoli (tel: 0575-556 130) and Campigna (tel: 0543-980 231; www.parks.it).

Parco Alpi Apuane

The park extends for over 20,000 hectares (49,000 acres) between the coastal plain and the rivers Magra, Aulella and Serchio. The Apuan Alps are different from the Apennines, with deep valleys, steep slopes and mountains of glistening white marble. Forests of chestnut and beech give cover to some 300 species of bird, while marmots can be spotted on the higher slopes.

Lago di Vaglia, in the heart of the mountains, is a reservoir containing a submerged medieval village that can be seen periodically. The underground landscape is equally inspiring, with caves often as deep as the mountains are high, and notoriously long and labyrinthine.

In Fornovolasco, east of Forte dei Marmi, the Grotta del Vento has the region's most fascinating network of caverns, riddled with steep gorges and secret passages, slowly revealing stalagmites and stalactites, fossils and alabaster formations, crystal pools and echoing chambers.

The visitor centre in Castelnuovo di Garfagnana (Piazza Erbe 1; tel: 0583-644 242; www.parcapuane.it; www.parks.it) provides help on hiking, climbing, cycling and horse riding. Park guides are available for hikes or visits to caves.

RIGHT: poppies brighten the fields of Tuscany in springtime.

Parco dell'Orecchiella

The mountains of the Orecchiella park in the Garfagnana region are higher than the neighbouring Apuan Alps, but the landscape is more tame and subtle, and crisscrossed by hiking trails.

The area is centred on the high broad plain of Pania di Corfino, overlooked by a dramatic limestone peak that dominates the Serchio valley. The wildlife includes deer, wild boar, mouflons, badgers, otters, weasels and wolves. San Pellegrino monastery offers fabulous views and houses a folk museum.

San Romano in Garfagnana visitor centre (tel: 0583-619 098; www.ingarfagnana.it) makes a good base for exploring.

Parco di Migliarino, San Rossore, Massaciuccoli

This park covers the coastal hinterland behind the beach resorts between Viareggio and Livorno, and includes the forest of San Rossore and Lake Massaciuccoli. Huge holm oaks and maritime pines grow right up to the beach and are home to wild boar, fallow deer and countless species of native and migratory birds. The San Rossore archaeological site, where a fleet of Roman ships was unearthed, can be visited by appointment.

There is a visitor centre at Coltano (Villa Medicea, Via Palazzi 21; tel: 050-989 084), while the Tenuta San Rossore organises walking and cycling tours (tel: 050-530 101; www.parcosanrossore.it). Boat tours of Lake Massaciuccoli depart from Torre del Lago.

Parco della Maremma

This beautiful, unspoilt wilderness, covering over 100 sq km (40 sq miles), stretches along the Tyrrhenian coast from Principina a Mare to Talamone. It is centred on the Monti dell'Uccellina, which rise up from the sea.

The rugged landscape is a mixture of marshland, mountains and coast backed by umbrella pines, interspersed with rocky outcrops and coves. There are no human settlements, and just one access road links Alberese, the park entrance, to Marina Alberese, a virgin seaside stretch that attracts migratory birds on their journey to Africa. The dense vegetation here provides the perfect habitat for wild boar, the symbol of the Maremma, while herds of Maremman cattle and horses of the *butteri* (local cowherds) roam on its plains.

The Alberese visitor centre (Via Bersagliere 7; tel: 0564-407 098; www.parco-maremma.it) works with Naturalmente Toscana, which offers walking, riding and canoeing trips – as well as free food and wine tastings onsite (tel: 0564-407 269; www.naturalmentetoscana.it).

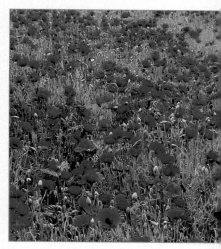

Parco dell'Arcipelago Toscano

This is Europe's largest marine reserve and is popular with diving enthusiasts. It covers the seven islands of the Tuscan Archipelago: Elba, Capraia, Gorgona, Pianosa, Montecristo, Giglio and Giannutri. The coastline and sea bed vary enormously from island to island, hence the variety of flora and fauna on show to curious visitors. Sea birds such as shearwaters and blackheaded gulls proliferate, while dolphins, sperm whales and even the rare monk seal may also be sighted.

The marine park is based in Elba (tel: 0565-919 428; www.isoleditoscana.it). ❏

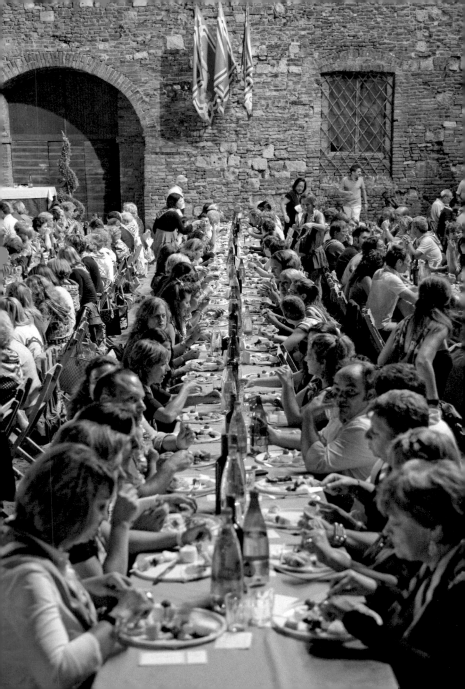

A TASTE OF TUSCANY

Traditional Tuscan cuisine is *cucina povera*, robust "peasant food" – but this deceptive simplicity is now valued as tasty authenticity, served straight from the land

Tuscany has everything to offer the foodie, with dishes designed to bring out the richness of the wine. From T-bone steaks to peasant soups, wild-boar stews, truffle sauces, hearty cheeses and divine cakes, this is as far from faddish "creative" cuisine as you can get.

What is immediately striking about Tuscan food is that it is rustic, simple but robust, nourishing the soul and the spirit as much as the body. The Tuscan monks who cultivated wine and oil estates knew what they were doing and, in some cases, are still doing. The cooking is never elaborate or excessive; there are no fussy finishing touches, complex reductions of sauces or subtly blended flavours. But there is a basic earthiness about the dishes that has made them popular the world over.

Tuscany produces its own inimitable versions of Italian staples: pasta dishes with gamey wild-boar sauce; *pici* pasta with fresh ceps; and *fagioli all'Uccelletto*, beans in tomato sauce. But along with a traditional attitude to food, the region also offers distinctive delicacies and seasonal dishes, such as truffles and wild mushrooms.

Bean-eaters rule

The Tuscans are known as *Toscani Mangiafagioli* – bean-eaters, because the pulse enriches so many dishes. Legumes are a mainstay in Tuscany, where *cannellini*, white kidney beans, add a smooth texture. Served in terracotta pots, thick soups and hearty bean stews are often

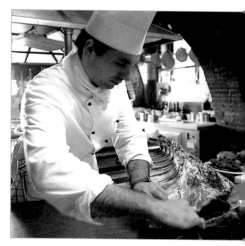

enhanced by a trickle of olive oil added at the table. Many chefs rate Tuscan oil the world's finest but rarely agree on which area, let alone which estate, produces the very best. As the locals are never impartial, foodie visitors are left to compare the virtues of oil from Lucca, the Chianti, the Maremma and Siena.

Soups are made of the ubiquitous beans, and include *acquacotta*, a vegetable soup with an egg added before serving, and *pappa al pomodoro*, a thick soup of bread and tomatoes. Even more typical is the Florentine winter speciality, *ribollita* ("reboiled"), which improves the flavour of the soup.

Elsewhere, the rugged Garfagnana region

LEFT: a Sienese celebratory feast during the Palio.
RIGHT: preparing *bistecca alla Fiorentina*.

favours tasty spelt soups, enriched by oil, onions and *borlotti* beans.

Coastal Livorno produces delicious *cacciucco*, a filling shellfish-and-fish soup that supposedly inspired the French *bouillabaisse*. The story goes that the soup originated in the port after a tremendous storm that left a widowed fisherman's wife desperately trying to feed her hungry brood. The children came home with handfuls of mussels, shrimps, half a fish and some fish heads – which the wily mother tossed into a pot with herbs and tomatoes to create the glorious *cacciucco*. While *zuppa di pesce* (fish soup) can be eaten all over Italy, *cacciucco* can be eaten only around Livorno, ladled over toasted, garlicky croutons.

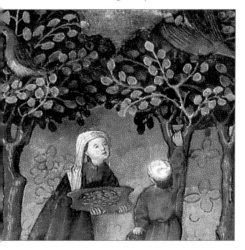

Bread and cheese

Tuscan bread is made without salt, supposedly because salt was once reserved for "precious" foods such as salami. Dante wrote of Florentine bread, comparing it favourably with the salty bread he was forced to eat in exile. The importance of bread is revealed in local expressions, such as "Bread cannot be made with flour alone", or "Better stale bread at home than a roast at someone else's house". In fact, stale bread finds its way into *panzanella*, a typical peasant dish made with tomatoes, onions, cucumber and basil, drenched in olive oil. You will also sample bread in the form of *bruschetta* or *crostini*, coated with olive oil or liver-based spreads.

Tuscan cheeses are varied and plentiful. There is a delightful overspill of cheeses from neighbouring Emilia Romagna, including Parmesan, *parmigiano reggiano*, which complements Tuscany's marvellous pasta dishes and soups. Other stalwarts include pecorino, a hard, healthy ewe's-milk cheese, produced since Roman times. Although ideally suited to grating, pecorino matures well and can also be used in pasta fillings. Lesser-known cheeses include *marzolino*, a ewe's-milk cheese made in March, when milk is most plentiful in the Chianti valley; *mucchino*, cow's-milk cheese made in and around Lucca by the same procedure as pecorino; and all the local rustic *cacciotte* and ricotta made with cow's, goat's and ewe's milk. Pienza is a key centre for artisan cheeses, especially *cacio pecorino*.

Hearty stews and barbecues

Tuscan cooks favour rustic, outdoor cooking – a grill over an open wood fire is not uncommon

---

TRUFFLE TROVE

"Truffles taste and smell of people and sweat," says chef Giorgio Locatelli. "Everything that life tastes and smells of is in there." Pungent and pricey, the white truffle is a paradox; a princely treat harvested by peasants since Roman times.

Dubbed "the white diamond", it is actually a dirty yellow-brown in colour. Emperor Nero called truffles "the food of the gods", while excitable food critics wax lyrical about truffles as "the sex of the gods". Truffles are underground fungi, developing close to the roots of oaks, poplars and hazelnut trees. But the exact location of a "truffle trove" is a well-guarded secret, with truffle-hunters regarding their talented dogs, who unearth the tuber, as important members of their families.

Although the most prized white truffles come from Piedmont, Tuscany also has its share, centred on San Miniato, which hosts a truffle festival in November. The precious white truffle is available from September to December, while variants of black truffle are available all year. Connoisseurs favour simplicity in use, with shavings of white truffle grated over pasta, fried egg, salad or risotto. Black truffles suit more complex dishes, but are equally delicious grated over a *crostini* (grilled bread) coated with *stracchino* cheese.

Set in a castle in San Giovanni d'Asso, the intriguing Truffle Museum provides information on truffle fairs, tours and inns (www.museodeltartufo.it; and www.assotartufi.it).

behind a chic Florentine restaurant or in the garden of a rural *trattoria*. Fresh sage, rosemary and basil are used, as they grow in abundance.

The Tuscan meat dish *par excellence* is the *bistecca alla Fiorentina*, a vast, tender, succulent T-bone steak – preferably from cattle raised in Val di Chiana. With expressive eyes and long-limbed grace, the beautiful white Chianina breed was used in Roman triumphal marches, or sacrificed to the gods in Etruscan times. The meat is brushed with the purest virgin olive oil and grilled over a scented wood fire of oak or olive branches, then seasoned with salt and pepper. In good Florentine restaurants, you will be able to see the meat raw before you order.

can times. The odd-looking pig is even depicted in Lorenzetti's famous 14th-century fresco of *Good Government* in Siena's Town Hall.

Hunting is a popular sport, resulting in plentiful offerings of *cinghiale* (wild boar), which comes in many guises. Despite conservationists' pleas, small birds, from sparrows to quail, are also still considered fair game.

Autumn harvest

The "fruits of the forest" are particularly prized in Tuscany, especially chestnuts, mushrooms and truffles. Chestnuts are a staple, particularly in mountainous regions, where they are made into flour, pancakes, soups and sweet cakes such as

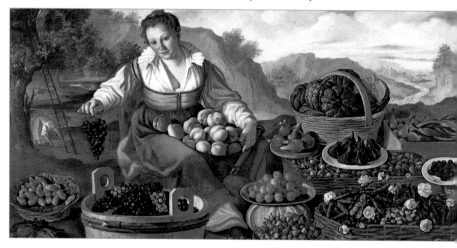

Another famous Tuscan meat dish is *arista alla Fiorentina*, pork loin highly seasoned with rosemary and ground pepper. The dish dates back to the 15th century, when the Greek bishops were served it at a Florentine banquet and pronounced it *"aristos"*, meaning "very good" in Greek. The name stuck, and it has become a feature of Tuscan cuisine ever since.

In the Sienese countryside, the white-striped Cinta Senese breed has been producing the region's finest pork and charcuterie since Etrus-

Left: picking olives, as depicted by a 15th-century artist.
Above: *The Fruit Vendor*, a 16th-century painting by Vincenzo Campi, celebrates the region's harvest.

EXTRA VIRGIN

Tuscans are passionate about olive oil, and cook with oil rather than butter. Tuscan olive oil has long been famous for its quality, flavour and texture, and is accorded DOC status, an equivalent to the French *appellation contrôlée* system for wine. Quality is measured by acid content, with *Extra vergine* the top quality, with less than 1 percent acid content. Excellent delicate, fruity oils include Extravergine di Scansano, Extravergine del Chianti, and Extravergine Badia á Coltibuono. The Badia dí Coltibuono is Tuscan perfection: a tranquil, medieval oil and wine estate set in landscape that has been cultivated since time immemorial. In Tuscany, it is hard to separate the oil from the landscape.

castagnaccio, flavoured with rosemary and pine nuts. The season peaks around mid-October, when chestnut lovers can travel on a restored 1920s steam train from Florence to Marradi's *Sagra delle Castagne*, or chestnut festival, to join the celebrations.

In the autumn, when the rains fall, the hills are awash with family outings. Long lines of cars park along the side of the mountain roads – particularly in the Maremma, Garfagnana and Mugello areas, where locals arm themselves with baskets and hooked knives, in search of *funghi*. The wild-mushroom season is eagerly awaited but if you want to join in, go with a local, since many types of mushroom are poisonous. Or

simply purchase *funghi* from a roadside market during the August–October season. The varieties of wild mushrooms depend upon the type of tree nearby – but the most sought after are the perfect *porcini (Boletus edulis)*, ceps that grow to enormous size and thickness.

Fresh wild mushrooms are best grilled in the Tuscan way, like a steak: rub each with a slice of lemon, season with slivers of garlic and sprigs of thyme – or, even simpler, just brush with olive oil and salt. Dried *porcini* are even tastier, as the dehydration concentrates the flavour. When regenerated by soaking in lukewarm water, they are ideal for use in risotto or pasta sauces. Mushrooms can also be used to flavour *pici*, the

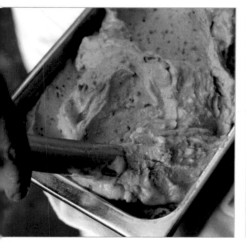

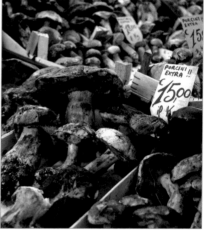

typical Tuscan spaghetti. But if there is one food that provokes more excitement than wild mushrooms, it is the *tartufo*, or truffle – particularly the white variety *(see page 74)*.

Saffron is another autumn harvest, cultivated around San Gimignano for over 800 years. The valuable spice was even used as a currency, given its prestige and transportability. In 1200, the Bishop of Volterra used saffron to bribe the counsellors to the Roman Curia. Saffron only flowers for a fortnight between October and November, and must be gathered at dawn when the purplish flower is closed. Over 500 hours of work are required to produce a kilo, since the rust-coloured filaments are picked by hand, then dried and "toasted", before finding their way into risotto and sauces.

Sienese sweetmeats

Siena is the most sweet-toothed city, famous for its pastries, biscuits and cakes. *Panforte*, a Sienese Christmas speciality, is unmistakable in its brightly coloured octagonal box. It is a rich, sweet cake of candied fruit, nuts, spices, honey and sugar, sandwiched between sheets of ricepaper. *Ricciarelli* are delightful, diamond-shaped almond cakes, also saved for Christmas, along with the rich, golden rice cake called *torta di riso*. Instead, *cavallucci* are hard biscuits served at the end of a meal and dipped in Vin Santo

Tuscan biscuits: Prato's version, *biscottini di Prato*, are made from almonds, eggs, flour and sugar, and are delicious dipped in Vin Santo. Castelnuovo della Garfagnana specialises in a simple chestnut cake called *torta garfagnina*, while closer to the Emilia Romagna borders, look out for a baked-apple cake, the *torta di mele*.

No visit to Florence would be complete without ice cream – the Florentines claim to have invented *gelato*. Always look for the sign *Produzione Propria* (home-made). The city produces *zuccotto*, a sponge-cake mould with a filling of almonds, hazelnuts, chocolate and cream. Once eaten, it is never forgotten. Literally translated as "small pumpkin", this dome-shaped Florentine

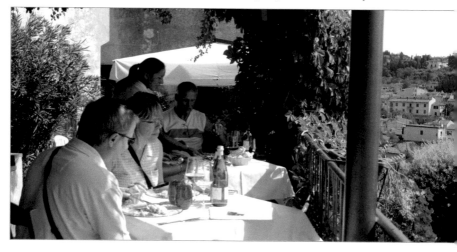

dessert wine. The local *pasticcerie* are filled with delectable varieties.

Siena faces stiff competition from the cake shops of Lucca, Pistoia, Prato and the Garfagnana. Lucca favours a plain, ring-shaped cake known as *buccellato*, and a sweet tart of spinach and chard with pine nuts. Pistoia produces the pretty *corona di San Bartolomeo* for the feast of St Bartholomew on 24 August, when mothers lead their children to church wearing this cake "necklace" to receive a blessing from the saint. *Cantuccini* are typical

speciality either alludes to the cathedral (Duomo) or to the clergy: in Tuscan dialect, a cardinal's skullcap is also called a *zuccotto*.

Tuscany is truly a food-lover's paradise, riddled with wine and food trails that invariably run through a patchwork of vineyards and olive groves or cornfields edged with sunflowers. The Chianti route is a chance to enjoy a T-bone steak and Chianti Classico wines. In the Tuscan capital, if you can stomach it, there is a trail that includes tripe, a Florentine delicacy. In the Garfagnana, book a Slow Food tour with Sapori & Saperi to savour, or even harvest, chestnuts, salami, wild mushrooms and bread baked in a wood-fired oven (www.sapori-e-saperi.com). ❑

FAR LEFT: it is claimed that Italy's famous *gelato* was invented in Florence. **LEFT:** fresh *funghi*. **ABOVE:** a meal with a view in Florence.

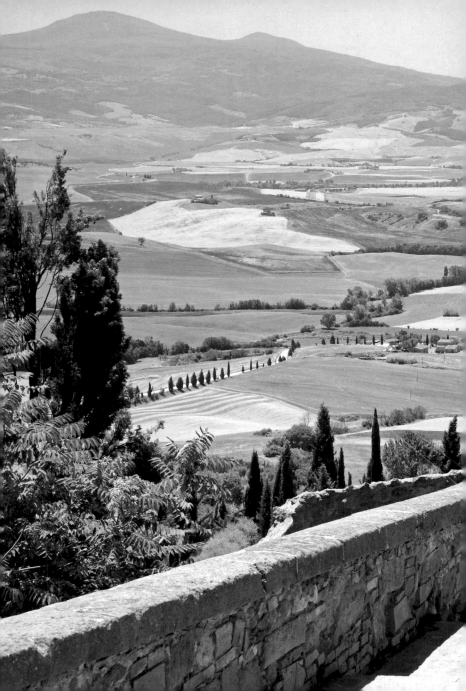

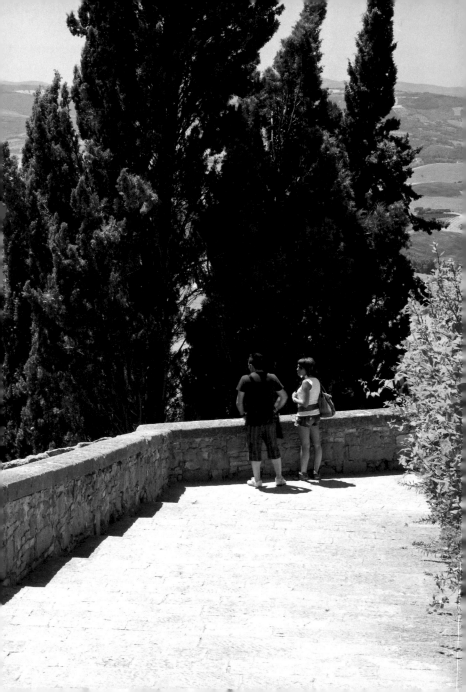

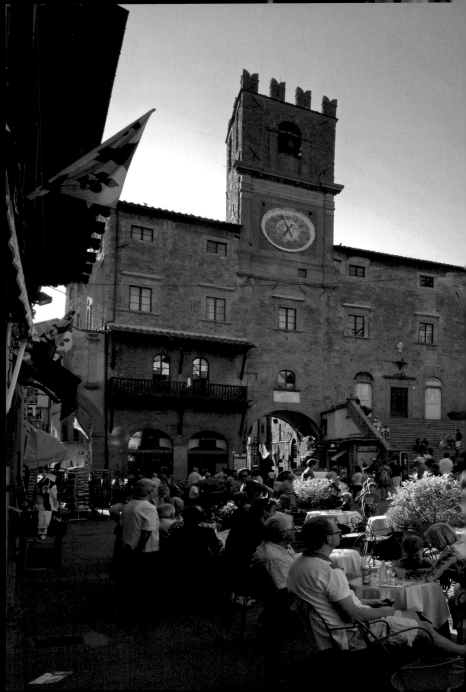

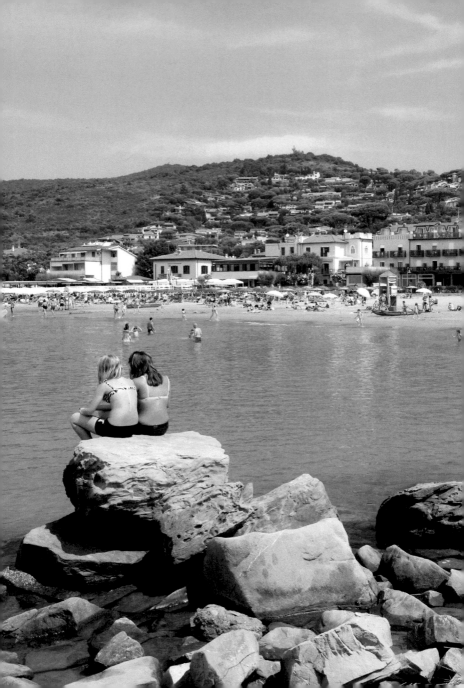

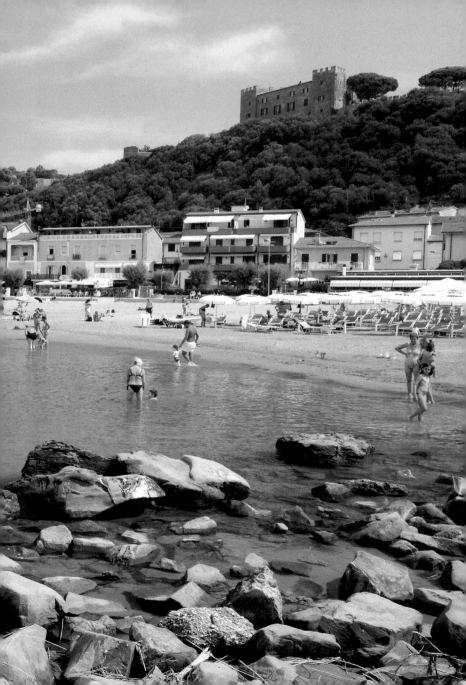

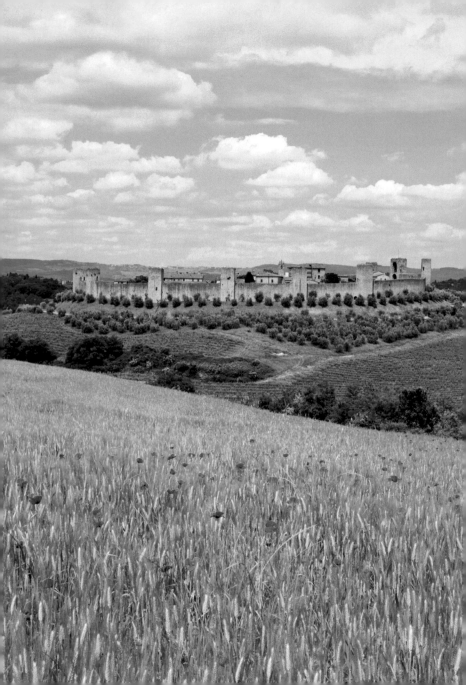

PLACES

**A detailed guide to the region, with the principal
sites clearly cross-referenced by number to the maps**

For many visitors, Tuscany is the true Italy – as conjured up by clichéd Merchant-Ivory film adaptations of E.M. Forster novels – a land of swaying cypress trees, olive groves and vineyards, scattered with medieval castles and Medici villas. Tuscans are more nuanced about their rural idyll. To them, Tuscany evokes the wild as well as the tamed, stretching from the Carrara-marble quarries to the Maremma wilderness, embracing the rugged coastline, rolling Chianti vineyards and the wooded slopes of Monte Amiata. Despite a deep relationship with the land, the heirs to the Etruscans recognise the tough realities of rural life. Tuscans are also innately sociable and will always prefer living in large villages or small towns to an isolated farmhouse, however idyllic.

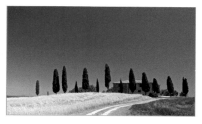

The appeal of Tuscan towns is their timelessness, civility and sense of ease with their past. Florence, the cradle of the Renaissance, retains a huge number of the artworks created in its honour. Gazing at the skyline from Piazzale Michelangelo reveals how little the cityscape has changed since its artistic heyday. Variety underpins Tuscan townscapes: from medieval hilltop eyries to Etruscan outposts; from *fin-de-siècle* spa towns to sophisticated beach resorts; from the splendour of a Renaissance palazzo to a stark Romanesque church. Medieval Siena and Renaissance Florence may be unmissable, but spare some time for Etruscan Volterra, genuine Massa Marittima or cyclist-friendly Lucca. Tuscan towns are built on a human scale. As for scenery, lap up the Unesco-protected Val d'Orcia countryside, mountainous Garfagnana, and wild, coastal Maremma.

For all Tuscany's artistic and architectural riches, however, most visitors would agree that as much pleasure can be derived from lunch on the shady terrace of a rustic trattoria and banter with its owner, as an encounter with Michelangelo's David and Botticelli's Venus. As Forster observed: "The traveller who has gone to Italy to study the tactile values of Giotto, or the corruption of the papacy, may return remembering nothing but the blue sky and the men and women who live under it." ❑

PRECEDING PAGES: wall trail in south Siena; watching the crowds go by in Cortona; Castiglione della Pescaia. **LEFT:** Monteriggioni in the Chianti region. **ABOVE:** a cypress-surrounded villa.

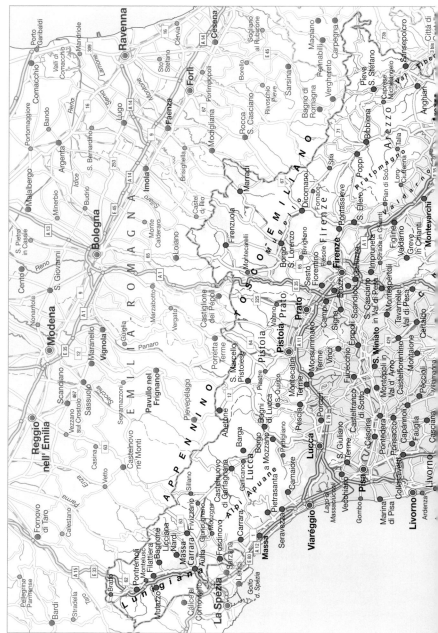

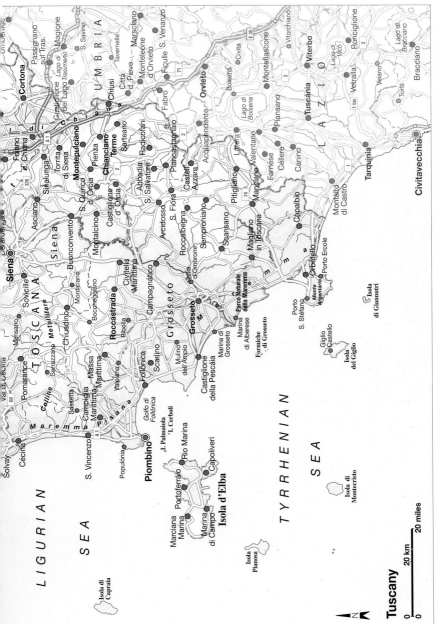

Tuscany

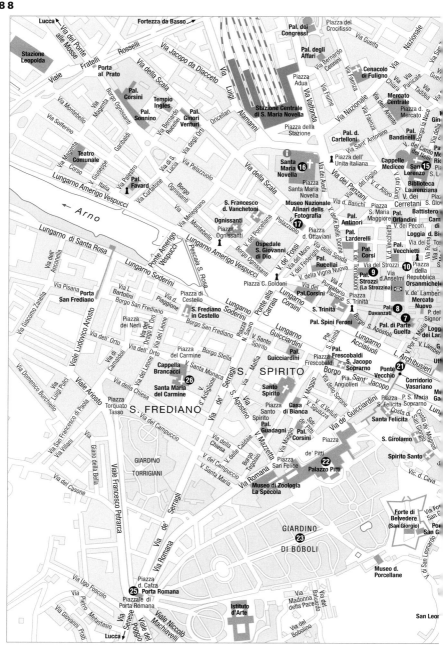

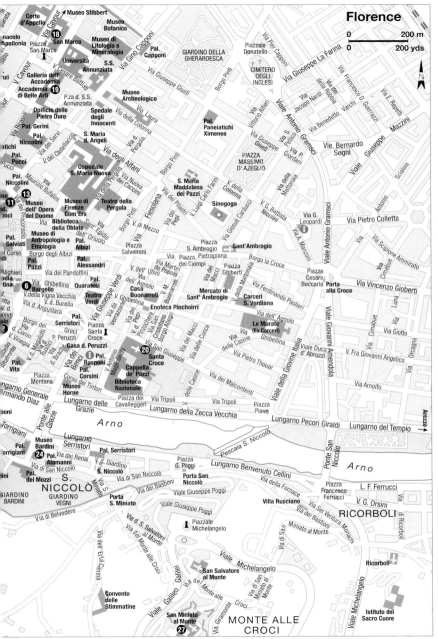

Florence

0   200 m
0   200 yds

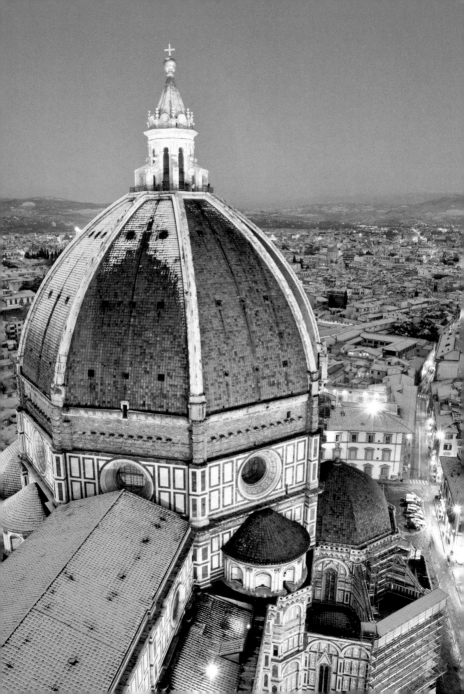

THE CITY OF FLORENCE

One of the world's architectural masterpieces, packed with palaces and art galleries, a revitalised Florence is an essential stop on any modern-day Grand Tour

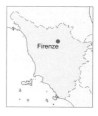

Firenze

More than any other Italian city, Florence is defined by its artistic heritage. The city is both blessed and burdened by a civic identity bound up with the Renaissance, and basks in its reflected glory. As the birthplace of the Renaissance, the city witnessed the Florentine miracle, a flowering of the human spirit that has left a lasting artistic imprint. The churches, palaces and galleries are studded with the world's greatest concentration of Renaissance art and sculpture. In 1743, Anna Maria Lodovica, the last of the Medici line, bequeathed her property to Florence, ensuring that the Medici collections remained intact forever. As a result, Florence is still awash with many of the treasures that Vasari, the first art historian, mentions in his *Lives of the Artists* (1550).

Although artistic treasures predominate, Florence is experiencing a revival that makes it far more than a Renaissance theme park. According to Matteo Renzi, the dynamic mayor, "Florence was on everyone's must-see list, and we got lazy. The sites were run for the benefit of bureaucrats. It is my duty to change this." True to his

word, he has pedestrianised swathes of the city, improved public transport, tackled pollution, sanctioned bicycle-friendly routes, extended museum opening times, and introduced a combined museum and transport pass.

Fortuitously, Florence is also experiencing a cultural resurgence, linked to the proliferation of new arts centres, theatre-dining clubs, cool bars, contemporary-art galleries and music venues, including a new opera, ballet and classical music

Main attractions

PIAZZA DELLA SIGNORIA
PALAZZO VECCHIO
GALLERIA DEGLI UFFIZI
BARGELLO
DUOMO AND BATTISTERO
MUSEO DELL'OPERA DEL DUOMO
CAPPELLE MEDICEE
SAN MARCO
GALLERIA DELL'ACCADEMIA
SANTA CROCE
PONTE VECCHIO
PALAZZO PITTI
GIARDINO DI BOBOLI
CAPPELLA BRANCACCI

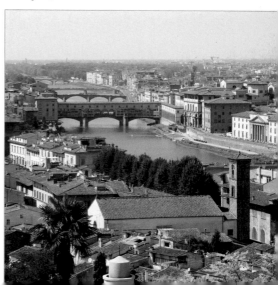

LEFT: the snow-capped dome of Florence's famous Duomo. **RIGHT:** a view of the River Arno running through the centre of Florence.

TIP

The Firenze Card (tel: 055 055; www.firenze card.it) is a 3-day museum and transport pass to Florence's museums, villas and gardens, plus all buses and trams (www.ataf.it). It covers 33 museums, including the major ones, plus the Medici villas beyond the city. The swipe card allows speedy access to museums, with no need for prior reservation, and free access to temporary exhibitions too. It costs €50 for 3 days, including all booking reservations, and is bought online or at 6 places in the city.

BELOW LEFT: Palazzo Vecchio at night. **BELOW RIGHT:** Medici lion, Loggia del Lanzi.

complex opening shortly.

To make the most of your stay, and to avoid the lengthy queues, either buy the three-day Firenze Card *(see Tip)* or pre-book the "blockbuster" museums, such as the Uffizi Gallery (tel: 055-294 883; www.firenzemusei.it).

Viewed from the surrounding hills, Florence seems to be floating in a bowl that, at dusk, is tinged violet. The honey-coloured walls and rose-coloured roofs combine to make a unity that is dominated by a single, vast building, the Cathedral, or Duomo. It is by far the biggest building for miles around, with its roof and dome in the same subtle colour-range as the surrounding smaller buildings, above which it also seems to float like a great liner among tugs.

There are few towers or spires to be seen in Florence. Giotto's multicoloured Campanile next to the Duomo, plain in outline but intricate in detail, and the thrusting tower of the Palazzo Vecchio, elegant and sombre, soar above a low-slung skyline. The overall impression is not that of a city, but of one single,

vast building, a majestic palace.

Close contact with the city can be initially disconcerting, even disappointing and claustrophobic. The streets are narrow, hemmed in by towering, plain buildings. There is no delicate filigree, as in Venice, or cheerful Baroque, as in Rome, to tempt the eye. Indeed, some of the city's buildings resemble 19th-century warehouses – grim structures that were erected at a time of social unrest, their primary function being that of fortresses. As for palaces, Florentine architectural taste runs to the monumental, macho and unembellished.

Here, the city has been grouped into four sections, starting with the area around Piazza della Signoria and the Palazzo Vecchio, followed by the Duomo area, and then by three important religious foundations (which, though physically scattered around the city, have been grouped together in this chapter). The final section is the River Arno and beyond. Many of the sights are within easy walking distance of each other – despite Florence's size, its historic centre is reasonably compact.

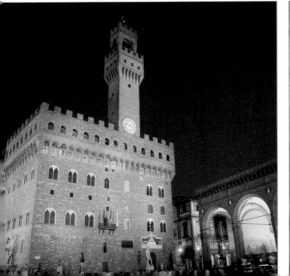

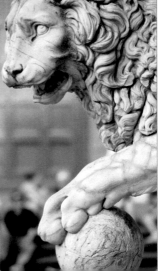

Piazza della Signoria: the civic centre

Florence is dauntingly monumental, nowhere more so than the **Piazza della Signoria ❶**, which is an open-air museum of sculpture, starring the so-called *déjà-vu David*, a copy of Michelangelo's famed heroic boy. More than any other square in Italy, the Piazza della Signoria evokes the ancient world and the overweening pride of the Renaissance city. Even so, of all the great city squares, Florence's is the most perversely irregular. There is nothing in the Piazza della Signoria to compete with the grace of Siena's curved Campo, or the simple majesty of Rome's Capitol. Tucked on one side is the **Palazzo Vecchio ❷** (tel: 055-276 8224; Fri–Wed 9am–midnight, Thur until 2pm; charge), the seat of government for the past six centuries.

The Medici administration was based in the Palazzo Vecchio, which remains the town hall, and which was redesigned during the reign of Cosimo I. The palace, under different guises, has been the emblem of Florentine power since the 14th century. With its bold swallowtail crenellations and asymmetrical bell tower, the Palazzo is the most evocative of city symbols.

The courtyard, with its copy of an enchanting fountain by Verrocchio, is a delight. Vasari's monumental staircase leads to the frescoed **Salone dei Cinquecento**, the Hall of the Five Hundred, where members of the Great Council met. Cosimo I set his stamp on the chamber by commissioning a series of vast frescoes, painted by Vasari, which glorified his military triumphs.

Beyond the art and the style, the palace reveals everyday Medici court life. It is also one of the few museums in conservative Florence to have moved into the 21st century in terms of presentation. The use of multimedia, "secret itineraries", and a children's perspective on great artworks has proved a resounding success. The **Museo dei Ragazzi** (Children's Museum) organises workshops with actors who bring the history to life.

The huge fountain in the centre of the piazza is the subject of affectionate

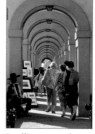

Strolling among the artworks for sale.

BELOW: the courtyard of Palazzo Vecchio.

Unfinished Masterpieces

The "finishing" of landmark buildings has always been controversial, particularly with regard to facades. Florentines will vote whether the facade of San Lorenzo should be finished according to Michelangelo's 500-year-old plans – his models and drawings still exist. Even in their heyday, the Florentines were notorious for not completing buildings, and 19th-century benefactors were happy to help. The foreign intelligentsia, in the grip of the Gothic Revival, set about dressing key city churches in evocative neo-Gothic facades, beginning with the Duomo and Santa Croce. The result is more atmospheric than authentic; critics describe the stripy green, white and pink marble facade as "a cathedral wearing pyjamas".

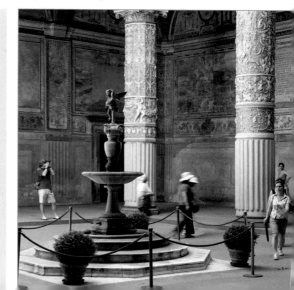

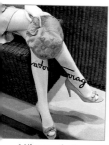

Milan may be the fashion capital, but Florence has its fair share of home-grown designers of international repute. Nearly all have their outlets at the southern end of Via de' Tornabuoni, including the shoemaker, Ferragamo.

mockery by Florentines themselves, and no two buildings in the piazza seem to have the same facade. With a despot's love of order, Cosimo I tried to impose an artificial unity on the square, but his schemes came to nothing, leaving the piazza as a perfect illustration of Florentine "unity in diversity".

The square has changed little over the centuries, as is evident in a contemporary painting (in the Museo di Firenze Com'Era) of the execution of Savonarola, the anti-Medici Dominican preacher, which took place here in 1498.

The **Marzocco**, the lion symbol of the city that prisoners were forced to kiss, can be found here, as well as a copy of Michelangelo's immense statue of *David* (the original is in the Accademia, *see page 118*), commissioned in 1501 to mark an important change in the constitution. Nearby is a statue of the first Medici duke, Cosimo I.

Next to the Palazzo Vecchio stands the elegant **Loggia dei Lanzi** ❸, crammed with statues. The loggia (named after the mercenaries employed by Cosimo) has an impressive statue of a triumphant Perseus holding the severed head of Medusa, which Cosimo commissioned from Cellini. Most stunning among the other statues in the loggia is Giambologna's *Rape of the Sabine Women* on the opposite side.

Galleria degli Uffizi

Adjoining the piazza are the immense galleries of the **Uffizi** ❹ *(see page 110)*. As the world's greatest collection of Italian art, the revamped Uffizi is both a feast for the senses and an indigestible banquet. What you choose to be moved by will depend on your mood. The Leonardo da Vinci room pays tribute to the greatest genius of the age, the master of the High Renaissance style.

Contemplation of great art is still possible, at least away from the Botticelli bottleneck, the Giotto genuflection, the Leonardo line and the Michelangelo muster station. Given the fickle nature of popular taste, Fra Angelico, Perugino, Pollaiuolo and Mantegna, to name but a few Renaissance peers, are often left to sleepy

Florence for Families

It's a myth that the city offers little to families sated with art and culture. You can now see the city **by bicycle**, by Segway (www.segway.it), or **by bicycle rickshaw** (Tre Rote, tel: 338-638 9245; www.pedicab-firenze.it). Pick up a "normal" bike on Piazza Santa Croce or opt for a ride in a **horse-drawn carriage** (from Piazza del Duomo or Piazza della Signoria). In summer, lounge on the Lungarno **urban beach,** a sandy affair on the banks of the Arno, or cruise along the river on *barchetti*, typical boats (embarkation near Piazza Mentana). Let off steam by exploring the grotesque statues and grottoes in the **Boboli Gardens**, retreating to a **Medici villa** or cycling through the Chianti countryside.

Child-friendly museums include the trailblazing Museo dei Ragazzi in the **Palazzo Vecchio** (tel: 055-276 8224; www.

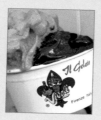

museoragazzi.it). Dress up in historical costume, learn about life at the Medici court, explore secret passages, or follow the nightwatchmen's rounds on the rooftops. In the **Leonardo da Vinci Museum**, get to grips with the designer's genius by studying the wooden models of his flying machines and armoured tanks, swing bridges and robots (tel: 055-282 966; www.mostredileonardo.com). With its chivalric mood and medieval armour, the **Stibbert Museum** is "culture lite" for kids (tel: 055-475 520; www.museostibbert.it). Jump into the cool **Palazzo Strozzi** for both arty children's tours and adult blockbusters. When all else fails, bribe the children with **ice cream** at Il Re Gelato (Piazza Strozzi), Grom (Via delle Oche) or Vivoli (Via Isola delle Stinche). As punishment, dare them to **eat tripe** ("awful offal") at San Lorenzo food market.

custodians and connoisseurs.

Just behind the Uffizi is the **Museo Galileo ⑤** (Mon, Wed–Sat 9.30am–6pm, Tue until 1pm; charge), formerly called the Museum of the History of Science. The revamped museum, housed in the 14th-century Palazzo Castellani, makes a refreshing change after an overindulgence in the arts. The collection of scientific instruments shows that Renaissance Florence was pre-eminent as a centre of scientific research. Amid the museum's prized collection of Galileo's instruments, the mathematician's middle finger of his right hand is displayed like the relic of a Christian saint.

Other rooms are devoted to astronomy, navigation, the science of warfare, and to the Medici who founded this scientific treasure trove.

The Bargello

Chronologically, the Palazzo Vecchio is the second city hall of Florence. Its predecessor, the **Bargello ⑥** *(see page 120)*, was built 50 years earlier in 1250 as the seat of the chief magistrate, the *Podestà*. The Bargello was, in effect, the police headquarters, and its courtyard witnessed public executions. The building is now a wonderful museum of sculpture, with a rich collection of works by artists such as Michelangelo, Cellini, Donatello – and is not nearly as bewildering as the Uffizi. The Bargello's tantalising calling card is Donatello's coquettish *David*, a rival to Michelangelo's more virile version in the Accademia.

Palaces and piazzas

Just west of the Piazza della Signoria is a loosely linked cluster of buildings that span four centuries of Florentine history, from the embattled Middle Ages to the era of ducal control. The **Palazzo di Parte Guelfa ⑦** (just off Via delle Terme) was the headquarters of the all-powerful Guelf Party, which, after

the defeat and expulsion of the rival Ghibellines, ruled the city.

For light relief, drop into the engagingly touristic **Mercato Nuovo** – the 16th-century covered market. Remember to stroke the *Porcellino*, the bronze boar whose snout is polished to gleaming gold: touching it supposedly guarantees your return to the city.

Also referred to as the Museo dell'Antica Casa Fiorentina, the **Palazzo Davanzati ⑧** (Tue–Sun 8.15am–1.50pm; charge) is the best-preserved example of a patrician home and provides an insight into life in medieval Florence.

Built in about 1330, its painted Trecento walls serve to soften and brighten the interior, turning the fortress into a home. The great Gothic halls on the upper floors are frescoed to give the semblance of fabrics and drapery. Other striking aspects include the vaulted entrance hall and the staircase supported by flying buttresses. In style and decor, the lofty, galleried palace bridges the medieval and Renaissance eras, making Palazzo Davanzati the most

BELOW: the Museo Galileo.

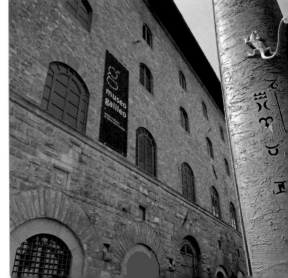

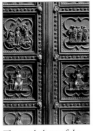

The south doors of the Baptistery were the work of Andrea Pisano (c.1270–1348) – goldsmith, sculptor and architect rolled into one.

BELOW: Piazza della Repubblica.

illuminating example of a patrician dwelling from the period.

From Palazzo Davanzati, Via de' Sassetti leads you to the grandiose **Palazzo Strozzi** (tel: 055-264 5155; www.palazzostrozzi.org; daily 9am–8pm; charge), an important cultural hub and the setting for blockbuster art exhibitions. This bombastic building is also a testament to the overweening pride of the powerful merchant banker, Filippo Strozzi, who dared to build a bigger palace than the Medici's. The monumental nature of the rusticated facade is echoed by the bold inner courtyard. As the quintessential 15th-century Florentine princely palace, Palazzo Strozzi was a model for centuries to come.

Situated in the restored cellars of the Palazzo Strozzi, **La Strozzina** (www.strozzina.org; Tue–Sun 9am–8pm; charge) is a challenging new exhibition space – which is exactly what it was until the "great flood" of 1966, when the River Arno inundated these cellars.

Worth a visit while you're in the vicinity is the Romanesque church of **Santa Trinita** (Mon–Sat 8am–

noon, 4–6pm, Sun 4–6pm), which features a fresco cycle of the life of St Francis painted in 1483 by Domenico Ghirlandaio.

East of Palazzo Strozzi, **Piazza della Repubblica** was laid out over the medieval market quarter and Ghetto, which were demolished in the 19th century. The plan to develop central Florence was conceived between 1865 and 1871, when the city was briefly the capital of Italy. The ancient and "squalid" buildings were to be swept away and replaced by broad avenues, symbolic of the new age of the United Kingdom of Italy. Thankfully, the scheme was abandoned. The self-important square, with its old-fashioned cafés, remains rather soulless, a modern intrusion into the heart of the city.

The Duomo: the religious centre

The street that links the two great monuments of the Palazzo Vecchio and the Duomo is still known as the Street of the Hosiers – Via dei Calzaiuoli – after the stocking-knitters who plied their trade here. The guilds were gathered in this area, hence the guild church of **Orsanmichele** (Tue–Fri 10am–5pm). It is, in effect, an open-air sculpture gallery, with an array of statues displayed in individual niches in the walls.

Holding up to 20,000 people, the enormous **Duomo** (daily 10am–5pm, winter until 4pm, Sun pm only; free) only serves to emphasise the smallness of the surrounding square, and the narrowness of the adjoining streets. At no point can one take in the whole. But now fully pedestrianised, the square is yours to wander freely, possibly even in a horse-drawn carriage, which can be picked up in the piazza.

The Baptistery

Despite the Duomo's dominating presence, the **Battistero** (Mon–

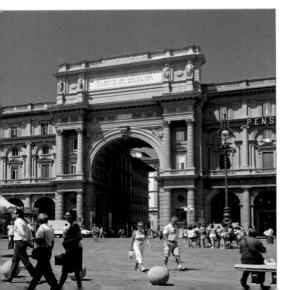

Sat noon–7pm, summer also Thur and Fri until 10.30pm; charge) easily holds its own. The oldest building in the city, it was built on, or reconstructed from, a 7th-century building sometime between 1060 and 1120 and served as the cathedral of Florence until 1228. Dante was among the eminent Florentines baptised there, and the wealthy Wool Guild (*Calimala*) lavished vast sums on the superb Venetian mosaics decorating the cupola.

The *Calimala* then turned its attention to the three great doors, first commissioning Andrea Pisano to create bronze doors for the south entrance, then initiating a competition for the other doors, which was won by Lorenzo Ghiberti. There is no mistaking the second pair (the east doors, facing the Duomo) – which took Ghiberti 27 years to create, and which Michelangelo described as the "Gates of Paradise". But the present panels are copies. The original panels are in **the Museo dell'Opera del Duomo** ⓭ on the east side of the Piazza del Duomo (Mon–Sat 9am–7.30pm, Sun 9am–1.40pm; charge),

while the competition panels are in the Bargello.

The two doors are divided into 10 panels, each representing a scene from the Old Testament. Round the panels are heads of the Sibyls and the Prophets. Seek out Ghiberti's self-portrait, halfway down on the right-hand side of the left-hand door: although minuscule, it is a perfect portrait – a small, balding man peering knowingly out.

It took the Florentines over 400 years to decide on the kind of facade they wanted for the west front of the Duomo, with the present, controversial facade designed in 1887.

Inside the Duomo

After the multicoloured splendour of the freshly restored exterior, the interior of **Santa Maria del Fiore** (the Duomo's official name) is muted, coming to life only at the time of religious festivals, when immense crimson banners adorn the walls. But the eye falls on two large murals high on the wall to the left of the entrance. The right-hand one is of an Englishman, John Hawkwood, a

TIP

Florence by bike: there are cycle-rental points at the main railway station, as well as on Piazza Santa Croce and Piazza Annigoni by Sant'Ambrogio market. Also contact Alinari (Via San Zanobi 38R; tel: 055-280 500; www. alinarirental.com). Or try a bicycle rickshaw with Tre Rote (tel: 338-638 9245; www.pedicab firenze.it)

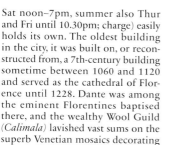

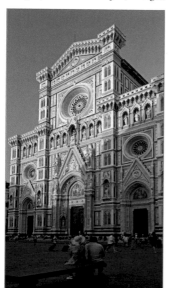

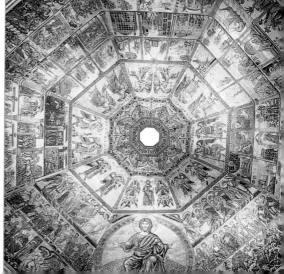

BELOW LEFT: the Duomo facade. **BELOW RIGHT:** the cupola mosaics of the Battistero.

The quiet cloister in the north of San Lorenzo, with its box-lined lawns and pomegranate bushes, leads to the Biblioteca Laurenziana (open for exhibitions or scholars only, hours variable; tel: 055-210 760). Designed by Michelangelo between 1524 and 1534, the Laurentian Library houses more than 10,000 manuscripts (including the famous 5th-century Virgil codex) from the Medici collection.

BELOW: the interior of Brunelleschi's dome.

mercenary soldier (*condottiero*) who first attacked Florence for his paymasters and then became the city's Captain-General in 1375.

Further along the aisle is the painting of *Dante Declaiming The Divine Comedy* by Michelino. On Dante's right, Hell and Purgatory are depicted, contrasted with a contemporary view of the city's major monuments.

The Duomo's greatest treasure is Michelangelo's unfinished *Pietà*, sculpted for his own tomb in 1550, and now in the museum collection. It is entirely different from his earlier, more famous *Pietà* in St Peter's, in Rome; where that is all calm, resigned acceptance, this is simply the utter defeat of death.

The dome and bell tower

It is still Brunelleschi's dome that defines Florence, over 500 years after it was built. Filippo Brunelleschi created the purest Renaissance architecture, buildings striking in their simplicity and pared-down loveliness. The cupola of the Duomo, which uses rigorous geometry based on classical forms, is the perfect expression of a rational use of space. His stroke of genius was to devise a cunning system of an inner shell and outer dome to distribute the weight of the cupola, with thick walls negating the need for further buttressing. Out of respect for Brunelleschi's achievement, the city forbade the construction of any building taller than the Duomo – to this day, the massive dome dominates the red rooftops, rising almost higher than the surrounding hills.

If you have a head for heights, ascend to the gallery of the dome (Mon–Fri 8.30am–7pm, Sat 8.30am–5.40pm; charge). It is not for vertigo sufferers: the gallery is narrow and the balustrade low, but only here can Brunelleschi's stupendous achievement be fully appreciated. The interior of the dome is covered in Vasari's bold allegorical frescoes, although the original plan was to cover the space with mosaics, which would have emphasised its soaring majesty. But its majesty is not in doubt.

Scarcely less tall, at 85 metres (278ft), is the **Campanile** (daily 8.30am–7.30pm; charge) alongside, begun by Giotto shortly after he was

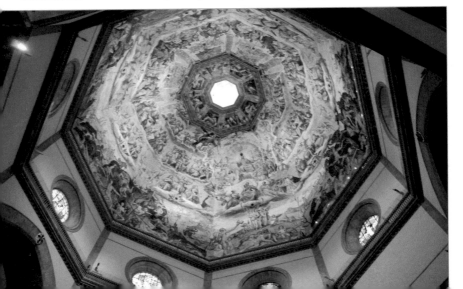

appointed chief architect in 1331, and finished off after his death in 1337 by Andrea Pisano and then Talenti. Work was eventually completed in 1359. The climb to the top is worth the effort for intimate views of the Cathedral's upper levels and the panoramic city views.

East of the Duomo is the **Museo di Firenze Com'Era** (closed for refurbishment). The historical-topographical museum of "Florence as it was" is best seen once you have familiarised yourself with the city, so you can recognise the buildings depicted in the collection.

Memories of the Medici

A few streets northwest of the Duomo is the heartland of Medicean Florence: the **Medici Palace** and the church of **San Lorenzo**, which is surrounded by a boisterous market. The palace – now known as the **Palazzo Medici-Riccardi** 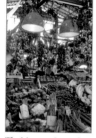 (Thur–Tue 9am–7pm; charge) – is dignified but not ostentatious. It still has the look of a fortress about it, particularly in the rusticated facade with its massive blocks of masonry. The Medici lived

here from its completion in 1452 until 1540, when they moved into the politically symbolic Palazzo Vecchio. While much of the palace is swathed in institutional gloom, the courtyard and loggia are striking, and the Cappella dei Magi revels in the most uplifting fresco cycle in Florence.

The museum contains various mementoes of the family, including the poignant death-mask of Lorenzo, but it is the chapel that displays the brightest jewels in the Medici crown, including the *Journey of the Magi* by Benozzo Gozzoli (*c.*1460). This painting breathes the spirit of the Florentine Renaissance in its mixture of real figures of identifiable people, historical recreation and delight in colour. The immense procession, winding its way through a vividly improbable landscape, is led by a handsome, richly dressed youth on horseback – the young Lorenzo. Behind him comes his grandfather, Cosimo, soberly dressed, attended by a black servant, but look out for the painter himself, with his name inscribed on his hat. In the distance is the Medici retreat, Villa Cafaggiolo

The Mercato Centrale, Florence's main food market.

BELOW: the church of San Lorenzo, with its unfinished facade.

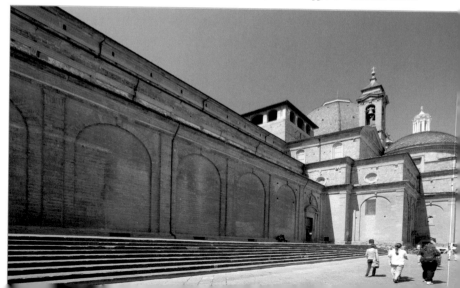

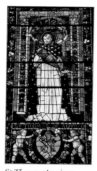

St Thomas Aquinas, depicted on one of the stained-glass windows of Santa Maria Novella.

BELOW: Giotto's *Crucifix* in Santa Maria Novella.

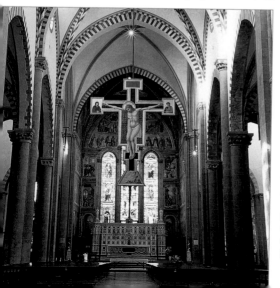

– and a couple of camels to remind the observer that the picture is set in the Middle East.

San Lorenzo

The church of **San Lorenzo** ⑮ (Mon–Sat 10am–5.30pm, summer also Sun 1.30–5.30pm; charge) is one of the earliest and most harmonious of all Renaissance churches, representing a break with French Gothic and a return to an older, classical style. The facade is rough and unfinished, though the Mayor has mooted a plan to complete it according to Michelangelo's designs.

The interior is outstanding, a gracious composition of the grey stone *pietra serena* and white walls. Giovanni, father of Cosimo de' Medici, commissioned Brunelleschi to design San Lorenzo in 1419, but neither lived to see it completed. Thereafter, successive members of the Medici family continued to embellish it, commissioning the greatest artists of their age to add frescoes, paintings and – ultimately – their mausoleum. Of particular note in the basilica are Donatello's pulpits with bronze reliefs of the Passion, and the Old Sacristy adorned with sculptures, also by Donatello.

The Medici chapels

The entrance to the **Cappelle Medicee** (Tue–Sun 8.15am–4.50pm; charge) is outside the church, in the Piazza della Madonna degli Aldobrandini. You go in via the crypt, where a floor slab commemorates Anna Maria Ludovica (died 1743), the last in the Medici line. Stairs lead to the opulent **Cappella dei Principi** (the mausoleum of the Medici grand dukes) and the **New Sacristy** (the Medici tombs), the latter Michelangelo's first architectural commission, and a chilly cocoon. The two New Sacristy tombs of Giuliano (son of Lorenzo the Magnificent) and Lorenzo (his grandson) are graced with the reclining figures of *Dawn, Evening, Day* and *Night,* conveying an unforgettable feeling of uneasiness, sadness and loss.

Santa Maria Novella, San Marco and Santa Croce: three influential churches

The three great buildings of Santa Maria Novella, San Marco and Santa Croce are some distance apart – the first near the Stazione Centrale, the second in the north, and the last on the far eastern side of the city. They are grouped together here because they illustrate a truth about Florence, that religion was a driving force – probably even stronger than commerce or the desire for self-aggrandisement – a force that nearly drove the city to destruction.

Santa Maria Novella

The church of **Santa Maria Novella** ⑯ (Mon–Thur 9am–5.30pm, Fri 11–5.30pm, Sat 9am–5pm, Sun noon–5pm) was designed by Dominican monks in 1246. Though dignified and indeed majestic, it reflects their gloomy preoccupations: striped like a tiger, the family chapels are sombre and overwhelming, their murals little more than illustrations of sermons. The **Spanish Chapel** carries this to extremes, with its murals dedicated to the 13th-century theologian, Thomas Aquinas, who was, of course, a Dominican. The chapel now lies within the **Cloister Museum** (Fri–Sun 10am–4pm; charge) adjoining the church, as do Uccello's frescoes. In the church itself is Masaccio's *Trinity*, and the chapel is frescoed by Fra Filippino Lippi and Ghirlandaio. Although Brunelleschi's decorative touches lighten the spirit, the church feels oppressive.

At the southern end of Piazza Santa Maria Novella, the **Museo Nazionale Alinari Fotografia ⑰** (www.alinarifondazione.it; Mon–Tue and Thur–Sat 10am–7.30pm, closed in Aug; charge) has one of the best photographic collections in Europe. Founded in 1852, the Alinari brothers' photographic studio supplied 19th-century Grand Tourists with prints, postcards and art books.

Long neglected, and once a gathering place for vagrants, **Piazza Santa Maria Novella** has recently returned to its former glory, prompted by renovation of the Dominican complex, with the finest facade in Florence, and by the pedestrianisation of the square. Helping to raise the tone are a cluster of chic boutique hotels, from JK Place to Palazzo dal Borgo, which overlooks the historic perfumery of the **Officina di Santa Maria Novella** (Via della Scala), where monks have been concocting precious potions since the 13th century.

San Marco

The convent of **San Marco ⑱** was almost entirely rebuilt with money provided by Cosimo de' Medici; the irony lies in the fact that San Marco became the headquarters of the friar Girolamo Savonarola, who was the greatest enemy of Cosimo's grandson,

Lorenzo. Cosimo engaged his own favourite architect, Michelozzo, who had designed the Palazzo Medici, to build San Marco, and endowed it with a magnificent library.

Savonarola was Prior of San Marco from 1491 until his execution in 1498. During those years he dominated Florence, nearly succeeded in overthrowing the Medici and even presented a challenge to the papacy. The vivid portrait of him by Fra Bartolomeo, which can be seen here, shows a man with a forceful but ugly face, a great beaked nose and burning eyes.

San Marco is now a **museum** (Tue–Fri 8.15am–1.50pm, Sat until 4.50pm, Sun and Mon until 1.50pm, closed alternate Sun/Mon; charge). The prize exhibits are the murals of Fra Angelico, himself a Dominican, but one who brought a delicacy to his work quite at variance with the austere tenets of that order. Each of the friars' cells is graced by one of his murals, and at the head of the stairs is Fra Angelico's masterpiece, the *Annunciation*. Savonarola's cell is laid out as he knew it, complete with desk

TIP

Beyond the remnants of the city wall is a reminder, though a rapidly fading one, that Florence is a country town: a brisk walk along Via di San Leonardo will take you from the very heart of the city out into vineyards, olive groves and maize fields.

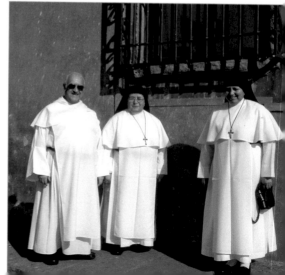

BELOW: San Marco nuns and priest.

Piazza Santa Croce is the lowest area in the city, and recorded water levels as high as 6.2 metres (20ft) in the 1966 flood. The watermarks are still visible today on some buildings.

and severe-looking chair.

Just south of San Marco is the legendary **Galleria dell'Accademia** ❶ *(see page 118)*, often identified by the enormous queues outside. Its star attraction – and the museum's *raison d'être* – is the colossal statue of *David*, which was carved between 1501 and 1504 from a single piece of marble, and established Michelangelo as the foremost sculptor of his time before the age of 30. The statue now standing in front of the Palazzo Vecchio is an impressive copy.

Near to the Accademia, on the Via Alfani, is the **Opificio delle Pietre Dure** (Tue–Fri 8.30am–7pm, Sat– Sun until 2pm; charge), where restoration of artistic treasures takes place. Exhibits include inlaid semi-precious stones used in *pietra dura*, as well as workbenches and instruments once used by the craftsmen.

Nearby, the **Museo Archeologico** (Tue–Fri 8.30am–7pm, Sat–Sun 8.30am–2pm; charge) in Piazza d. S.S. Annunziata features an important collection of Greek, Egyptian, Etruscan and Roman art. The highlights include the recreation of an

Etruscan tomb and bronzes of Etruscan mythological beasts.

Santa Croce

The great **Piazza Santa Croce** was a favoured place for processions, horse races and tournaments. *Calcio Storico*, an historic football match, is still staged here every June. The square, dominated by a statue of Dante, is also home to the fascinating Santa Croce Leather School, a testament to Florentine craftsmanship.

Although the facade of **Santa Croce** ❷ (Mon–Sat 9.30am–5.30pm, Sun from 1pm; charge) dates from the mid-19th century, Arnolfo di Cambio began work on the church in 1294. With the lightness and elegance associated with Franciscan churches, it is the Pantheon of Florence – and, indeed, of Italy, since this is where so many of the country's illustrious dead were laid to rest, from Galileo to Ghiberti.

The tomb of Michelangelo, designed by Vasari, invariably has a little bunch of flowers laid upon it, unlike the grave of Machiavelli, who died in 1527. Crowning the whole

BELOW: charming Ponte Vecchio.

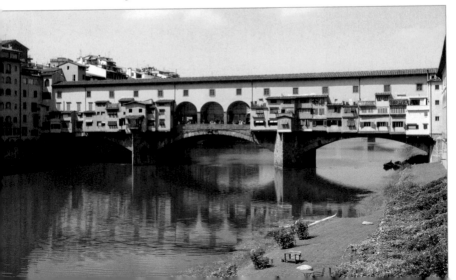

are the frescoes painted by Giotto and his school.

The cloisters, designed by Brunelleschi, lead to the recently restored **Cappella de'Pazzi**, which contains 12 terracotta roundels of the Apostles by Luca della Robbia.

The **Museo dell'Opera di Santa Croce** (Mon–Sat 9.30am–5.30pm, Sun opens at 1pm; charge) houses the beguiling *Tree of the Cross* by Taddeo Gaddi and Cimabue's iconic 13th-century *Crucifix*, which was badly damaged in the 1966 flood. It has only been partially restored since then as a poignant reminder of the city in peril.

Oltrarno: across the river

The Florentines regard their river with mixed feelings. It has brought both wealth and disaster in its unpredictable wake. The Arno becomes a raging brown torrent in winter, although it can shrink to a trickle along a dried-up bed during summer. Recently, sun-worshippers have become fond of its enjoyable urban beach.

The **Ponte Vecchio** ㉑ was erected by Taddeo Gaddi sometime after 1345 and has become a symbol of Florence itself. Fortunately, the Germans spared it when they blew up every other Florentine bridge during World War II. It bears the same appearance that it has borne for six centuries. Even the goldsmiths and jewellers who throng it today were established there in the mid-16th century. Before the goldsmiths, the shops on the bridge were occupied by butchers and tanners, who used the river as a dumping ground until they were evicted in 1593.

It was for Ferdinando's father, Cosimo I, that Vasari built the extraordinary **Vasari Corridor** in 1565. Running from the Uffizi to the Pitti across the Ponte Vecchio, the private walkway made a physical as well as symbolic link between the two centres of Medicean power. In his film *Paisà*, Roberto Rossellini shot an unforgettable sequence of the fighting that took place along this gallery during the German retreat. (The corridor is currently undergoing full refurbishment and will re-open in 2014.)

> ❝
>
> *Whoever desires to found a state and give it laws must start with assuming that all men are bad and ever ready to display their vicious nature, whenever they may find occasion for it.*
>
> Niccolo Machiavelli
>
> ❞

The Contemporary City

If sleepy Florence has finally woken up, much credit is due to two Prince Charmings. Canadian James Bradburne put the city on the contemporary art map with Palazzo Strozzi and its inclusive yet international approach to culture *(see page 96)*. Not that he takes credit for it: "Florence has the highest concentration of intellectual, creative and business firepower that I have ever seen. It punches way above its weight. Here everyone from art historians to plumbers is able to carry on extraordinary conversations about art and literature. The question is, why doesn't Florence do more with this firepower?"

Mayor Renzi has followed suit, supporting a host of creative projects, including the Nuovo Teatro del Maggio, the city's new opera house and concert hall. New festivals, art galleries and *aperitivi* bars have sprung up, along with vibrant theatre-dining clubs, such as the Teatro del Sale. Disused stations, convents and fortesses have been turned into multimedia libraries and events centres. Le Murate, a former nunnery and prison on Via Ghibellina, now offers live music, arty bars and an outdoor cinema. The Universale, once a run-down cinema, has been reborn as a designer-chic club with cinematic screens. Stazione Leopolda, a reconverted neoclassical station, now stages fashion shows, concerts and exhibitions. Symbolically, Norman Foster's avant-garde railway hub, opening in 2014, will strengthen the city's international links. Only the controversial Uffizi expansion project is on hold, considered too cutting edge for traditionalists. Franco Zeffirelli, the Florentine-born film director, decries it as a form of "being blackmailed by progressivist culture". And many agree. But most other "grand projects" command popular support. Damien Hirst's diamond-encrusted skull has even been displayed in the Palazzo Vecchio. Bizarre, but Florence can finally claim to be about more than Renaissance art.

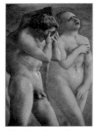

The Expulsion from Paradise *by Masaccio (c.1427) in the Cappella Brancacci. They are among the most powerfully emotive figures ever painted in Western art.*

Below: the facade of San Miniato al Monte.

The Pitti Palace

The part of Florence south of the river, the **Oltrarno**, has a bohemian character all of its own, with its charm enhanced by the gradual pedestrianisation of this area. Yet in the 15th century, this area was the centre of opposition to the Medici, spearheaded by the Pitti family. It was they who built the **Palazzo Pitti** ㉒ *(see page 114)*, the most grandiose of all Florentine residences, which, by the irony of history, eventually became the seat of government for the Medici dukes themselves. Today it is home to Medici museums and art galleries, notably the **Galleria Palatina**, adorned by masterpieces by artists such as Raphael, Rubens, Van Dyck and Titian.

Adjoining the gallery are the **Appartamenti Monumentali** or **Reali** (State Apartments), lavishly decorated with impressive works of art. The palace also contains the **Galleria d'Arte Moderna**, the **Galleria del Costume** and the **Museo degli Argenti**.

An excellent antidote to the overwhelming splendours of the Pitti are the beautiful adjoining Boboli Gardens, the **Giardino di Boboli** ㉓ *(see page 115)*.

Also included in the Boboli ticket is the **Giardino Bardini**, accessible from Via dei Bardi 1r or Costa San Giorgio 2 (tel: 055-263 8559; www.bardinipeyron.it; 8.15am–sunset). The recently restored park offers stunning vistas, a café and quiet spots for meditation, as well as access to the **Villa Bardini** (contact as above ; Fri–Sun 10am–4pm; charge).

Once owned by antiquarian Stefano Bardini, the villa is now home to a fine restaurant and small museums dedicated to the modern artist Annigoni and fashion maestro Roberto Capucci. But Bardini's heart belonged to his Renaissance art collection down the hill in **Museo Bardini** ㉔ (Via dei Renai 37; tel: 055-234 2427; Fri–Mon 11am–5pm; charge). The newly reopened collection mixes works by Donatello with eclectic finds, such as the original *Porcellino*, the wild-boar bronze created for the Mercato Nuovo.

Alternatively, from Villa Bardini, continue up Costa San Giorgio to the **Forte di Belvedere** (Tue–Sun 3–7pm), a 16th-century fortification designed by Buontalenti for the Grand Duke Ferdinando I de' Medici. The fort, which commands breathtaking views over Florence, hosts modern-art and photography exhibitions.

The Porta Romana

The **Via Romana**, which begins just past the Palazzo Pitti in Piazza San Felice, goes to the **Porta Romana** ㉕, stretching from the city centre, via the Ponte Vecchio, to the outside world. The larger gates of Florence were, like the 14th-century Porta Romana, both a garrison and a customs post, collecting dues on all the goods that came into the city. You can now walk a section of the ramparts near Porta Romana.

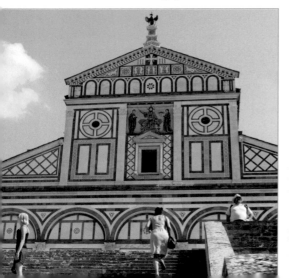

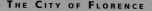

Oltrarno churches

Several churches of note lie on this south side of the city. The first, not far from the Ponte Santa Trinità, is **Santo Spirito** (Thur–Tue 10am–12-.30pm, 4–5.30pm; free), its modest 18th-century facade masking the harmonious interior designed by Filippo Brunelleschi.

Just west is **Santa Maria del Carmine 26**, which contains one of the greatest treasures of Italian painting – the **Cappella Brancacci** frescoes (tel: 055-276 8224; www.firenzemu-sei.it; Mon, Wed–Sat 10am–5pm, Sun 1–5pm; charge; reservation required). Considered by many to rival even Michelangelo's Sistine Chapel in Rome, the work of Masolino (including *The Temptation of Adam and Eve*), Masaccio (*The Expulsion from Paradise* and *The Tribute Money*) and Filippino Lippi is truly magnificent. Unfortunately, due to the popularity of the frescoes, visitors are only allowed 15 minutes to see them.

Further east, dominating a hilltop, awaits **San Miniato al Monte 27** (daily 8am–12.30pm, 3–5.30pm). A building stood on this site as early as the 4th century, but the present complex dates from 1018 and is a fine example of Florentine Romanesque. Inside, seek out the **Cappella del Crocifisso**, a tiny vaulted temple, and the 11th-century crypt, which houses the relics of St Minias. You can hear the monks chanting here each afternoon at 4.30pm.

San Miniato towers above the **Piazzale Michelangelo**, reached from the Porta Romana along the enchanting Viale dei Colli, or else by climbing up from the river, past the Porta San Niccolò, taking the winding paths through the gardens to the piazzale.

Adorned with bronze copies of Michelangelo's various works of sculpture, this touristic terrace is a Florentine pilgrimage destination that entwined lovers feel obliged to visit. Even if the views are far lovelier from **Bellosguardo**, above Porta Romana, Piazzale Michelangelo is picture-postcard Florence – from the sheepish couples and nude *David* souvenirs to the city at sunset decked out below. ❏

It was in Florence Cathedral that Boccaccio's seven young maidens met in the spring of 1348, where they were joined by three young men and launched the comedy of The Decameron.

BELOW: view of the city from Piazzale Michelangelo.

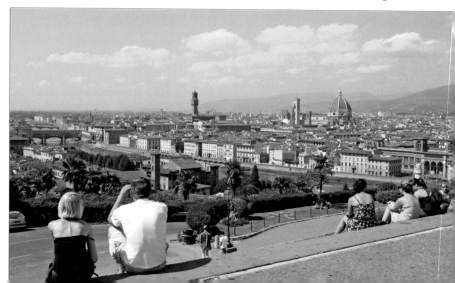

BEST RESTAURANTS, BARS AND CAFÉS

Restaurants

Prices for a three-course meal per person with a half-bottle of house wine:
€ = under €30
€€ = €30–45
€€€ = €45–65
€€€€ = over €65

Acqua al Due
Via della Vigna Vecchia 40r
Tel: 055-284 170
www.acquaal2.it €€
A popular dining experience, so book ahead for a chance to dine at this atmospheric spot. Try the *assaggio di primi* (five pasta dishes as chosen by the chef) followed by the *assaggio di dolci* (a selection of the desserts of the day).

Alle Murate
Via del Proconsolo 16r.
Tel: 055-240 618
www.allemurate.it €€€€
Romantic, dinner-only spot in a historic guildhouse with original frescoes, including one of Dante, and a Roman cistern. Superb Tuscan-meets-Southern gastro cuisine in a relaxed but stylish setting. Led by top restaurateur Umberto Montano, this is one of the city's best restaurants. Cheaper snacks in the bar. Closed Mon.

Benedicta
Via della Scala 33
Tel: 055-264 5429 €€
Dependable Tuscan dishes, from steak to pasta, with a quietly creative touch in a contem-

porary-looking setting, despite being in a former Franciscan convent. It is close to Santa Maria Novella.

Buca Lapi
Via del Terbbio 1r
Tel: 055-213 768
www.bucalapi.com €€€
Set in the wine cellars of the Antinori palazzo, this claims to be the oldest restaurant in town. Highly traditional Tuscan cuisine. Eve only Mon–Sat.

Cantinetta Antinori
Piazza Antinori 3
Tel: 055-292 234
www.antinori.it €€€
Restaurant in a 15th-century palazzo, serving typical Tuscan snacks and meals with wines from the well-known Antinori estates. A good

place for a light lunch at the bar or a fuller meal in the elegant dining room. Closed weekends and Aug.

Cantinetta da Verrazzano
Via de' Tavolini 18–20
Tel: 055-268 590
www.verrazzano.com €
Old-fashioned wood-panelled wine bar serving rustic lunch sandwiches and wines from the owners' Chianti estate; closed Sun, and closed after 9pm.

La Casalinga
Via del Michelozzo 9r
Tel: 055-218 624 €
One of the best-value eateries in town, close to Piazza Santo Spirito. Plentiful helpings of home cooking attract

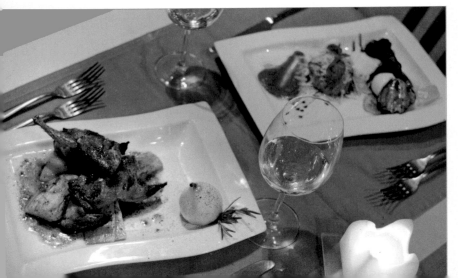

locals as well as visitors. It is family-run and highlights include the *bollito misto* and the Limoncello sorbet. Closed Sun.

Il Cibrèo
Via Andrea del Verrocchio 8r
Tel: 055-234 1100
www.cibreo.com €€€€
Justly famed, elegant but relaxed restaurant, one of the most popular in the city. Pure Tuscan cuisine, with a creative twist. No pasta, but a selection of superb soups and other *primi* (first courses). Closed Sun and Mon.

Coco Lezzone
Via del Parioncino 26
Tel: 055-287 178 €€
Traditional bustling trattoria of the highest quality, especially the meat dishes. The menu is seasonal. Closed Sun and Aug.

Enoteca Pinchiorri
Via Ghibellina 87
Tel: 055-242 777
www.enotecapinchiorri.com €€€€
Elegant dress and a jacket are required at "Italy's finest restaurant" (three Michelin stars). It occupies a 15th-century palace with a fine courtyard for alfresco meals. Expect excellent nouvelle-meets-Tuscan cuisine, rare wines, and a hefty bill. Reservation essential. Closed Sun, and Mon–Wed lunchtime.

Dei Frescobaldi
Via de' Magazzini 2r
Tel: 055-284 724
www.deifrescobaldi.it. €€
Tasty Tuscan cuisine off Piazza della Signoria, including grilled Tuscan meats and pumpkin ravioli, washed down with Frescobaldi wine. Or snack on Tuscan "tapas" (salami, cheese, salads) in the adjoining wine bar.

Golden View Open Bar
Via dei Bardi 58r
Tel: 055-214 502
www.goldenviewopenbar.com €€€
Touristic by day, fashionable jazz bar by night. Great view of Ponte Vecchio, with live jazz almost every night and good food, although not cheap.

Gustavino
Via della Condotta 37r
Tel: 055-239 9806
www.gustavino.it €€
Stylish contemporary restaurant with an open kitchen so you can watch the chefs in action. The food is creative without being too fussy and is beautifully presented, with a fine choice of wine. You can also just have a drink in the wine bar. Closed Mon.

Mario
Via delle Rosine 2r
Tel: 055-218 550
www.trattoriamario.com €
Intimate and down to earth, this is a great place to experience earthy Tuscan food,

from *ribollita* soup to grilled chicken and a variety of steaks. Only lunch Mon–Sat. Closed Aug.

Le Mossacce
Via del Proconsolo 55r
Tel: 055-294 361 €
Trattoria between the Duomo and the Bargello, serving pasta dishes and basic Tuscan fare. Popular with office workers at lunchtimes. Closed Sat–Sun.

Napoleone
Piazza del Carmine 24
Tel: 055-281 015
www.trattorianapoleone.it €€
This trattoria in the trendy Oltrarno neighbourhood features simple Tuscan fare with Mediterranean influences. Same owners as the popular Da Zà Zà. Open for dinner.

Da Nerbone
Mercato di San Lorenzo
Tel: 055-219 949 €

Authentic, very good market eatery as old as the market itself. Dishes such as tripe and *lampredotto*, as well as the usual trattoria fare. There are few tables. Closed evenings and Sun.

Omero
Via Pian dei Giullari 11r
Tel: 055-220 053
www.ristoranteomero.it €€
Located in the hills just outside the city centre, this restaurant specialises in Florentine cuisine. Great view and good wine selection. Closed Tue.

Opera et Gusto
Via della Scala 17r
Tel: 055-288 190 €€
Eclectic new dining club where you can listen to opera, blues or jazz while tucking into Tuscan cuisine. The setting is a theatrical red-and-black "stage".

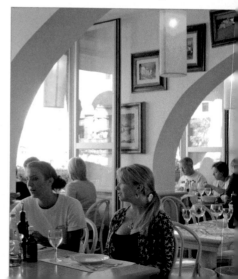

LEFT: a meal at stylish Gustavino.
RIGHT: enjoying food and wine at Golden View.

Prices for a three-course meal per person with a half-bottle of house wine:
€ = under €30
€€ = €30–45
€€€ = €45–65
€€€€ = over €65

Osteria Caffè Italiano
Via Isole delle
Stinche 11/13r
Tel: 055-289 368/289 080
www.caffeitaliano.it €€€
Under the same management as Alle Murate (above). Short menu but high standards and superb Tuscan cuisine near Santa Croce. 10am "till late", closed Mon.

Osteria de' Macci
Via dei Macci 77
Tel: 055-241 226 €
Typical, dependable Tuscan trattoria with no frills, good food but perfunctory service.

Pane e Vino
Via di Cestello 3r
Tel: 055-247 6956
www.ristorantepaneevino.it €€
Situated close to the river, on the Oltrano side, this is a pleasant, informal restaurant with an interesting menu (including a daily tasting menu) and excellent wine. Closed Sun.

La Pentola dell'Oro
Via di Mezzo 24–26r
Tel: 055-241 808
www.lapentoladelloro.it €€
As well as being unique, this is one of the friendliest restaurants in the city. Chef Giuseppe Alessi is more than willing to explain the dishes; the recipes – published in the restaurant's book – are inspired by medieval and Renaissance cookery. Closed Sun.

Il Pizzaiuolo
Via dei Macci 113r
Tel: 055-241 171 €
The pizzas are wonderful, but there's plenty more besides. Try the *antipasto della casa*. Popular. Closed Sun and Aug.

Relais Le Jardin, Hotel Regency
Piazza Massimo d'Azeglio 3
Tel: 055-245 247
www.regency-hotel.com €€€€
Top-notch but light interpretations of Tuscan cuisine in an exclusive hotel restaurant, overlooking a garden. Dine on the summer veranda. Elegant dress and reservation required.

Ristorante Le Carcere
Piazza Madonna della Neve
Tel: 055-247 9327
www.ristorantelecarcere.it €
An amiable pizzeria, trattoria and wine bar set in the former prisons of Le Murate, which are now a cultural complex off Via Ghibellina.

Ristorante Terrazza Bardini
Costa San Giorgio 4a
Tel: 055-200 8444
www.moba.fl.it €€€
Set in a panoramic spot in the Villa Bardini complex, this elegant fish restaurant is matched by La Terrazza, which serves cocktails and light Tuscan meals on the summer terrace. Art exhibitions and jazz. Tue–Sun evenings only.

Da Ruggero
Via Senese 89
Tel: 055-220 542 €€
Excellent restaurant just outside the Porta Romana. Popular with the locals, so best to reserve. Great *ribollita* and other Tuscan fare. Closed Tue, Wed and 3 weeks in July/Aug.

Santa Lucia
Via Ponte alla Mosse 102r
Tel: 055-353 255 €
Authentically Neapolitan, no-frills trattoria, serving the best pizzas in town. Good seafood, too. Booking essential. Closed Wed and Aug.

Il Santo Bevitore
Via Santo Spirito 64r
Tel: 055-211 264 €€
Moody, mid-priced, stylish wine bar and restaurant with great appeal, atmosphere and sound creative cuisine; worth waiting for a table as it's deservedly popular.

Da Sergio
Piazza San Lorenzo 8r
Tel: 055-281 941 €
Big, airy trattoria, hidden behind a row of stalls. A haunt of market workers and discerning tourists. There's a short, simple, seasonal menu. Try the spelt soup (*minestra di farro*) and the steak. No desserts served. Lunch only; closed Sun.

Targa Bistrot
Lungarno Cristoforo Colombo 7
Tel: 055-677 377
www.targabistrot.net €€€€
Very pleasantly situated restaurant on the north bank of the Arno, some way from the centre, with a wood-panelled interior. Imaginative take on Tuscan dishes. Closed Sun and 3 weeks in Aug.

Taverna del Bronzino
Via delle Ruote 25/27r

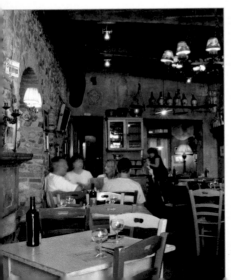

LEFT: the dining room at Da Zà Zà.

Tel: 055-495 220 €€€€
Classically comfortable restaurant in a quiet side street, some way from the centre. Elegantly served traditional food. The black tortellini, flavoured with truffle, is a must. Closed Sun and Aug.

Il Teatro del Sale
Via de Macci 111r
Tel: 055-200 1492
www.teatrodelsale.com €€
Hedonistic dining club run by celebrity chef Fabio Picchi (of Cibrèo, below). A filling Tuscan buffet is offered before live blues, jazz or theatre; membership essential but cheap, as is the good-value buffet dinner, which includes wine and entertainment.

Trattoria Cibrèo (Il Cibreino)
Via de Macci 122r
Tel: 055-234 1100
www.cibreo.com €€
Annexe of Il Cibrèo (see page 107), but with meals at half the price. Few frills, but the food is basically the same as in the main restaurant. No bookings. Closed Sun and Mon. Caffè Cibrèo (Via del Verrocchio) is even cheaper, for snacks.

Il Vegetariano
Via delle Ruote 30r
Tel: 055-475 030 €
The imaginative use of fresh vegetables in its dishes makes Il Vegetariano the city's best vegetarian eatery. The laid-back, informal atmosphere is halfway between a diner and a cafeteria. Closed Mon, weekends at lunch.

Le Volpi e le Uva
Piazza de Rossi 1r
Tel: 055-239 8132 €
Welcoming and well-run wine bar for a light lunch or supper of superb wines, cheeses, cold cuts and bruschetta; closes 9pm.

Da Zà Zà
Piazza del Mercato Centrale 26r
Tel: 055-215 411
www.trattoriazaza.it €€
Good quality, earthy food and delicious *pasta e fagioli* soup and puddings. The riotous atmosphere is enjoyed by locals and tourists alike, along with the warm, rustic brick-and-beam dining rooms.

Bars, Cafés and Ice-cream Parlours

A hot chocolate or *aperitivo* at **Rivoire** (Piazza della Signoria) is worth experiencing just once. **Dei Frescobaldi**, at the end of the square, has a moody bar that is perfect for relaxing over Tuscan "tapas" and wine from one of the most famous *vino* dynasties. Piazza della Repubblica, the rival major square, is the place for people-watching in the grand, time-warp cafés of **Paszkowski**, **Gilli** or **Giubbe Rosse**. Alternatively,

Café Giacosa (Via della Spada 10) is a historic café that's had a makeover by designer Roberto Cavalli, whose own estate wines feature highly.

Far more relaxed, **Le Volpi e le Uva** (Piazza de Rossi 1r) is an addictive wine bar for a light supper of cheeses, cold cuts – and superb wines. **Fusion Bar** in Gallery Hotel Art (Vicolo dell'Oro) is for posing while nibbling on Asian finger food. **Cibrèo Caffè** (Via del Verrocchio 5r) is a peaceful café for delicious, but inexpensive, Tuscan treats from the celebrated restaurant over the road. Satisfy your sweet tooth at **GROM** (Via delle Oche), whose *gelati* reflect the seasons. **Vivoli** (Via delle Stinche), between the Bargello and Santa Croce, is another popular ice-cream parlour. Towards the Arno, **Moyo** (Via de Benci) is a slick *aperitivi* bar. The elegant bars lining the river are where Florentines go to be seen. On the south bank, sip wine at **Caffè Pitti** (Piazza Pitti) or have a cocktail at the ever-popular **Il Rifrullo** (Via San Niccolò). **Zoe** (Via dei Renai) is an all-day (and late-night) arty café in Oltrarno that takes a trendy crowd from brunch to cocktails and beyond. **Negroni**, in the same street, attracts a quieter, more sophisticated set. End the evening in ostentatious style at **Cavalli Club** (Piazza del Carmine 7r), a flashy club and disco bar founded by, yes, Florentine fashion supremo, Cavalli.

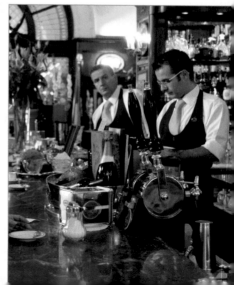

RIGHT: grand charm in Gilli on Piazza della Repubblica.

THE UFFIZI

The greatest collection of Renaissance art to be found anywhere in the world

This is Tuscany's foremost gallery (tel: 055-294883; www.firenzemusei.it; Tue–Sun 8.15am–6.50pm, Tue late opening till 10pm in summer; charge). Pre-booking is advisable, and you can do this through the Firenze Card, which covers all museums and transport, www.firenzecard.it.

The Uffizi was the administrative nerve centre of the grand duchy, reinforcing the chain of command between the Palazzo Vecchio, the Medici power base, and the court at the Pitti Palace. Founded by the Medici, this is now the greatest art gallery in Italy. Francesco de' Medici (1541–87) decided to transform the second floor of the Uffizi into a museum, coincidentally paying tribute to the Medici's dynastic glory. For the introverted ruler, the gallery was essentially his private playground "for walking, with paintings, statues and other precious things".

On display are paintings by masters from Giotto to Botticelli, Piero della Francesca, Michelangelo, Leonardo da Vinci, Raphael, Titian and Caravaggio. Although Tuscan art reigns supreme, the panoply of Italian art is also well represented, particularly painters from Umbria, Urbino, Emilia and the Veneto. Since most visitors come to see the Early Renaissance works, the High Renaissance rooms are far more peaceful and, by the time Titian and Veronese finally make way for Caravaggio and Tiepolo, Rubens and Rembrandt, the crowds have faded away as miraculously as a Tiepolo trompe l'oeil. By the same token, the wonderful classical and cinquecento statuary in the gallery corridors is often overlooked in the lemming stampede to see specific Renaissance paintings.

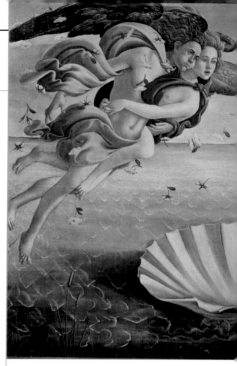

ABOVE: the Botticelli Rooms (10–14) are the most popular in the Uffizi, containing the world's best collection of work by the artist. Here are the famous mythological paintings, which fused ideas of the spiritual and the secular: the *Birth of Venus*, painted around 1485, and *La Primavera (Spring)* painted some five years earlier. The meaning of the latter work remains a subject of fervent discussion, while Venus has overtones of the Virgin Mary.

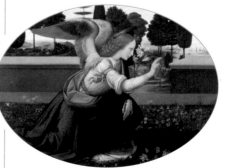

ABOVE: Room 15 exhibits Leonardo da Vinci's early works – including the *Annunciation* (1475) and the unfinished *Adoration of the Magi* (1481) – and also paintings by Perugino and Signorelli.

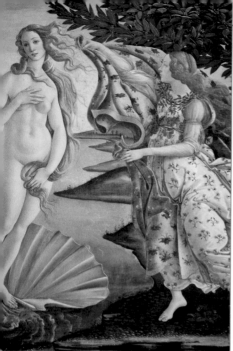

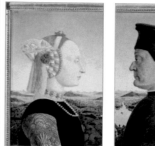

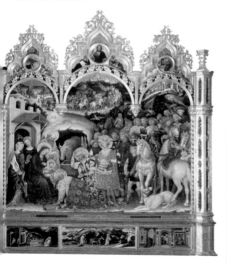

BELOW: Rooms 5–6 form the International Gothic Rooms, whose paintings exhibit a more conservative and less lavish approach, in keeping with the medieval mindset. Lorenzo Monaco's *Crowning of Mary* provides a good example of this by one of the main practitioners of the era.

THE EASTERN CORRIDOR

The two corridors from which the 45 rooms lead off are filled with sculptures, while the strip connecting the sides allows magnificent views down the river and towards the Ponte Vecchio. Rooms 2–4 are dedicated to works from Siena and Florence during the duecento and trecento (13th and 14th centuries), exhibiting the decorative and iconographic pre-Renaissance style. Notable works are the interpretations of the Madonna by Giotto and Duccio, as well as that of Cimabue, Giotto's master.

Room 7 is dedicated to the early Renaissance period and its founders and leading exponents, who include Masaccio and Uccello and, later, Fra Angelico. The Filippo Lippi Room (8) holds the Franciscan monk's lovely *Madonna with Angels*, as well as a number of other celebrated works, and is worth visiting to see Piero della Francesca's portraits of the Duke and Duchess of Urbino I *(pictured above)*. Room 9 holds works by the Pollaiuolo brothers, whose paintings display no distinctive style as such but are nonetheless decorative.

After a room of sculpture, the newly restored Tribuna (Room 18) is an octagonal room lit from above, with a beautiful mother-of-pearl-encrusted ceiling, that was designed by Buontalenti. This room's structure and decor was designed to allude to the four elements and previously exhibited the objects that were most highly prized by the Medici. It holds a collection of portraits and sculpture, as well as Rosso Fiorentino's ubiquitous *Putto che Suona*, or *Angel Musician (pictured opposite)*. The circular route visitors must take around the room unfortunately renders it somewhat difficult to either appreciate the art from a good distance or to linger in front of the portraits.

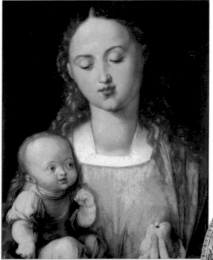

THE WESTERN CORRIDOR

The western corridor starts with the Michelangelo Room and his vivid *Holy Family* tondo (below). This prelude to Mannerism was produced for the wedding of Angelo Doni to Maddalena Strozzi, and the depth of the figures betrays Michelangelo's penchant for sculpture. Early works by Raphael – such as the glowing *Madonna of the Goldfinch* – and Andrea del Sarto's *Madonna of the Harpies* can be seen in the next room. Room 27 is the last room to focus on Tuscan art before moving on to other regions of Italy.

ABOVE: the High Renaissance continues in Room 19, which exhibits Perugino and Signorelli's work. These Umbrian artists worked during the 15th and 16th centuries, and the latter's tondo (circular painting) *Holy Family* is reputed to have inspired Michelangelo's version. Room 20 is a break from Italian art, with work by Dürer, including his *Madonna and the Pear (pictured above)*, and Cranach. The last few rooms on the eastern corridor hold works from the 15th and 16th centuries: the Venetian school in Room 21, followed by Holbein and other Flemish and German Realists (22) and more Italian work by Mantegna and Correggio in Room 23. Room 24 contains a collection of miniatures.

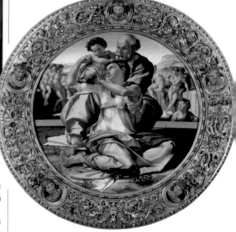

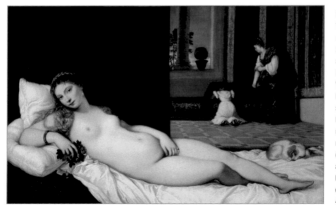

LEFT: Room 28 displays work by Titian, including the erotic *Venus of Urbino (pictured left)*. Rooms 29–30 focus on Emilia Romagnan art and the Mannerists Dosso Dossi and Parmigianino. Veronese's *Annunciation* is in Room 31, while Tintoretto's sensual *Leda and the Swan* hangs in Room 32. A number of rooms are now dedicated to minor works of the cinquecento (16th century), before the Flemish art of Rubens and Van Dyck in Room 41. The Sala della Niobe celebrates sculpture, while Room 44 has works by Rembrandt.

On the first floor are five rooms of paintings, as well as the Verone sull'Arno – the bottom of the U-shaped corridor that looks over the Arno and the Piazza degli Uffizi the other side.

The Sala del Caravaggio holds three paintings by the troubled artist, whose style is characterised by his realism and use of light *(see his* Sacrificing of Isaac, *right).* His method inspired the works by other artists contained in the same room and the next three: the Sala di Bartolomeo Manfredi, the Sala di Gherardo delle Notti, and the Sala dei Caravaggeschi.

The Vasari Corridor, the picture-lined overhead passageway connecting the Uffizi to the Palazzo Pitti via the Ponte Vecchio, is closed until 2014.

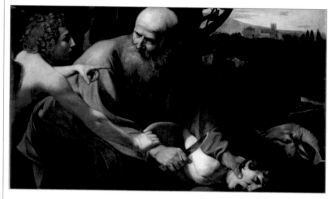

BATTLE FOR THE UFFIZI

While retaining the original Medici layout, the Uffizi's ground floor and labyrinthine offices are being remodelled to make the museum facilities more user-friendly. So rich is the Uffizi's collection that many masterpieces are kept in storage for lack of space, which the curators are keen to remedy. However, proposals for major expansion *(see plans right)* are currently stalled, including the controversial new loggia entrance designed by cutting-edge architect Arata Isozaki. Traditionalists, who see the city solely as "the cradle of the Renaissance", are pitted against progressives who sense a lack of nerve symptomatic of Florentine lethargy.

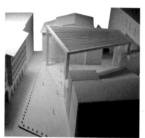

Galleria degli Uffizi

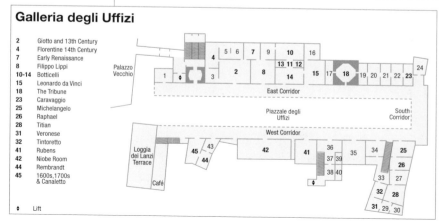

2	Giotto and 13th Century
4	Florentine 14th Century
7	Early Renaissance
8	Filippo Lippi
10-14	Botticelli
15	Leonardo da Vinci
18	The Tribune
23	Caravaggio
25	Michelangelo
26	Raphael
28	Titian
31	Veronese
32	Tintoretto
41	Rubens
42	Niobe Room
44	Rembrandt
45	1600s,1700s & Canaletto
✦	Lift

PALAZZO PITTI AND GIARDINO DI BOBOLI

The gigantic Palazzo Pitti and the Boboli Gardens were once the royal residence

Set in a massive Renaissance palace that dominates the Oltrarno, the Pitti houses seven museums, and provides access to the splendid Boboli Gardens that became a model for Italian landscaping. To appreciate the sumptuous Medici art collection and the lifestyles of the Grand Dukes, the Royal Apartments and Palatine Gallery (Galleria Palatina) are the obvious choices. The Silver Museum (Museo degli Argenti) comes a close second, more for the magnificently decorated rooms than for the contents. In terms of art history, the Modern Art Museum (Galleria d'Arte Moderna) takes up the story where the Uffizi leaves off, and gives a sense of the lavish but somewhat dubious decorative tastes of the last residents, the rulers of the houses of Lorraine and Savoy. By comparison, the Porcelain Museum and the Costume Museum are more for connoisseurs.

For light relief, a museum visit should be combined with a stroll in the beguiling Boboli Gardens, once a pastoral Medici pleasure-dome. The gardens' landscaping, following the slope of the hill, provides the perfect complement to the sumptuous palace, with longer walks leading to Forte Belvedere and the Bardini Gardens. The Palazzo Pitti museum ticketing deals are confusing but pre-booking is advisable, tel: 055-294883; www.firenzemusei.it; or through the Firenze Card, www.firenzecard.it.

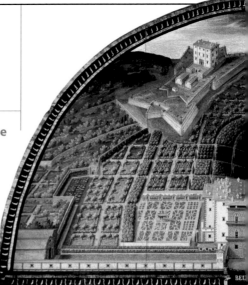

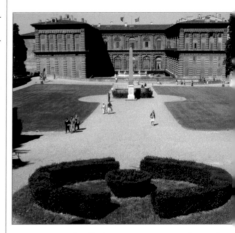

Above: at the end of the Medici reign in 1737, the palazzo became the home of the Lorraines, and its elongated cubic form was further extended by the wings that curve round to frame the paved square at its front. Work on the outside was paralleled by alteration to the interior decor, which exhibits the ostentatious tastes of the period of the Lorraines and the Savoys, the next to take up occupancy within its walls. The history of the palazzo includes brief tenure by the Bourbons and the Emperor Napoleon before the last ruling monarch, Vittorio Emmanuel III, transferred the house to the public.

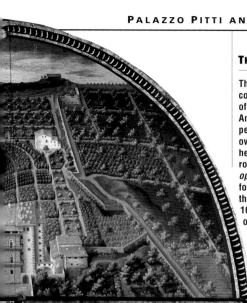

THE GARDENS

The gardens (daily 8.15am–sunset; charge) were commissioned by Cosimo I and created by a range of prolific figures of the day, from Vasari and Ammannati to Buontalenti. One of the most compelling characteristics of the Boboli is the shadowy dark-green colour of the cypress and box hedges that serve to highlight the statues of amorous nymphs, satyrs and statuesque deities *(see opposite and below)*, as well as the grottoes and fountains. The steps lead up to the terrace behind the palace and in front of Susini's fountain of 1641. The amphitheatre surrounding the fountain occupies the site of a quarry used to obtain much of the stone for the palace, and contains an Egyptian obelisk. A series of terraces leads up the hill to the Neptune Fountain, round to the Rococo Kaffeehaus and up to the statue of *Abundance*. At the summit lies the Giardino del Cavaliere, or Knight's Garden. This delightful garden – with its low hedges, rose bushes and little cherub fountain – gives open views of San Miniato to the left and the village of Arcetri to the right, rising above a valley dotted with villas and olive groves. This is where the Museo delle Porcellane is located.

The cypress-statue-lined avenue known as Il Viottolone leads to the Vasca dell'Isola (Island Pool) with its Oceanus Fountain by Giambologna *(pictured left)*, murky green water, ducks, fish, strange mythical creatures and circular hedge. The route from here to the exit leads past the Grotta di Buontalenti, named after the sculptor who created this cavern in 1583–8. Copies of Michelangelo's *Slaves* (the originals are on display in the Accademia; *see page 118*) are set in the four corners.

Finally, on the right as one exits and nestling below the wall of the corridor, is the naked, potbellied statue of Pietro Barbino, Cosimo I's court dwarf, seated on a turtle.

ABOVE: the Palazzo Pitti was commissioned in the 15th Century by Luca Pitti, and was designed by Brunelleschi, although he never lived to see the final results. The Medici family took over ownership in 1549, when Eleonora di Toledo, wife of Cosimo I, purchased the palazzo when the Pitti family ran into financial trouble. She transferred her family from the Palazzo Vecchio to this more tranquil location, though still close to the political heart of the city. This link was strengthened by the Vasari Corridor, which directly connects the residence with Piazza della Signoria by way of the Uffizi and the Palazzo Vecchio. Under the Medici family, work on the palazzo continued, substantially increasing its size and grandeur. Ammannati was given architectural control, and he constructed the inner courtyard and redesigned the outer facade, which was later further extended.

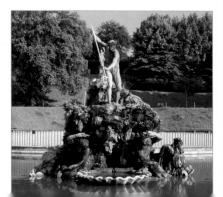

Palazzo Pitti

First Floor

14 Prometheus Room
19 Ulysses Room
21 Education of Jupiter Room
23 Iliad Room
24 Saturn Room
25 Jupiter Room
26 Mars Room
27 Apollo Room
28 Venus Room
29 Room of the Niches

Palatine Gallery

Royal Apartments

Empress Marie Louise's Bathroom

Poccianti Staircase

Chapel of the Relics

Del Moro Staircase

Entrance Hall

Ammannati Staircase

Piazza de' Pitti

♦ Lift

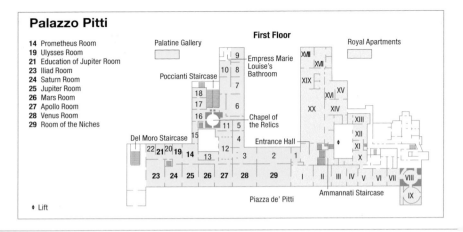

The **Galleria Palatina** (Palatine Gallery) on the first floor (Tue–Sun 8.15am–6.50pm, closed Jan; charge) houses an extraordinary range of paintings collected by the Medici family. In the west wing of the building are the rooms comprising the **Royal Apartments** (same times as the gallery). They are garish and ostentatious, decked out in heavy carpets, wallpapers, fabrics and furnishings, and over-stuffed with treasures. Several of the rooms are named after the colour in which they are themed, and contain paintings and portraits fitting with the mood, followed by the Queen's Apartments, the King's Apartments and a ceremonial room, all filled with ponderous period furniture.

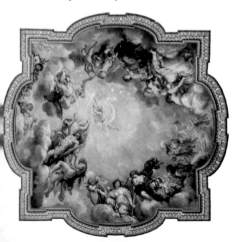

ALLEGORICAL FRESCOES

The most important rooms, named after the planets, are frescoed by Pietro da Cortona (see Sala di Giove ceiling detail, left) to allegorise the stages of Prince Ferdinando's education: Sala di Saturno, Sala di Giove, Sala di Marte and Sala di Venere. These contain works such as Rubens' The Consequences of War (Sala di Marte), Raphael's Portrait of a Lady (Sala di Giove). Other important paintings, such as Raphael's The Pregnant Lady (Sala dell'Iliade), Lippi's tondo of The Madonna and Child (see above: Sala di Prometeo) and Sleeping Cupid by Caravaggio (Sala dell'Educazione di Giove) are found in the smaller rooms.

SILVER AND PORCELAIN

On the ground floor, the Museo degli Argenti (Silver Museum) is in the left-hand corner of the courtyard, while the Museo delle Porcellane (Porcelain Museum) is situated in the Boboli Gardens (daily 8.15am–sunset; closed 1st and last Mon of the month). The former contains much more than silver, ranging from antique vases much loved by Lorenzo the Magnificent to baubles encrusted with semi-precious stones and jewellery. The frescoed rooms alone make a visit worthwhile – in particular the Sala di San Giovanni, which formed part of the summer apartments. The frescoes by the artist after whom the room is named depict the reign of Lorenzo de' Medici, portrayed as a great patron of the arts. The latter museum displays porcelain as well as objets d'art.

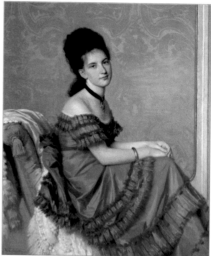

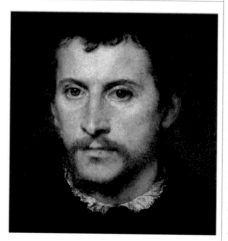

The Galleria d'Arte Moderna (Modern Art Mueum; Tue–Sun 8.15am–6.50pm) contains mainly Italian works from the neoclassical and Romantic movements, dating from the 18th century to the period after World War I, including *Portrait of Alaide Banti* by Michele Gordigiani (*pictured above*). The most notable feature of the second-floor collection is its holding of paintings by the Macchiaioli, 19th-century Italian Post-Impressionists. Also situated on the second floor is the **Galleria del Costume** (Costume Museum; Apr, May, Sept, Oct daily 8.15am–6.30pm, June–Aug until 6.50pm, rest of the year until 5.30pm; charge), which is an intriguing display of Italian costume and fashion, especially from the Medici to the modern period, including creations by designers such as Capucci.

ABOVE: one of the finest rooms is the Sala di Apollo, in which hang important works by Andrea del Sarto (including his *Lamentation of Christ*, 1522–3). The Sala di Venere includes works by another master of the High Renaissance, Titian; notably his *The Interrupted Concert* and *Portrait of a Man (above)*.
RIGHT: the ornate Prometheus Room in the Galleria Palatina.

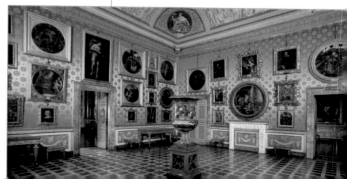

THE ACCADEMIA

Originally the world's first school of art, the gallery is now home to Michelangelo's most famous work, *David*

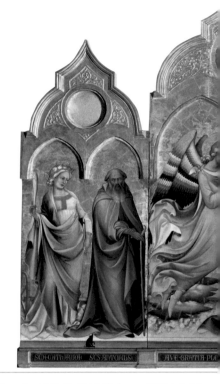

Michelangelo's *David* is the main attraction of the Galleria dell'Accademia (entrance at No. 60; tel: 055-294883; www.firenze-musei.it; Tue–Sun 8.15am–6.50pm; Tue, Thur open till 10pm in summer; charge, the Firenze Card can be used).

Most visitors dutifully come to gasp over the famous statue and then call it a day, scarcely realising that this is one of the city's finest galleries, despite its stifling intensity. The collection dates back to a school of fine arts founded by Cosimo I de' Medici in 1563. Although many treasures have moved to the Uffizi and San Marco, the remaining array of Florentine Byzantine and Gothic art justifies a visit, without the added inducement of a certain Michelangelo. The foremost sculptor of his age, or arguably of all time, is well represented by the authentic *David*, and by his magnificently unfinished *Four Slaves*. *David*, the city's most deified statue, was produced in a heroic age of sculpture. It was, in public-minded Florentine fashion, placed in front of the Palazzo Vecchio as a civic lesson. In keeping with the rulers' dissimulation of power, ostentation and self-aggrandisement were publicly frowned upon in Florence, as was the glorification of the individual. Yet the statue became both the symbol of liberty and a symbol of the artistic aspirations of the city.

David may be the centrepiece,

ABOVE LEFT: Botticelli's delightful *Madonna and Child* is in the Sale del Quattrocento Fiorentino. **ABOVE:** Lorenze Monaco's *Anunciation* Triptych is also in the gallery.

but the so-called *Nonfiniti* (unfinished) *Slaves* illustrate the magnitude of Michelangelo's talent and ambition. In the brooding intensity of his figures one can sense the laying bare of the innate idea, the eternal truth that his art strove to attain. More clearly than in other masterpieces, these works reveal Michelangelo's philosophy: the genesis of a sculpture is not the classic shaping of art out of chaos but the struggle to free a creature that already exists. Even if his paintings have a rare sculptural quality, only the sculpted naked body can express Michelangelo's most sublime concepts.

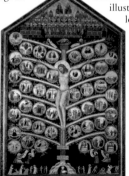

RIGHT: Pacino di Bonaguida's *Tree of Life*, dating from the 14th century.

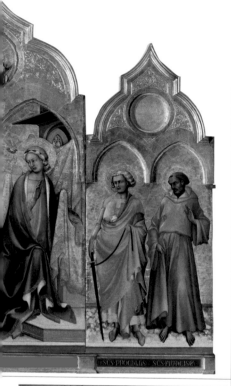

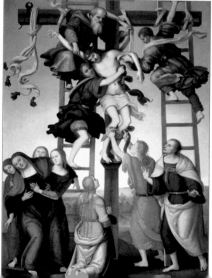

DAVID

As the most famous sculpture in Western art, *David (pictured below)* has immediate appeal, both thanks to the sculpture's recognition factor and to its accessibility. When criticising the gigantism of the work, it has to be remembered that the statue was intended for a large civic space, not designed to be cooped up in a corner of an airless museum. Michelangelo's statue was installed, with much pomp, in a specially created Tribune here, in the Accademia, in 1873.

To most modern visitors, *David* is a celebration of the nude, stripped of his original cultural and political significance. It is therefore remarkable that, even without any artistic background, the average high-school student is still awed enough to be drawn into an appreciation of Renaissance art through Michelangelo's boyish ambassador. Giorgio Vasari, Michelangelo's reluctantly admiring contemporary, concurred, praising its grace, serenity, proportion and harmony: "This figure has overshadowed every other statue, ancient or modern, Greek or Roman."

But this timeless icon of virility is under threat and may yet be on the move again. After the discovery of cracks in the 500-year-old marble, the statue has been declared at risk of toppling over. The cracks in the statue's ankles are believed to have developed after *David* spent over a century leaning forward dangerously from his proud perch on Piazza della Signoria. The weight of the marble, bearing down on *David*'s left ankle, is also partly to blame, as are the vibrations from the traffic and roadworks outside the gallery. Fortunately, the experts have declared that Florence's most famous statue is not in danger of imminent collapse, but as a precaution, there is perennial talk of transferring the symbolic statue to a purpose-built site on the outskirts of the city.

LEFT: among the most notable pieces is Filippino Lippi's striking *Deposition from the Cross*, which was finished by Perugino on the former's death. Other highlights are *Christ as a Man of Sorrows* – a poignant fresco by Andrea del Sarto – and Fra Bartolomeo's *Prophets*.

THE BARGELLO

The Bargello holds Florence's most important collection of sculpture from the Medici and private collections

The **Bargello** is open daily (tel: 055-294883; www.firenzemusei.it; 8.15am–1.50pm, closed 1st, 3rd, 5th Sun of the month and 2nd, 4th Mon; charge). Unlike the Accademia, the Bargello would be a major site even without its art treasure trove. As the oldest surviving seat of government in Florence, the Bargello preceded the Palazzo Vecchio. The collection clearly shows the transition from statuary that was flaunted as public symbols to sculpture that was appreciated as private treasures.

The Bargello is also the best place in which to gain a sense of the interconnectedness of Florentine Renaissance sculpture. It provides a clear overview, with works of art by the greatest masters. Moreover, despite the virtuosity of Michelangelo, the Bargello is more of a shrine to his predecessor, Donatello, the only sculptor to lay claim to equal gifts. Unlike Michelangelo's work, Donatello's sculpture betrays little sign of creative torment and virtuosity for virtuosity's sake, which accounts, at least in part, for Donatello's less glittering reputation. However, in the Bargello at least, Donatello is the undoubted star. Those single-mindedly in pursuit of Renaissance sculpture would do well to head straight for the Donatello gallery, followed by the Verrocchio and della Robbia rooms, set on the floor above. To fully appreciate the sculpture, avoid being waylaid by the distracting displays of unrelated decorative arts.

Above: the Bargello contains works by Andrea della Robbia, a Renaissance sculptor specialising in glazed terracotta, including *Bust of a Woman*.

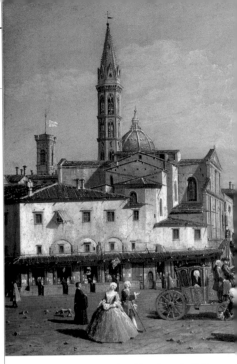

Below: the Bargello museum is situated in an impressive Gothic palazzo constructed in the mid-13th-century on Via del Proconsolo, in the heart of the ancient city. The building has previously been used as a barracks and a prison.

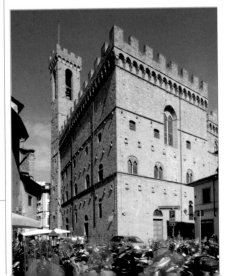

THE DONATELLO AND BRONZE GALLERIES

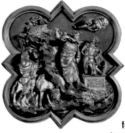

The Salone del Consiglio Generale is often nicknamed the Donatello Gallery. Apart from *David*, other works by Donatello in the room are *Saint George*, designed for the Orsanmichele church, and *Cupid*. You can also see the bronze panels submitted by Ghiberti and Brunelleschi *(pictured above)* for the Baptistery doors here. The walls of the room feature several glazed terracotta works by Luca della Robbia, while the first floor chapel (Cappella Maddalena) features frescoes depicting Hell: look out for the figure on the right dressed in maroon thought to be a depiction of Dante. Also on the first floor is a corridor displaying an eclectic group of 5th- to 17th-century objets d'art, including ivories and Islamic treasures.

Upstairs (currently open afternoons only), the Verrocchio Room displays Tuscan sculpture from the late 15th century, including portrait busts of notable Florentines and an interpretation of *David* by the artist who lends his name to the room, Andrea del Verrocchio. The adjoining rooms are filled with work by members of the della Robbia family – predominantly Andrea and Giovanni – dominated by the often overbearing large reliefs coloured in yellow, green and blue.

The last major room in the museum is the Bronze Gallery. This has one of the most rewarding displays in the Bargello. The sculptures generally depict mythological tales or Greek history, in the form of both models and more functional articles such as candelabra. The model for Giambologna's *Rape of the Sabines* (on display in the Loggia dei Lanzi) stands out, as do two others of his statues: *Kneeling Nymph* and *Hercules and Antaeus*.

Completing the second floor is a collection of medals.

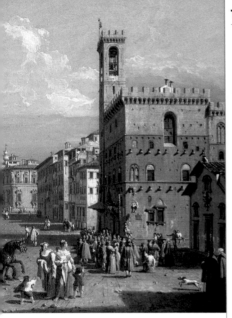

ABOVE: the museum building can be seen on the right of this 18th-century painting by Florentine artist Giuseppe Zocchi.

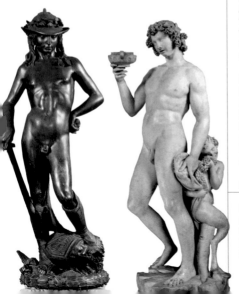

LEFT: statues in the Bargello include Donatello's recently restored *David* (far left, of 1430–40) – a small bronze most renowned for being the first nude since antiquity. It differs dramatically from Michelangelo's masterpiece not just in size and material, but also in its coyness and melancholy.

AROUND FLORENCE

Along with vineyards, the Medici villas are one of the glories of the Florentine countryside, even if the encroaching nature of the suburbs sometimes tarnishes their allure

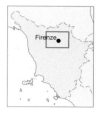

nder the Medici, villa building became a form of self-exaltation and self-indulgence, allied to bucolic pleasures and property speculation. Perched on a scenic hill, the patrician villa became not just a rural estate and glorified hunting lodge, but also a place for feasting and festivities, and an escape from the summer heat. The picture of rural harmony extends to hamlets perched on steep, cypress-covered hills and to vineyards that have been producing famous wines since the Renaissance. Chianti country is close by, while, north of Florence, lies the Mugello, the fertile Apennine region bordering Tuscany and Emilia Romagna. Indulge in a little wine tasting before exploring the harsher Mugello, the Medici homeland.

Hilltop retreat

The best view of the mountains is a seat in the Roman theatre of **Fiesole** ❶, a delightful hill town 8km (5 miles) northeast of Florence. Fiesole was first settled by Etruscans probably in the 8th century BC. The Romans later named the place Faesulum – praising it for its freshwater springs and strategic location. During the 15th century Fiesole became a city suburb where wealthy Florentines built their villas. Today, a villa on the slopes of Fiesole's verdant hill is one of the most sought-after addresses.

The main route from the centre of Florence is the Via San Domenico (the No. 7 bus goes from Piazza Stazione or Piazza San Marco), which climbs up to Fiesole's centre. The views on the way up reveal a landscape of extraordinary beauty, dotted with Renaissance villas perched on the slope of the hill.

Main attractions
FIESOLE
MUGELLO VALLEY
CASTELLO DEL TREBBIO
MEDICI VILLAS
PRATO
SAN MINIATO

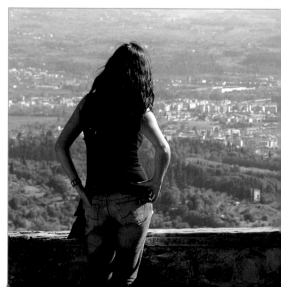

LEFT: attractive villas cling to the hillsides above the city. **RIGHT:** view from Sant Alessandro, Fiesole.

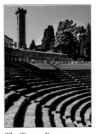

The Teatro Romano, with its numbered seats, could originally accommodate an audience of up to 2,000 people. It is in a remarkable state of repair, and is still used for dances and shows during the summer festival season.

Everything you will want to see in Fiesole lies a short distance from the Piazza Mino da Fiesole, the main square. A lane leads north to the **Teatro Romano**, where you can buy tickets for Fiesole's **Zona Archeologica** (winter Thur–Mon 10am–4pm, summer daily until 7pm), entered from the ticket office and comprising the city's 1st-century BC Roman theatre, public baths of the same era, and an Etruscan temple, built in the 4th century BC and dedicated to Minerva, goddess of wisdom and healing. Also within the complex, the **Museo Archeologico**, built in the style of a Roman temple, is packed with finds from excavations in Fiesole. Included in the ticket is entry to the **Museo Bandini**, behind the cathedral on Via Duprè – a small art gallery with a fairly wide and representative selection of paintings from the early and middle Renaissance.

On the square, the huge **Cattedrale di San Romolo** (daily) is almost completely unadorned except for four frescoes, including a serene portrait of St Sebastian by Perugino (early 16th century). The Cathedral's jewel is the marble funerary monument to Bishop Leonardo Salutati, by Mino da Fiesole (1429–84), with a realistic bust of the smiling bishop.

From the southwest corner of the square, Via Vecchia Fiesolana leads to the **Villa Medici** (entrance along Via Beato Angelico). Any of the downhill paths from this point can be taken to reach the hamlet of **San Domenico**, about a 15-minute walk. The church of San Domenico (1406) contains a restored *Madonna with Angels and Saints* (1430), an early work of Fra Angelico who began his monastic life here before transferring to San Marco.

Opposite, the Via della Badia dei Roccettini descends to the **Badia Fiesolana** (Mon–Fri 9am–5pm, Sat 9am–noon; free), once a monastery and now home to the European

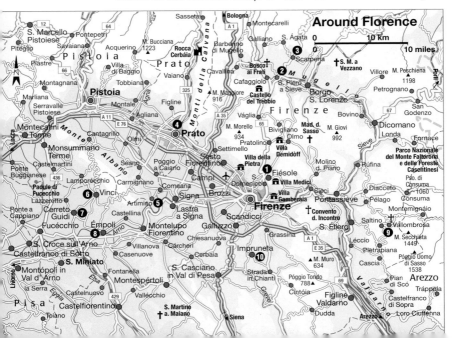

University Institute. The unfinished brick facade of the huge church (dull inside, so don't worry if it is closed) incorporates the lovely green-and-white Romanesque facade of an earlier and smaller church. The No. 7 bus can be caught in San Domenico for the return journey to Florence.

The Mugello valley

Just a few kilometres north of Florence, the Apennine foothills and Sieve river basin form the Mugello region (www.mugellotoscana.it). Like the Chianti, only less well trodden, it is characterised by bluish-green hills, brooding oak and chestnut woods, silvery olive groves and well-tended vineyards. The landscape is at its most picturesque in the western Sieve valley.

The Mugello has great associations with the Medici, who originated from here and lavished a lot of attention on the region. In 1451, Cosimo il Vecchio had Michelozzo alter the old fortress of Cafaggiolo just west of **San Piero a Sieve ❷** to create a country retreat, where Lorenzo il Magnifico spent part of his childhood, and writers and artists were lavishly entertained. The

palace was modified by the Borghese family, who acquired it in the 19th century. Although recently restored, this original Medici seat, known as the **Castello Mediceo di Cafaggiolo** (tel: 055-844 685; www.castellodicafaggiolo.it) is closed for the forseeable future but used for weddings, events and a cookery school.

A little further south, **Castello del Trebbio** (tel: 055-830 4900; www.vino turismo.it; guided visits Tue and Thur 10.30am and other times; booking essential; charge) received similar treatment at the hands of Michelozzo, and, more than any other 15th-century Tuscan villa, retains the feudal atmosphere of a Medici villa. Deservedly popular for Chianti wine tastings, welcoming cookery classes and gourmet feasts in the vaulted cellars, this castle-like retreat is a place that celebrates all these activities in one day.

Overlooking San Piero a Sieve, high on a thickly wooded outcrop, is the **San Martino** fortress built in 1569 by Lanci and Buontalenti to enable Cosimo I to defend the Florentine state. This massive pentagonal castle is currently being restored, although

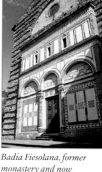

Badia Fiesolana, former monastery and now home to the European University Institute. From the terrace in front of the church there are views down the Mugnone River valley back to Florence.

BELOW: Villa Medici.

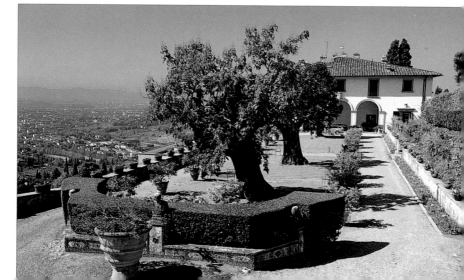

Villa Country

The Medici villas reflect Florentine fine taste during the Renaissance, when these retreats were a haven for philosophers, artists – and the Medici rulers themselves

The idea of a country retreat, so popular in Tuscany today, originated with the Romans. The villas were either working farms or were planned purely for pleasure. In the 15th century, the idea of the country villa was revived by the Medici family, who commissioned magnificent residences and elaborate gardens, modelled on classical principles. In 1452, Leon Battista Alberti decreed that a truly well-appointed country retreat had to be on a slope, full of light and air, with rooms grouped round an inner hall. The villas and gardens described here are all easily accessible from Florence, but it's wise to call ahead.

The **Villa Medici** (Via Beato Angelico; tel: 055-59417; Sat–Sun 9am–1pm; gardens appointment only; charge) at Fiesole, described as "the first true Renaissance villa", was designed by Michelozzo for Cosi-

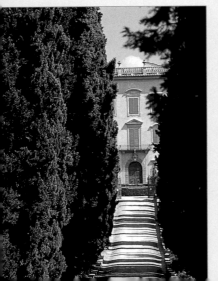

mo il Vecchio between 1458 and 1461. It commands a superb view of Florence.

On the outskirts of Florence, the 15th-century **Villa la Pietra** (tel: 055-5007 210; www.nyu.edu/global/lapietra; guided tours Fri pm, advance booking necessary; charge) was the home of the writer Sir Harold Acton. He bequeathed the villa and his Renaissance art collection to New York University.

Another American-owned villa in the Florentine hills is the historic **Villa i Tatti** (tel: 055-603 251; www.itatti.harvard.edu; by appointment; charge), beside the pretty village of Settignano. Formerly the home of art collector Bernard Berenson (1865–1959), who restored the villa to house his Renaissance art collection, it is now the Harvard University Center for Renaissance Studies.

Nearby, the **Villa Gamberaia** (tel: 055-697 205; www.villagamberaia.com; daily 9am–6pm but by appointment only; charge) is another fine Renaissance villa whose original garden survives.

The **Villa Medicea Poggio a Caiano** is often dubbed the perfect villa. The facade was modelled by Sangallo on a Greek temple to satisfy the tastes of Lorenzo the Magnificent. In the 19th century, the gardens were converted according to the fashionable English style, with romantic temples, fountains, an aviary and a mock-Gothic ruin.

Set on a steeply sloping hill, the **Villa Medicea della Petraia** (Via della Petraia; tel: 055-452 691; daily 8.15am–sunset; villa by guided tour only; free) was designed by Buontalenti for Ferdinando de' Medici as an elegant villa suitable for sumptuous entertaining. The interior is marred by the pretentious taste of the house of Savoy, but the Italianate gardens are a delight.

Only the gardens of the **Villa Medicea di Castello** (Via di Castello; tel: 055-452 691; daily 8.15am–sunset; free) can be viewed. Grottoes and statuary abound.

Another villa with attractive surroundings is the **Villa Demidoff** and **Parco di Pratolino** (Apr–Sept Thur–Sun, Mar and Oct Sun, 10am–sunset; charge), whose Mannerist gardens were remodelled in the English romantic style. ❑

LEFT: cypress avenue leading to Villa la Pietra.

you can walk along its walls.

Just north of San Piero a Sieve is the town of **Scarperia ❸**. **Palazzo de Vicari**, in the main street, is one of the finest examples of 13th-century civil architecture in Tuscany, similar in style to Florence's Palazzo Vecchio. The outer facade, decorated with the coats of arms of local notables, carved in stone or worked in della Robbia terracotta, faces the **Oratorio della Madonna della Piazza** in the small square, which features a *Madonna and Child* by Taddeo Gaddi. At the bottom of the main street, near the entrance to the town, is the **Oratorio della Madonna dei Terremoti**, dedicated to Our Lady of Earthquakes, which contains another fresco of the *Madonna and Child*, said to be by Filippo Lippi *(see right)*.

Scarperia is famous as a centre of knife-making. In local workshops traditional methods are still used to fashion knives by hand. There is even a museum dedicated to the craft, the **Museo dei Ferri Taglienti** (Museum of Cutting Tools) in the Palazzo dei Vicari (summer Tue–Sat 3.30–7.30pm, winter Sat only 10.30am–1pm, 3–6pm; charge), and in September the town hosts an international knife exhibition.

Scarperia is also known for the racetrack on its outskirts. The scenic "Mugello" circuit is used as a Ferrari F1 test centre and hosts the Italian motorbike grand prix in June.

A turning on the left of the southern approach to Scarperia wends its way through dense woodlands to the remote **Bosco ai Frati** Franciscan convent (tel: 055-848 111; daily; ring the bell and one of the monks will usually be happy to let you in; free). This retreat retains the peace and solitude of the Franciscan ideal that places such as Assisi lack; no touring hordes, no postcard-sellers, only the peace and quiet offered by a church and its convent in a clearing in the woods. The monastic buildings were remodelled by Michelozzo around 1440 for Cosimo il Vecchio. They house a little-known, large wooden *Crucifix*, attributed to Donatello, one of the greatest masters of the Italian Renaissance.

Prato

Prato ❹, to the northwest of Florence, is the third-largest city in Tuscany, and long-time rival of Florence. Refreshingly, Prato doesn't depend on tourism but on trade, and revels in its confident, mercantile personality. The city is renowned for its textile-manufacturing industries, with numerous factory outlets selling fine fabrics, cashmere and designer clothes. Although the trade has made contemporary Prato a rich city, it was already a leading textile town in the 12th century and its magnificent monuments are evidence of its former wealth. Amid the industrial estates, and factories dominated by Chinese immigrants, lies a compact *centro storico*, contained within medieval walls. But Prato is also a cosmopolitan city, drawn to contemporary art, as witnessed by the Henry Moore

While painting the fresco cycles in Prato's Cathedral, Fra Filippo Lippi famously seduced a nun, Lucrezia Buti, who was modelling for his Madonna. The nun and friar ran away together and had a son, Filippino Lippi, who became an important fresco painter in his own right. It is said that the face and figure of Salome dancing at Herod's feast in the John the Baptist cycle are those of Lucrezia.

Glorious Gardens

The centrepiece of any Medici villa was the garden, which provided a harmonious link with the wild countryside beyond the walls. The enclosed medieval garden, the *giardino segreto*, survived at first, with vegetable and herb gardens planted nearby. However, Renaissance landscape gardeners embellished the concept of enclosure and, in keeping with humanistic ideals, it became a symbol of tamed nature.

The villa and garden were considered an organic whole, linked by loggias, porticoes and new perspectives. Emphasis was placed on geometrical rigour and the laws of perspective were used to create terraced gardens with straight avenues lined by cypresses or lemon trees in tubs. Semicircular ponds, adorned with sculpture, closed the line of vision.

The Mannerist era witnessed a profusion of allegorical fountains and grotesque sculpture, much of which remains. The main players were Buontalenti, who brought architectural rigour to garden design, and Il Tribolo, a pupil of Michelangelo who was responsible for the Boboli Gardens. Four of the best gardens are at: Villa Gamberaia; Villa Demidoff; Villa Medicea della Petraia; and Villa Medicea di Castello.

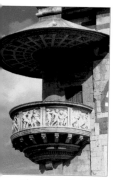

The Pulpit of the Holy Girdle on Prato's Duomo.

sculpture that greets most visitors.

The city possesses an extraordinary relic: in the delightful green-and-white **Duomo** (daily 7.30am–7pm; free) is what is believed to be the girdle of the Virgin Mary. The legends surrounding this relic have been celebrated by Agnolo Gaddi, whose frescoes cover the walls of the Chapel of the Holy Girdle. Above the high altar are fresco cycles of *The Life of St Stephen* and *The Martyrdom of St John the Baptist* by Filippo Lippi. Outside the Duomo is the Pulpit of the Holy Girdle, decorated with dancing cherubs by Donatello, where, on Christmas Day and several other holy days in the year, the girdle is displayed. The **Museo dell' Opera del Duomo** (Mon, Thur–Sat 9am–1pm, 2.30–6.30pm, Wed 9am–1pm; charge) in the cloister contains paintings, sculptures and reliefs by Donatello, Fra Lippi and others.

Other notable monuments include the church of **Santa Maria delle Carcere** (daily 7am–noon, 4–7pm; free), built by Giuliano Sangallo in typical no-frills Brunelleschian style. In front of the church is the **Castello dell'Imperatore** (Sat–Sun 10am–1pm, 4–7pm, Mon–Fri 4–7pm; charge), built by Frederick II Hohenstaufen in the first half of the 13th century, and unique in Tuscany, taking as its model the Norman castles of Puglia. A walk along its ramparts offers a good view of Prato.

In Via Rinaldesca is the 14th-century frescoed **Palazzo Datini** (Mon–Fri 9am–12.30pm, 3–6pm, Sat am only; charge), former home of Francesco Datini (1330–1410), better known as the Merchant of Prato. Datini, a successful wool merchant, died one of the richest men in Europe, leaving his money to city charities, and is commemorated in statues around the town.

For a break from Renaissance art, the **Centro per l'Arte Contemporanea Luigi Pecci** (tel: 0574-5317; www.centropecci.it; Wed–Mon 4–11pm; charge) lies on the edge of town. The museum's attitude and energy are currently more important than the collection of contemporary works on display.

Outside the historic centre is the more engaging **Museo del Tessuto** (Via Santa Chiara 24; Mon, Wed–Fri 9.30am–2.30pm, Sat 10am–6pm, Sun 4–7pm; charge), dedicated to the fine textiles that made Prato's fortune. Gorgeous masterpieces of antique cloth are on display, and the skills that led to their production are not lost, as the section on contemporary textiles clearly demonstrates.

Leonardo country

A gentle meander into the countryside due west of Florence takes in some lovely views, a few small towns and Leonardo's alleged birthplace of Vinci. Head west out of Florence on the SP66 (in the direction of Pistoia), and turn south at **Poggio a Caiano**, site of Lorenzo the Magnificent's favourite retreat, built by Sangallo (1480–85). It is one of the most magnificent and best preserved of Florentine rural retreats (daily

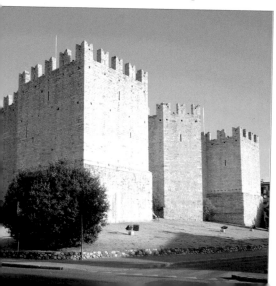

8.15am–sunset; villa by guided tour only, hourly from 8.30am; closed 2nd and 3rd Mon of the month; charge).

The walled village of **Artimino** ❺, about 11km (7 miles) from Poggio a Caiano, is a classic case of a *borgo* reborn as a villa, wine estate and medieval residential complex. It is also the setting for another huge Medicean villa (tel: 055-875 1427; www.artimino.com; open by appointment only; charge), this one built by Bernardo Buontalenti as a hunting lodge for Ferdinando I in 1594 and curious for the number of tall chimneys on the roof. It has been beautifully restored, and converted into a distinguished hotel, complete with a restaurant specialising in dishes with Medici origins. Part of the villa is open to visitors, including a small Etruscan museum. After wandering round Artimino *borgo*, consider dining in the Biagio Pignatta *(see page 131)* in the villa stables, or in the rustic Cantina dei Redi (tel: 055-875 1408) overlooking the villa.

A tortuous road leads through olive groves and vines from Artimino to **Vinci** ❻, alleged birthplace of Leonardo. Here, the 13th-century castle in the centre of town is home to the **Museo Leonardiano** (summer daily 9.30am–7pm, winter 9.30am–6pm; charge), which has a vast selection of mechanical models built to the exact measurements of Leonardo's drawings. In neighbouring **Anchiano**, a revamped Leonardo museum reopens in late 2012 (tel: 055-933 251).

Five kilometres (3 miles) southwest of Vinci is the hill town of **Cerreto Guidi** ❼. Once owned by the Guidi counts, it now produces a good Chianti Putto wine and boasts yet another Medici villa, the austere **Villa di Cerreto Guidi** (daily 8.15am–7pm; closed 2nd and 3rd Mon of the month; charge), built in 1564 for Cosimo I as a hunting lodge. It contains some fine portraits of the Medici family. Isabella, daughter of Cosimo I, is said to have been murdered here by her husband for her infidelities.

West of Florence

West of Florence, the first major stop along the *superstrada* is **Empoli** ❽, a prosperous, modern market town

Prato is home to Italy's largest Chinese community, who make up to 25 percent of the population and increasingly dominate the city's textile industry. Since the 1990s, Chinese migrants have been setting up their own factories, along with a Chinatown. There is now some tension between Italian craftsmanship and quality, and Chinese "fast fashion" (pronta moda), but the medieval Merchant of Prato would probably have seen it as a business opportunity.

BELOW LEFT: ancient San Miniato.

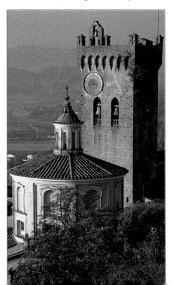

San Miniato

The ancient town of San Miniato, whose origins go back to Etruscan times, is set on the top of three hills, equidistant from the important historical cities of Pisa, Florence, Lucca, Pistoia, Siena and Volterra. On the proverbial fine day you can gaze as far as Volterra and the Apuan Alps. High on the hillside are the two towers of the **Rocca** (Thur–Sun 11am–6pm), rebuilt in the 12th century by Frederick II. The older tower, the Torre di Matilde, was converted into a bell tower when the **Duomo** (daily 8am–6pm, winter until 4.30pm) was added, with its Romanesque brick facade. The **Museo Diocesano d'Arte Sacra** (Thur–Sun 10am–6pm; charge), in the old sacristy of the Duomo, displays art and sculpture, including works by Lippi, Verrocchio and Tiepolo. Built by the Lombards in the 8th century, the magnificent church of San Francesco (daily 8am–12.30pm, 3–7pm) is the oldest building in San Miniato.

But to most Italians, San Miniato means one thing only: white truffles. The town produces a quarter of Tuscany's crop, which are best tasted during the November truffle fair. The Association of Trufflers of the San Miniato Hills issues a map showing where to find the aromatic fungus, which is dug out of the ground with a type of pole called a *vangheggia*.

TIP

The New Museum Card provides access to 12 small museums in the Valdarno and Chianti, including: Barberino Val d'Elsa; Bagno a Ripoli; Figline Valdarno; Greve in Chianti; Impruneta; Incisa in Val d'Arno; Reggello; Rignano sull'Arno; San Casciano in Val di Pesa; Tavarnelle Val di Pesa. For details, see: www.chiantimusei.it and www.verditerre.org

with a small *centro storico* and a superb Romanesque church, the **Collegiata Sant'Andrea**. The green-and-white-striped facade is reminiscent of Florence's San Miniato, and the small **museum** (Tue–Sun 9am–noon, 4–7pm; charge) contains a surprising amount of precious Florentine art.

A few kilometres west of Empoli is **Fucecchio**, noted for the **Padule di Fucecchio**, to the north of town. Now Italy's biggest inland marsh, covering 1,460 hectares (3,600 acres), this was a Medicean fishing ground in the 16th century, and Cosimo I had a bridge and weirs built to facilitate the sport. It is now home to rare birds and a variety of flora. The land is privately owned, but the wetland centre in **Castelmartini di Larciano** (tel: 0573-84540) organises guided tours.

Valdarno

East of Florence, off the SS70, a narrow pass climbs up the western slope of the Pratomagno hills to the monastery of **Vallombrosa** , founded in the 11th century, but remodelled over the centuries, and its **Museo d'Arte Sacra** (tel: 055-862 251; July–Aug only, Mon–Sat 10am–noon, 3–6pm; charge). The reward for making the journey is not so much the monastery itself as the splendid beech wood that surrounds it. Romanesque churches worth visiting in the vicinity are **San Pietro in Cascia** and **Sant'Agata in Arfoli**. Nearby, the tiny village of **Saltino** is handy in the winter for the ski runs of **Monte Secchieta**.

Towards Chianti

Not far south of Florence, towards Chianti, is the town of **Impruneta**, an important sanctuary in the early medieval period when a shrine was erected here to house an image of the Virgin Mary, thought to have been the work of St Luke and believed to be capable of performing miracles. This shrine, the **Basilica di Santa Maria** (daily 7.30–11.30am, 4.30–7pm), with its terracotta tabernacle by Luca della Robbia in Michelozzo's Chapel of the Cross, underwent alterations over the centuries, and was bomb-damaged in World War II.

Subsequent restoration and repair to this and to other pre-17th century buildings has meant that Impruneta has retained a great deal of its early character, though without the patina of age. Brunelleschi insisted that the tiles for the roof of the Duomo in Florence be supplied by Impruneta, which is still an important centre for terracotta production. Call into the **Tesoro,** the cathedral treasury, too (tel: 055-203 6408; Sat–Sun 9am–1pm, 4–7pm; free).

West of Impruneta, **San Casciano in Val di Pesa** is a quiet old Chianti town, enlivened every February by carnival. The town's reputation today rests solely on the art displayed in the Collegiata church, the convent, the church of St Francis and the church of the Misericordia, including paintings by Simone Martini, Ugolino di Neri, Taddeo Gaddi and Fra Bartolomeo.

We are now in the Chianti region covered on pages 199–209. ❑

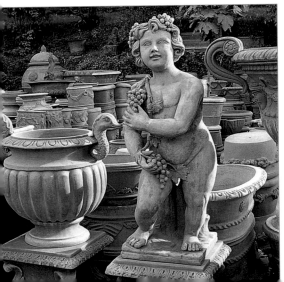

BELOW: Impruneta, just south of Florence, is an important centre of terracotta production.

BEST RESTAURANTS

Restaurants

Prices for a three-course meal per person with a half-bottle of house wine:
€ = under €25
€€ = €25–40
€€€ = €40–60
€€€€ = over €60

Artimino

Biagio Pignatta
Paggeria Medicea, Viale Papa Giovanni XXIII
Tel: 055-875 1406 €€–€€€
This restaurant is part of a four-star hotel, Paggeria Medicea, which occupies the former stables of a Medici villa. Dishes with historical origins a speciality. Closed Wed evening and Thur lunch.

Da Delfina
Via della Chiesa 1
Tel: 055-871 8074
www.dadelfina.it €€–€€€
High-quality ingredients served in an elegant setting, overlooking the Medici villa. Tuscan food, often with a twist. Closed Mon, Tue lunch, and Oct–May Sun evening.

Barberino di Mugello

Cosimo de' Medici
Viale del Lago 19
Tel: 055-842 0370 €€
A well-respected restaurant, serving Tuscan and international food of a consistently high standard. Closed Sun evening and Mon.

Borgo San Lorenzo

Ristorante degli Artisti
Piazza Romagnoli 1
Tel: 055-845 7707
www.ristorantedegliartisti.it €€€
Not far from Scarperia, this restaurant in the hills features delicious Tuscan fare. Traditional dishes include wild hare, wild boar, served with fresh, seasonal vegetables. Closed Wed, most of Jan, 3rd week in Aug.

Cerbaia, Val di Pesa

La Tenda Rossa
Piazza del Monumento 9/14
Tel: 055-826 132
www.latendarossa.it €€€€
One of the best restaurants in the Florence area, serving elegant and creative food in modern, refined surroundings. Excellent wine list. Worth the trek. Closed Mon lunch, Sun and Aug.

Fiesole

La Reggia degli Etruschi
Via San Francesco 18
Tel: 055-59385
www.lareggia.org €€–€€€
The patio of this restaurant has a wonderful view over Florence. The food, if not quite as breathtaking as the view, is reliable, from the cold cuts to the handmade spaghetti, risotto and steaks. Oct–May closed Tue.

Pizzeria San Domenico
Piazza San Domenico 11
Tel: 055-59182 €–€€
This is a simple spot for pizzas, pastas and friendly service. Also recommended are the big salads followed by a *coppa della casa*, the house dessert. Closed Mon outside summer months.

Vinandro
Piazza Mino 33
Tel: 055-59121
www.vinandrofiesole.com €
Tiny rustic wine bar that offers simply prepared meals and good wine. Reservations recommended. Open air seating. Closed Mon.

Galluzzo

Bibe
Via delle Bagnese 1r
Tel: 055-204 9085
www.trattoriabibe.com €€
Above-average rustic trattoria in this typical suburb, with a delightful garden for alfresco meals. Closed Mon–Fri lunch and all day Wed.

Prato

Il Baghino
Via dell'Accademia 9
Tel: 0574-27920 €–€€
This traditional establishment in the historic heart of Prato serves local specialities to a faithful clientele. Closed Aug, Sun, and Mon lunchtime.

Osvaldo Baroncelli
Via Fra Bartolomeo 13
Tel: 0574-23810 €€€
Acclaimed restaurant that mixes traditional and innovative choices. Has a good wine list. Booking advised. Closed Sat lunch and Sun.

San Casciano in Val di Pesa

Trattoria Mamma Rosa
Via Cassia – Loc. Calzaiolo
Tel: 055-824 9454 €–€€
Off the beaten track, this unpretentious but elegant trattoria serves some of the best Tuscan food, using locally sourced ingredients. Excellent wines. The proprietor-chef also runs a cooking school in the Il Borghetto hotel. Closed Wed.

San Miniato

Il Convio – San Maiano
Via San Maiano 2
Tel: 0571-408 114
www.ristoranteilconvio.com €€
A pleasant, rustic restaurant with views over the hills and outdoor seats in summer. Traditional Tuscan fare. Closed Wed.

Firenze Settignano

La Capponcina di Settignano
Via San Romano 17r
Tel: 055-697 037
www.capponcina.com €–€€
Set in the hills just outside Florence, this restaurant has great, reasonably priced food. The terrace offers an outstanding view of Florence. Closed Mon in autumn/winter.

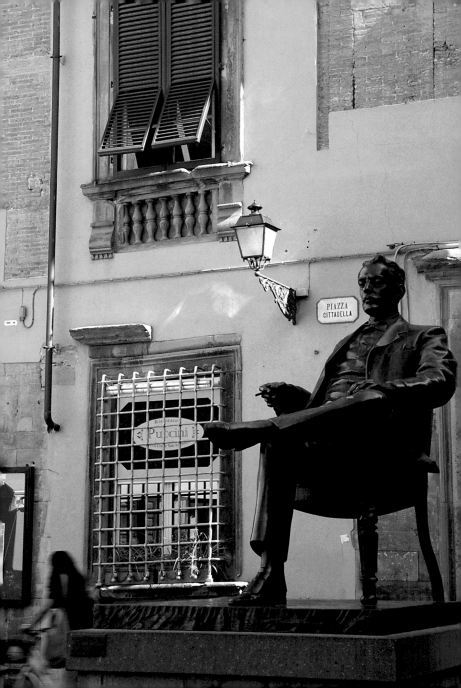

LUCCA AND PISTOIA

Take some mountains and spas, add a scattering of grand villas, blend in two underrated cities full of character, and you begin to paint a picture of Lucca and Pistoia provinces – where you can swim, ski, shop or soak in the spas to your heart's content

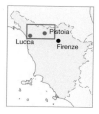

Perfectly proportioned Lucca, and its harmonious, villa-studded countryside, occupy the alluring heart of this region. Lucca, like Siena, is a city built on a human scale, designed to be savoured slowly, and on foot. To the west of the walled city is the Tuscan Riviera, known as Versilia, a broad strip of land between the sea and the Apennines – and, to the north, are the steeply mountainous Garfagnana and Lunigiana regions.

Despite its charms, neighbouring Pistoia always feels marooned in a historical backwater. Pistoia province, sandwiched between Lucca and Florence, and fought over for centuries by both, has yet to make its mark. Its lower profile is partly due to its bewildering diversity. Part-fertile plain and part-mountains, the province is bordered, in the north, by the Apennines, where Abetone is Tuscany's premier ski resort. Further south, spa country rules, with Montecatini Terme playing the dowager to Grotta Giusti's laid-back younger sister.

Miniature cultural capital

Often bypassed by fans intent on ticking off the Leaning Tower of Pisa,

Lucca ❶ is Tuscany's self-deprecating star. In spite of this, it is the only Tuscan city to see tourism expand exponentially in recent years. Its perfectly preserved walled heart, quiet sophistication and peaceful pace of life are all credited with winning over visitors. And that's before talking about its pinky-gold palaces, pedestrian-friendly bastions, crowd-pleasing concerts, enchanting churches, and its renowned olive oil and wine estates. To jaded urbanites, Lucca represents life as it should be led.

Main attractions

LUCCA
CASA MUSEO PUCCINI
VILLA REALE
MONTECATINI TERME
MONSUMMANO TERME
CATTEDRALE DI SAN ZENO, PISTOIA
ABETONE

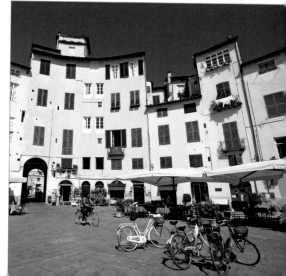

LEFT: statue of composer Giacomo Puccini in Lucca. **RIGHT:** cycling in the sunshine in Lucca's Piazza Anfiteatro.

A jewellery shop in Lucca.

Sitting on a marshy plain between the Apennines and Monte Pisano, Lucca has been inhabited since ancient times. Little remains of Etruscan Luk, but Roman Luca survives in the grid design of streets, and in the elliptical Piazza Anfiteatro, around which houses were subsequently built. As an independent city-state, 11th-century Lucca spent the next 400 years defending itself against an ever more belligerent Florence. Even though the Florentines won the title of capital of the region, Lucca never ceded its political and economic autonomy. It remained an independent republic, apart from a brief period of Pisan rule, until the Napoleonic invasion of 1796.

This graceful and prosperous provincial capital, 77km (48 miles) west of Florence on the A11, is a city of many charms, not least the walls encircling the city. They were built after 1500 to keep Lucca's enemies at bay. In 1817, the massive ramparts were planted with a double row of plane trees, which shade the broad avenue running along the top of the walls, now used by Lucca's citizens as a playground, promenade, jogging trail and cycle route.

The Cathedral square

A path from the walls leads directly to the **Duomo di San Martino** Ⓐ (Mon–Fri 9.30am–5.30pm, Sat until 6.45pm, Sun 9.30am–10.45am, noon–6pm, winter closes 1hr earlier; free). The Cathedral's striking facade is decorated with a sculpture of St Martin dividing his cloak (the original sculpture is now just inside the church). The inlaid marble designs typify Tuscan Romanesque style: hunting scenes figure large, with dogs, boars, and huntsmen on horseback. Flanking the central portal are scenes of the *Labours of the Months* and the *Miracles of St Martin*.

Inside is the octagonal *tempietto* that contains a larger-than-life

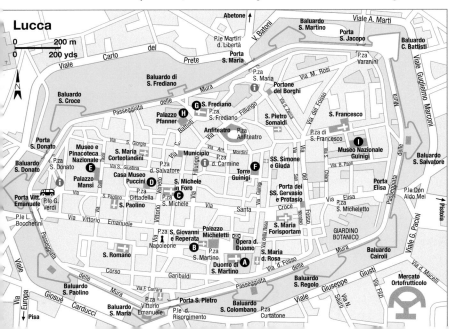

Crucifixion in carved and painted wood. Known as the *Volto Santo* (Holy Face), the Romanesque carving was once believed to be a true portrait of Christ, carved by Nicodemus, who witnessed the Crucifixion (in fact, the highly stylised figure is probably a 13th-century copy of an 11th-century copy of an 8th-century original). Each year, on 13 September, this revered relic is paraded through the streets at dusk. Off the south aisle is the **Sacristy** (Mar–Oct daily 10am–6pm, Nov–Feb Mon–Sat 9.30am–5.45pm; Sun 9.30am–10.30am, noon–6pm; charge). This contains the greatest treasure: Jacopo della Quercia's tomb of Ilaria del Carretto, who died in 1405. It's a tender effigy, depicting a faithful dog at her feet, waiting for his mistress to awake. As the wife of Paolo Guinigi, Lord of Lucca, Ilaria died at the age of 24, following the birth of their second child.

Across the square is the church of **Santi Giovanni e Reperata** Ⓑ (mid-Mar–2 Nov daily 10am–6pm, 3 Nov–mid-Mar Sat–Sun only 10am–5pm; charge). Originally Lucca's cathedral, the church has been excavated

to reveal a wealth of Roman and Romanesque features. The earliest is a 1st-century BC mosaic floor, superseded by a 2nd-century Roman bathhouse, which itself gave way to a 5th-century baptistery, later joined by a series of churches, culminating in the present 12th-century building. Highlights include the Roman font, Romanesque pavements and the coffered ceiling.

Via del Duomo leads west of the Cathedral to Piazza del Giglio, home to the theatre and opera house. Adjoining the square is Piazza Napoleone, shaded by tall plane trees and lined by restaurant terraces.

Pisan Romanesque to Puccini

Heading north out of the square takes you to Piazza San Michele, ringed by Renaissance arcades. At the centre of the square, the church of **San Michele in Foro** Ⓒ (daily 9am–noon, 3–5pm; free), built on the site of the Roman forum, has one of the most spectacular Pisan Romanesque facades in Italy. Flanked by Lucca's loveliest bell tower, the tiered arcades

BELOW: buskers in Piazza San Michele.

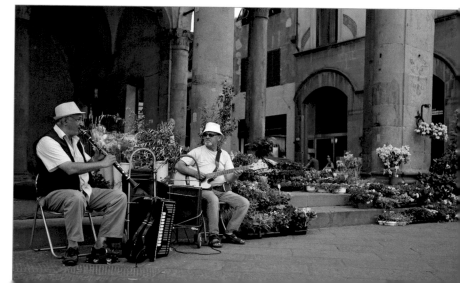

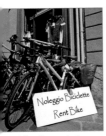

Bikes for rent in Lucca.

BELOW: bird's-eye view of Lucca and the Apuan Alps beyond.

are decorated with delicate motifs and allegories; hunting scenes carved in green and white marble, with creatures both exotic (bears, dragons and elephants) and domestic (a rabbit, a duck and a crow eating grapes). The church is topped by a huge gilded statue of Archangel Michael slaying the dragon, flanked by two angels.

Turning your back on the facade, take Via di Poggio, which leads to the newly revamped **Casa Museo Puccini** (www.fondazionegiacomo puccini.it; Apr–Oct daily 11am–5pm; charge), the birthplace of Lucca's celebrated composer, Giacomo Puccini (*see box on page 137*).

Heading west, feel your way through Lucca's maze of medieval alleys to Palazzo Mansi, in Via Galli Tassi, which houses the **Museo e Pinacoteca Nazionale** (Tue–Sat 8.30am–7pm, Sun 8.30am–1pm; charge). Deities and allegorical figures romp across the ceilings of the splendidly furnished 17th-century home of Cardinal Spada (1659–1724). Upstairs, at the end of a sequence of rooms decorated around the theme of the Four Elements is a

sumptuous bedchamber dedicated to Fire. This fire is not a destructive one, but the flame that burns when Eros strikes with his arrow. The room features a gorgeous double bed, its lovely hangings decorated with birds and flowers.

Remnants of medieval wealth

The wealth of Lucca, like that of Florence, was based on banking and its silk industry. As early as the 12th century, bankers were plying the Mediterranean or travelling north to Bruges, Antwerp and London, buying and selling silk and woollen cloth. Successful bankers, such as the Guinigi family, built ostentatious tower-houses, although only one of these remains, the 14th-century **Torre Guinigi** (daily Mar–Sept 9am–8pm, Oct 10am–6pm, Nov–Feb 9am–5.30pm; charge). As in San Gimignano (*see page 199*), such fortified homes were both medieval status symbols and retreats in times of trouble. Climb the tower to admire rural views, and to make out the outline of Lucca's Roman Amphitheatre

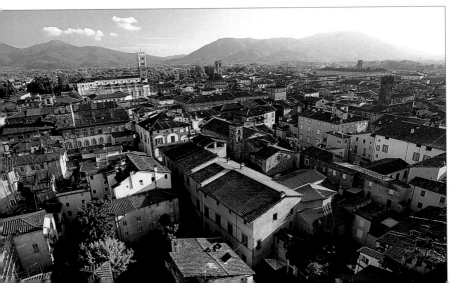

(Anfiteatro), perfectly preserved in the buildings that were constructed against it in the Middle Ages.

For a closer look at the resulting egg-shaped piazza, turn right out of the tower, and first right in Via delle Chiavi d'Oro. Passing the Art Deco baths (now a cultural centre), keep going until you reach the curving wall of the **Anfiteatro**. Ringed by pavement cafés, restaurants and souvenir shops, the Amphitheatre is an atmospheric place in which to enjoy an ice cream or linger until the evening for dinner.

Leave through the opposite archway, following the curve of the Amphitheatre to Via Fillungo, Lucca's main shopping street and **San Frediano** ❻ (Mon–Sat 9am–noon, 3–5pm, Sun 9am–noon, 3–5pm; free), with its huge gold-and-blue facade mosaic of *Christ in Majesty*. The treasure of this church is its Romanesque font carved with scenes showing Moses and his entourage of camels, leading his people (dressed in medieval armour) through the divided Red Sea.

To the rear and left of the church is the **Palazzo Pfanner** ❼ (daily Mar–Oct 10am–6pm; charge), a delightful 17th-century residence. Without paying, you can catch a glimpse of the wonderful garden and external staircase at the rear by climbing on to the city walls behind San Frediano church and walking left for a short distance. Highlights inside include swathes of 17th-century Lucchese silk in the bedrooms and beer-making equipment in the cellar – the palace was used as a brewery until 1929.

The Guinigi were not the only ones to flaunt their wealth by creating towers. A picture hanging in the **Museo Nazionale Guinigi** ❶ (Tue–Sat 8.30am–7.30pm, Sun 8.30am–1.30pm; charge) shows that the city was once, like San Gimignano, a forest of towers, and illustrates just how wealthy medieval Lucca was. Among the artistic treasures here is a *Madonna and Child* in bas-relief by Matteo Civitalli, a contemporary of Donatello, and Lucca's most renowned sculptor.

Lucchesi villas

The area surrounding Lucca is rich in villas: the patrician Villa Torrigiani,

A variety of delicious biscotti on sale.

Giacomo Puccini

Both a giant of 19th-20th-century opera and a crowd-pleasing showman, Giacomo Puccini (1858–1924) was a musical master of erotic passion, pathos and despair. His lush operas are characterised by soft harmony, gentle orchestration and an emotional sensitivity that is very modern. Ever the populist, Puccini was the composer with the most in common with musical theatre, and conceived of opera as drama set to music.

Puccini was born into a musical family in **Lucca**, where his newly restored home is now a museum in his honour. The young Puccini womanised at **Torre del Lago**, where his villa, set between the sea and reedy **Lake Massaciuccoli**, welcomed bohemian painters, beautiful women, gamblers and hunters as keen as himself. As Puccini boasted, "I am a mighty hunter of wildfowl, beautiful women and good libretti." He was deeply attached to the lake where he went poaching as a boy and would even compose at the piano, dressed in breeches and riding boots, with a loaded gun and hunting dogs ready by his side. Here, in this villa overlooking the Luccan hills, Puccini's jealous wife would lace her husband's wine with an aphrodisiac antidote if she felt any female guests were too alluring. The raffish playboy was reckless with women, fast cars and yachts called *Mimi*, naturally named after the heroine of *La bohème*. Puccini's music is of more lasting allure, despite his scandalous private life. "Nessun Dorma" from *Turandot* even became the theme music for the 1990 Football World Cup. Although Stravinsky dismissed *Madama Butterfly* as "treacly violin music", director Jonathan Miller disagrees: "I'm made to cry by Puccini and I never am by Verdi."

The Spa Renaissance

The new breed of thermal spas marks a return to Roman roots: these are both pampering and restorative spas that bathe body, mind and spirit

Taking the waters has become fashionable once more. Water cures, popular since Etruscan and Roman times, have always been part of local culture. In the 1st century AD, Emperor Augustus's physician issued a prescription to the poet Horace to visit the Tuscan spas, one of the first medical prescriptions on record. The Romans saw spas as both curative and civilising, distinguishing their citizens from the Barbarians, who didn't know how to combine warm water with warm company and well being. Thermal spas were also recreational in the days of the Tuscan Grand-Dukes, when resorts such as Bagni di Pisa welcomed the crowned heads of Europe to wallow in the waters, gamble in the casino and dance in the ballrooms. But somewhere along the line, the spas languished, and lost out to "liver-boosting

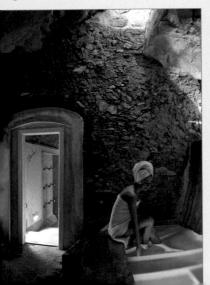

water cures" in echoing marble halls.

However, the scary white-coat brigade has been banished from the best Tuscan spas, such as Chianciano's **Terme Sensoriali**, one the most approachable yet seductive day spas. Neighbouring **Fonteverde**, floating on a sea of hills in Val d'Orcia, is a terraced spa resort clustered around a late Renaissance villa. The stylishly simple estate is dotted with thermal pools but, as a destination spa, also delivers oriental massage, skin consultations, dietary advice, yoga, spiritual healing – all presented clearly, without pushiness or psychobabble.

While not throwing the baby out with the bathwater, spas such as **Grotta Giusti**, in Monsummano Terme, manage to combine gracious 19th-century living with superb massage, thermal pools, sprawling grounds, and steamy grottoes dubbed "the eighth wonder of the world" by the composer Giuseppe Verdi. Health-seekers don bizarre boiler suits to follow the Dantesque route into "Inferno", where grottoes named Purgatory, Paradise and Hell induce a surreal detox. After sweating in Hell, there's floating under the thermal jets in the giant pool, Ayurvedic massage or sneaky golf sessions.

Set at the foot of low-slung mountains, **Bagni di Pisa** is a delightful retreat with a view of the Leaning Tower. This romantic 18th-century resort is charmingly nostalgic, with vaulted bedrooms, a winter garden, frescoed halls, and a folly Byron was fond of. The hammam is a steamy, couples-only cavern and stone-clad pool with a 38-degree temperature conducive to chilling out, detoxing and lowering the blood pressure.

In the Maremma, **Saturnia Terme** is a sophisticated affair, as befits a spot that has provided rest and recreation to Romans, ancient and modern. Fed by historic springs, a beguiling thermal pool is matched by an indoor recreation of Ancient Roman baths, outdoor cascades and timeless views of the Etruscan countryside.

For a full list of spas offering health and beauty treatments, see page 301. ❑

LEFT: the Grand Duke hammam at Saturnia Terme.

the Baroque Villa Mansi and the Villa Reale at Marlia are all surrounded by beautiful parks. Most of these villas are still in appreciative private hands, but often the gardens can be visited even if the house is not open to the public. Wandering through fragrant shrubbery and cool grottoes, past whimsical statuary and fountains, is a delightful diversion on a hot summer's afternoon.

Leave Lucca on the SS12 in the direction of the Garfagnana, and after passing through Marlia, turn off at **Villa Reale ❷** (gardens open to the public with guided tours every hour on the hour Tue–Sun Mar–Nov 10am–6pm, Dec–Feb by appointment only; charge). It was built in the 17th century by the noble Orsetti family, and substantially remodelled by Elisa Bacciocchi, Napoleon's sister. There is a lush park with a lake, which surrounds the formal Italian gardens. Most wonderful of its many fine features is the *teatro verde*, an outdoor theatre surrounded by clipped yew hedges, a key setting for concerts during Lucca's summer festival.

Continue on through a fairly built-up area to Segromigno in Monte and the charming **Villa Mansi** (tel: 0583-920 234; Mar–Sept Mon–Sat 10am–noon, 3–5pm, best to call first; charge), with beautifully landscaped gardens. Just 2km (1.2 miles) away in Camigliano, **Villa Torrigiani** (Mar–2nd Sun in Nov daily 10am–1pm, 3pm–1hr before dusk; charge) is a fine example of Baroque architecture. Also consider **Villa Bernardini** in Vicopelago just outside Lucca (tel: 0583-370 327; www.villabernadini.it; visits by request; charge).

Equally splendid is the **Villa Garzoni** (villa closed for renovation; gardens: Mar–2 Nov daily 9am–sunset; charge) in the town of **Collodi ❸**, with a glorious Baroque garden full of mythical monsters modelled in terracotta, fountains and topiaried animals. The steep terraces of the 17th-century garden lead to some memorable viewing points.

If you were entranced as a child by the adventures of a wooden puppet with a remarkable nose, you may recognise the name of this town as being that of the author of *The Adventures*

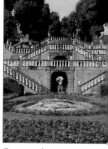

Ornate staircases at Villa Garzoni.

BELOW: the grand Villa Torrigiani.

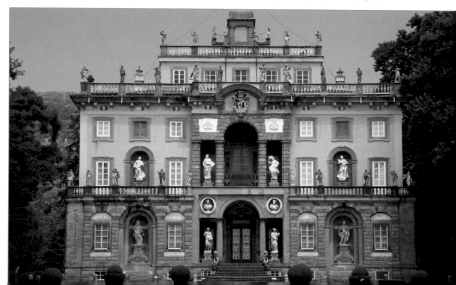

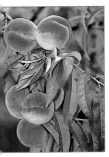

In the spring, the peach blossoms of Pescia are outstanding; every September in even-numbered years, Pescia hosts the colourful Biennale del Fiore – Festival of Flowers.

of Pinocchio (1881). Carlo Lorenzini adopted Collodi as his pen-name because he had fond memories of staying here as a child. The town now has **Parco di Pinocchio** (same hours as Villa Garzoni gardens) devoted to Pinocchio, consisting of mosaics, mazes and statues based on scenes from the story. Contemporary children, accustomed to virtual reality and adrenalin-fuelled theme parks, may find it rather tame, but there are plans to enhance the attractions at the nearby Villa Garzoni.

En route to the spa resorts

Where Lucca's villa country ends, Pistoia Province begins, as does the route east to the thermal-spa resorts of Montecatini Terme and Monsummano Terme. Just south of Collodi is **Pescia ❹**, cradled in the plain of the Valdinievole. Pescia is famous for its flower production and has the largest flower market outside the Netherlands. Prosperous Pescia

is surrounded by nurseries, greenhouses, olive groves and hills dotted with gracious villas. Divided by a river, the medieval town boasts several fine churches, including the cathedral and Sant'Antonio, as well as a crenellated town hall. In the hills above town is the Convento di Colleviti, a Renaissance monastery, accessible by footpath from Pescia.

Just south of Pescia are two appealing villages, notably the shabbily scenic **Uzzano**, which has a curious church on the crest of the hill, and well-tended **Buggiano**, with an interesting church and lovingly restored palazzo.

Further east awaits **Montecatini Terme ❺**, once famed throughout Europe for its elegance and luxury. It was remodelled by Grand Duke Leopold of Tuscany in the 18th century and became a destination spa resort before the term was invented. Belle Epoque nostalgia is still the order of the day, even if many foreign

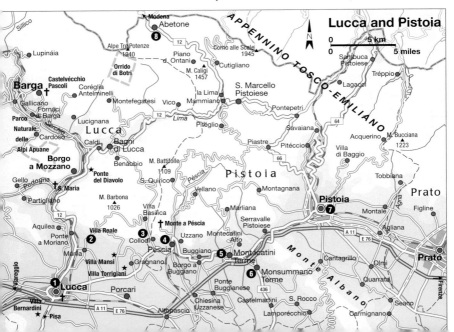

spa-goers feel more comfortable in the purely pampering spas. Avenues of neoclassical spa pavilions dispense health-giving waters to drink and offer treatments ranging from inhalation to mudbaths. With its fountains and Art Nouveau flourishes, Tettuccio is the grandest and most languid. Cast aside your wariness and dip a toe in the waters: whether sipping them in marble pavilions, strolling through the magnificent parks, or committing yourself to a complete cure.

Montecatini Alto is the original medieval fortified town above the thermal springs, and can be reached by funicular or by road. Although over-popular in high season, it is still a restful place to visit, with a shady chestnut-tree walk along the lower terrace, and panoramic views over Valdinievole, "valley of the mists". Drink something stronger than water in the main square, Piazza Giusti, and cast your eye over the ruined fortress and equally ruined Romanesque church, unfortunately marred by an ill-judged restoration.

Montecatini represents a crossroads, from where you can continue east to Pistoia, make a brief foray north, or collapse in a superb spa just south. Driving north of Montecatini along the N633, you arrive at **Marliana** via a scenic mountain road, and can meditate over views from Marliana's castle and campanile. A little further on, medieval **Vellano** makes a good lunch stop, with rustic inns overlooking the valley slopes and olive terraces. Alternatively, south of Montecatini, **Monsummano Terme** ❻ is home to an extraordinary spa, Grotta Giusti Spa Resort *(see page 138)*, where you can bathe in thermal pools or sweat it out in a bizarre steamy grotto, best savoured on an overnight stay.

Cycling in Lucca

Lucca is full of lanes too narrow for cars, so the locals often get about by bicycle. This, combined with Lucca's reputation for culture and intellectual pursuits, has earned the city the nickname of the "Cambridge of Tuscany".

The old walls are equally popular with walkers and joggers. Every now and again, you can take the sloped

BELOW: cheeky decorative tiles at Tettuccio Terme, Montecatini.

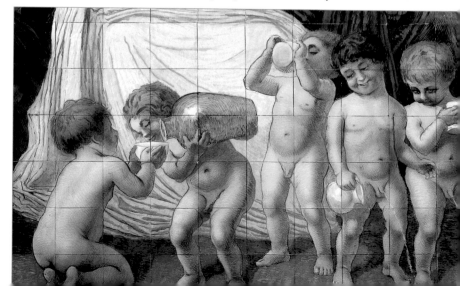

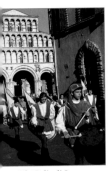

The Palio di San Paolino – a medieval celebration of Lucca's patron saint, with costume parades, flag-throwing and crossbow-shooting competitions.

exit down into the town and cycle around the key sites, locking the bike up to a gate when entering a museum or walking around a piazza.

You can hire a bike at one of the two tourist offices, either at the East Gate or the West Gate. Current bike hire for half a day costs from €7.50 per person. Cycling is also a healthy alternative to a day on the beach. Near Lucca, one leisurely coastal route runs from the Viareggio seafront to Lido di Camaiore, Marina di Pietrasanta and Forte dei Marmi. Another 20km (12.4-mile) trail links Viareggio with Torre del Lago Puccini. To book a short bike trip, or a bigger cycling holiday in Tuscany, contact Gusto Tours (www.gustocycling.com) or consult Love Italy (www.loveitaly.co.uk).

Unsung Pistoia

The path most travelled from Montecatini leads east to **Pistoia** ❼. The provincial capital tends to be overshadowed by its glittering neighbour, Florence, only 37km (22 miles) distant, and is rather unfairly neglected as a result. Its historic heart is delightful, and it has a profusion of elegant shops, inns and hotels tucked away in the medieval streets. What's more, the citizens of Pistoia take great pride in their monuments and churches, and when dusk falls, the shadowy, lamplit streets have an authentic atmosphere. Church bells peal, Franciscan monks stride along in their unmistakable brown habits and rope belts, and the stone slabs outside the shops are laid out with goods for sale just as they might in the Middle Ages.

Pistoia was originally a Roman town, founded as a staging post on the Via Cassia. It flourished as a banking centre during its medieval heyday, but was constantly buffeted between Florence and Lucca, eventually falling under the dominion of Florence. The impressive

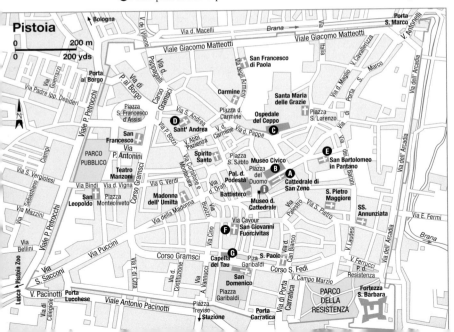

trapezoid walls that encompass the city are part of the bastion built by the Medici during the 15th century. Much of the area around the **Piazza del Duomo** has been pedestrianised, and, when not full of market stalls (Sat and Wed), the piazza is a peaceful place for taking stock of Pistoia's riches.

The **Cattedrale di San Zeno Ⓐ** (Mon–Sat 8am–12.30pm, 3.30–7pm, Sun 8am–1pm, 3.30–7pm; free) originated in the 5th century, but was rebuilt in Romanesque style with a splendid Pisan-style facade of green and white marble stripes. A marble porch was added later and decorated with an exquisite blue-and-white Andrea della Robbia bas-relief.

Inside are many medieval frescoes, an impressive Crucifix (1274), Renaissance paintings and – most glorious of all – the massive, ornate silver altar in the **Chapel of Saint James** (contact the sacristan; charge), decorated with bas-reliefs and statues over a period of two centuries by many different artists, including Brunelleschi. Next door in the Palazzo dei Vescovi (Bishops' Palace), above the helpful

tourist office (tel: 0573-21622), is the **Museo della Cattedrale** (Tue, Thur and Fri; guided tours only 10am–1pm, 3–5pm; charge).

Beside the Duomo is the soaring **Campanile**, originally a watch-tower, naturally adorned with three tiers of green-and-white Pisan arches, echoing the Duomo facade. You can climb the bell tower for magnificent views over the town (Sat–Sun by reservation at the tourist office). Opposite is the 14th-century octagonal **Battistero** of San Giovanni in Corte, designed by Andrea Pisano (daily 10am–6pm).

The piazza is lined with Renaissance palaces, including the **Palazzo del Podestà,** still the city's law courts, with a finely decorated inner courtyard. Opposite is the **Palazzo del Comune** (Town Hall), with a harmonious facade of arches and delicately pointed windows, decorated with the ubiquitous Medici crest and a grim black-marble head. Inside is a courtyard and sweeping stairway, and sculptures by local artist Marino Marini (1901–80), many of them based on his favourite

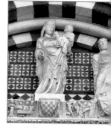

Detail from the entrance to the Cattedrale di San Zeno.

BELOW: Della Robbia's majolica frieze above the Ospedale del Ceppo loggia.

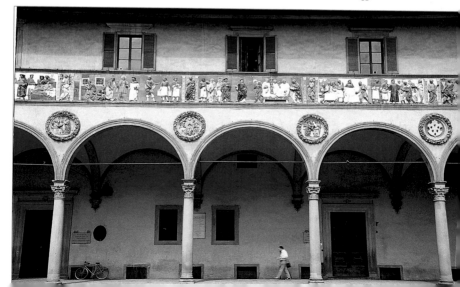

In 1996, the province was hit hard by floods and subsequent landslides. Although many areas were affected to some extent, worst hit were the small villages high up in the hills, where people lost homes, businesses, even families. Scars are still clearly visible around the province today.

BELOW: Pistoia's market is set up on the pretty Piazza della Sala.

theme of riders and horses. Upstairs in the first- and second-floor rooms is the impressive art collection of the **Museo Civico** ❸ (Tue, Thur–Sat 10am–6pm, Wed 4–7pm, Sun 11am–6pm, winter Tue, Thur–Sat 10am–5pm, Wed 3–6pm, Sun 11am–5pm; charge), which includes a rare 13th-century painting of St Francis.

To the north of the Duomo, in Piazza Giovanni XII, is the **Ospedale del Ceppo** ❸. It was founded in 1287 and still functions as a hospital. Above the loggia is a brilliantly coloured majolica frieze by Giovanni della Robbia that depicts the *Seven Works of Mercy*: worthy citizens handing out food to the poor, comforting prisoners and washing the feet of dusty travellers. The figures are realistic, often humorous, despite the gravity of their occupations.

A congregation of churches

Pistoia's striped churches encircle the historic centre like zebras – with the Pisano pulpits the great pride of the town. **Sant'Andrea** ❸ (8am–6pm), in the Via Sant'Andrea, has

an arcaded facade and reliefs above the central door. Inside is a richly painted wooden ceiling and narrow nave, well lit from the upper clerestory. Here is Giovanni Pisano's hexagonal pulpit (1297), modelled on the Nicola Pisano pulpit in the Pisa Duomo. The sharply carved marble reliefs border on the melodramatic in their depiction of *The Life of Jesus* and *The Last Judgement*.

San Bartolomeo in Pantano ❸ (St Bartholomew in the Swamp; 8am–7pm), in the Piazza San Bartolomeo, is one of Pistoia's oldest churches, built in the 12th century with a five-bay facade. Inside there is a pulpit by Guido da Como (1250) depicting *Christ's Nativity*, with the edifice resting on the backs of men and lions carved out of marble.

In the pedestrianised **Via Cavour** is the 12th-century church of **San Giovanni Fuorcivitas** ❸ (7.30am–noon, 5–6.30pm) adorned with an almost psychedelic green-and-white striped marble facade in Pisan style. The treasures inside include a pulpit created in 1270 by Fra Guglielmo da Pisa, a pupil of Nicola Pisano, a

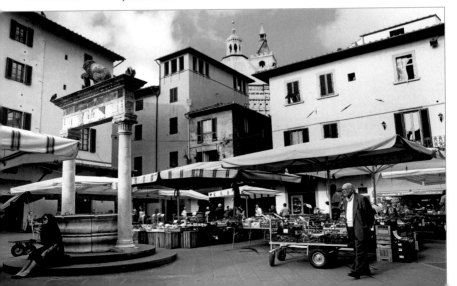

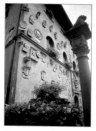

water stoup by Giovanni Pisano, and a touchingly beautiful white-glazed terracotta of *The Visitation* by Luca della Robbia.

In Piazza Garibaldi, the monastery of **San Domenico** (Mon–Sat 8–11.50am, 4.30–6pm, Sun 8am–12.30pm, 4.30–7pm) was insensitively restored after damage in World War II, but seek out the Renaissance tombs, cloisters and the colourful Benozzo Gozzoli fresco.

Opposite San Domenico is **Cappella del Tau** 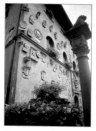 (Mon–Sat 8.15am–1.30pm). This former chapel is now an artistic monument, with darkly dramatic Gothic frescoes and vaulted ceilings, including a fine fresco of *The Fall*. The Palazzo del Tau is now home to the **Museo Marino Marini** (Mon–Sat 10am–5pm; charge), named after Pistoia's most famous 20th-century son. Marino Marini (1901–80) made his native city an important bequest of his sculptures, etchings, prints and drawings based on the recurring theme of horses and riders.

Recover from an overdose of art and churches in a café on the Piazza della Sala, where the fruit-and-vegetable market is set out around an old well. At night the piazza is home to a number of lively bars. If still in need of light relief, browse the shops for embroidery, shoes, leather and jewellery on Via Cavour, Via Cino, Via Ateo Vannucci and Via d. Orafi. Ever earnest, Pistoia can even turn shopping into a dutiful museum experience. The city is famous for its embroidery, fine examples of which can be seen in the **Museo del Ricamo**, set in the Palazzo Rospigliosi (via Ripa del Sale 3; Tue–Thur 10am–1pm, Fri–Sat 10am–1pm, 3–6pm; charge).

Alternatively, consider visiting **Pistoia Zoo**, which is set in a pine forest in Via Pieve a Celle about 5km (3 miles) outside town (www.zoodipistoia.it; Mon–Sat 9am–6pm, Sun until 7pm; charge).

From Pistoia, clear your head in the mountains, going via **San Marcello Pistoiese**, the main town, traditional **Cutigliano**, and the lofty, all-year-round resort of **Abetone** 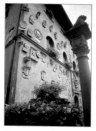, which is only 90 minutes' drive from Pistoia (*see box below*). ❑

The grand Palazzo Pretorio in Cutigliano.

BELOW LEFT: Pistoia's Cattedrale di San Zeno and campanile, built in the 12th century.

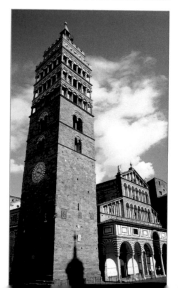

Mountain Pursuits

The drive into the mountains north of Pistoia is stunningly beautiful, especially in autumn. But winter-sports enthusiasts will prefer it with a good covering of crisp snow. The main town is **San Marcello Pistoiese**, traditionally known for the *Mongolfiera*, or hot-air balloon, launched on 8 September to mark the end of summer. Near San Marcello, at Mammiano, is a spectacular suspension footbridge, 220 metres (720ft) long, connecting to the road across the River Lima. **Cutigliano**, further down the valley, is surrounded by fir trees, but has limited skiing on its 13km (8 miles) of pistes, so serious skiers will prefer Abetone.

Abetone, set 1,400 metres (4,660ft) above sea level, is the most popular ski resort in the Apennines. It offers a wide range of pistes served by 25 ski lifts; has three ski schools and some fine new hotels, designed in "Swissified" mountain style. In the absence of good snow, the snow machines can cover 40km (25 miles) of slopes. In summer, Abetone makes an invigorating centre for climbing and walking expeditions in the surrounding pine and chestnut woods. *Rifugi*, or mountain shelters, are dotted around the area, often combining basic accommodation with an inn serving rustic fare.

BEST RESTAURANTS

Restaurants

Prices for a three-course meal per person with a half-bottle of house wine:
€ = under €25
€€ = €25–40
€€€ = €40–60
€€€€ = over €60

Abetone

Da Pierone
Via Brennero 556
Tel: 0573-60068 €€
Rustic restaurant. Good cooking based on traditional mountain fare. Closed Mon, 15–30 June, 20 Oct–early Nov.

Lucca

Buca di Sant'Antonio
Via della Cervia 1/3
Tel: 0583-55881
www.bucadisantantonio.it €€€
Renowned restaurant serving Lucchese and Garfagnana classic dishes (try the fettuccine with pigeon sauce), alongside dishes with a more modern slant. Closed Sun evening, Mon and periods in Jan and July.

Cantine Bernardini
Palazzo Bernardini, Via del Suffragio 7
Tel: 0583-494 336 €€
Feast on chickpea soup, steak, wild-boar terrine, Pecorino cheese, and pasta stuffed with artichokes. The dishes represent the best of Lucca and Garfagnana. These vaulted cellars, along with the restaurant, wine bar and deli,

belong to the patrician Bernardini family, who also sell wines from their estates.

Gli Orti di Via Elisa
Via Elisa 17
Tel: 0583-491 241
www.ristorantegliorti.it €
Good choice for a quick lunch: a busy trattoria with a wide choice of pasta and pizzas, plus a self-service salad bar. Closed Wed dinner and Sun.

La Mora
Via Sesto di Moriano 1748, Località Sesto di Moriano
Tel: 0583-406 402
www.ristorantelamora.it €€€
The 15-minute drive north of Lucca (on the Barga road) is worth the

effort for the superb food. Seasonal local ingredients are inventively prepared and beautifully presented. Closed Wed.

Ristorante Giglio
Piazza del Giglio 2
Tel: 0583-494 058
www.ristorantegiglio.com €€
Charming restaurant specialising in fish and Tuscan meat dishes. Tables spill out on to the piazza. One of Lucca's best restaurants, and very popular with locals. Closed Wed lunch, Tue and 2nd half of Nov.

San Colombano Ristorante/Caffetteria
Baluardo San Colombano 10

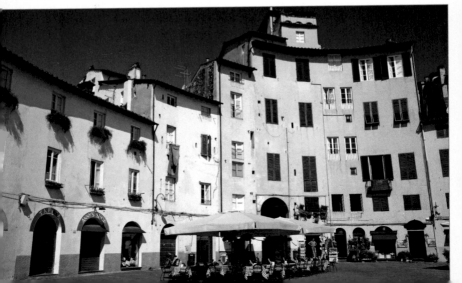

BELOW: alfresco dining on Piazza Anfiteatro, Lucca.

Tel: 0583-464 641
www.caffetteriasancolombano.it
€€€
Excellent restaurant on the city walls with superb views over the city. Typical Lucchese dishes change with the season. The café serves good snacks throughout the day and is a lovely spot for an *aperitivo*. Closed Mon. Reservations recommended.

Montecatini Terme
Enoteca Da Giovanni
Via Garibaldi 25
Tel: 0572-73080 €€€–€€€€
The wine list is extensive, but the food is the main attraction. Excellent meat and fish. The annexe, known as the Cucina da Giovanni, serves more traditional Tuscan fare and is cheaper. Closed Mon

and last 2 weeks in Feb and Aug.

Pescia
Cecco
Via Forti 84
Tel: 0572-477 955
www.ristorantececco.com €€
Mushrooms, asparagus and truffles feature here, and the fish is also good in this historic and welcoming trattoria. Closed Mon in winter.
Monte a Pescia
Località Monte a Pescia
Tel: 0572-490 000 €€
This trattoria specialises in meats grilled over an open fire. Lovely terrace overlooking olive trees and hills.
Closed Wed.

Pistoia
Al Posto Giusto
Via Mammianese 399
Tel: 0572-69247 €

Outside Pistoia, this non-touristic restaurant offers excellent food at a moderate price. The drive out takes you along winding country roads. Very friendly owners. Closed Wed.
La Limonaia
Via di Gello 9a
Tel: 0573-400 453
www.osterialalimonaia.it €
Appealing, rustic trattoria a little way from the centre of town. Unusual herbs and flavourings pep up the Tuscan food. Closed Mon and Tue.
Lo Storno
Via del Lastrone 8
Tel: 0573-26193 €
A tiny eatery, with a few tables on the street, just off Piazza della Sala. Local Pistoian dishes are the speciality here. Closed Sun.
Osteria Boccon di Vino
Corso Gramsci 83

Tel: 0573-358 765 €
A central, pleasant restaurant serving simple but very tasty food. Closed Mon.
Ristorante San Jacopo
Via Crispi 15
Tel: 0573-27786
www.ristorantesanjacopo.it €€
One of the best restaurants in Pistoia, set in the *centro storico*. It serves dishes from Pistoia and elsewhere in Tuscany, with particularly good seafood and juicy *bistecca alla fiorentina*. Closed Mon.
Trattoria dell'Abbondanza
Via dell'Abbondanza 10–14
Tel: 0573-368 037 €€
Traditional restaurant focusing on recipes from the surrounding region, including the delicious *farinato* (a hearty Tuscan soup). Closed Wed and Thur lunch.

BELOW: a *caffè* in Lucca's backstreets.

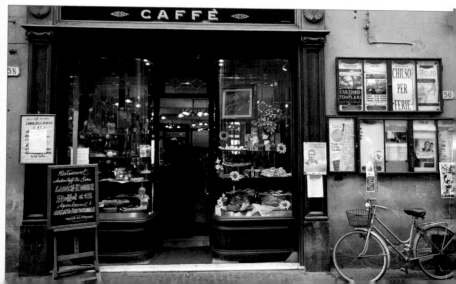

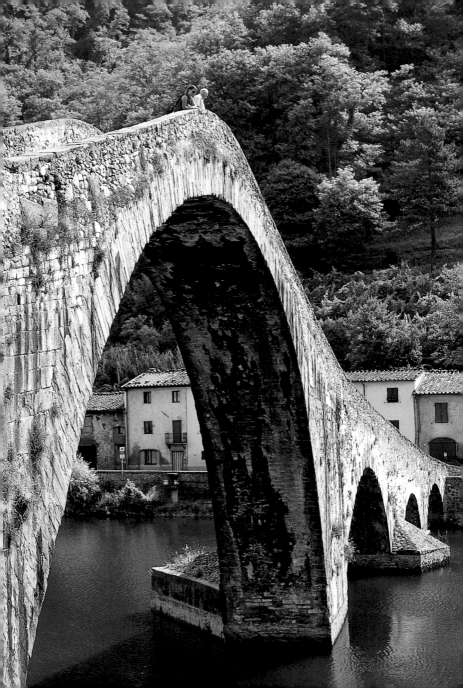

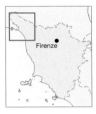

VERSILIA, GARFAGNANA AND LUNIGIANA

Tuscany's northern corner is one of its wildest, loveliest, yet least explored areas – from the Versilia coast to a dramatic landscape of pine-covered mountains, craggy ravines, remote castellated villages and marble peaks. And all this with the famous beach resorts of Forte dei Marmi and Viareggio attached

Versilia is renowned for its sociable beach resorts, which range from sophisticated Forte dei Marmi to laid-back Viareggio. But beyond the seaside bustle lies an elemental landscape that challenges popular perceptions of Chiantishire. The coastal lowlands of the Versilia give way to a dramatic hinterland of snowcapped mountains, terraced hillsides, deep gorges and mountain streams, populated by deer, wild boar, badgers, stone martens and wolves, not to mention walkers, rock climbers, cavers and canoeists. Tuscany's northernmost tip is an untamed rocky region known as the Lunigiana, bordered by the Apuan Alps in the south, Liguria in the west and Emilia to the east. Bordering it to the south is the Garfagnana, cut through by the Serchio River, which flows between the Apuan Alps and the Apennines. Together they make up one of the wildest, most beautiful, yet least explored parts of Tuscany.

Versilia

This coastal region lies west of Lucca, squeezed between the Apuan Alps in the east, and Lago di Massaciuccoli

in the south. Michelangelo built a road from the marble quarries to transport the marble to waiting ships – and inadvertently created a summer playground. Once pine-covered, the coast has succumbed to rampant development, but in the place of rustic charm it offers fine seafood restaurants, a sense of fun, and beach entertainment, Italian-style – all against the backdrop of the Apuan Alps. Whereas Forte dei Marmi is the resort for socialising and being seen, Viareggio is for everyone.

Main attractions
VIAREGGIO
TORRE DEL LAGO PUCCINI
PIETRASANTA
FORTE DEI MARMI
CASTELNUOVO DI GARFAGNANA
PARCO DELL'ORECCHIELLA
BARGA
GROTTA DEL VENTO
BAGNI DI LUCCA
CARRARA MARBLE QUARRIES
PONTREMOLI

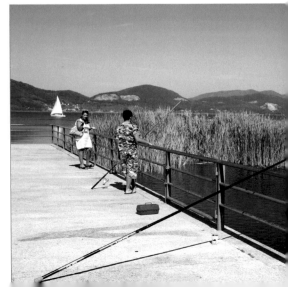

LEFT: the dizzying Devil's Bridge spanning the River Serchio. **RIGHT:** fishing at Torre del Lago Puccini.

TIP

In Viareggio, a carnival museum, the **Museo della Cittadella** (Via Santa Maria Gorretti 16; tel: 058-4511 76; Mon, Wed, Fri 10am–noon; free), on the site where the floats are made, tells the story of the origins and characters of the famous Carnival.

Viareggio ❶ is the oldest resort in the Versilia, and famous for its Carnival as well as for its beaches and boat-building tradition. The pre-Lent Carnival, one of the biggest and boldest in Italy, sees thematic floats spiced up with political satire. The resort enjoyed its heyday at the beginning of the 20th century, as testified by a handful of seafront cafés, beach clubs and historic hotels, such as the Plaza de Russie, originally built for the pre-Revolution Russian aristocracy. Today's Russian tycoons much prefer Forte dei Marmi, where their opulent villas nestle between the beaches and the Alps. Instead, unpretentious Viareggio offers pockets of genteel charm, seafood restaurants and leisurely cycle rides. The seafront boulevard, the **Passeggiata Margherita**, is at the heart of the action, especially since cycling has taken off on this stretch of the coast. For a stylish meal, seek out the Art Nouveau **Gran Caffè Margherita** (Viale Margherita 30) – Puccini's favourite.

On the downside, the beach clubs have a regimented feel: the sea can be reached only if you pay an entrance fee and wish to lie on a sunbed

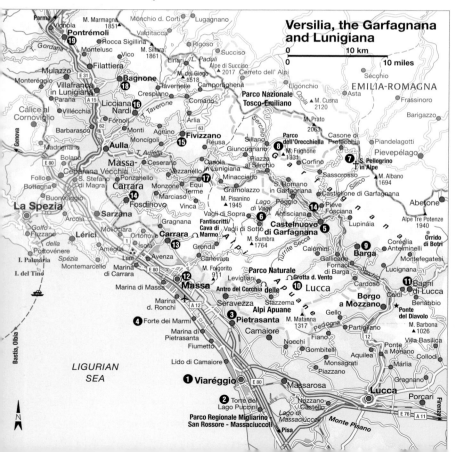

among rows of others, on sand carefully raked and flattened.

Lakeside retreats

An operatic pilgrimage just south of Viareggio takes you to **Torre del Lago Puccini** ❷, best reached through the deep Macchia Lucchese pine groves. Here, on **Lago di Massaciuccoli** is Giacomo Puccini's villa, where all his operas save *Turandot* were composed. This pleasant but over-popularised retreat was a peaceful backwater in Puccini's day. **Puccini's villa** (Tue–Sun, June–Oct 10am–12.30pm, 3–6.30pm, winter until 5.30pm; guided tours; charge) displays his musical instruments – as well as his guns. Puccini is buried in the nearby chapel. In August, a summer opera festival takes over the atmospheric lakeside stage beside Puccini's villa – the maestro would have approved.

The lake and neighbouring wetlands form a nature reserve and haven for birdlife – the **Parco Regionale di Migliarino-San Rossore-Massaciuccoli** (tel: 050-525 500) is best explored on a boat trip around the lagoon.

Seaside resorts

Continuing north from Viareggio, the resorts fall into line in quick succession. **Lido di Camaiore** is slightly downmarket, but access to the beach is easier – and virtually free of pay-as-you-enter stretches of sand. From this part of the shore it is easy to reach **Camaiore** (to the Romans, Campus Maior), which is about 7km (4 miles) to the east.

Pietrasanta ❸ is about 8km (5 miles) inland from the sea; its name, "Holy Stone", refers to the town's chief product, marble. This is the Tuscan centre for stone sculptors, who come here in droves to work the marble, ever since the days of Henry Moore and Joan Miró. As a result of all this artistic intensity, a fine white dust covers everything in Pietrasanta, even the wine glasses in the bars of the Piazza Carducci. Fortunately, there is some public sculpture on display, often presented to the town by the resident artists themselves.

This is the case with Colombian sculptor Fernando Botero, who lives in the resort for part of the year: "I like Pietrasanta, a beautiful town

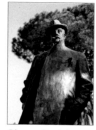

Giacomo Puccini, composer of La Bohème, Tosca *and* Madama Butterfly, *lived and died at Torre del Lago, where his villa is now a museum dedicated to his life and work.*

Tuscany's Best Beaches

Tuscan beaches deliver both romance on the rocks and the regimented lines of beach umbrellas that most Italians consider to be beach-break heaven. In Forte dei Marmi, Versilia boasts the best-known beach resort for the chic set, while Viareggio remains the most popular big beach resort in Tuscany. The romantic, rocky cove of Cala Piccola, on Monte Argentario, arguably has the most aquamarine waters. Yachties will prefer to swim off chici Porto Santo Stefano and glitzy Porto Ercole. As for privacy and a back-to-nature remoteness, nothing beats Marina di Alberese, within the Parco della Maremma.

In the annual "beach charts", Tuscany is triumphing. Every year Italian beaches get ranked by Green organisations, notably Legambiente's *Blue Guide*, which measures the cleanliness of the water, safety, quietness, eco-friendliness and sustainability. In 2011 Tuscany was judged to have a superbly clean coastline, second only to Liguria's.

In Versilia, the resorts awarded the best "blue flags" were chic Forte dei Marmi and bustling Viareggio. Near Pisa, family-friendly Tirrenia is a winner. Further south, on the Etruscan Riviera, the beaches do even better, with blue flags going to Castiglioncello, Bibbona and Antignano. In the Maremma, the best beaches include family-friendly Castiglione della Pescaia, remote Marina di Alberese, and most of the chic Monte Argentario peninsula's "Silver Coast". As usual, the region's best beaches were deemed to be Capalbio and Castiglione della Pescaia, in the Maremma, followed by beaches on the islands of Capraia and Giglio. Elba also fared very well, with awards for the popular beaches of Campo nell'Elba, Porto Azzurro, Marciana Marina and Capoliveri.

All of the winning Tuscan beaches mentioned tend to be firm favourites whose Green credentials are sound. (For more information see: www.bandietblu.org; and www.legambienteturismo.it.)

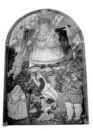

Fresco by the 20th-century Colombian artist, Botero, in Pietrasanta's church of Sant'Antonio.

with a unique square, a cathedral worthy of a great city, and the Apuan Alps as a backdrop. What mountains, what greenery, what shade, what rivers, what fresh streams flow beneath chestnut trees and olive groves and orange orchards, all framed by marble quarries along the green." At the Enoteca Marcucci *(see page 161)* you can eat alongside sculptors and painters, feasting on Tuscan *ribollita* soup, grilled meats and fine wines.

Luxurious villas

Further north, **Forte dei Marmi** ❹ is the favoured retreat of Italian celebrities and captains of industry, from the Agnelli dynasty, who helped to launch this chic resort, to Giorgio Armani and celebrity tenor Andrea Bocelli. Forte *is* snooty and cosmopolitan but also charming and old-fashioned: the *dolce vita* is cultivated according to time-honoured tradition, despite the influx of a brasher set ready to pay a fortune to sit under the right beach awnings.

Forte dei Marmi grew up around a fort built in 1788 by Leopold I of Tuscany – these remains dominate the main square today. The surrounding sleek boutiques and cafés manage to combine cosmopolitan chic with a small-town atmosphere, enhanced by a lack of high-rise buildings. The parasol pines are still the tallest markers around, framing discreet villa gardens overflowing with bougainvillea.

While catering to an elite, with its exorbitantly priced beach clubs and tropical-style bars, Forte still retains something of the seductive mood that once captivated bohemian writers and artists, from Thomas Mann to Henry Moore. When the gently sloping beaches pall, today's celebrity visitors happily hop on to vintage bicycles to potter down the coast to Pietrasanta.

Into the mountains

Given the mountainous nature of the interior, any inland trek along minor roads will inevitably be a leisurely trail along narrow, switchback roads, but with dramatic views and chance discoveries as compensation. This is "Slow Tuscany" so take Garfagnana and Lunigiana at a leisurely pace, ideally staying there – forays from

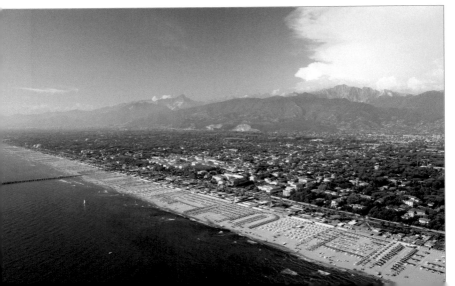

the coast can also make a delightful diversion from the beach scene. If time is short, then bear in mind that it is quicker and easier to reach the area via Forte dei Marmi, Pietrasanta, Viareggio or Lucca than to travel as the crow flies.

Garfagnana

Castelnuovo di Garfagnana ❺, about 64km (40 miles) north of Lucca, is a convenient stepping stone to the Garfagnana. This fortress town once controlled the route from Genoa to Lucca and Pisa, and was ruled by the Este dukes of Ferrara until Italian unification. The town suffered during World War II, even if the Duomo survived, as did the town walls, and the church of San Michele, containing a 14th-century *Madonna*.

Other highlights are the **Rocca,** or governor's palace, which is now the town hall, and the medieval fortress at the top of the hill. But beyond the sights is the sense of a Tuscany off the tourist trail. This is exemplified by Il Vecchio Mulino, an engaging Slow Food inn run by the cherubic Andrea. If you prove *"simpatico"*,

Andrea will lead you through a tasting of local dishes *(see page 160)*.

Scenic routes

Northwest of Castelnuovo di Garfagnana, a scenic road runs from Poggio to Vaglia alongside the river Edron and **Lago di Vagli ❻**. The old stone houses and parish church in Vagli di Sotto are worth seeing, but the real draw is the partially submerged medieval village of **Fabbrica di Carregine**, covered by the creation of a dam in the 1940s. Sometimes seen peeking through the surface, the village is fully visible every 10 years when the lake is drained to service the dam. The next emptying is scheduled for 2014.

The road winds its tortuous way through mountain scenery for about 18km (11 miles) to **San Pellegrino in Alpe ❼**, an ancient monastery housing the **Museo Etnografico Provinciale** (Tue–Sun, Apr–May 9am–noon, 2–5pm, summer until 7.30pm; charge), whose display of peasant life is less compelling than the mountain views.

San Romano in Garfagnana

TIP

At almost every turn there are more medieval villages, more castles, more breathtaking views. One of the best ways to see this rich and varied region is to take the little train between Aulla and Lucca on its slow journey through the mountains.

BELOW: Castelnuovo di Garfagnana.

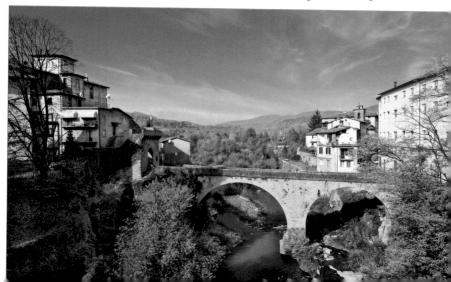

TIP

Barga's best bar is the historic Caffè Capretz (Piazza Salvo Salvi), a favourite meeting place for poets and politicians at the end of the 19th century. It has a terrace with a view at the back and tables laid out under the loggia at the front.

offers a medieval castle and the stark peaks of the Alta Garfagnana, whose barren beauty is best appreciated with a visit to the **Parco dell'Orecchiella** ❽ *(see page 71)*, now part of the Parco-Tosco-Emiliano (www.appennino park.it). This wilderness, laced with waymarked trails and cycling paths, is framed by the grandiose peaks of the Apennines.

A scenic route to the coast from Castelnuovo di Garfagnana goes along the spectacular Túrrite Secca through the Parco Naturale delle Alpi Apuane, via the **Marmitte dei Giganti** ("Giants' Cooking Pots") – 23 huge hollows (20 metres/65ft in diameter) made by Ice Age glaciers – and through the Galleria del Cipollaio, a long tunnel carved out of the marble. From here the road winds down to Seravezza and Forte dei Marmi on the Versilia coast.

Barga

To the south, pretty, arty, medieval **Barga** ❾ is by far the most beguiling town in the district. This quaint, surprisingly cosmopolitan place battles the problem of the rural exodus in its own way: many of those who left to make their fortunes abroad have returned, or keep a summer place here, including the Scots. The returning émigrés have brought a broader outlook to Barga, as seen in the kind of art galleries rarely found in a rural Tuscan outpost. The annual opera festival also brings the old town to life in July and August.

The sights, such as they are, are mostly about atmosphere, charm and stunning location, with lovely views at the very top. Leave your car outside the old city walls and head through the gate to explore the old town, with its narrow, winding streets lined with Florentine-style palazzi overlooked by the Romanesque Duomo, which commands wooded views of the Garfagnana from its hilltop position.

The Apuan Alps

From Barga, cross the Serchio valley to Gallicano. Just after the village, look out for signs to the 13th-century **Eremo di Calomini**, a gleaming white hermitage clinging to a rocky slope between the trees. Another 9km (5.5 miles) of steep and

Slow Food in 'Slow Tuscany'

Garfagnana is not just a hiking paradise. It is the domain of Slow Food. The best place to start a tasting session is in Il Vecchio Mulino (tel: 058-3621 92), a rough-and-ready inn and a temple to Slow Food. Here, as in other welcoming Garfagnana villages, you can taste *biroldo*, the local blood sausage, and a protected Slow Food delicacy. The popularity of salami and blood sausages is also linked to the proximity of Emilia Romagna and its penchant for pork products.

The most typical ingredient is spelt (*farro*), one of the oldest known grains, dating back to Roman times. While spelt has disappeared from most regions, it takes pride of place in Garfagnana dishes, and finds its way into spelt soup, made with sage, garlic, red wine and pork rind. Spelt is also used to make local bread, pasta and savoury tarts and pies. Whether roasted or boiled, chestnuts are also a feature of local cooking and are used in the so-called "paupers' bread". As in many mountain areas, polenta is a typical base for hearty rural dishes and is often combined with mushroom dishes. Polenta is also the base of chestnut cakes and in *castagnaccio*, the sweet local dessert. Instead, neighbouring Lunigiana specialises in *panigacci*, chestnut-flour pancakes cooked over an open fire and served with creamy cheese and home-cured meats.

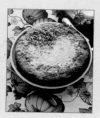

To meet the cheese-makers and craftsmen, weavers and wine-makers, book a day's tour with Sapori & Saperi (tel: 339-7636 321, www.sapori-e-saperi.com). This small, local company runs food and craft adventures, introducing visitors to anything from ricotta-making to sourcing the best inns, the places that only insiders know. These are culinary experiences, to meet Slow Food and wine producers and get a taste of their lives, far from the Chiantishire stereotypes.

winding road brings you to **Forno-valasco** and the **Grotta del Vento** ⑩ (Cave of the Wind; daily 10am–7pm; guided tours only, departing on the hour; charge), in the Apuan Alps, a labyrinthine system of tunnels, caves and secret passages full of dramatic stalactites and stalagmites, underground lakes and echoing chambers. There are guided tours of one, two and three hours, with the three-hour itinerary (10am or 2pm only) the most dramatic. The cave complex, one of over 1,300 in the Apuan Alps, is chilly, even in summer.

Bagni di Lucca ⑪, once a fashionable spa town, played host to Shelley, Byron and the Brownings, who all bathed in these warm, sulphurous waters. Today, the **Bagni Caldi**, the "hot baths", are scenically shabby, including an intriguing time-warp spa, with maze-like passages carved into the rock, and steam-vapour grottoes. Rugged walking country beckons, including the white-water gorge of **Orrido di Botri**, an authentic wilderness with a canyon.

From Bagni di Lucca, the road winds along the banks of the River Serchio to **Borgo a Mozzano**, and the splendid, lofty five-arched bridge of Ponte della Maddalena, also known as the **Ponte del Diavolo** – Devil's Bridge *(see right)*.

Massa-Carrara

Bordering on Liguria, the province of Massa-Carrara has only been part of Tuscany since the mid-19th century, and still feels out on a limb, particularly in Lunigiana. Many of the locals talk of "going to Tuscany" as if it were a foreign land, which it is, in some ways. While Massa-Carrara's main towns and resorts are disappointing, the marble trails make up for it, as does the jagged backdrop. Expect pine-covered mountains, craggy ravines, remote castellated villages – and the majestic marble peaks of the Apuan Alps glittering deceptively like snow in bright sunshine.

The towns of Massa and Carrara have both prospered from the marble trade, but their Faustian pact leaves them blighted by industrial eyesores. **Marina di Massa** is a popular resort, with fine wide, sandy beaches interspersed with groves of

The impressive Ponte della Maddalena which spans the Serchio just south of Bagni di Lucca, is also known as the Ponte del Diavolo, or Devil's Bridge. Legend has it that the bridge-builder appealed to the Devil for assistance. The Devil agreed, but in return demanded the soul of the first to cross the bridge. The shrewd builder kept his promise by sending a dog across.

BELOW: the colourful facades of Barga's backstreets.

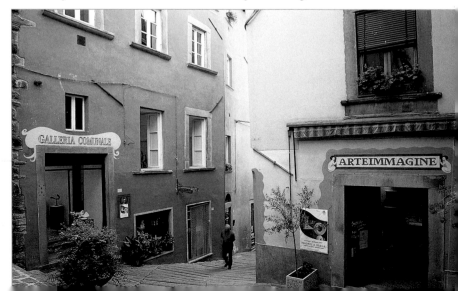

TIP

Between Carrara and Marina di Carrara is a marble museum, the Museo Civico di Marmo (Oct–Apr Mon–Sat 9am–5pm, May, June and Sept Mon–Sat 10am–6pm, July and Aug 10am–8pm; closed Sun; charge). Displays include many varieties of marble and granite, geographical and historical exhibits and some modern sculptures.

BELOW: Eremo di Calomini in the Apuan Alps.

pine trees and a promenade of pretty pastel-shaded holiday villas. Ribbon development swallows up the port, from where ships carry marble all over the world.

Although somewhat lacklustre, **Massa** ⑫ has a well-preserved medieval centre, built by the dukes of Malaspina, who ruled Massa for three centuries, and were entombed in the cathedral. Massa is dominated by the magnificent Renaissance **Castello Malaspina** (mid-June–Sept Tue–Sun 10.30am–12.30pm, 5.30–8pm, 18 Sept–Dec 2.30–6pm; charge). Beyond the narrow old streets of the town, walk on up through leafy lanes past decaying villas dotted over the mountainside. The fortress walls provide marvellous views, and welded on to them is a graceful Renaissance palace, its delicate marble pillars providing a powerful contrast to the grim towers of the original castle.

The main evidence of the famous marble quarries in **Carrara** ⑬ is the river of white mud that flows through the town, which has a dusty, disaffected air about it. It is a working town, not a monument to marble; there are few fine marble statues to be seen, even in the Pisan-style Duomo.

If time is short, ignore the town centre in favour of a visit to the marble-working quarries looming above the city. From the Carrara roundabout, decorated with a lofty marble sculpture, follow signs to **Fantiscritti.** The Vara bridges signal your arrival and are a striking sight, either in full sunlight or in moonlight, when the moon intensifies the shadows and the marble glows. After your marble tour (*see page 158*), the descent back to the coast is via hairpin bends, viaducts and gorges, and a crawl through the marble tunnel, once part of the "marble railway" linking the three main quarrying fields.

Finally, in a scruffy area off the Via Aurelia, north of Carrara, there is **Luni,** the original Roman settlement from which marble was shipped. Beyond the amphitheatre and museum, excavations have revealed columns, capitals, mosaic floors and tomb fragments.

Just over the Ligurian border is

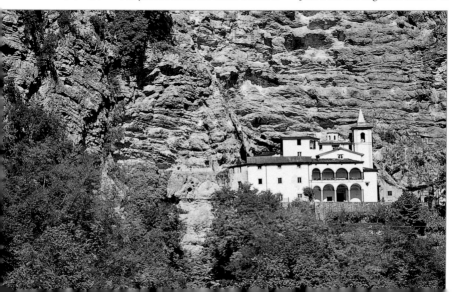

Sarzana, a thriving market town colonised by artists. There is a large market in the Piazza Matteotti, which is surrounded by Romanesque arcades sheltering smart little cafés.

Lunigiana

Luni gave its name to **Lunigiana**, "the land of the moon", an inward-looking, virtually undiscovered part of Tuscany. Lunigiana has always been a main trading route, however, and its many castles were built by the powerful Malaspina family who controlled the region to extract tolls from pilgrims and merchants.

Lunigiana was in the front line of fighting at the end of World War II, and this has left its mark. Since then there has been inevitable rural depopulation, with many people emigrating to the United States. Now, an enlightened attitude to tourism promises new hope for the area, with villages and castles being restored and the roads in a good state of repair.

It is a mountainous region of steep, winding roads, deep wooded valleys and sparkling streams. On the lower slopes of the hills, vines and olives grow. Narrow valleys are dotted with tiny villages; higher up are forests of oak and the chestnut trees that have provided a staple of the local diet for centuries, and there are deer and wild boar *(cinghiale)* in abundance. The terrain sweeps from the River Magra valley to the profound silence of deep river gorges.

The region's Romanesque churches, medieval villages and castles also attract an arty community of outsiders, with some castles taken over by eclectic sculptors, or turned into cultural centres. The inhabitants are notoriously proud and insular, in rural areas still growing most of their own food, wine and olives, and regarding other produce with suspicion. The locals will even buy in grapes from the Chianti, to make the wine themselves rather than buy a ready-made product from "foreigners".

Fortified villages

From Sarzana, **Fosdinovo ⓮** is the first fortified village en route to Aulla. Its squares are shaded by chestnut trees, and the steep streets

BELOW: the Serchio River at Bagni di Lucca.

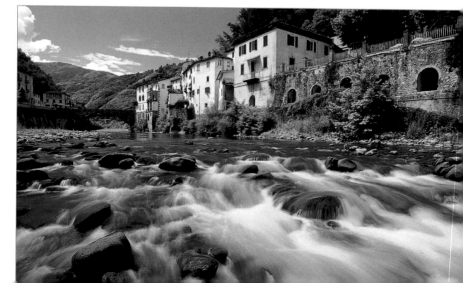

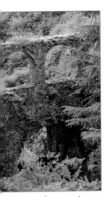

Ruins of an aqueduct near Barga.

are dominated by the magnificent 13th-century Malaspina castle. It is one of the best-preserved castles in the region, despite wartime damage. The Germans had a command post here, exploiting its superb strategic position with views from all sides. Networks of corridors and loggias reveal beautiful frescoed walls (guided tours Wed–Mon: summer 11am, noon, 3.30pm, 4.30pm, 5.30pm, 6.30pm; charge).

Aulla itself is the gateway to Lunigiana, where the rivers Magra and Taverone meet. The brooding 15th-century fortress was restored earlier last century by Montagu Brown, the British consul in Genoa.

Fivizzano ⓰, a few kilometres east, is an attractive market town full of elegant Renaissance palaces. Nearby is the enchantingly restored castle of **Verrucola**, a fortified settlement on the banks of the river. Red-roofed houses cluster around the castle keep, with geraniums spilling from window boxes and gardens full of courgette, beans and tomatoes crammed right down to the river's edge.

To the northwest of Fivizzano is **Licciana Nardi** ⓰, a fortified town dating from the 11th century. Much of the town wall is still visible, with narrow passageways running through immensely thick walls into the village. In the Piazza del Municipio, the imposing 16th-century castle dominates the square, and is joined to the graceful Baroque church by a small bridge.

Comano is an important base for walking and riding, and nearby is the Castello di Comano, a ruined, malevolent-looking tower surrounded by a tiny farming community, with ducks and chickens wandering the streets, and steep steps up to the tower.

At the end of the valley is **Camporaghena,** the last outpost before the Apennines, where there is a sad war memorial in the church. When German soldiers came hunting for escaped prisoners of war and partisans, the priest rang the church bell as a warning and was summarily shot for his brave deed.

A 16km (10-mile) drive south of Fivizzano brings you to **Equi Terme** ⓱, a popular, if sulphurous, spa

Marble Mountains

The fine-grained pure white marble for which Carrara is renowned has been quarried here since Roman times. Italian medieval churches are decorated with it, and it has supplied artists from Michelangelo to Henry Moore with raw material.

Marble is formed from limestone, hardened by great pressure and heat, and Carrara is still the world's single largest and most important source of the stone. About 200 of over a thousand original quarries are still functioning. They are scattered across three steep valleys: the Colonnata, Fantiscritti and Ravaccione. Here the villages cling to the mountainside that has been sliced away like a chunk of cheese. There are extraordinary views down into the quarries, where precarious-looking staircases are strung across the sides, and massive trucks trundle across the marble surface far below.

The best way to appreciate the majesty of the marble mountains and Carrara's "white gold" is to visit a couple of quarries and do a short marble tour, ideally at the **Fantiscritti historic quarries** that Michelangelo favoured. The master-sculptor apparently spent three years looking for just the right block of marble to make Pope Julius II's tomb and found it here.

The Ravaccione section of Fantiscritti pioneered quarrying in the heart of the mountain and now runs fascinating guided tours into the mountain (11am–6pm daily; follow signs to Fantiscritti from Carrara, via Miseglia; tel: +39 339 765 7470; www.marmotour.com; charge). The main chamber in this working quarry genuinely feels like a "marble cathedral" so it is no surprise that it has featured in glamorous Maserati and Lamborghini advertisements.

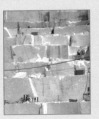

resort, with a lovely walk through a gorge, to the vaulted caves called **Buca del Cane** (tel: 0585-948 269; tours daily June–Sept, Sun only Oct–May or by appointment; charge), where the remains of paleolithic men, dogs and even lions and leopards were found.

The Magra valley

A string of pretty castles and villages lines the main route (SS62) up the Magra valley between Aulla and Pontrémoli.

Bagnone ⑱ is an attractive town of Renaissance palaces, shady arcades and a honeycomb of houses, arches and passageways leading down to the river bank. Nearby **Filetto** is a symmetrical, square-walled village where almost every street is linked by covered overhead passages or bridges. Originally a defensive structure, it is now quite cosy, with cats snoozing in corners and village women passing the time of day.

Sleepy **Pontrémoli** ⑲ gives a good flavour of the Lunigiana, offering some of Italy's finest honey and mushrooms, not to mention

testaroli, the typical pancakes, served with local pesto or cheeses. There are rich medieval town houses, and the Church of the Annunziata has a 16th-century octagonal marble temple by Sansovino. The town was once divided in two to separate the warring factions of the Guelfs and Ghibellines, and the Castruccio fortress, built in 1332, similarly divides the town.

The hulking **Castello del Piagnaro** houses the fascinating **Museo delle Statue-Stele** (May–Sept Tue–Sun 9am–12.30pm, 3–6pm, winter 9am–12.30pm, 2.30–5.30pm; charge). Some 20 prehistoric statues or menhirs found in the area are on display, the oldest of which date from 3,000 BC.

Don't leave town before sampling the local pastries in **Antica Pasticceria degli Svizzeri** (Piazza della Repubblica), a charming Art Nouveau café serving almond cake and *spongata*, a rich and tasty honeyed nut and raisin cake. The rustic specialities are low-key, quirky, old-world and engaging – much like Lunigiana itself.   ❑

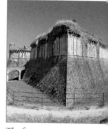

The fortress at Fosdinovo is one of the region's best-preserved castles.

BELOW: a Carrara marble quarry in the Garfagnana.

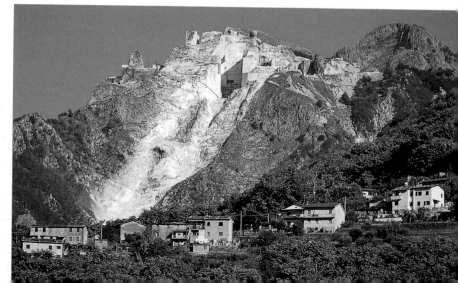

BEST RESTAURANTS

Restaurants

Prices for a three-course meal per person with a half-bottle of house wine:
€ = under €25
€€ = €25–40
€€€ = €40–60
€€€€ = over €60

Bagni di Lucca
Corona
Via Serraglia 78
Tel: 0583-805 151
www.coronaregina.it €€–€€€
Overlooking the Lima River, this restaurant specialises in local cuisine and seafood. Outdoor terrace. Closed Wed and mid-Jan–mid-Feb.

Barga
Caffe Capretz
Piazza Salvo Salvi
Tel: 0583-723 001 €
A traditional café, bar and pastry shop in the centre of Barga, with a terrace view over the countryside.

Carrara
Il Trillo
Via Bergiola Vecchia 30, Località Castegnetola
Tel: 0585-46755
www.iltrillo.net €€
A restaurant in the hills above industrial Massa, 7km (4 miles) south of Carrara, set in a lemon grove with sea views. The food is traditional and plentiful. Closed Sun and Mon lunch in summer, Mon in winter.
Ninan
Via Lorenzo Bartolini 3
Tel: 0585-74741 €€€€

Sophisticated gourmet dining. The chef, Marco Garfagnini, has won a Michelin star for his excellent Tuscan cuisine. Must book. Closed Mon.

Castelnuovo di Garfagnana
Osteria Il Vecchio Mulino
Via Vittorio Emanuele 12
Tel: 0583-62192 €
Run by Andrea Bertucci, the local leader of the Slow Food movement, the inn has hams hanging from the beams and shelves piled with spelt. Lunch on local salami and cheese before sampling one of the 10 varieties of coffee on offer.

Marina di Massa
Blue Inn
Via Fortino di San Francesco 9, Località Partaccia (4km/2.5 miles from Massa)
Tel: 0585-240 060 €€€
Modern creative cuisine from a young chef whose speciality is fish. The extensive wine list includes regional offerings, as well as the great Tuscan reds. Closed Sun, Mon in summer, 2–15 Jan and 1–15 Nov.

Forte dei Marmi
Lorenzo
Via Carducci 61
Tel: 0584-84030 €€€€
Expensive, chic Michelin-starred restaurant specialising in fish. Popular

BELOW: laid tables at the sophisticated Ninan.

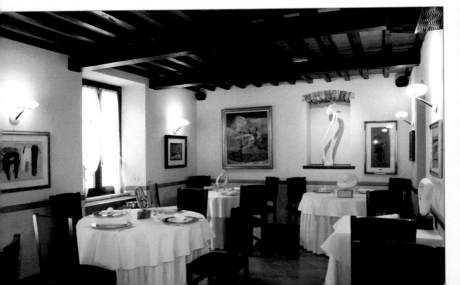

with well-heeled Milanese. Must book. Closed Mon and lunch July–Aug.

Enoteca Marcucci
Via Garibaldi 40
Tel: 0584-791 962 €€–€€€
Fashionable wine bar and inn with a vast choice of wines. The food is simple but superb, and is British fashion designer Paul Smith's favourite restaurant. Must book. Closed Mon, lunchtime (except July–Aug) and Nov.

Cà del Moro
Via Casa Corvi 9
Tel: 0187-832 202
www.cadelmororesort.it €€–€€€
Charming restaurant serving Tuscan specialities. Popular with golfers. Also has rooms. Closed Sun evening and Mon,

BELOW: dining alfresco at Enoteca Marcucci.

two weeks Jan and Nov.
Osteria da Busse
Piazza Duomo 31
Tel: 0187-831 371 €€
Owned by a local farmer, the inn features his vegetable tarts, home-cured salami and lasagna made from local chestnut flour. Try the *zuppa con ragu*, the filling house soup.
Osteria Oca Bianca
Via Cavour 27
Tel: 0187-833 219 €
The menu is short but tempting in this cosy inn. Try the local speciality: *testaroli*, pancakes served with a pesto sauce, the stuffed ravioli or the roast cooked in a terracotta pot. Lunch only Mon–Fri, but lunch and dinner at the weekend.

Butterfly
Belvedere Puccini 24/26

Tel: 0584-341 024 €€
A restaurant with rooms overlooking the lake. Sardinian dishes feature alongside Tuscan and fish specialities. Good value. Closed Fri.

Cabreo
Via Firenze 14
Tel: 0584-54643 €€
Pleasant family-run restaurant with an emphasis on the "catch of the day". Closed Mon and Nov.
Gran Caffè Ristorante Margherita
Via Regina Margherita 30
Tel: 0584-581 143 €€
This legendary Art Nouveau café has moved with the times and serves versions of classic Tuscan dishes, either in the historic dining room, or the garden. Also a bookshop.
Il Puntodivino
Via Mazzini 229
Tel: 0584-31046 €€–€€€

Young and buzzing atmosphere; serves meals and snacks. Wine tastings in the wine bar. Closed Mon.
L'Oca Bianca
Via Coppino 409
Tel: 0584-388 477
www.oca-bianca.it €€€–€€€€
Possibly Viareggio's finest restaurant, with a creative seafood menu. Exquisite service; exceptional wine list. Near the port. Closed Tue (except July–Aug) and lunch Fri–Sun.
Osteria Giordano Bruno
Viale Europa 7
Tel: 0584-392 201
www.osteria-giordanobruno.com €€€
Enoteca with good wine selection, and modern cuisine with Italian, French and Japanese influences. Great desserts. Daily for dinner, Oct–May also for lunch.

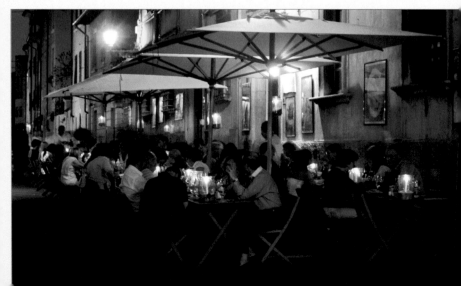

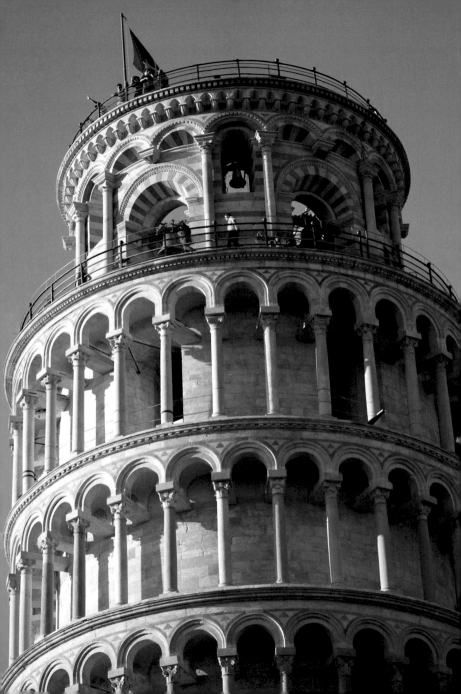

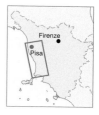

PISA AND THE ETRUSCAN RIVIERA

Beyond the iconic Leaning Tower and "Field of Miracles", Pisa province has much to offer, from spa centres to family-friendly beach resorts. Further south, unsung Livorno province offers Etruscan ruins, scenic coastal stretches, forgotten hill towns and great fish restaurants – but give Livorno itself a wide berth

With barely enough Renaissance art to enliven an over-cast beach holiday, Livorno should be on the defensive. However, the province is as varied as its famed fish soup, *cacciucco*. The ingredients, a little of everything in the right proportions, apply to Livorno's seascapes. Captured in moody canvases by the Tuscan Impressionists, the rocky northern coast is as dramatic as the southern coast is soothing. The mainland stretches from wild, marshy Maremma to the rugged, hilly interior, or the Elban mountains.

Instead, Pisa province, despite its spas and beach resorts, means only one thing in the public imagination. The Leaning Tower draws tourists to Pisa like a magnet, many of them pausing to appreciate the religious architecture, others to enjoy the glorious art and history of this Tuscan city. Once a thriving Roman port, Pisa's harbour had silted up in the 15th century, and it now stands on the Arno River, 10km (6 miles) from the coast. Great sea battles were fought during the Middle Ages, with the city-state of Pisa becoming first an ally then a rival of a number of other states, including Genoa, Lucca, Venice and Florence.

At its height, Pisa's power extended to Sardinia, Corsica and the Balearic Islands. Trade with Muslim Spain, North Africa and Lebanon meant that Pisa even had a kasbah district for Arab and Turkish merchants. Arabic numerals were introduced to Europe through Pisa, and the city's major architectural monuments – the Leaning Tower, the Duomo and Baptistery – show the clear influence of Islamic architecture.

Pisa ❶ is split in two by the gently curving River Arno, its steep stone

Main attractions
CAMPO DEI MIRACOLI
TORRE PENDENTE
BORGO STRETTO QUARTER
BAGNI DI PISA
CERTOSA DI PISA
COSTA DEGLI ETRUSCHI
CASTIGLIONCELLO
BOLGHERI
SUVERETO
POPULONIA

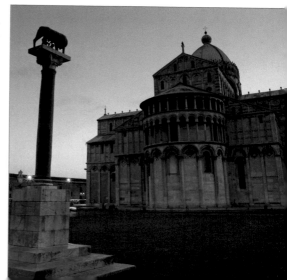

LEFT: the top of the Leaning Tower of Pisa.
RIGHT: the Duomo in the "Field of Miracles".

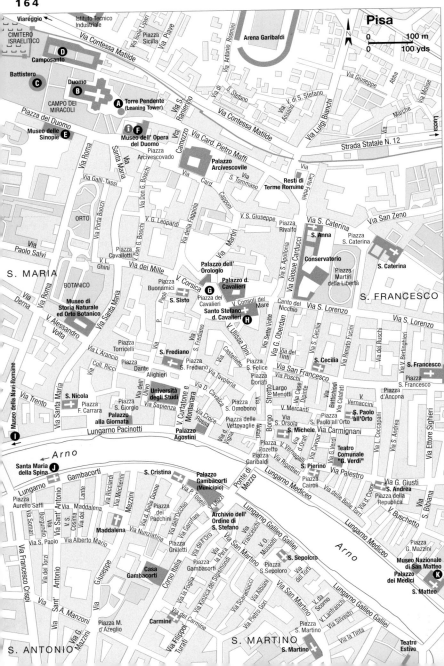

banks coloured by floating green algae. Elegant 16th-century palazzi along the banks hide the dilapidated areas in the narrow alleys behind.

The city's trump card is the budget airlines' choice of Galileo Galilei airport as their regional hub; but the town doesn't want to be Tuscany's airport lounge – Pisa needs visitors to come for more than just a photo of the Tower. No city in the world is as closely associated with one single monument as Pisa is with her tower. Even during the 1990s, when the marble miracle was in architectural intensive care and out of bounds to visitors, most still failed to notice that there was life outside the Campo. But after centuries of Pisan twilight, there are signs of a resurgence, especially around the arcaded Borgo Stretto area and the Arno, an area aspiring to a Left Bank feel. Centred on the prestigious university, a large student presence brings energy to the area, as does the enthusiasm of Pisan cyclists, who are among the most dedicated in Tuscany.

Crossing the original city bridge, Ponte della Citadella, the Via Nicola Pisano leads to the **Campo dei Miracoli** (Field of Miracles), a green swathe of manicured grass in the northwestern corner of the city walls – with perhaps the most perfect assemblage of religious buildings in Tuscany. The Campo dei Miracoli ticket office (daily 9.30am–30 min before last Leaning Tower climb), to the north side of the Leaning Tower, sells tickets to all the sites.

The Leaning Tower

Visitors flock from all over the world to marvel at the phenomenon of the **Torre Pendente A** (advance bookings www.opapisa.it; daily Apr–Sept 8.30am–8pm, Mar 9am–5.30pm, Oct 9am–7pm, Nov–Feb 9.30am–5pm, Dec–Jan 10am–4.30pm; it may be possible to buy tickets on the day from the Campo dei Miracoli ticket office on the north side of the Tower, daily 9.30am–6.30pm; no entry to children under eight, and children between eight and 12 must be held by the hand; charge). The best place to catch your first sight of the 12th-century Campanile is through the archway of the Porta Santa Maria, otherwise

BELOW LEFT: souvenir stalls near the Tower.

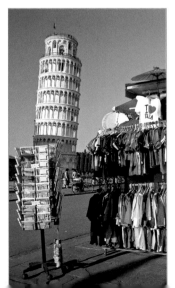

Halting the Tilt

Pisa's Torre Pendente really does lean to a frightening degree, though less than it used to. The unstable subsoil that underlies the Piazza dei Miracoli has caused all the buildings to tilt and subside to dizzying effect. Just to the right of the entrance to the Tower is a date stone inscribed ANDMI MCLXXIII (standing for Anno Domini 1173), the year in which building work started on the Campanile. But work stopped at the third stage because the building was already collapsing. A century later, three more stages were added, deliberately constructed to tilt in the opposite direction, so the Tower has a decided kink as well as a tilt. By 1989, the Tower was leaning to such a perilous degree that it was in danger of collapse. It was promptly closed to the public, and an international team of engineers spent the next two decades in a battle to save it. During the first phase, completed in 2001, the tower was straightened by 40cms to avoid imminent collapse. In 1992 it was given a girdle of steel braces that were attached to a cunning counterweight system. A year later, the bells were silenced because of the damaging effect of vibration on the edifice. In 2011, work to stabilise the Leaning Tower was pronounced a success, and it was reopened to the public.

TIP

Pisa's annual Anima Mundi festival is a celebration of sacred music, with concerts by world-class musicians staged in the Duomo. This acclaimed event runs from mid-Sept to the mid-Oct. For information and bookings tel: 050-387 2229/2210; or visit www.opapisa.it.

BELOW: the Duomo and exterior of the Camposanto.

known as the Porta Nuova. When the sun is shining, the whiteness dazzles; when raining, it glistens.

The Cathedral

The Duomo B (daily Nov–Feb 10am–1pm, 2–5pm, Mar 10am–6-pm, Apr–Sept 10am–8pm, Oct 10am–7pm; charge, free Sun and hols), built between 1068 and 1118, is one of the major monuments of Italy. The beautiful white-marble facade, the model for the Pisan Romanesque style, is set with mosaics, inlaid marble and glass pieces.

The tomb of Buscheto, the architect of the building, is above eye level on the left of the facade, designed by Rainaldo and built in the early 12th century. The 16th-century bronze doors are surrounded by frames enlivened by animals. The main entrance to the Duomo was intended to be through the bronze transept doors of the Porta di San Ranieri, near the Tower. The work of Bonanno Pisano, dating from 1180, they are decorated with 24 New Testament vignettes, including such delightful scenes as shepherds in their conical

caps playing their pipes to soothe the newborn child, and the figures of the Apostles under rows of swaying palm trees.

The rich complexity of the Cathedral interior is created by the forest of pillars rising to arches of banded white and grey stone, and the colourful mix of altar paintings and Cimabue's apsidal mosaic, from 1302. The beautiful marble pulpit by Giovanni Pisano (1301–11) is a masterpiece. Supported by figures representing prophets, sibyls and allegorical figures, its crowded and dramatic marble panels depict scenes from the *Life of Christ*.

Hanging from the westernmost arch of the great dome is Galileo's Lamp, so called because its pendulum movement is said to have inspired Galileo to discover the rotation of the Earth (in reality, the lamp wasn't here in Galileo's time).

The Baptistery

Across from the Rainaldo facade is the third building of the Duomo complex: the **Battistero C** (daily, Apr–Sept 8am–8pm, Oct 9am–7pm,

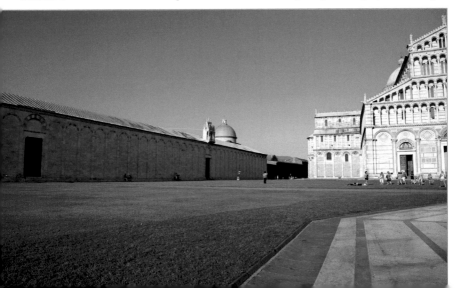

Nov–Feb 10am–5pm, Mar 9am–6pm; charge), the largest baptistery in Italy, with richly decorated exterior niches and statues of saints. The interior is far plainer, but it has one great treasure: Nicola Pisano's pulpit of 1260, carved with scenes from the *Life of Christ*, clearly influenced by Ancient Roman art (the source for which we shall see next, in the Camposanto). Mary, for example, has the long neck, veil and ringlets typical of middle-aged matrons in Roman portraiture. You may be lucky enough during your visit to hear one of the attendants demonstrate the Baptistery's remarkable acoustics. As four or more individual notes are sung, the long echo allows them to build up to a complete chord that rings eerily round the dome.

Camposanto

The fourth element of the Duomo group is the **Camposanto** **Ⓓ** (hours same as the Baptistery; charge), one of the world's most beautiful cemeteries. The graceful white-marble cloister is paved with the grave slabs of medieval Pisans, carved with coats of arms or tools of their trade. Roman sarcophagi, imported from the Holy Land and reused as coffins for wealthy Pisans, line the walls, carved with the mythological scenes that inspired the pulpits of Nicola and Giovanni Pisano. Frescoes damaged by incendiary bombs during World War II have been restored to their original positions. They include a grim series of images (1360–80) inspired by the Black Death, on the themes of the *Last Judgement* and the *Triumph of Death*.

On the opposite side of the Campo dei Miracoli is the **Museo delle Sinopie** **Ⓔ** (hours same as the Baptistery; charge), where you can learn more about the Camposanto frescoes and how they were created by laying down a sketch on the plaster undercoat using red paint (called *sinopia* because the pigment came from Sinope on the Black Sea). When the final thin layer of white plaster was applied, the *sinopia* sketch showed through and guided the artists as they completed the fresco in full colour.

The fire that followed the bombing of the Camposanto destroyed some

BELOW: inside the Camposanto.

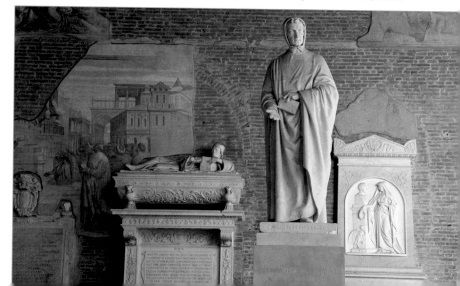

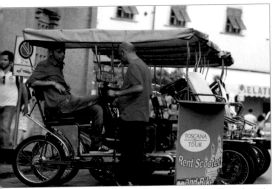

Bike and scooter rental in Pisa.

BELOW: the Arno cuts Pisa in two.

of the frescoes and left the others in so precarious a condition that it was necessary to remove them – but that was how the immense *sinopie* lying beneath the frescoes came to light and were salvaged, and are now carefully restored.

The Cathedral Museum

The final piece of the jigsaw is the **Museo dell'Opera del Duomo** ❻ (hours same as the Baptistery; charge) – the Cathedral Museum. Room 1 contains casts of the foundation stones of each of the buildings and a chronology, which begins in 1064 with the start of work on the Cathedral, followed by the Baptistery in 1154, the Campanile in 1173, and the Camposanto a century later, in 1277. This short burst of fireworks was followed by swift decline as the city's harbour silted up. (Recent excavations have revealed Roman and medieval boats, complete with cargoes, preserved in the waterlogged silt, now exhibited in the maritime museum). By 1406, the city had been conquered by Florence and was about to be eclipsed culturally by that city's dogged determination to build even bigger and bolder monuments.

The museum is packed with 12th–15th-century sculptures and paintings: Giovanni Pisano's ivory *Virgin and Child* (1299) is one of the highlights, using the natural shape of the ivory tusk to give the Virgin her naturalistic stance. There are models to show the construction techniques used to build the domed Baptistery, and to explain the marble-inlay technique used to give all the buildings their intricate exterior decoration.

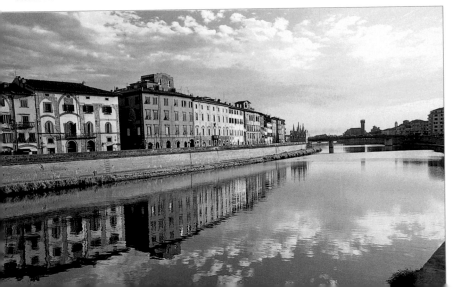

Best of all, the rooms of the museum open out on to a quiet shady cloister, with a spectacular view of the Leaning Tower and the Cathedral.

New life in the old town

Students often congregate on the **Piazza dei Cavalieri** **G**, one of the most attractive squares in the city. This was the centre of activity in the Pisan Republic. It was in one of the towers of the Palazzo dell'Orologio (the building with the clock to the north of the square) – so we learn from Dante's *Inferno* – that Count Ugolino, wrongly convicted of treason in 1284, was left to starve to death with his sons.

The square is named after the order of knights *(cavalieri)* founded by Cosimo I (1561), to fight the Turks in the Mediterranean. The duke gave its members the Palazzo della Carovana, the former council chambers of the Pisan Commune. The magnificent *sgraffito* decoration (floral patterns, coats of arms, symbols) and the next-door church of **Santo Stefano dei Cavalieri** **H** (Mon–Sat 10am–7pm, Sun

1–7.30pm; charge) were based on plans by Vasari (1511–74). In 1606 Giovanni de' Medici added the marble facade and placed the knights' emblem above the great doorway. Displayed inside are trophies and spoils of war from Pisan naval victories against the Ottomans. Just south, you can dine in an authentic early 13th-century tower-house in the **Osteria dei Cavallieri** (Via San Frediano 16; tel: 050-580 858; www. osteriacavallieri.pisa.it). This atmospheric "chivalric" inn serves hearty local dishes such as T-bone steak, cheese pie or beef with beans.

The lively warren of alleyways and shopping streets between the square and the Arno is known as the **Borgo Stretto quarter** and is the most elegant part of town. Lined with cafés and shops, the arcaded Borgo Stretto opens out at Piazza Garibaldi and the Ponte di Mezzo. Call into the **Pasticceria Federico Salza** (Borgo Stretto 46), the city's most delectable bar and pastry shop, set under the porticoes. It makes a tempting place for a light lunch, an afternoon coffee and cake, or evening cocktails.

Pisa's Museo di San Matteo displays a collection of antique armour used in the Gioco del Ponte medieval tug-of-war festival held on the last Sunday in June. The displays include breastplates, helmets and other pieces dating from the 15th and 16th centuries.

BELOW: attractive Piazza dei Cavalieri.

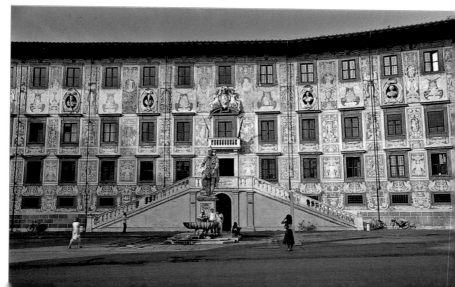

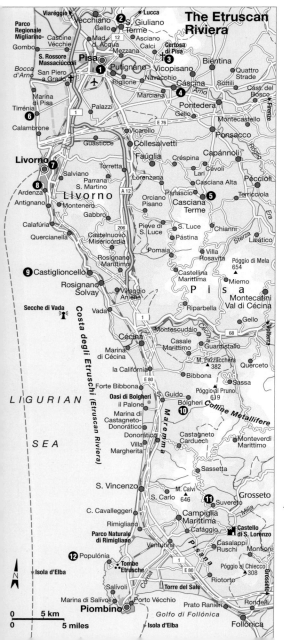

Off the southern end of the Borgo Stretto, the arcaded **Piazza delle Vettovaglie** market area has been revamped, making it the haunt of Pisa University students who are drawn to the reasonably priced bars. Just beyond, the Arno River, with its boat tours and festivals, is being touted as the Pisan "Left Bank".

Banks of the Arno

To the west, some distance along the river, the **Museo delle Navi Romane** ❶ (Lungarno Simonelli; www.cantiere-navipisa.it; closed for restoration) in the Medici Arsenale, the old Medici shipyards, houses the finds from the ongoing excavation of Pisa's ancient port, buried by silt in the 15th century. In 1998, workers expanding the railway station stumbled on the site, where the remains of 10 Ancient Roman ships and their contents (including the skeleton of a sailor) have been unearthed. These docklands, where the sea met the Arno, were probably composed of marshy flatlands and lagoon, very similar to Venice. Proclaimed a "marine Pompeii", excavations and restorations continue so this remarkable archaeological site is called an "exhibition in progress".

On the opposite bank of the Arno, across the Ponte Solferino, stands the church of **Santa Maria della Spina** ❶ (Mar–Oct Tue–Sun 10am–1.30pm, 2.30–6pm, Sat–Sun until 7pm, Nov–Feb Tue–Sun 10am–2pm; charge). Don't worry if it is closed when you visit: it is the vivacious exterior that is the most important feature, a *tour de force* of Gothic pinnacles and niches, crowded with statues of saints carved by members of the Pisano family from 1230. Back in the days when Pisa was a port, before its harbour silted up, seafarers came to pray here before setting sail.

The chapel once guarded what was believed to be a thorn (*spina*) from the "crown" of Jesus, but that relic, plus the original statues, is now housed downriver, in the **Museo Nazionale di San Matteo** ⓚ (Lungarno Mediceo; daily Tue–Sat 9am–7pm, Sun 9am–12.30pm; charge). Set in rooms around the cloister of a medieval church, the museum contains such treasures as Masaccio's *St Paul* (1426), a contemplative man with a high brow, hooked nose and patriarchal beard; Donatello's bust reliquary for San Rossore; and a whole room of glowing Renaissance paintings by artists of the calibre of Gozzoli and Ghirlandaio.

Pisan country retreats

The Pisan countryside ranges from pretty to unprepossessing, with the magnificent Certosa di Pisa the main attraction, along with several charming spa resorts. Midway between Pisa and Lucca, at the foot of the Pisan mountains, is the charmingly faded spa town of **San Giuliano Terme** ❷. Olives, chestnuts and pines grow in the surrounding fertile countryside, wild horses roam the hills and ruins dot the valleys. San Giuliano is renowned for the curative powers

of its thermal springs. Here, the best place to try out a thermal spa treatment, or simply indulge in some pampering, is the atmospheric **Bagni di Pisa** spa resort, which, in its heyday, played host to the Romantic poets *(see page 301)*. These spa waters have been famous since Roman times, and are especially good for the treatment of rheumatism and arthritis. Montaigne, Byron and Shelley were among famous Grand Tourists.

Set in lush countryside, near Calci, 10km (6 miles) east of Pisa, stands the imposing **Certosa di Pisa** ❸ (Tue–Sat 9am–6.30pm, Sun 9.30am–noon; charge). The Charterhouse of Pisa was founded in 1366, but the finishing touches were only put to this Carthusian monastery in the early 18th century. The Carthusians were one of the strict new orders who believed that the increasing prosperity of the Cluniac orders was accompanied by a decline in religious observance. Their architecture reflected this stance; the monks lived in separate cells within a main enclosure. The

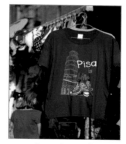

Souvenirs on sale to satisfy the many tourists who visit Pisa.

The Pisan Paradox

Since the glory days of the "Field of Miracles", some critics feel that Pisa has rested on its laurels, overwhelmed by the burden of its great history. It is as if, after pouring all its creative genius into one square, Pisa then slumbered for the next 500 years. Nor does it help that the Leaning Tower is so iconic that most visitors to the city see virtually nothing else.

There are no easy solutions because Pisa, unlike its Tuscan rivals, has no real centre. The Field of Miracles is set on the northern edge of the city, thus distorting the geography of tourism. Pisans themselves set great store by the River Arno as a dividing line, and a defining line, between different districts. But, unfortunately, much of the river is nondescript, with the Lungarno presenting a procession of blank, ochre facades that all merge into one another, matched by an equally unappealing and muddy-coloured river.

Pisa is not picturesque, and, for outsiders, simply

doesn't tug the heartstrings like many other towns and cities in Tuscany. But there is a warmer side to the city. On the north bank, Piazza delle Vettovaglie welcomes a bustling daily market, while the neighbouring arcaded Borgo Stretto is the most beguiling place for a coffee.

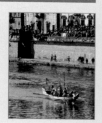

Visitors can best appreciate the Pisan sense of belonging at one of the heartfelt festivals held in the city, such as the Gioco del Ponte, the medieval tug-of-war fought on the Ponte di Mezzo. Also in June are the celebrations in honour of Saint Ranieri. Known as the Luminaria, the night before the medieval regatta is a mesmerising festival that sees the banks of the Arno bathed in candlelight.

The original spa building at Casciana Terme was designed in 1870 by Poggi, but a direct hit from a bomb in World War II left only the facade and the hall intact. In 1968 the spa was completely rebuilt around the remains of the original structure.

centre of monastic life was the Great Cloister, of which the Certosa di Pisa has a particularly fine example. Work on the frescoes of the church walls began in 1701, and in 1718 workmen from Carrara carved the marble and renovated the church facade. In 1981 a part of the Charterhouse was allotted to the University of Pisa to house the **Museo della Storia Naturale e del Territorio** (Tue–Sun 10am–6pm, summer until 7pm; charge).

Lined with plane trees, the route to **Cascina** 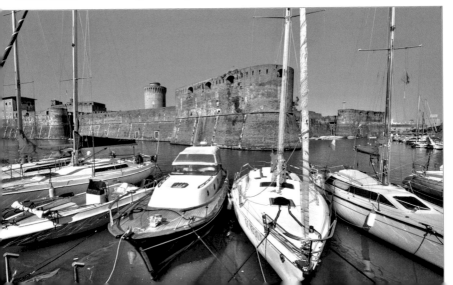 passes fields of sunflowers, grapevines and maize. Cascina is proud of its solid stone walls, dating from 1142, which are depicted in Vasari's energetic painting of the *Battle of Cascina*, now hanging in the Palazzo Vecchio in Florence. On Corso Matteotti, the tiny chapel of **Suore di Carmelitane di Santa Teresa**, on the left, has beautifully detailed frescoes. The nearby church of the saints Casciano and Giovanni, *c.*970, is a graceful building with a simple interior.

Casciana Terme ❺, less than 40km (25 miles) southeast from Pisa, is surrounded by vineyards, olive groves and peach orchards. The

Below: a view of Fortezza Vecchia.

appeal of the area lies in the gentle hills, mild climate, leisurely pace of life – and the spa culture. Casciana is a dedicated spa town, with its thermal waters attracting both earnest Italians "taking the cure" and holiday-makers seeking a break. At certain times, you can even try a "spa by night" experience, including a light dinner and drinks (tel: 0587-644 608; www.termedicasciana.it).

The Pisan coast

The pretty road from Pisa to the coast pauses here and there at railway crossings as it follows the Arno to the sea. About 6km (4 miles) southwest of Pisa, it passes **San Piero a Grado**, a magnificent basilica that would once have overlooked the sea. Legend has it that this is the spot where St Peter first set foot on Italian soil. The fresco cycle in the nave shows scenes from the Apostle's life.

The road reaches the sea at **Bocca d'Arno**, with moody views of fishing nets. Just south, the pleasant resort of **Marina di Pisa** makes a good stop for a stroll along the café-lined promenade. On a clear day, the islands of

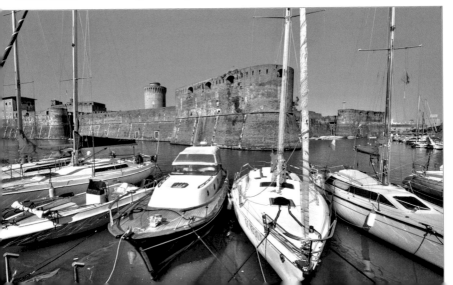

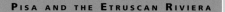

Gorgona and Capraia can be made out in the distance.

At **Tirrenia ❻**, 5km (3 miles) further down the coast, lies a stretch of Mediterranean pine forest – the one place where building has been prohibited. The trees act as a natural barrier against the *libeccio*, a strong southwesterly wind, reducing it to a light, scented breeze of pine and juniper that cools the air on hot summer days. Despite the appeal of this patch of coast, Tirrenia is a pleasant but underwhelming resort. The seafront stretch beyond the sand dunes is currently undergoing major development, with new residential areas, restaurants and a shopping and entertainment complex all centred on **Calambrone**. While rather charmless compared with more upmarket Forte dei Marmi or Marina di Pietrasanta, this emerging holiday resort is perfect for families looking for an active holiday, centred on the beach. Reasonably priced restaurants line the main route, while golf, tennis, horse riding, fishing, windsurfing, sailing and rowing are readily available. Each year colourful regattas and boat races are held, and the training centre for the Italian National Olympics is in Tirrenia.

Livorno city

The central coastal area of Tuscany is dominated by the busy comings and goings at the port of **Livorno ❼**, just south of Pisa. This is the Tuscan gateway to the sea and a city crossed by canals. As Italy's second-largest port after Genoa, it owes its existence to the silting up of Pisa in the 15th century; the Livornese joke that, unlike their rivals, the Pisans, they will never be so careless as to let the sea slip away from them. The rivalry between Pisans and Livornese is legendary and very much alive today. There is a saying in Livorno: *"Meglio un morto in casa che un Pisano all'uscio"* – "It is better to have a dead body in your house than a Pisan on the doorstep."

In 1421 the Florentines paid the Genoese 100,000 florins for Livorno, a vast sum for such a mosquito- and hence malaria-plagued village. It was the enlightened Cosimo I who, in 1575, transformed Livorno into the greatest Medicean port.

TIP

Trips to the sleepy volcanic island of Capraia are worth considering if you want to discover somewhere new. It's 64km (40 miles) off the coast of Livorno – a 2½-hour boat ride from the port. Ferry services are run by Toremar (www.toremar. it). For more information on the seven islands of the Tuscan Archipelago, see box on page 186.

BELOW: early morning fish market in Livorno port.

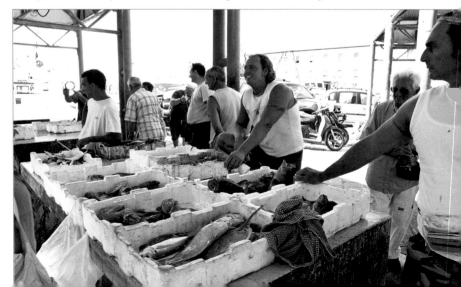

Livorno is the birthplace of painters and composers, including Amedeo Modigliani, Pietro Mascagni, Giovanni Fattori and the Macchiaioli School, who influenced the development of art all over the world. It was also popular with British expatriates, such as Byron and Shelley, who anglicised the city's name to Leghorn.

Cosmopolitan salons and elegant avenues made it a fashionable port of call for the Grand Tourists. But after 80 bombing raids in World War II, Livorno resembles a modern necropolis. Visitors soon realise that the city lives on commerce, not tourism. Few linger unless en route to the islands or the hills, but attractions there are. The Medicean port is unchanged. The red-brick **Fortezza Vecchia** is a patchwork of Livornese history, including Roman remains, medieval Pisan walls and a Romanesque tower. The **Fortezza Nuova** (daily 8am–8pm; free), built in 1590, completed the ambitious Medici fortifications. The murky canals encircling it once led to Pisa. Now restored, the New Fortress is landscaped as a park and is a popular spot for children's romps and summer festivals. The other main attraction is neighbouring **Piccola Venezia**, dubbed "Little Venice" for its network of quiet canals.

From 2013, the **Navicelli canal**, between Pisa and Livorno, will once again be fully navigable, with weekend cruises connecting the two cities,

allowing visitors arriving in Livorno to reach the historic centre of Pisa. The canal through the marshes was opened in 1575 by the Medici, but fell into disuse and was partly destroyed in World War II. In the meantime, you can still do day and evening cruises on the Arno (contact Pisa tourist office, tel: 050-42291).

The Etruscan Riviera

South of here is the area known as the Maremma Pisana – once a mosquito-infested swampland but now transformed – and the **Costa degli Etruschi**, the Etruscan Riviera. This is clever branding, even if it does conjure up incongruous images of beady-eyed Etruscans lounging under beach umbrellas, much as they do on their funerary urns.

Over 60 miles of coastline, Etruscan sites, medieval villages, hills, valleys and wild woods make this lesser-known part of Tuscany unique. The coast is no architectural desert: a coastline of Pisan watchtowers and Medicean fortresses hides the occasional Roman villa or Etruscan necropolis.

Tuscany by Train

The region abounds in scenic rail trips so do consider doing the occasional leg by train, including sampling the minor branch lines. These routes are not designed for speed but for savouring the countryside.

For arty sights and romantic scenery, the Pisa to Orvieto route is perhaps the finest introduction to the Tuscan and Umbrian landscape, which is dotted with hill towns and scenery depicted by the Renaissance masters. The route travels through the heart of Tuscany, revealing green hills striped with olive groves and vineyards, as well as historic towns studded with Renaissance art and architecture. Domesticated Tuscany melds with the hazy spirituality of Umbria's green hills. A variant on this rewarding route could take you from Pisa to Lucca, then Florence, Siena, Chiusi and possibly on to Orvieto.

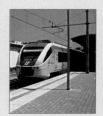

Also from Pisa, you can follow the coastal route all the way to Liguria, stopping off at the resort of Viareggio for the beach, and Massa di Carrara for the striking marble quarries. From Chiusi, there is a delightful branch line that takes you on a plucky two-carriage train to sleepy Asciano, Siena and Buonconvento, with views of sunflowers, Montalcino shimmering in the distance, and a Sienese landscape straight out of a fresco by Lorenzetti.

Lucca also makes a lovely rail base, with good onward services to Pisa (25 minutes), Viareggio (20 minutes) and Florence (1 hour 20 minutes). From Florence, the scenic journey into mountainous Garfagnana is also recommended. Welcome to Slow Tuscany. Many of the best itineraries and rail holidays can be planned through Railbookers (www.railbookers.com).

The high coastal road from **Ardenza** ❽ to Castiglioncello offers some delightful scenic stretches as it hugs the cliffs' edge and dips in and out of tunnels. Ardenza, a fashionable resort flanked by palms and Art Nouveau villas, was home to what the Livornese called "Leghorn's British Factory". The sea views and the dramatic summer storms revived Shelley enough to enable him to write his famous *Ode to a Skylark*. Byron, also devoted to Ardenza, was a frequent visitor.

The coast becomes progressively more rugged, and the road winds past Medici castles, watchtowers and follies. Castello del Boccale, encircled by gulls and rocky paths to the shore, is a Medicean fort converted into a private villa. At **Calafuria**, an isolated Medicean tower and distorted rock formations provided the Italian Impressionist painters with a dramatic setting. After Romito, the coastline becomes wild and wooded. As the small resort of **Quercianella** comes into view, pine woods run down to the water's edge; small coves, shingle beaches and a narrow harbour vie for space.

Quercianella is followed by the popular rocky resort of **Castiglioncello** ❾, which the Livornese seem to favour above the monotonous stretches of sand below Cecina. The Livornese also know that there are sandy bays tucked into the rocks. Cosimo's fort, built on the pine-clad promontory, was designed to keep pirates at bay, but since the 19th century it attracted all the great Italian Impressionists. In the 1930s, Castiglioncello was also very popular with film stars. It may not have much cachet today, but it's nice enough for a dip and a cheap lunch at one of the dockside bars.

For sightings of flamingos sheltering under umbrella pines, the **Parco Naturale di Rimigliano**, hugging the coast between San Vincenzo and Populonia, is where to head.

Rural hinterland

But for a rewarding wine-tasting foray, leave the coast at **Cecina** and

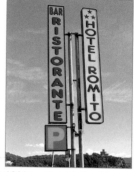

For a fabulous fish lunch with a sea view, this truck stop on the coast road a few kilometres north of Quercianella is worth knowing about (see page 178).

BELOW: Castiglioncello beach.

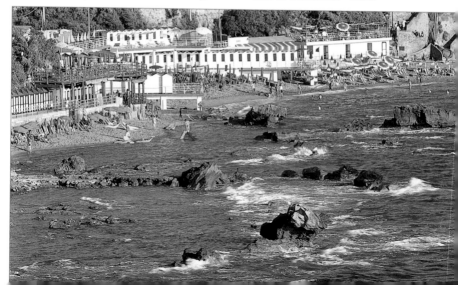

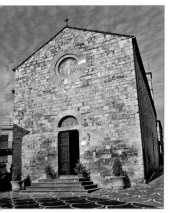

The church of Santa Maria della Pietà in the pretty inland village of Bibbona.

take the inland road to higgledy-piggledy **Bibbona** and wine-growing Bolgheri via **Casale Marittimo**. Quiet lanes trace through marshy countryside dotted with red farmhouses and occasional herds of placid white Maremman cattle, and spiral up into the hills.

The sun-baked hill town of Casale Marittimo offers views across the Livorno coast and out to Elba. Just south, medieval **Bolgheri** ⑩ is a pocket of the Maremma fashionable for the so-called Super Tuscans, wines such as Sassicaia, Ornellaia and Antinori Solaia. To many wine experts, this is the future of Tuscan wine-making. Continue winding south through **Castagneto Carducci**, where the flatness is broken by low farmhouses, olive trees and the village vineyards, part of the wine trail bordering the Etruscan Riviera.

Sassetta, a bird's nest of a *borgo*, with a medieval castle, waits in the hills slightly further south. From here a winding road through olive groves, oleanders and woodland leads to **Suvereto** ⑪, another well-preserved village, with a crenellated town hall, an early Romanesque church, and a steep ascent through a rabbit warren of covered passageways. Many buildings are vividly decorated with the local red, brown or grey variegated marble, which has been quarried since medieval times. Suvereto's urban design, based on rising concentric circles, is simple but effective: each level corresponds to a street, from the church to the towering castle above. The sedate village pours on to the streets for the evening *passeggiata* and, in season, for the *sagra del cinghiale*, a wild-boar feast combining food and folklore. This area is **Val di Cornia**, an enchanting region of gently wooded hills, hot springs, lush valleys and old quarries.

The winding route south, towards the coast, leads to **Campiglia Marittima**, a hilly market and mining town known for its imposing castle and rustic cuisine based on sausages, chestnut polenta and bean soups.

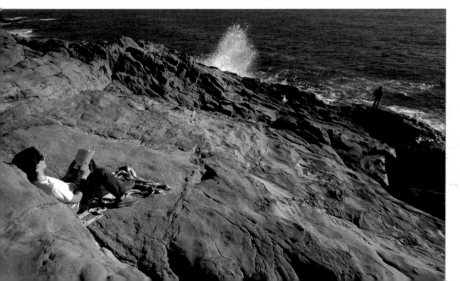

Populonia

If the coast beckons, San Vicenzo's metallic sands and monotonous strip of beach bungalows can be sacrificed to **Populonia** ⑫, and the scenic ruins of the last of the 12 Etruscan cities to be founded, located behind the sweep of Baratti Bay (Tue–Sun 10am–6pm; free). The Etruscans, very considerately, had themselves buried beside a pine-fringed beach, reason enough to visit the only Etruscan city built on the coast. The ancient city was divided into two parts: the acropolis – the religious centre clustered high around the village – and the maritime and industrial centre around the bay. The necropolises cover the slopes that sit between the two centres.

Thanks to its proximity to Elba and to the metal-bearing Campigliese hills, Populonia became a rich industrial city. While Elban iron ore was smelted and then traded within the Etruscan League, minerals from Campiglia were shipped to Corsica, Sardinia and France. In the ancient "industrial zone", excavations have uncovered a blast furnace and sophisticated metalworking equipment dating back to the 6th century BC. Foreign slave labour was used to dig water channels, operate the furnace and mint coins. In the 6th century BC, Populonia was the first Etruscan city to mint gold, silver and bronze coins. Sadly, many tombs lie buried or collapsed under the weight of ancient slag heaps. Before setting out, check the Populonia archaeological park online (tel: 0565-226 445; www.parchivaldicornia.it) and also find time for the medieval village of Populonia. If catching a ferry to Elba from gritty Piombino, call in at the archaeological museum there, which displays the best Etruscan finds from Populonia (Piazza della Cittadella; tel: 0565-221 646; www.parchivaldicornia.it; Tue–Sun 10am–1pm, 3–6pm; charge).

From Populonia there are smoky views of **Piombino**, a grimy, gritty city, where you can catch a ferry to **Elba** *(see page 181)*. Best seen on foot, Piombino's genteel, down-at-heel charm lingers on in quiet squares and Art Deco bars. ❏

October in Sassetta is a month of celebrations. A costumed Palio is held on the first Sunday of the month. The second sees a giant polenta cooked in the main square. The third Sunday is the Sagra del Tordo, a celebration of the thrush – this is a place where hunting is both a religious cult and a hobby, carried out in all seasons, legally or otherwise. A torchlit procession is followed by a banquet of roast thrush served with chestnut-flavoured polenta.

BELOW: the village of Suvereto.

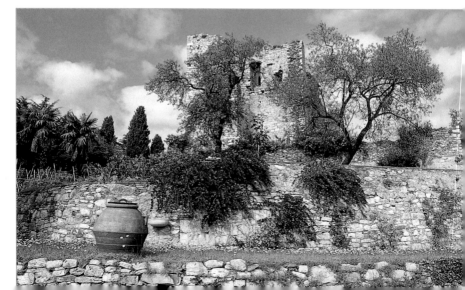

BEST RESTAURANTS

Restaurants

Prices for a three-course meal per person with a half-bottle of house wine:
€ = under €25
€€ = €25–40
€€€ = €40–60
€€€€ = over €60

Pisa

A Casa Mia
Via Provinciale Calcesana 10, Ghezzano (just outside Pisa)
Tel: 050-879 265
www.acasamia-pisa.com €€
Very pleasant, family-run restaurant set in a little villa. Freshest ingredients form the basis of the traditional Tuscan cuisine, but with creative flourishes. Closed Sat lunch and Sun, 1–7 Jan and Aug.

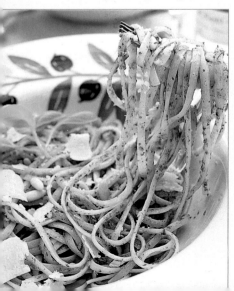

Al Ristoro dei Vecchi Macelli
Via Volturno 49
Tel: 050-20424 €€€
Famous restaurant on the north bank of the Arno, near Ponte Solferino. Cosy ambience. Try the fish and the *Menu di Primi*, which involves a succession of pasta dishes. Must book. Closed Sun lunch and Wed.

Da Bruno
Via Bianchi 12
Tel: 050-560 818
www.anticatrattoriadabruno.it
€€–€€€
Tuscan and Pisan flavours are the hallmarks of the cuisine in this atmospheric and popular restaurant. Closed Mon evening and Tue.

Il Campano
Via Cavalca 19
Tel: 050-580 585 €€
Set in a quiet spot beside the marketplace, this restaurant dating back to medieval times specialises in fish, seafood and pasta. In summer its terrace is a pleasant setting for dining alfresco. Good wine list. Closed Wed and Thur lunch.

La Clessidra
Via del Castelletto 26/ 30
Tel: 050-540 160 €€
Typical Tuscan flavours feature at this pleasing and popular restaurant in an elegant part of town. Booking advised. Closed Sat lunch, Sun, Christmas–early Jan and Aug.

Osteria dei Cavalieri
Via San Frediano 16
Tel: 050-580 858
www.osteriacavalieri.pisa.it €€
Modern restaurant near Piazza dei Cavalieri where fish is the speciality. A simpler menu is offered at lunchtime. Excellent value. Booking essential. Closed Sat lunch, Sun and Aug.

Osteria del Porton Rosso
Vicolo del Porton Rosso 11
Tel: 050-580 566
www.osteriadelportonrosso.com
€€
A brother-and-sister team create excellent fish dishes in the centre of Pisa. Booking recommended for this rustic and gastronomic find. Closed Sun.

Marina di Pisa

Da Gino
Via delle Curzolari 2
Tel: 050-35408
www.daginoamarina.it €–€€€
Excellent fish restaurant near the sea; dishes simply prepared and delicious. Popular with both locals and tourists. Closed Mon and Tue and Sept.

Foresta
Via Litoreana 2
Tel: 050-35082
www.ristoranteforesta.it €€€
Overlooking the sea, this little family-run restaurant serves gourmet cuisine. The speciality is fish and other seafood. Must book as covers are limited. Closed Sun evening and Thur.

Antignano

Il Romito
Via del Littorale 274, 3km (1.7 miles) from Antignano
Tel: 0586-580 520 €€
Roadside restaurant suspended above the sea, with fabulous views from its spacious semi-circular terrace. Service is brisk, but the dishes, predominantly fish-based, are presented with pride. Closed Wed in summer.

LEFT: fresh pasta, fresh pesto – the simpler the better.

Trattoria in Caciaia
Piazza del Castello 9
Tel: 0586-580 403 €–€€
Set on a quiet piazza, this pleasing trattoria offers a great selection of typical Livornese fish dishes. Closed Mon and Tue, weekday lunchtimes and 1 week in Sept.

Ardenza
Ciglieri
Via Ravizza 43
Tel: 0586-508 194
www.ristoranteciglieri.it €€€€
The warm, inviting decor is matched with excellent cuisine using only seasonal specialities. Must book. Closed Wed.
Oscar
Via Oreste Franchini 78
Tel: 0586-501 258 €€€
Historic restaurant with modern "designer" ambience and a pleasant garden for alfresco dining. Fish predominates, with *cacciucco* a speciality (must be ordered in advance). Extensive wine list. Closed Mon and 20 days from 27 Dec.

Castagneto Carducci
Da Ugo
Via Pari 3/A
Tel: 0565-763 746 €€
Family-run restaurant that lives up to its reputation. Robust dishes feature wild boar, wood pigeon, rabbit and *porcini*, and there's an excellent choice of local wines from their well-stocked cellar. Closed Mon.

Livorno
Da Galileo
Via della Campana 20
Tel: 0586-889 009 €€
Trattoria specialising in fish and authentic Livornese cuisine at very reasonable prices. Book ahead. Closed Sun evening and Wed, and last two weeks in July.
Ristorante Montallegro
Piazza Montenero 3
Tel: 0586-579 030 €€–€€€
Set in a spot with panoramic views near the Sanctuary of Madonna di Montenero. *Cacciucco* features every day of the year, with other traditional specialities. Pleasant frescoed dining room and terrace for warmer weather. Closed Tue in winter. Book ahead.
Trattoria Antica Venezia
Via dei Bagnetti 1
Tel: 0586-887 353 €
A typical Tuscan trattoria in the heart of Livorno's Venezia neighbourhood. Offers traditional *Livornesi* recipes including possibly the best *cacciucco* (seafood soup) in town.

San Giuliano Terme
Dei Lorena
Hotel Bagni di Pisa, Largo Shelley
Tel: 050-88501
www.bagnidipisa.com
€€€–€€€€
Set in a lovely resort between Pisa and Lucca, this restaurant is a celebration of Tuscan cuisine. Enjoy distant views of the Leaning Tower while tucking into giant Pisan steak, Tuscan bouillabaisse (*cacciucco*), truffled pasta and Antinori wines. Separate menus for vegetarians and dieters – resist. Do have a drink in the bar, once a stylish salon frequented by Shelley.

San Vincenzo
Gambero Rosso
Piazza della Vittoria 13
Tel: 0565-701 021 €€€€
Elegant restaurant overlooking the sea; one of Tuscany's best. Fish is prominent. The wine list is around 100 pages long. Closed Mon–Tue.

Tirrenia
Dante e Ivana
Via del Tirreno 207c
Tel/fax: 050-32549
www.danteeivana.com €€€
Pleasant fish restaurant with an open kitchen and a tank from which to choose your feast. Closed Sun and Mon, 20 Dec–end Jan.
Green Park Resort
Via dei Tulipani 1, Calambrone 56018
Tel: 050-313 5711 €€–€€€
www.softlivingplaces.com
Behind the dunes, dine either in the romantic, candlelit Lunasia gourmet restaurant (creative cuisine, including seafood in a pot, or prawn, pecorino and broad bean salad), or in the family-oriented Le Ginestre (reinterpretations of classic Tuscan dishes). Both places are excellent. Charming staff.
La Terrazza
Viale del Tirreno 313
Tel: 050-33006 €
Bustling, reliable, family-friendly pizzeria that is packed in summer; service is slow.

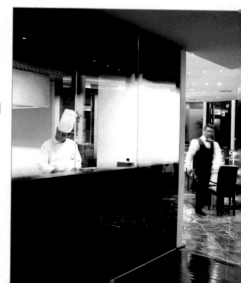

RIGHT: open kitchen at Lunasia, Green Park Resort.

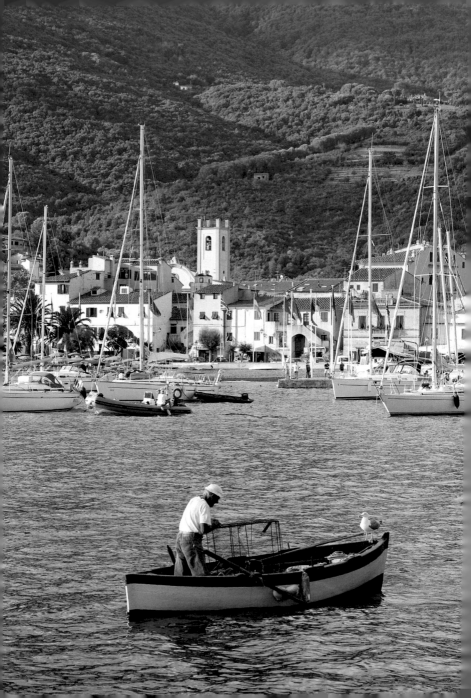

ISOLA D'ELBA

Every August, the beaches of "Tuscany's island" are invaded by sun-worshipping Italians. For the rest of the year, its rocky roads, wooded slopes and sandy bays belong to intrepid tourists who make the short sea crossing in search of unspoilt nature, crystal-clear waters, Napoleonic landmarks and good food and wine

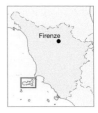

Firenze

K nown to the Etruscans as Ilva ("Iron") and to the Greeks as Aethalia ("Soot Island"), Elba has exploited its mineral wealth for more than 3,000 years. As the European powers occasionally took an interest in the island's attractive strategic position, waves of Romans, Pisans and Genoese were followed by Spanish, Turkish and French invasions. In 1548, the powerful and vainglorious Medici duke, Cosimo I, fortified the capital and named it Cosmopolis, after himself. His great military architect, Giovanni Camerini, designed the star-shaped defensive system and the two Medicean forts, Forte della Stella and Forte Falcone, to keep the Saracens at bay. Today, Portoferraio's horseshoe harbour, backed by a cluster of sun-baked pastel houses, is more welcoming than forbidding, as ferries, fishing boats, yachts and pleasure cruisers glide in and out of its embrace.

Napoleon's Elba

Portoferraio ❶ is inextricably linked to that other great imperialist, Napoleon Bonaparte. He made his official home in two converted windmills above the charming Forte

della Stella. Under the terms of the Congress of Vienna in 1814, Elba became a principality of the fallen sovereign. Napoleon's great empire shrank to his faithful "old guard", pragmatic mother and libertine sister Pauline. Most Elbans were proud to have him improve the administration, build new roads, develop the mines and expand the island's fleet. The foreign commissioners, however, rightly feared that the "Eagle" might spread its wings: after nine months, Napoleon flew, with the connivance

Main attractions
PALAZZINA DEI MULINI
MARCIANA MARINA
MARCIANA ALTA
MONTE CAPANNE
CAPO SANT'ANDREA
CAPOLIVERI
PORTO AZZURRO
RIO MARINA

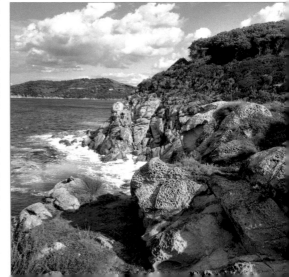

LEFT: fisherman with fish trap, Marciana Marina. **RIGHT:** the rugged coastline of Isola d'Elba.

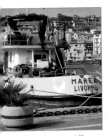

Fishing boat on Elba.

of the Elbans. He escaped with no less than 1,000 troops, the Elbans' affection, his sister's diamond necklace and his mother's curt blessing: "Go and fulfil your destiny." His **Palazzina dei Mulini** (Mon–Sat 9am–7pm, Sun 9am–1pm; charge) was lined with silver and books from Fontainebleau, and furniture from his sister Elisa's house in Piombino. Most of its charm lies in the period furnishings and Italianate gardens.

The 17th-century Misericordia church on the Via Napoleone, a broad stairway nearby, displays one of Napoleon's bronze death-masks.

A few kilometres inland from Portoferraio is the emperor's country residence, **San Martino** (Tue–Sun 9am–7pm, joint ticket with the Palazzina), purchased with one of Pauline's handy diamond necklaces. The villa's classical facade was installed in 1851 by the Russian emigré Prince Demidoff. However, after the grand cypress-lined avenue and grandiose

facade, the house itself seems a spartan affair. In one room, Napoleon's Nile campaigns of 1798–9 are recalled in the Egyptian-style frescoes, painted in 1814. In another, his tiny bed is a reminder of just how short he was. Information on the emperor's life and times is thin on the ground here (though souvenir stands are not), but the fine garden, shaded by evergreen oaks and terraced vineyards, is pleasant to stroll through.

Portoferraio to Marciana

The scenic drive westward from Portoferraio to Marciana Marina passes a number of popular beaches. **Le Ghiaie**, the nearest beach to the town, is noted for its multicoloured pebbles, but it's worth going the extra distance to **Capo d'Enfola ❷**. The road to the cape ends at Porto di Sansone, a tiny isthmus flanked by two small pebble beaches and a couple of restaurants. Formerly restricted for military use, the cape

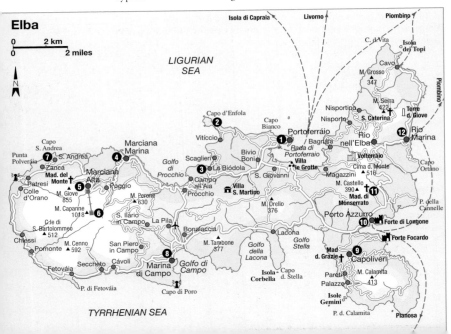

itself remains closed to traffic, but is popular among walkers. Viticcio is another pretty cove, but sand-seekers head for **La Biodola ❸**, considered the chicest beach on Elba, dominated by expensive resort complexes filled with rich bronzed Florentines in Valentino swimwear. At La Biodola and **Procchio**, a more egalitarian paradise, the rocky ocean bottom means clear, sediment-free water.

Between Procchio and Marciana Marina is "La Paolina", an islet named after Napoleon's sister, whose passion for nude sunbathing would scandalise the natives.

Marciana Marina ❹ has evolved smoothly from fishing village to elegant resort, set amidst magnolias, palms and oleanders at the end of a long valley. The thin, pastel-coloured houses in the old quarter are reminiscent of those on the Ligurian coast. On 12 August the port explodes in a firework display to honour Santa Chiara, the patron saint.

Marciana Alta ❺, perched above, is Elba's best-preserved medieval town, where chestnut woods frame red-tiled rooftops, narrow alleys and

the crumbling fortress. The local "Antiquarium" displays Etruscan sacred objects, Roman oil lamps and ivory statues found in shipwrecks.

Twin peaks

From the foot of Marciana, a cable car, the **Cabinovia del Monte Capanne** (mid-Apr–mid-Oct 10am–12.15pm, 2.30–4.45pm, June–Aug until 6.30pm) lurches over crags and chasms up to the summit of **Monte Capanne ❻**. When not misty, the views are all-encompassing. Even in high summer, this wooded mountain area is wonderfully quiet and breezy. Depending on the season, patches of orchids, snapdragons and helianthemums are as common as the cedars and chestnuts. Even the coastal vegetation is more exotic than in the east: eucalyptus and magnolia rather than vines or maquis.

The high road from Marciana to the south side of the island winds past the quiet, neglected village of **Poggio** to Monte Perone nature reserve (for a scenic walk on the mountain, stop off at Poggio and follow the waymarked trail), vineyards

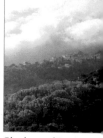

Cloud-covered Poggio.

Elba's Iron Heart

Elba is a mineralogist's paradise and the island's metal heart creates a mysterious landscape that makes a lasting impression on most visitors. Its mineral wealth has been fully exploited since Etruscan times and continues to this day: the swords wielded by countless Roman legionaries were famously made from Elban iron.

In the Copper Age, colonisers mined copper, followed by the making of bronze and the mining of iron by Etruscan and Greek settlers. While ruling Elba, Napoleon reorganised the iron mines and was a serious steward of the island. But the last mine closed in 1984, and since then the island's economic mainstays have instead been tourism, agriculture and fishing.

To the east of Portoferraio is the scar across Elba's iron heart, where most of the mines and forges were located. In the hills around Rio nell'Elba, signs of Etruscan mining camps can still be seen. Neighbouring Rio

Marina, now home to the mineralogical museum, was the set-off point where the cargoes of metal were shipped overseas. Further south, in Capoliveri, the black, iron-bearing lodestone still plays havoc with the compasses aboard passing ships.

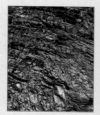

In this eastern part of the island, colourful semiprecious stones abound, from green quartz to black onyx and pink or pale-green beryl. The proper mineral name for most gem tourmalines is, in fact, "Elbaite".

In the resorts and mineralogical museums there are ample opportunities for picking up pieces of rock or clunky jewellery that are now the last link with Elba's mining past.

TIP

Capo Sant'Andrea makes a good base for hiking, mountain biking, birdwatching, sea kayaking, snorkelling and other outdoor activities in the northwest of the island. For more information, go to www.visitelba.com, a useful website run by the owner/manager of the Hotel Ilio, who is a keen promoter of eco-tourism on the island. The tourist office produces a booklet, *Walking in the National Park*, which describes walks in the area.

BELOW: smooth rocky platforms attract sunbathers.

and the plains behind Marina di Campo, the only part of the island flat enough for an airport.

The "Other Elba"

The northwestern corner of Elba is a protected area of wild, natural beauty, with granite cliffs, thick holm-oak and chestnut woods, and dense maquis. Dubbed the "Other Elba", this craggy corner attracts the active and eco-conscious. The sea here is ideal for snorkelling, diving and kayaking, while the mountains are exploited by mountain bikers, birdwatchers, trekkers and climbers. A long, winding road leads down past houses and hotels to **Capo Sant'Andrea** ❼, a tight bay with a small port protected from westerly winds by the surrounding cliffs. This is an ideal base for exploring the area, starting with the walk from Capo Sant'Andrea to the next bay at Cotoncello.

The coastal road from Sant'Andrea to Marina di Campo clings to the edge of the island, an exhilarating and occasionally heart-stopping drive. Wherever you see a cluster of parked cars, chances are there's a

rocky cove below, where those in the know gather to swim and sunbathe. This section of the coast is good for diving and snorkelling; most of the diving schools can be found in and around Pomonte.

As you round the southwestern corner, the first visible stretch of sand at **Fetovaia** comes into view – a pretty, child-friendly sweep of beach, edged by trees, that gets very crowded in summer. Between Fetovaia and Cavoli, another small, pleasant enough resort, the low rocks make perfect sunbathing platforms.

The south

With its expanse of golden sand, **Marina di Campo** ❽, in the south, is the largest, most buzzing resort on the island. While often overrun by German package tours in summer, it is still a good springboard to the medieval hamlets in the hills behind. Fortified by the Pisans in the 12th century, the hamlets of **San Piero in Campo** and San Ilario conceal Romanesque churches and hermitages.

Capoliveri ❾ is a traditional

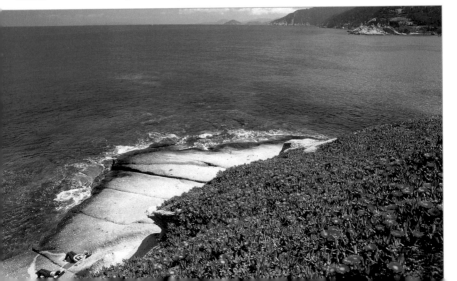

inland village, with a Roman and medieval past as dramatic as its location high on the southern promontory. Carved into the iron mountain of Monte Calamita, Capoliveri is also an ancient mining village, where the mineral-rich soil is ideal for the production of sweet red Aleatico, reputedly the favourite wine of Napoleon Bonaparte. Often independent, Capoliveri was the only village to reject Napoleon in 1814. The story is that only the intercession of a local beauty saved the village. It soon became part of Napoleon's hunting estate, and to this day is noted for its dishes of woodcock, pheasant and hare.

The hills are covered with heath, fern and juniper; the scent of thyme and rosemary are never far away. Roads from the hills to the sea often turn into cart tracks but are worth pursuing unless specifically marked *strada privata*; this is often the only access to the loveliest beaches.

Innamorata is a sandy inlet linked to the romance between a nymph and a fisherman. Believing her lover drowned in a shipwreck, the nymph drowned herself; he survived and asked the gods to turn him into a seagull so he could seek her out.

From the east to the interior

Capoliveri also surveys fashionable **Porto Azzurro** 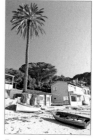, the main town on the east coast of Elba and once part of the Spanish protectorate. The vast Forte Longone, constructed in 1603 as a Spanish naval base, is now a top-security prison. Forte Focardo, its sister fortress across the bay, has uninviting ramparts running down a sheer cliff. By day, Porto Azzurro has a rather uninspiring seafront. In the evening, however, it comes to life with a leisurely promenade (the famous *passeggiata*), designer shopping and people-watching. It is also a top place for sampling seafood, including *cacciucco*, a seafood soup of octopus, scorpion fish, prawns and *riso nero* or "black rice" (risotto with dark cuttlefish ink), perhaps followed by *schiaccia briaca* ("drunken cake"), made with hazelnuts and Aleatico wine. After enough Elban wine, one's impressions of Porto Azzurro are of harbour lights, cheerful bustle and

Forno beach, on the Biodola Bay.

BELOW: the pretty resort of Marciana Marina.

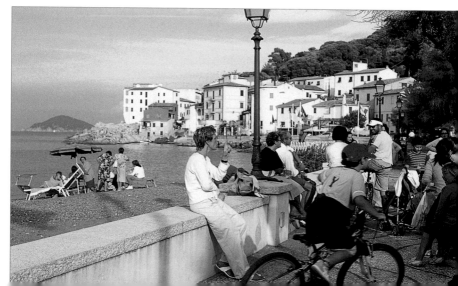

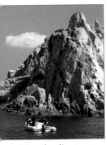

Divers heading to sea.

BELOW RIGHT: Portoferraio Lighthouse.

gently bobbing boats.

Behind Porto Azzurro is the most mystical spot on the island, the remote sanctuary of **Madonna di Monserrato** ⓫ (daily mid-July–mid-Sept, closed noon–3pm). It was built in the Toledan style by a Spanish governor, Ponce de León, in 1606. A steep, rocky track leads high up the mountain to the tiny red-domed church precariously balanced among the crags. Despite mountain goats cavorting on impossible ledges, the place has great solemnity and few visitors, and is the most important shrine on Elba. The Spanish facade and bell tower find echoes in the *Black Madonna* inside, which is a copy of an early Spanish painting. Every September, an Elban pilgrimage celebrates the Festa della Madonna with a walk past ravines and isolated grottoes to the church.

East of Portoferraio, the workaday town of **Rio Marina** ⓬ was once the centre of the mining activity. Surrounded by hills rich in ferrous oxide, the whole port has a pinkish hue, including the octagonal Pisan watchtower overlooking the harbour.

More than 700 mineral exhibits are on display in the **Museo Mineralogico** (tel: 0565-962 088; www.parcominelba.it; daily 9.30am–12.30pm, 4.30–6.30pm; charge). Only dedicated rock-hunters will continue to the **Parco Minerario**, set in a disused mine, where you can book a train tour or a hunt for minerals (book as above).

Inland, **Rio nell'Elba** is a strange, rather wild village perched on a couple of ledges among desolate mountain slopes and scattered remains of mines. A few kilometres west, on the road to Portoferraio, a steep road leads uphill to Volterraio and the ruins of an 11th-century Pisan fortress, perched on a rock.

From Rio nell'Elba to the small beach resort of **Cavo** in the northeast, the picturesque road cuts through woods and moorland. Paths trail through gorse, heather and the wild flowers of the maquis. Like the northwestern corner of the island, Elba's northeastern tip has quiet, unspoilt stretches of coast. Just north of Cavo, the remains of a Roman villa can be seen at Capo Castello. ❑

Archipelago

Elba is the largest island in a chain of seven between the Ligurian and Tyrrhenian seas, all loosely protected as part of the Arcipelago Toscano marine park. On a clear day, Pianosa, Gorgona, Montecristo and Capraia are visible from the island's highest reaches. Pianosa, just 14km (9 miles) from Elba, was a maximum-security prison until 1997 but is now a marine reserve. Gorgona, the smallest and most northerly island in the archipelago, is still a prison. Montecristo, 34km (21 miles) away, is a nature reserve, uninhabited but for its four guardians. So as not to disturb the fragile ecosystem, visitor numbers are restricted, but day trips are available from Porto Azzurro on Elba. Capraia, a miniature Elba without its history or architecture, is a two-hour ferry ride from Livorno and draws divers and those wishing to explore the marine grottoes.

Giglio, the second-largest island, and Giannutri are the southernmost islands. Giglio is popular with weekending Romans and divers. Both can be reached from Porto Santo Stefano on the Argentario peninsula. Frequent hydrofoils to Elba run from Piombino, on the mainland, to Rio Marina (45 minutes) or to Portoferraio (1 hour). See Toremar ferries at www.toremar.it and www.arcipelago.turismo.toscana.it.

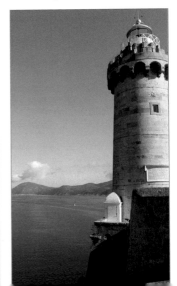

BEST RESTAURANTS

Restaurants

Prices for a three-course meal per person with a half-bottle of house wine:
€ = under €25
€€ = €25–40
€€€ = €40–60
€€€€ = over €60

Capo d'Enfola

Da Giacomino
Localita Viticcio
Tel/fax: 0565-915 381
www.ristorantedagiacomino.it
€–€€
A small, family-run trattoria, a short drive from the island capital. Sunsets from the terrace across the bay are memorable. Pizzas served in the evening. Closed Tue lunch, Oct–Easter.

Ristorante Emanuel
Porto di Sansone
Tel: 0565-939 003 €–€€
The road to Capo d'Enfola promontory ends at a pebble beach with a couple of restaurants. Emanuel is a good option for a snack lunch, and one of few places to offer a vegetarian menu. Closed Wed Sept–Oct and Nov–Easter.

Marciana Marina

Affrichella
Via Santa Chiara, 7
Tel: 0565-996 844 €€–€€€
Intimate restaurant, tucked down a backstreet away from the seafront

bustle, offering an inventive fish-based menu.

Borgo al Cotone
Via del Cotone 23
Tel: 0565-904 390 €€–€€€
Romantic harbourside restaurant where fish and shellfish come grilled and gratinated, or in more adventurous concoctions such as lasagne with chickpeas and clams. Closed Oct–early Mar.

Ristorante Capo Nord
Localita La Fenicia
Tel: 0565-996 983 €€€–€€€€
The island's top restaurant, where you will be fed exquisite Tuscan food by impeccably dressed and deferential waiters. Dress up and book. Ask for table 5 or 6. Closed Mon in autumn and Nov–Easter.

Marina di Campo

La Lucciola
Viale degli Eroi
Tel: 0565-976 395
www.lalucciola.it €€€
Brush the sand off your feet and step on to the wooden-decked terrace of this relaxed beach bar/restaurant, where you can enjoy a drink, a big summer salad, or go for the catch of the day. Closed Tue and mid-Apr–Oct. Booking recommended.

Poggio/Marciana Alta

Publius
Via della Madonna 18

Tel: 0565-901 284 €€–€€€
Nestled on the mountainside, Publius has a well-established reputation on the island, and offers fine views from the terrace. Elban wines, fish and game dishes. Closed Mon.

Porto Azzurro

I Quattro Gatti
Piazza del Mercato 4
Tel: 0565-95240 €€–€€€
A cosy and convivial restaurant decorated with copper pots, beaded lamps, old wirelesses and other knick-knacks. The menu is equally eclectic, with offerings such as herrings with apple, carpaccio of cod and fish ravioli. In a resort town full of bright

and brash restaurants, this is a real find. Closed Mon in low season.

Portoferraio

Da Lido
Salita Falcone 2
Tel: 0565-914 650 €€
Set back from the port area, this consistently good and constantly bustling trattoria is one of Portoferraio's best. Closed Sun in low season, mid-Dec–mid-Feb.

Osteria Libertaria
Calata Matteotti 12
Tel: 0565-914 978 €–€€
Traditional inn overlooking the marina. Grab one of the two outdoor bench tables and watch the boating bustle over a pasta or fish dish. Daily Apr–Nov. Best to book.

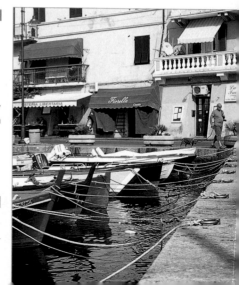

RIGHT: boats moored at Isola d'Elba.

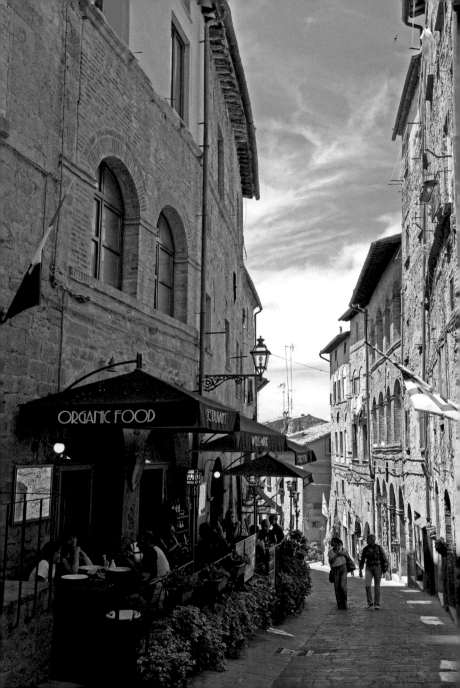

VOLTERRA AND MASSA MARITTIMA

Perched on a windy plateau overlooking the Sienese hills, Volterra remains the most Etruscan of cities. The scenery sweeps from dry and desolate crags to the dense, eerie forests of the "Metal-bearing Mountains" – south to engaging Massa Marittima, the gateway to the Maremma

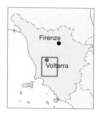

One of the most important towns in Tuscany is **Volterra ❶**, which has a richly layered history with abundant evidence of its 3,000 years of civilisation. It commands a majestic, windswept position on a steep ridge 545 metres (1,780ft) above sea level. Walking round the ancient fortifications is an excellent way to view the medieval town, the Roman and Etruscan walls, and the wide sweep of countryside below.

Volterra was the Etruscan city-state of Velathri, one of the confederation of 12 city-states that made up Etruria. It became an important Roman municipality (Volterrae) when Rome annexed Etruria in 351 BC. It followed the new faith of Christianity, and at the fall of the Roman Empire, AD 476, it was already the centre of a vast diocese.

The modern city of Volterra sits within the walls of a much larger Etruscan predecessor. Wherever archaeologists dig in the city, they turn up new treasures. Sometimes they do not even need to dig, since parts of the city, built on tufa and undermined by subterranean springs, have been slipping slowly down the hillside for centuries, revealing the remains of an extensive necropolis.

Exploring Volterra

The **Porta all'Arco** (the Arch Gate) is the best-preserved Etruscan gateway in Italy, dating from the 4th century BC (though partly rebuilt by the Romans in the 1st century BC), with sides of huge rectangular stone blocks and three mysterious carved basalt heads above the gateway, thought to represent Etruscan gods.

From the arch, a pretty road winds its way uphill to the **Piazza dei Priori**. Evidence of the Middle Ages is to be found both in Volterra's

Main attractions

PIAZZA DEI PRIORI, VOLTERRA
PALAZZO INCONTRI-VITI, VOLTERRA
MUSEO ETRUSCO GUARNACCI, VOLTERRA
TEATRO ROMANO, VOLTERRA
LE BALZE
COLLINE METALLIFERE
PIAZZA GARIBALDI, MASSA MARITTIMA
MASSA MARITTIMA DUOMO
CITTA NUOVA, MASSA MARITTIMA
MUSEO DELLA MINIERA, MASSA MARITTIMA
ABBAZIA DI SAN GALGANO

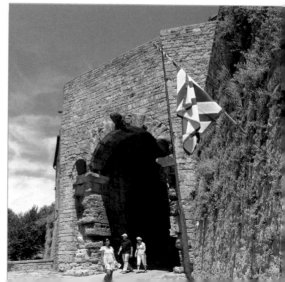

LEFT: restaurants on Via d'Arco, Volterra.
RIGHT: Porta all'Arco

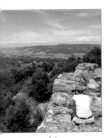

A view of the countryside from Volterra's walls.

BELOW: a 13th-century lion stands guard outside the Palazzo dei Priori.

urban structure and in its buildings, the most important of which are clustered around the main square. It is dominated by the tall **Palazzo dei Priori** (1208), the oldest town hall in Tuscany, and said to be the model for Florence's Palazzo Vecchio. Across the square is the 13th-century **Palazzo Pretorio**, with its crenellated Torre del Porcellino (Tower of the Little Pig), named after its decorative relief of a boar. On the square, call into the wonderfully helpful tourist office (tel: 0588-87257) to pick up the Volterra audioguide. It is a model of its kind, providing judicious background on all the main sights, visited at your own pace.

To the south of the square, Via Turrazza leads to the 12th-century **Duomo** (Piazza San Giovanni; daily 7am–12.30pm, winter 2–6pm, summer 7am–7pm; free), which boasts works of art from the Middle Ages to the Renaissance. The sculpture of *The Deposition* is an extremely rare Romanesque woodcarving, simple in execution but bursting with pathos and drama.

The bishop's palace next door is now the **Museo d'Arte Sacra** (Via Roma; daily 9am–1pm, 3–6pm, Nov–mid-Mar 9am–1pm; charge), a collection of gold reliquaries, church bells, illuminated manuscripts and some 13th-century sculptures of the Sienese school. The octagonal **Baptistery** opposite has an elegant marble doorway with a fine baptismal font sculpted by Sansovino.

As you head back towards the square, take Via Roma to Via Buonparenti and the Pisan-style **Casa Torre Buonparenti**, a pair of Gothic tower-houses.

At the top of Via Buonparenti, the **Pinacoteca e Museo Civico** in Palazzo Minucci-Solaini (daily 9am–7pm, winter 8.30am–1.30pm; charge) displays valuable paintings of the Sienese and Florentine schools, including an *Annunciation*

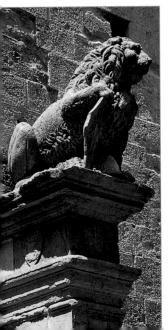

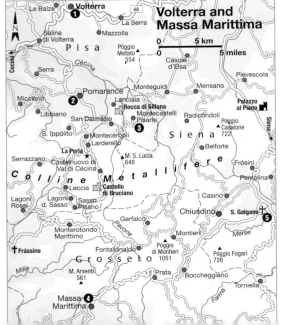

by Signorelli and *Christ in Glory* by Ghirlandaio. The most famous painting in the collection is a masterly *Deposition from the Cross* by Rosso Fiorentino (1495–1540).

The **Palazzo Incontri-Viti**, on Via dei Sarti (tel: 0588-84047; Apr–Oct 10am–1pm, 2.30–6pm, winter by appointment only; charge), is an impressive mansion whose facade is attributed to Ammannati, who worked on the Palazzo Pitti in Florence. Each salon is grander than the one before, adorned with art, porcelain and alabaster objects, a reminder that the palace once belonged to an alabaster merchant, whose heirs still live here. Renaissance buildings like these blend in surprisingly gracefully with the medieval Volterran houses. After exploring the patrician palaces, retreat to **Le Cantine**, the ancient cellars below Palazzo Incontri-Viti, for a drink in a cavern-like bar that contains a Roman cistern *(see page 197)*.

The Etruscan museum and Roman theatre

The best of the city's ancient treasures are displayed in the **Museo Etrusco Guarnacci** (Via Don Minzoni; daily 9am–7pm; 8.30am–1.30pm Nov–mid-Mar; charge). This is packed with ancient Etruscan funerary urns, proof that Volterra has some of the best Etruscan art outside Rome. The alabaster sarcophagi run the gamut of Etruscan demonology and Greek mythology, featuring sea monsters, Greek gods, griffins and sirens. *The Married Couple* urn is a masterpiece of realistic portraiture, but even more stunning is the bronze statuette known as *L'Ombra della Sera* (*The Shadow of the Evening*). Resembling a Giacometti sculpture but cast in the 5th century BC, this enigmatic elongated figure does indeed resemble the shadow of a boy thrown by the low beams of the setting sun. It blurs immortality and mortality in true Etruscan fashion.

After focusing so much on death, it's definitely a case of *carpe diem*: feast on Tuscan dishes in **Del Duca** *(see page 197)*. Naturally, the restaurant terrace is built below the walls of the Etruscan acropolis. The spirit of the enigmatic Etruscans will accompany you throughout your stay in Volterra. Like the mystical *Shadow of the Evening* sculpture, the Etruscans knew how to live as well as how to die.

Volterra is dominated at its highest point by the **Fortezza Medicea**, a magnificent example of Renaissance military architecture – today it serves as a top-security prison. Intriguingly, the prisoners perform plays of a professional standard every summer but, to watch them, visitors need a certificate stating that they have no criminal record, which is not easily come by.

Nearby, on the site of the former Etruscan acropolis, the **Parco Archeologico** (summer daily 10.30am–5.30pm, winter weekends only 10am–4pm; charge) is an ideal spot for a picnic.

On the north side of town, just

TIP

Walk along the remains of Volterra's Etruscan walls, at the northwestern edge of town, for lovely views at sunset.

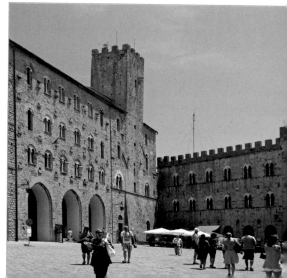

BELOW: Piazza dei Priori.

The mountains south of Volterra are rich in metal ores, and for centuries provided Tuscany with the precious commodities of silver, copper, lead and zinc. However, by the end of the 19th century, mining and related industries had fallen into decline and now these hills are a remote and lonely region. The ruins of mines and factories engulfed in thick forest littered with heaps of coloured metals present a surreal picture.

below the city walls, is the excavated **Teatro Romano** (summer daily 10.30am–5.30pm, winter weekends only 10am–4pm; free), the impressive remains of a complex built during the reign of Augustus, behind which lie the ruins of a 3rd-century Roman bathhouse. One of the loveliest walks runs along the city walls, from Porta Fiorentina to Piazza Minucci, and affords compelling views of the theatre below.

Le Balze

The countryside around Volterra is one of gentle, undulating hills, interrupted in the west by the wild and awe-inspiring spectacle of abrupt crevasses known as **Le Balze** (The Crags). Over the centuries, these deep gullies, created by the continual erosion of layers of sand and clay, have swallowed up churches and settlements along with Etruscan and early Christian remains. Today, an 11th-century abbey, the Badia, sits on a precipice, awaiting its inevitable fate. For the perfect view of this dramatic landscape, exit through the western San Francesco Gate, passing

the Borgo San Giusto and its remains until you reach Le Balze campsite (a 20-minute walk).

Metal mountains

The terrain south of Volterra goes from the crags of Le Balze to the dense, eerie forests of the "Metal-bearing Mountains". The wide vistas of the dry, desolate terrain just south of town seem a world away from the cosy green hills of Chianti. In a remote area without significant sights, it is the journey that counts, an elemental voyage through a disconcertingly untamed Tuscany of gullies, mining gashes and belching fumaroles. Geothermic geeks will be in their element, but so, too, will open-minded adventurers. Fortunately, at either end of this surreal journey, whether Volterra or Massa Marittima, the cities are as beguiling and warmly welcoming as any in Tuscany.

At Saline di Volterra, an industrial suburb that developed around its salt mine, the SS439 leads south to Massa Marittima and the coast, cutting through the **Colline Metallifere**,

Alabaster Workshops

Like everything in Volterra, alabaster carving is an Etruscan legacy. It is one of the many gifts the Etruscans have passed on to their descendants in this most Etruscan of cities. The ancient craftsmen made great use of alabaster from the 5th century BC onwards, primarily for their beautifully sculpted funerary urns.

Visit the Etruscan Museum before looking at alabaster *objets d'art in situ*, beginning with the grand collection created by Giuseppe Viti, the city's foremost alabaster merchant in the 19th century. Viti travelled the world to present his wares and, in India, sold his alabaster to the local rajah and, bizarrely, was then made Emir of Nepal. **Palazzo Incontri-Viti** displays superb pieces, including the grand candelabra in the ballroom, made for Emperor Maximilian, who was shot in 1867 before he could collect them.

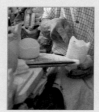

Alabaster is sold in Volterra's workshops, as well as being exported. One of the most respected alabaster-crafting firms is the family-run **Alabastri Lavorati Italiani** (Ali, Piazza Martiri della Liberta; tel: 058-8860 78; www.alabastro.it). Its showroom is the most elegant in town. Choose from lamps, sculpture, figurines, chess pieces, table tops, picture frames: so much can be carved from alabaster. Prices depend on the type, colour and veining of the alabaster, with colours ranging from creamy white to murky yellow. Visit one of the last remaining traditional alabaster craftsmen in his cramped workshop; **Giuliano Ducceschi** (Via Porta all'Arco 59) has been carving owls and fish, his favourite subjects, since the 1950s, and will continue until he drops. Also call in at the alabaster museum, the **Ecomuseo dell'Alabastro** (Piazzetta Minucci, 11am–5pm, winter until 1pm; tel: 058-8875 80; charge).

or Metal-bearing Hills. Beyond the Upper Cecina valley, dense forests of chestnut, beech and oak are punctuated by fumaroles, cooling towers and gleaming silver pipelines, making for a strange and distinctly un-Tuscan picture.

The first noteworthy town on this surreal route is **Pomarance ❷**, which retains vestiges of its prosperous past, including medieval town gates and the Romanesque church of San Giovanni. A short walk away, Via Roncalli is home to the **Bicocchi Museum** (summer Thur and Sun 3.30–6.30pm; charge), a lavish early 19th-century home, whose decorations evoke the lifestyle of the wealthy mine-owning families. A little further along the road is the hamlet of **San Dalmazio**, and a short but steep walk (2km/1¼ miles) that culminates in commanding views from the ruins of the 11th-century castle, **Rocca di Sillana**.

Across the valley, the medieval hamlet of **Montecastelli Pisano ❸** is dominated by the Torre dei Pannocchieschi. Like the Rocca Sillana, this fortified settlement was a pawn on the Tuscan chessboard, finally won by the Florentines in the 16th century. Follow the signs to **Castelnuovo Val di Cecina** and the "Buca delle Fate", a small but well-preserved 6th-century BC Etruscan tomb, just outside the village.

The road south from Montecastelli Pisano offers the best views of the medieval village of Castelnuovo Val di Cecina, which commands a steep ridge surrounded by woodland. A short walk east of the village leads through chestnut groves and down to the River Pavone, where you can swim in the rock pools, overlooked by two medieval bridges.

Steaming fumaroles

At the heart of this vast geothermic area, the industrial village of **Larderello** has been valued for its healing spring waters for centuries. But unless you're into industrial archaeology, move swiftly on to see geothermal activity in its more elemental form.

South along a back road from Larderello lie the hamlets of **Leccia** and **Sasso Pisano**, the latter of which commands a rocky outcrop

TIP

There are some excellent walks in the Forestali Berignone-Tatti, near Pomarance, especially in the autumn, when the leaves of the sweet chestnut turn golden-yellow and the forest becomes carpeted with bright pink cyclamen. Bicycle tours and horse-riding excursions can be booked through Pomarance's tourist office (in the car park on the SS439).

BELOW: the ruins of the Roman theatre.

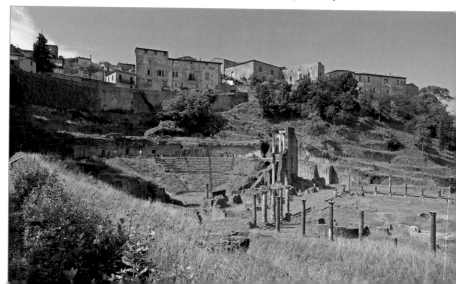

TIP

A memorable experience – and a lot easier to see than Siena's Palio – is the traditional Balestro del Girifalco, every last Sunday in May and every second Sunday in August. The *terzieri* of Massa (old city, new city and the outer Borgo) hold a shooting contest using mechanical falcons with ancient crossbows.

above the Cornia River. The hamlets are linked by a narrow, winding route that cuts through a landscape of steaming fumaroles. Just outside Leccia are the ancient baths of **Bagnone**, a vast Etruscan-Roman complex from the 3rd century BC. The craggy medieval village of **Sasso Pisano** is a strangely appealing place, often shrouded in clouds of steam from the surrounding fumaroles, and the air is heavy with the smell of sulphur. The road through the village leads back to the SS439.

As the main road winds south towards Massa Marittima, it climbs up steeply wooded hillsides to the summits of the Colline Metallifere. It is an area of outstanding natural beauty, with dense forest and large open views across to Maremma and the Gulf of Follonica; on a fine day, the islands of Elba and Corsica can be clearly seen.

Massa Marittima

Massa Marittima ❹ is about 24km (15 miles) inland, despite its maritime name. It is one of the most astounding Tuscan cities, perched

on top of a high hill on the edge of the Colline Metallifere. Although its relative remoteness from "picture-postcard Tuscany" has resulted in far fewer visitors than it deserves, Massa Marittima is finally coming into its own. This underrated gem has preserved its gorgeous medieval core as well as gracious palaces, authentic regional restaurants, and a clutch of fine museums.

Massa Marittima grew up in the 10th century, after the decline of ancient Populonia *(see page 177)*, which was too exposed to coastal malaria and plundering by pirates.

Massa, once the second city of the Sienese Republic, prospered from copper and silver mines exploited since Etruscan times. Although the proud city spiralled into centuries of decline when the mines failed and malaria returned, its stagnation has proved a joy for visitors today. Massa feels authentic, harmonious, a picture of urban refinement.

The city's old republican pride is reflected in the concentration of public buildings around the cathedral. In the main square – the

BELOW LEFT: Larderello, at the centre of geothermic activity. **BELOW RIGHT:** Campanile della Cattedrale, Massa Marittima.

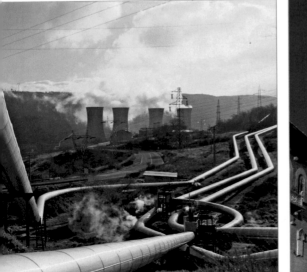

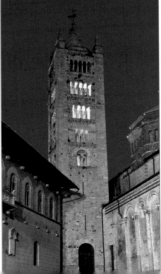

spectacular **Piazza Garibaldi**, one of the finest squares in Tuscany – are Palazzo Vescovile (seat of the bishop); Palazzo del Podestà (seat of the governor, now an archaeological museum); Palazzo del Comune (town hall); Zecca Cittadina (the mint); Fonte Pubblica (public fountain); and Palazzo dell'Abbondanza (the public granary). Set on a pedestal, the Pisan-Romanesque **Duomo** boasts Gothic windows and marvellous reliefs of the *Madonna delle Grazie*, ascribed to Duccio di Buoninsegna (1316), as well as the *Arca di San Cerbone* (St Cerbone's Ark), a Sienese sculptural masterpiece. Return to the theatrical square in the evening, when you can drink or dine while admiring the cathedral facade by moonlight.

Leave the old **Citta Vecchia** area around the Cathedral for the so-called **Citta Nuova**, hardly new despite its name. The quaint **Via Moncini** climbs to this Gothic quarter clustered behind Sienese fortifications, and ends in Piazza Matteotti, beside the medieval clock tower, the **Torre del Candaliere**. Nearby, on

Corso Diaz, is the **Museo di Arte Sacra** (Apr–Sept Tue–Sun 10am–1pm, Oct–Mar 11am–1pm, 3–5pm; charge). This delightful museum of sacred art is in the equally lovely complex of San Pietro all'Orta, a frescoed Romanesque-Gothic monastery. The art reflects Massa's period of medieval glory, with the highlight being Lorenzetti's *Maesta*, the Madonna in Glory. Sculptures taken from the cathedral facade are also on display here. Virtually next door is the intimate church of **San Agostino** and the **Museo Santa Cecilia** (tel: 05669-40282; variable opening times; charge), which is more engaging for its mood and architecture than for its treasures on display.

There are two mining-related museums in town, with the best being the **Museo della Miniera** in Via Corridoni, a short walk from the cathedral (tel: 0566-902 289; Tue–Sun, Apr–Sept 10am–5.30pm; guided tours; charge). Set in natural galleries and medieval mineshafts, this atmospheric mining museum saw service as an air-raid shelter in World War II. The child-friendly

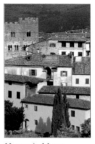

Houses in Massa Marittima.

BELOW: the landscape around Volterra.

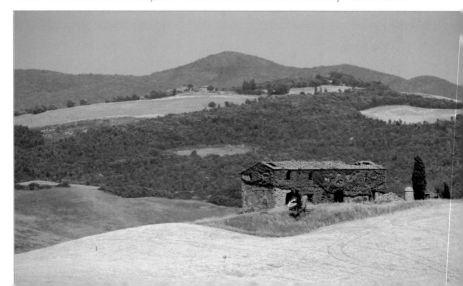

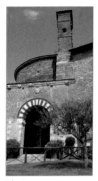

The Romanesque Cappella di Montesiepi.

tour passes wagons, pneumatic drills and munitions stores as it burrows deeper into the rock. The small display of minerals is a reminder that medieval Massa grew prosperous thanks to the discovery of silver and copper deposits nearby, followed by the mining of pyrites, found in veins of quartz.

Gothic ruin

Heading east from Massa Marittima along the Siena road leads to the Gothic ruins of **Abbazia di San Galgano 5** (8am–11pm), best seen when the setting sun sends shafts of light through its windows. This roofless abbey, with grass for a nave and fragments of frescoes clinging to crumbling walls, feels a mystical spot. Once the finest French Gothic abbey in Tuscany, San Galgano is now a noble ruin, albeit one tended by Olivetan nuns, who allow concerts to be staged here in summer. Consecrated in 1288, the abbey of San Galgano was the Cistercian mother abbey that held sway over central Italy. Its abbot arbitrated in disputes between city-states, while

its monks oversaw the building of Siena Cathedral. In the mid-14th century, the abbey was ransacked by the English mercenary Sir John Hawkwood – an attack sanctioned by the Pope, who was fearful of the Order's influence. Decline set in and by 1576, San Galgano was occupied by one solitary monk "who didn't even wear a robe". A lightning strike during Mass in 1778 saw the collapse of the campanile and signalled the last service at San Galgano. Although it sounded the death knell for the abbey, San Galgano, like its mystical founder, never gives up the ghost.

On the neighbouring hillock is the circular Romanesque **Cappella di Montesiepi**, built on the spot where St Galgano had a vision and renounced soldiering to become a hermit, thrusting his sword into a rock. The sword remains in the church, protruding from the rock. The bizarre event is illustrated by the frescoes of Ambrogio Lorenzetti that adorn the adjoining chapel walls.

Siena is about 35km (22 miles) distant on the SS73.   ❏

The "Twilight" Tour

Ever since Stephanie Meyer set her bestselling vampire novel in Volterra, droves of "vampire-ologists" have been visiting. The *Twilight* saga has sold millions of copies worldwide and *New Moon*, the second in the series, depicts the fictional home of the Volturi, a coven of elite vampires. Even if neighbouring Montepulciano was chosen for the filming (it has a larger main square), Volterra was the inspiration for the melodrama. Wildly popular vampire tours now visit the Piazza dei Priori where the heroine, Bella, rushes to save Edward, her vampire love. With its stern clock tower, the vampires' den can seem suitably chilling after dark.

The tour is not just for impressionable teenage girls, but is also a surreal way of discovering the dark side of Volterra, including candlelit caverns where you come face to face with cloaked vampires. In a secret wine bar with an Etruscan well you can drink local red wine masquerading as blood. Even if Volterra is probably vampire-free, a particular bronze in the Etruscan Museum would suggest otherwise – *The Shadow of the Evening* is reminiscent of the long shadow cast by a person at twilight.

(Book a vampire tour through the tourist office or tel: 058-8860 99; www.newmoonofficialtour.com; and www.volteratur.it).

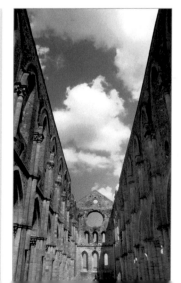

BEST RESTAURANTS

Restaurants

Prices for a three-course meal per person with a half-bottle of house wine:
€ = under €25
€€ = €25–40
€€€ = €40–60
€€€€ = over €60

Volterra

Le Cantine del Palazzo
Via dei Sarti
Tel: 0588-80033 €–€€
The moody wine cellars below Palazzo Viti are used for wine tasting and light meals (of Sienese salami, pecorino cheese and bruschette) in a labyrinth that includes an Etruscan well and a Roman cistern. The adjoining (slightly overpriced) restaurant has a courtyard overlooking the Roman theatre.

Del Duca
Via di Castello 2
Tel: 0588-81510 €€–€€€
The city's best restaurant is in a medieval building at the foot of an Etruscan acropolis, with wine cellars carved into the tufa walls. The menu celebrates Volterran specialities and features local truffles, stuffed pasta, Tuscan T-bone steaks. Barbecue in the courtyard garden every Wed.

Il Pozzo Degli Etruschi
Via delle Prigioni 28-30

Tel: 0588-80608
www.ilpozzodeglietruschi.com €
The simple medieval backdrop of this appealing eatery is echoed in the unpretentious and delicious Tuscan fare. In summer the shady inner courtyard is also open for dining. Closed Fri.

Osteria Il Ponte
Via Massetana, San Lorenzo (5km/X miles southwest of Volterra)
Tel: 0588-44160 €
Good, traditional home cooking in this welcoming inn that also serves snacks. Closed Tue.

La Vecchia Lira
Via Matteotti
Tel: 0588-86180 €–€€
Justifiably popular rustic-looking spot on the main street: it's a good quality self-service place at lunchtime but a proper restaurant in the evening. Friendly staff and a varied selection of regional dishes, ranging from grilled meats to *cacciucco* and *baccala alla livornese* (dried salted cod Livorno-style).

Massa Marittima

Il Brillo Parlante
Vicolo del Ciambellano 4
Tel: 0566-901 274 €€€
The best way to approach a meal in this tiny restaurant – there are just four tables – is to ask what's available. The dishes are

lovingly prepared and seasonal, and there's a good selection of fine wines. Booking essential. Closed Wed.

Le Mura
Via Norma Parenti 7
Tel: 0566-940 055 €€€
This large and busy restaurant has panoramic views towards Follonica and Elba, from both inside and out. The extensive menu incorporates typical Tuscan ingredients from the nearby wooded hills and fresh seafood from the coast beyond. Closed Tue.

Osteria Da Tronca
Vicolo Porte 5
Tel: 0566-901 991 €€
A reasonably priced and popular family-run restaurant offering simple,

well-prepared dishes cooked to traditional recipes. Booking recommended. Closed Wed.

I Tre Archi
Piazza Garibaldi
Tel: 0566-902 274 €
Gaze at the cathedral and medieval mansions from the terrace. In winter, retreat to the vaulted brick interior. A straightforward Tuscan menu that includes good pizzas.

Trattoria Dei Cavalieri
Via Norma Parenti 35
Tel: 0566-902 093/395 €€
This friendly restaurant is both value for money and a joy to be in. Local dishes such as *tortelli maremmani*, pasta and seafood, predominate. Booking advisable.

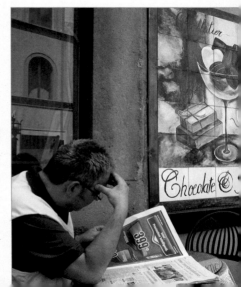

RIGHT: outside a café in Volterra.

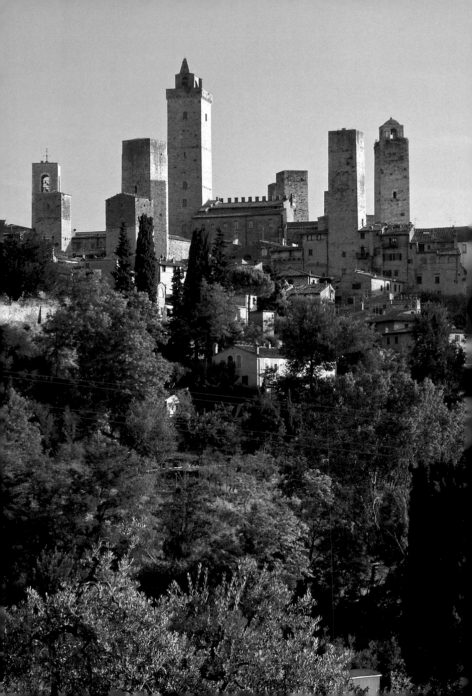

SAN GIMIGNANO AND CHIANTI COUNTRY

This is quintessential Tuscany, taking in the medieval "skyscrapers" of San Gimignano, the quaint hill town of Certaldo, and the rolling hills between Siena and Florence – the harmonious vineyards, villas and wine estates dotted along the Chianti trail

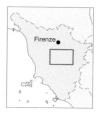

Famous for the sculptural quality of its skyline, **San Gimignano ❶** is a spectacular sight. It may be a cliché to call this hill town a "Medieval Manhattan", but the famous towers do resemble miniature skyscrapers. Seen from inside, it is the unspoilt townscape that bowls you over: almost nothing seems to have changed since the Middle Ages. In its heyday, the city had a total of 76 towers, only 14 of which remain. After San Gimignano fell under Florentine control, it became an economic backwater, bypassed by the Renaissance – for which we are eternally grateful.

Exploring San Gimignano

The towers are concentrated around the **Piazza del Duomo** and **Piazza della Cisterna**, which is teeming with tourists all year round. The towers alone make a visit here worthwhile, but the town abounds in quirky sights, even if staying overnight is the only way to appreciate this medieval time capsule in peace.

The Romanesque **Collegiata** (Apr–Oct Mon–Fri 10am–7pm, Sat 10am–5pm, Sun 12.30–7pm, Feb–Mar Mon–Sat 10am–4.30pm, Sun 12.30–4.30pm but no visits during Mass;

closed otherwise; combined ticket for most town attractions) will detain you longest, as every inch of wall space is covered in frescoes. The north aisle has Bartolo di Fredi's dramatic scenes from the Old Testament (1367), while the opposite aisle has Lippo Memmi's *Life of Christ* (1333–41) and the nave the *Last Judgement* by Taddeo di Bartolo (1393–6). Contrast these Gothic-style narrative paintings with Ghirlandaio's lyrical Renaissance frescoes (1475) on the life of a local saint, in the chapel of Santa Fina.

Main attractions

SAN GIMIGNANO CITYSCAPE
COLLEGIATA, SAN GIMIGNANO
MUSEO CIVICO, SAN GIMIGNANO
CERTALDO
MONTERIGGIONI
GREVE
RADDA IN CHIANTI
BADIA A COLTIBUONO
GAIOLE IN CHIANTI
CASTELLO DI BROLIO

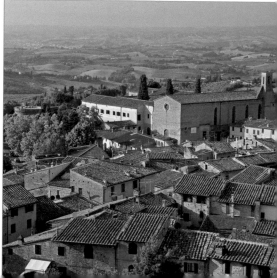

LEFT: San Gimignano's towers. **RIGHT:** Chiesa di Sant'Agostino, San Gimignano.

TIP

To see San Gimignano at its best, stay overnight in one of the characteristic hotels. Then you can savour the peaceful beauty of the town in the evening and early morning, after the coach-trippers have gone.

Four museums

Next to the Collegiata, the **Museo d'Arte Sacra** (Apr–Oct Mon–Fri 9.30am–7pm, Sat 9.30am–5pm, Sun 12.30–5pm, Nov–Mar Mon–Sat 9.30am–4.30pm, Sun opens at 12.30pm; closed late Jan and late Nov; combined ticket) contains a variety of sacred art from the 13th to the 15th century.

Alongside is the **Museo Civico** (daily Mar–Oct 9.30am–7pm, Nov–Feb 10am–5.30pm; combined ticket), housed in the Palazzo del Popolo, a forbidding fortress that served as the town hall. Completed in 1311, its tower, the **Torre Grossa** (daily 930am–7pm), is the tallest in the town (54 metres/175ft) and the only one you can climb; the views of the Val d'Elsa from the top are spectacular. Among the museum's many good paintings is a set of early 14th-century frescoes by Memmo di Filippucci – rare in that they depict secular rather than religious scenes. Known as the

Wedding Frescoes, they show a young bride and groom sharing a bath and climbing into their nuptial bed – an intimate glimpse into the private life of medieval Italy.

On Via Folgore, the former convent of Santa Chiara is now home to the **Museo Archeologico** (daily 11am–5.45pm; combined ticket). Fascinating exhibits range from Etruscan finds to a 16th-century pharmacy displaying ceramic and glass vessels designed for herbal remedies and healing lotions and potions.

The nearby **Piazza della Cisterna** is a lovely triangular space with a 13th-century well and medieval palazzi. East of the square, on Via di Castello, is the **Museo della Tortura** (daily 9.30am–7.30pm, winter Sat–Sun 10am–6pm; charge), with a gruesome collection of medieval instruments of torture.

Every church in San Gimignano offers some reward, but perhaps the best is **Sant'Agostino** (Apr–Oct

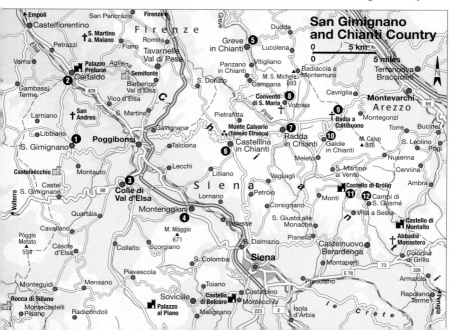

daily 7am–noon, 3–7pm, Mar, Nov–Dec until 6pm, late Jan–Feb Tue–Sun 10am–noon, 3–6pm, Mon pm only; free) to the north of the town (near Porta San Matteo). Here, in Gozzoli's faded frescoes on the *Life of St Augustine* (1465), you will find the same love of colour, rich clothing and exact portraiture as in Gozzoli's other frescoes, notably in *The Journey of the Magi* in the Palazzo Medici Riccardi in Florence.

On Via Berignano, call into the **Museo di San Gimignano** (tel: 057-7941 078; 8am–8pm but times can vary; charge). The museum seeks to show how the city was in its 13th-century heyday, with reconstructions of the 72 tower-houses, fortifications, churches and convents. But what is remarkable is how much of this medieval cityscape remains in San Gimignano today.

A short walk along the city walls to the 14th-century fortress before leaving is worthwhile. This semi-derelict **Rocca** has views over tiered gardens and olive groves winding down to the Vernaccia vineyards, which produce the famous white wine that was even mentioned in Dante's *The Divine Comedy*. Just beyond the fortress, the **Museo del Vino** (tel: 057-7941 267; daily 11.30am–6.30pm; free) is the place to sample a range of local wines.

The Val d'Elsa

A few kilometres north of San Gimignano, the windswept medieval hill town of **Certaldo ②** straddles the summit of a steep hill. To reach it, park in the unprepossessing lower town, Certaldo Basso, and take the funicular up the steep slope to the delightful upper town, which is closed to traffic. Certaldo Alto is a literary landmark as it was the home of Giovanni Boccaccio (1313–75), author of *The Decameron*, who died here in 1375. What is thought to have been his home was restored in 1823, bombed during World War II, and has now been rebuilt as the recently restored **Casa di Boccaccio** (daily summer 10am–1.30pm, 2.30–7pm, winter closes at 4.30pm; charge). An allegorical garden, inspired by *The Decameron*, has recently been created here. Featuring a marble fountain, and dotted with references to

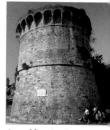

One of five circular towers along San Gimignano's city walls.

BELOW: Piazza del Duomo at dusk.

Medieval Manhattan

San Gimignano's towers were built in the 12th and 13th centuries by the *magnati*, or nobles, during the Guelf-Ghibelline conflicts. As well as defending the city, they served as status symbols: the higher the tower, the richer and more powerful its owner. The local 14th-century poet Folgore described the "earthly pleasures" he encountered in the city, including "silk sheets, sugared nuts, sweets and sparkling wine". The arrival of the Black Death in 1348 put an end to silk sheets in San Gimignano until the 20th century. While more civilised cities were exchanging towers for palazzi, this medieval backwater destroyed nothing and built nothing. The city's misfortune has made it the best-preserved medieval city in Tuscany.

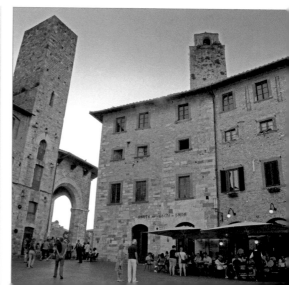

The Nectar of the Gods

Delightfully torn between tradition and creativity – like the contradictory Tuscans themselves – the wine scene allows for a duality between provenance and personality

"The know-how in the vineyards today compared with even a decade ago, is phenomenal," claims Lamberto Frescobaldi, whose Florentine family has been in the wine business for 700 years. For all its history, Tuscany remains at the forefront of the wine industry, which is still dominated by many of the original noble families. Wine-growing dates back to Etruscan times, as evidenced by the goblet found in an Etruscan tomb at Castellina in Chianti, and surviving Etruscan frescoes that depict Bacchus, the Roman god of wine. Medieval monasteries established viticulture here – where Badia a Coltibuono and Antinori's Badia a Passignano remain beguiling wine estates today.

In the mid-19th-century, Barone Bettino Ricasoli capitalised on improvements in production and spearheaded the modernisation of wine-making, with the establishment of the Chianti Classico brand. Since then, a consortium, the Consorzio Chianti Classico, controls production, with the *gallo nero* (black cockerel) emblem guaranteeing quality. (Try Barone Ricasoli Castello di Brolio Chianti Classico 2006.)

To some outsiders, Tuscany is still synonymous with Chianti – to the chagrin of the region's other fine red-wine producers. Situated between Florence and Siena, the Chianti Classico heartland includes Barberino Val d'Elsa, Castellina, Greve, Gaiole, and San Casciano. However, the top Tuscan red is arguably Brunello di Montalcino, made from Sangiovese grapes grown on hillsides south of Siena. Brunello is a powerful yet refined red that ages superbly, with Rosso di Montalcino its more approachable younger sister, and the "princely" Vino Nobile di Montepulciano, loved by princes and popes since Medici times. Brunello is bouncing back after the "Brunellogate" scandal in 2008 that saw certain producers illegally blend in non-Sangiovese grapes.

The wines of the Maremma are increasingly fashionable, and mostly made with Bordeaux varieties such as Cabernet Sauvignon, Franc and Merlot. These elegant wines have a crispness rarely found in New World Cabernets or Merlots. Around Bolgheri, look out for great names such as Sassicaia and Ornellaia. Antinori Solaia, Frescobaldi Giramonte, Sette Ponti Oreno and d'Alessandro Syrah are other superb "Super-Tuscans". Detractors claim that Super Tuscans lack a sense of place and are overpriced. Fans retort that these wines express the true creativity of the wine maker. The debate between native and French varieties pits provenance against personality, a sense of place against the creativity of the wine maker.

Follow your nose: if Bordeaux blends don't appeal, there is ample choice among native grape varieties. That's without mentioning Vernaccia di San Gimignano, the characteristic white wine – crisp, full-bodied, golden-hued, and popular since Dante's day. Or dipping almond cantuccini biscuits into Vin Santo, Tuscany's amber-hued dessert wine: nectar of the gods indeed.   ❑

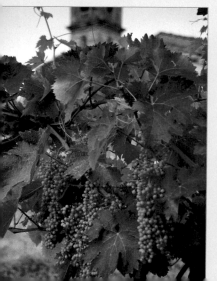

LEFT: vineyard below San Gimignano.

Boccaccio, the garden is used for concerts and film screenings.

The red-brick town is crowned by the castellated **Palazzo Pretorio**, whose 15th-century facade is studded with terracotta coats of arms. Any wandering will reveal impressive medieval gateways that lead down to steep, narrow-approach lanes. If hungry, stop at the **Palazzo del Vicario** (summer daily 9.30am–2pm, 2.30–7pm, winter until 4.30pm; charge). This frescoed, former monastery is now a delightful hotel and a Michelin-starred restaurant. Also be sure to drop into **Giuseppina** (Via del Castello 34, tel: 057-1650 242; www.cucinagiuseppina. com) to sample and buy local produce. It's worth booking a taster class in the eponymous owner's authentic cookery school, where you can learn how to make *ribollita* soup, Sienese *pici* pasta or crunchy almond cantuccini biscuits. The chef, Giuseppina herself, is helped by her wine-specialist son, who guides tastings at local vineyards or sets up truffle-hunting experiences for interested visitors.

South of San Gimignano, **Colle di Val d'Elsa** ❸ is split between two sites. The lower "new" town is a busy, haphazard sprawl, whose centre of activity is the crystal factory – Colle is Italy's largest producer of crystal and fine glass, and there are plenty of shops selling it. The **Museo del Cristallo** (Via dei Fossi; May–Sep Tue–Sun 10.30am–noon 4.30–7.30pm, Oct–Apr Tue–Fri 3.30–5.30pm, Sat–Sun 10am–noon 3–7pm; charge) tells its story. Follow the signs up to the ancient upper town. Here the main street is lined with 16th-century palazzi of unusual refinement, and, at one point, the stately procession of buildings is interrupted by a viaduct from which there are splendid views of the surrounding landscape.

More spectacular sights await in nearby **Monteriggioni** ❹, just off the N2 to Siena. The fortified town, encircled by walls and 14 towers, was built in 1213 to guard northern Sienese territory. Like Montepulciano, this little hill village is emblematic of the Tuscan landscape. It is seen at its best first thing in the morning, when you can enjoy a coffee on the main square before the coach parties arrive.

In 1716, a decree issued by the Grand Duke of Tuscany defined the boundaries of the Chianti area and established the laws governing the production and sale of wine. Today, this region is the world's oldest wine-producing league. The Chianti Classico area includes the communes of Barberino Val d'Elsa, Castellina, Greve, Gaiole, San Casciano and Tavernelle Val di Pesa.

BELOW LEFT AND RIGHT: all the elements of a classic Tuscan landscape.

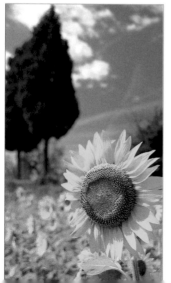

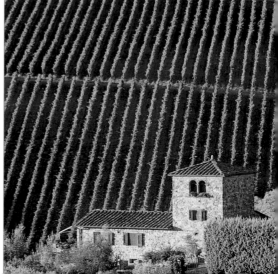

TIP

Cycling is an immensely popular way of touring Chianti country, and countless companies organise group or family holidays for people of all ages and abilities. You can also organise bike rental by the day or week through any of the Chianti tourist offices.

BELOW: driving the Chiantigiana.

The Chiantigiana

Spanning the hills between Florence and Siena, "Chiantishire" is a gentle vision of cypresses, vineyards and Medicean villa gardens. The rolling slopes are planted with olive groves that shimmer dark green and dusty silver. The Chianti is a spiritual rather than a geographical location. Its shifting borders reflect the fluctuations in Florentine and Sienese power, but, although it lies in Siena province, its soul remains where it has always been: on Florentine soil. It is a place whose turbulent history has shaped a scene of utter tranquillity, a harmony of tame hills and gentle people. In a place where nothing is essential viewing, everywhere is a glorious detour.

The SS222, known as **the Chiantigiana**, or Chianti Way, winds its picturesque way from Florence to Siena, through the heart of the region, offering archetypal scenes of cypress trees, olive groves and vineyards. First stop is the market town of **Greve ❺**, with an impressive arcaded square, Piazza Matteotti, topped with wrought-iron balconies dripping with geraniums. The shops under the arcades are crammed with the usual assortment of local foods, crafts and wines. The annual September Mostra Mercato del Chianti draws a large crowd.

An oft-missed jewel just five minutes' drive west of Greve is the tiny medieval walled town of **Montefioralle**, which was originally built as a feudal castle. Its narrow streets, stone houses and underpassages are beautifully preserved and splendid views are to be had from the various trattorias in the town.

Next on the SS222 is **Castellina in Chianti ❻**. Castellina overlooks symmetrical vineyards and wooded groves, a landscape dotted with low stone houses and Renaissance villas. New wine estates have been built from the remains of medieval castles. Villas have lazily domesticated the original castle or tower, but names like "La Rocca" or "La Torre" reveal the original function.

Castellina's name also reveals its medieval function as a Florentine outpost. In the late 13th century it was the first site of the Chianti League, a group of three Florentine feudal castles, each responsible for

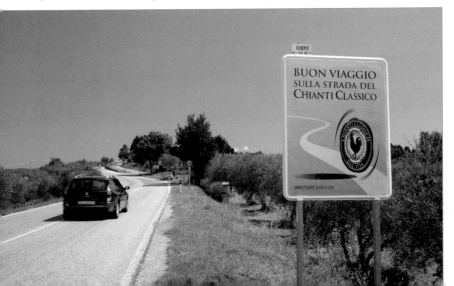

BUON VIAGGIO
SULLA STRADA DEL
CHIANTI CLASSICO

www.chianticlassico.com

a third of the territory. The castle is now a fortified town hall hiding a small Etruscan museum and a warren of atmospheric backstreets with half-glimpsed views of the Chianti hills.

Radda in Chianti

East of Castellina, **Radda in Chianti** 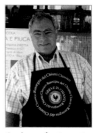 ❼ retains its medieval street plan and imposing town hall. As in Castellina, the spontaneous rural architecture is more rewarding. Classical Medici villas with 16th-century windows and wells compete with romantic villas, constructed from castles or Etruscan ruins. One 17th-century masterpiece is Villa Vistarenni, a white beacon of sophistication. The elegant loggias and the openness of the architecture symbolise the increasing wealth of the countryside and its proximity to urban Florence. In the tranquil Chianti, the country is richer and more civilised than the town.

From Radda a tortuous road climbs to **Volpaia** ❽, a pretty medieval village with a ruined castle and Brunelleschi-style church. If Chianti villages and towns have little sense of identity and few artistic treasures,

it is because they came into being with fully fledged Florentine and Sienese identities, while military outposts such as Radda had no time to develop artistically. Only the Chianti abbeys, which were endowed separately, had the independence to shape their own culture.

Abbey of the Good Harvest

Between Radda and Gaiole is the aptly named **Badia a Coltibuono** ❾ (Abbey of the Good Harvest; tel: 057-7744 832; www.coltibuono.com; May–Oct, closed am and Aug), set among pines, oaks, chestnut trees and vines. Since the Dissolution of the Monasteries in 1810, this medieval abbey has belonged to one family. The lovely 15th-century cloisters, chapel and frescoed ceilings can be viewed as a guest of the cookery school or the bed and breakfast, while the 12th-century walls and bell tower are open to all. The cellars are filled with Chianti Classico, the abbey's traditional living. No less famous are the aromatic chestnut honey and olive oil, which can be bought on the premises.

A wine maker promotes his produce at the Chianti wine festival held in Greve every September.

BELOW: a fountain in Radda in Chianti.

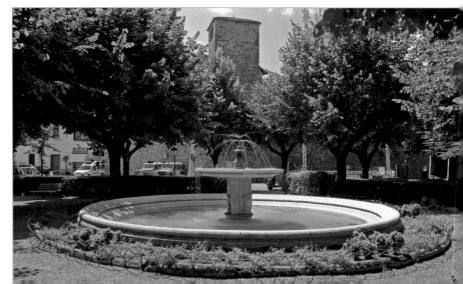

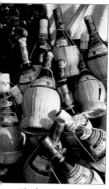

The famous Chianti flask is no longer mass-produced for export. However, the nostalgic will be pleased to find rustic wicker fiaschi *for sale throughout the region.*

BELOW: San Gimignano through the early morning mist.

Chianti castles

Gaiole in Chianti is a newer riverside settlement in a wooded valley. It is a popular summer escape for hot Florentines in search of family-run hotels, home cooking and the familiar *gallo nero* (black cockerel) wine symbol. History lies in wait at Meleto and Vertine, unusual castles, and Barbischio, a medieval village, is nearby. Tempting footpaths marked Sentieri del Chianti lead all the way to Siena. With vineyards rising up gentle slopes, tranquil Gaiole and sleepy Greve are traditional Chianti.

The countryside from Gaiole south to Siena and east to Arezzo is higher, wilder and wetter. The wooded peaks are green and fresh, with scents of thyme, rosemary and pine. Deep chestnut woods provide ideal cover for wild boar, recently reintroduced.

Of the many Florentine castles in the woods, **Castello di Brolio** (daily, times and tours vary; charge) is the most impressive – not least because of its views over the original Chianti vineyards stretching as far as Siena and Monte Amiata. On the medieval chessboard, every Florentine castle faced its Sienese shadow. If the surviving castles are Florentine, it is because Siena lost the match and all its pieces. While Sienese Cereto and Cettamura are small heaps, Florentine Brolio and Meleto are resplendent. As a Florentine outpost, Castello di Brolio's past spans Guelf-Ghibelline conflicts, sacking by the Sienese in 1529, and German occupation and Allied bombing in World War II. The medieval walls are the castle's most striking feature, along with the 14th-century chapel. Brolio has long been controlled by the Ricasoli, Chianti landowners since the 8th century. Baron Bettino Ricasoli, Italian premier in 1861, founded the modern Chianti wine industry, a business continued by the present family. (To visit the cellars, tour the estate, taste the wines, and see the family museum, tel: 057-77301/77302 20; www.ricasoli.it).

The Chianti is a place for pottering and chance encounters, one of which could be tiny **Campi di San Gusmé** , just south of Brolio. A short climb leads to a Romanesque church and views of tumbledown castles and vineyards. ❑

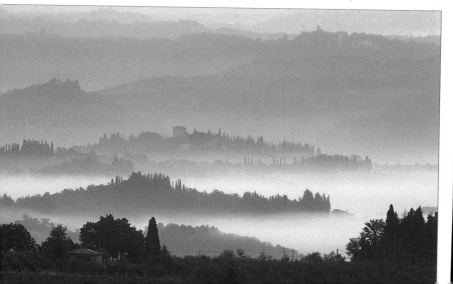

BEST RESTAURANTS

Restaurants

Prices for a three-course meal per person with a half-bottle of house wine:
€ = under €25
€€ = €25–40
€€€ = €40–60
€€€€ = over €60

Also try the restaurants at wine estates on the Chianti Trail (see page 208).

Castellina in Chianti

Albergaccio
Via Fiorentina 63
Tel: 0577-741 042
www.albergacciocast.com €€
The dishes change, but the quality of the food – which is Tuscan with flair – remains the same. Booking advisable. Closed Sun, summers also Wed at lunch.
La Torre
Piazza del Comune
Tel: 0577-740 236 €€
Restaurant with terrace outside the fortress. Extensive menu of predictable Tuscan fare, but reasonable. Closed Fri.

Certaldo Alto

L'Antica Fonte
Via Valdracca 25
Tel: 0571-652 225
www.tavernaanticafonte.it €€
Small, simple restaurant offering Tuscan specialities in a friendly and relaxed atmosphere. In summer there's additional seating in the garden, with views across the Val

d'Elsa. Booking essential. Closed Jan and Feb.
Osteria del Vicario
Via Rivellino 3
Tel: 0571-668 228
www.osteriadelvicario.it €€€
Charmingly set in Romanesque cloisters, this Michelin-starred restaurant serves inventive variations on Tuscan cuisine, including dishes inspired by ancient recipes. Closed Sun dinner, Mon.

Gaiole in Chianti

Badia a Coltibuono
Loc. Badia a Coltibuono
Tel/fax: 0577-749 031
www.coltibuono.com €€€
Part of a glorious rural wine estate, complete with 11th-century abbey. Specialities include home-made pasta with wild-duck sauce and antipasto della Badia. Popular stop on the Chianti trail. Closed Mon except May–Oct.
Il Carlino d'Oro
Località San Regolo
Tel: 0577-747 136 €
Family-run trattoria, far removed from typical underperforming restaurants on the well-beaten Chianti trail. Lunch only; closed Mon.
Ristorante della Pieve (Castello di Spaltenna)
Località Spaltenna 13
Tel: 0577-749 483
www.spaltenna.it €€€€
Magnificent restaurant in a hotel converted from a

fortified monastery. Dishes use fresh local ingredients, and food is cooked in a wood-burning stove. Closed Nov–Mar.

Greve in Chianti

Bottega del Moro
Piazza Trieste 14r
Tel: 055-853 753
www.labottegadelmoro.it €€
Restaurant serving good-quality traditional Tuscan fare. Try the coniglio (rabbit) or trippa alla Fiorentina (tripe) after a fresh pasta dish. Closed Mon.

Monterrigioni

Il Pozzo
Piazza Roma 20
Tel: 0577-304 127
www.ilpozzo.net €€
Famous restaurant full of foreigners in summer, but deservedly popular, in a gem of a tiny walled town. Closed Sun evening, Mon, most of Jan and period in Aug.

Panzano in Chianti

Enoteca Baldi
Piazza Bucciarelli 25
Tel: 055-852 843 €
Enoteca (wine bar/inn) with impressive wine selection. Open for a light lunch or afternoon snack.

Radda in Chianti

Le Vigne
Podere le Vigne Est (1km/0.6 miles outside town)
Tel: 0577-738 301 €€–€€€
Located among vineyards, and serving great

food, this is a treat. Reasonably priced rooms for rent above the restaurant. Closed mid-Nov–Feb.
Vignale
Via Panigiani 9
Tel: 0577-738 094 €€–€€€
Restaurant in a converted farm, serving refined and imaginative Tuscan cuisine. However, prices are high and tourists abound. Must book.

San Gimignano

Dorandò
Vicolo dell'Oro 2
Tel: 0577-941 862
www.ristorantedorando.it €€€€
Stylish restaurant specialising in recipes from the past. Closed Mon (except Easter–Nov) and 9 Dec–20 Feb.
Osteria delle Cantene
Via Mainardi 18
Tel: 0577-941 966
www.sangimignano.com/osteria catene €€
New-wave trattoria where traditional and contemporary ideas successfully co-exist. Try the local Vernaccia wine. Closed Wed and Jan.

Volpaia

La Bottega
Piazza della Torre 2
Tel: 0577-738 001
www.labottegadivolpaia.it €€
Gorgeous lunch spot with a maple-shaded terrace and valley views. Quality varies, but the service and location make up for it. Closed Tue.

THE CHIANTI WINE TRAIL

The Chianti Classico wine trail explores some of the most ancient and imposing wine estates, an experience combining countryside, castles, cuisine – and wine

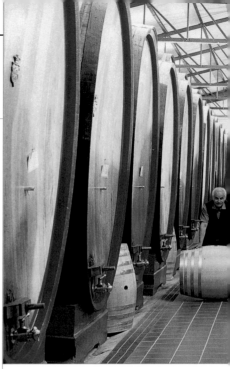

The Chianti covers an enormous region, spanning seven different wine "zones". At its heart, in the hills between Florence and Siena, is Chianti Classico, with the remainder – the Colli Fiorentini, Colli Senesi, Colline Pisane, Colli Aretini, Rufina and Montalbano – spread out over central Tuscany. The main centres in Chianti Classico are Greve, Panzano, Castellina, Gaiole, Fonterutoli and Radda. Easily accessible off the picturesque route SS222, the grandest, castle-like estates have often been run by the same families since medieval times, as is the case with the aristocratic Antinori, Frescobaldi, Mazzei and Ricasoli dynasties. Their vaulted castles, rolling vineyards and gastronomic restaurants encourage you to linger.

Contact the Chianti Classico consortium (tel: 055-82285; www.chianticlassico.com) for links to their producers. For a memorable experience, book a tasting *(degustazione)* combined with a tour of the vineyards and cellars.

BELOW: the hills of Chianti are blanketed with vineyards; many of the wine estates are hundreds of years old and have been run by the same families for generations.

ABOVE: although chestnut was the traditional wood of the region, Chianti *normale* is now usually kept in oak barrels for several months to mature.

BELOW: estate owners are usually proud to show off their wines and explain their particular methods of wine-making.

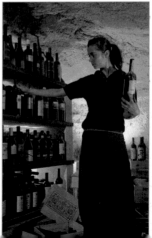

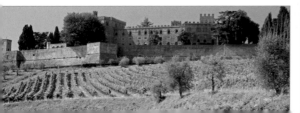

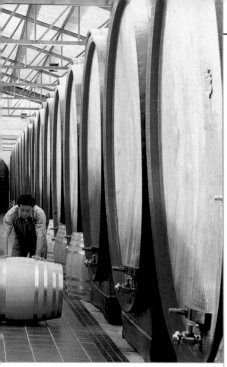

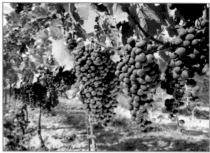

RECOMMENDED WINE ESTATES

Badia a Coltibuono
Gaiole in Chianti; tel: 0577-74481;
www.coltibuono.com
This wine estate, run by the Stucchi Prinetti family,
markets itself as a "wine resort" – stay overnight;
dine in the stables; do a cookery course – within
the former Romanesque abbey. Visits 2–5pm
April–October; tastings 5pm or by appointment.

Badia a Passignano
Tavarnelle Val di Pesa; tel: 055-807 1278;
www.osteriadipassignanano.com
Book a tour at this estate and sample iconic Antinori wines, such as Tignanello, Guado al Tasso
and Solaia, as well as Chianti Classico Riserva
Badia a Passignano. After the cellar visit, enjoy
an oil tasting, followed by lunch in the Michelin-
starred Osteria.

Castello di Brolio
Gaiole in Chianti; tel: 0577-730 220;
www.ricasoli.it
Baron Ricasoli, whose descendants now
run the castle (daily 9am-7pm), first designated the grape mixes to be used in
Chianti wine. Explore the castle gardens
and cellars before a tasting and
lunch (best to book).

Castello di Fonterutoli
Castellina in Chianti;
tel: 0577-741 385;
www.mazzei.it
Owned by the Mazzei family since
1435, Fonterutoli's award-winning
wines are matched by their grappa,
olive oil and Tuscan cuisine. Wine
tours at 3pm, reservations are recommended.

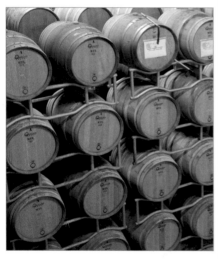

ABOVE: the smaller barrels used to store the wine produced in the
Chianti region are known as *barriques*; the larger barrels are
known as *botti*.

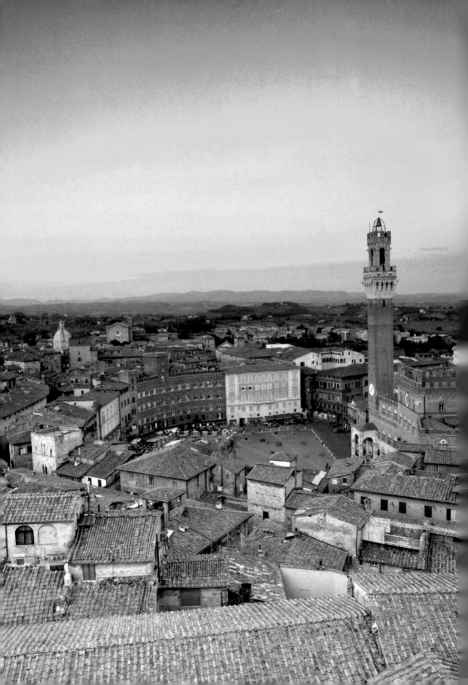

SIENA

Siena is a classic case of a city that Italians call *"a misura d'uomo"* – meaning a city "made to the measure of man". Siena is, indeed, a Gothic city built on a human scale, and is effortlessly civilised, harmonious and at ease with itself

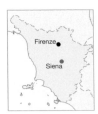

From its striped marble Cathedral to its tunnelled alleys, brilliant Campo and black-and-white city emblem, Siena is a chiaroscuro city. In its surging towers it is truly Gothic. Where Florence is boldly horizontal, Siena is soaringly vertical; where Florence has large squares and masculine statues, Siena has hidden gardens and romantic wells. Florentine art is perspective and innovation, while Sienese art is sensitivity and conservatism. Siena is often considered the feminine foil to Florentine masculinity.

For such a feminine and beautiful city, Siena has a decidedly war-like reputation, nourished by sieges, city-state rivalry and Palio battles. The pale theatricality in Sienese painting is not representative of the city or its inhabitants: the average Sienese is no ethereal Botticelli nymph, but dark, stocky and swarthy.

A brief history

In keeping with Sienese mystique, the city's origins are shrouded in myths of wolves and martyred saints. According to legend, the city was founded by Senius, son of Remus, hence the she-wolf symbols you

will encounter throughout the city. St Ansano brought Christianity to Roman Siena and, although he was promptly tossed into a vat of hot tar and beheaded, he has left a legacy of mysticism traced through St Catherine and St Bernardino to the present-day cult of the Madonna. The power of the Church came to an end when the populace rose up against the Ecclesiastical Council and established an independent republic in 1147. The 12th century was marked by rivalry in which the Florentine

Main attractions
IL CAMPO
PALAZZO PUBBLICO
DUOMO
MUSEO DELL'OPERA
   METROPOLITANA
SANTA MARIA DELLA SCALA
PINACOTECA NAZIONALE
FORTEZZA MEDICEA

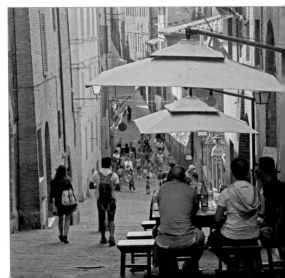

LEFT: Palazzo Pubblico and the Piazza del Campo glowing pink at sunset, Siena. **RIGHT:** a Sienese backstreet café.

The city is divided into three districts or terzi *(thirds) – The Terzo di San Martino, Terzo di Città and Terzo di Camollia. But this is purely an administrative division; Siena's true identity is inextricably linked to the* contrade, *the 17 medieval districts from which its social fabric is woven.*

Guelfs usually triumphed over the Sienese Ghibellines.

In 1260, the battle of Montaperti routed the Florentines and won the Sienese 10 years of cultural supremacy, which saw the foundation of the University and the charitable "fraternities". The Council of the Twenty-Four – a form of power-sharing between nobles and the working class – was followed by the Council of Nine, an oligarchy of merchants that ruled until 1335. Modern historians judge the Nine self-seeking and profligate, but under their rule the finest works of art were either

commissioned or completed, including the famous amphitheatre-shaped Campo, the Palazzo Pubblico and Duccio's *Maestà*.

The ancient republic survived until 1529, when the reconciliation between the pope and the emperor ended the Guelf-Ghibelline feud. The occupying Spanish demolished the city towers, symbols of freedom and fratricide, and used the masonry to build the present fortress. The final blow to the republic was the long siege of Siena by Emperor Charles V and Cosimo I in 1554.

After the Sienese defeat, the city

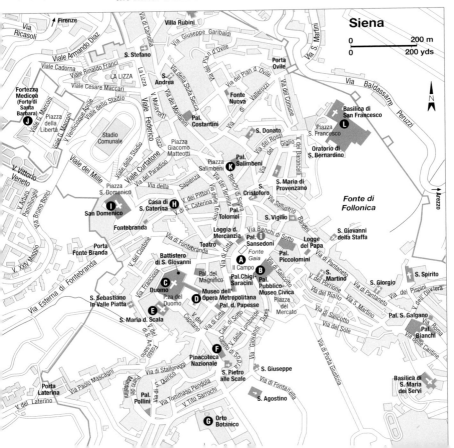

of Siena became absorbed into the Tuscan dukedom. As an untrusted member of the Tuscan Empire, impoverished Siena turned in on itself until the 20th century. Still today, Siena's tumultuous history as arch-rivals of Florence is written in the streets and squares, and resonates in the passionate souls of the Sienese. Of all Tuscans, the Sienese have the longest memories and there are local aristocrats who still disdain to visit Florence.

Change is anathema to the city: traditional landowning, financial speculation, trade and tourism are more appealing than the introduction of new technology or industry. Siena has made a virtue of conservatism; stringent medieval building regulations protect the fabric of the city; tourism is decidedly low-key; old family firms such as Nannini, Siena's most famous café, do a roaring trade with locals (and also produced Gianna Nannini, one of Italy's best-known female singers). Siena is Italy's last surviving city-state, a city with the psychology of a village and the grandeur of a nation.

Il Campo

All roads lead to **Il Campo A**, the huge main central square, shaped like an amphitheatre – the Sienese say that it is shaped like the protecting cloak of the Virgin, who, with St Catherine of Siena, is the city's patron saint. From the comfort of a pavement café on the curved side of the Campo, you can note the division of the paved surface into nine segments, commemorating the beneficent rule of the "Noveschi" – the Council of Nine that governed Siena from the mid-13th century to the early 14th, a period of stability and prosperity when most of the city's main public monuments were built.

The Campo is tipped with the Renaissance **Fonte Gaia** (Fountain of Joy). The marble carvings are copies of the original sculptures by Iacopo della Quercia, which are on display in Santa Maria della Scala *(see page 217)*. Beneath the fountain lies one of Siena's best-kept secrets – a

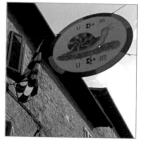

Chiocciola contrada; traditionally, its residents worked as terracotta makers.

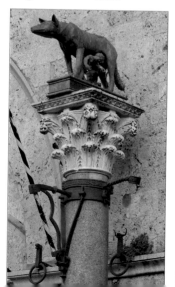

BELOW LEFT: Romulus, Remus and the she-wolf; Remus' son is said to have founded Siena.

"Contrade" Passions

Siena's cultural aloofness owes much to the *contrade*, the 17 city wards designated for now-defunct administrative and military functions during the Middle Ages, which continue to act as individual entities within the city. To outsiders, the only real significance of the *contrade* seems to be in connection with the Palio *(see page 222)*, but their existence pervades all aspects of daily life. Despite its public grandeur, parts of Siena are resolutely working class and attach great weight to belonging to a community. Events such as baptisms are celebrated together, while traditional Sienese will only marry within their *contrada*.

All over the city, the importance of the various *contrade* is evident. Little plaques set into the wall indicate which *contrada* you are in (such as snail unicorn, owl, caterpillar, wolf or goose). Each neighbourhood has its own fountain and font, as well as a motto, symbol and colours. The last are combined in a flag, worn with pride and seen draped around buildings for important *contrada* events, notably a Palio triumph. To gain an understanding of this secret world, book a private Palio tour (tel: 057-7280 551) that takes you to the individual museums, churches and stables associated with individual *contrade*, all in the heart of the city.

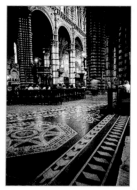

The interior of the Duomo, a magnificent Gothic structure of banded black-and-white stone, with a superb floor of inlaid marble depicting biblical and pagan themes.

BELOW: a backstreet leading towards the Duomo.

labyrinth of medieval tunnels extending for 25km (15½ miles), constructed to channel water from the surrounding hills into the city. The undergound aqueduct has two main tunnels: one leads to the Fonte Gaia and the other to the Fonte Branda, the best preserved of Siena's many fountains. Parts of this subterranean system can be visited and explored on a guided tour (enquire at the tourist office for more information).

At the square's base is the **Palazzo Pubblico** ❸, the dignified Town Hall with its crenellated facade and waving banners, surmounted by the tall and slender tower. The Town Hall, which has been the home of the commune since it was completed in 1310, is a Gothic masterpiece of rose-coloured brick and silver-grey travertine. Each ogival arch is crowned by the *balzana*, Siena's black-and-white emblem representing the mystery and purity of the Madonna's life.

The distinctive **Torre del Mangia** (daily 10am–7pm, until 4pm Nov–mid-Mar; charge) – named after the first bell-ringer, Mangiaguadagni, the "spendthrift" – is 87 metres (285ft) high, and it's a 500-step climb to the top to enjoy glorious views of the pink piazza and Siena's rooftops. At the bottom of the tower, the Cappella in Piazza (Chapel in the Square) was erected in 1378 in thanksgiving for the end of the plague.

The city museum

Although bureaucrats still toil in parts of the **Palazzo Pubblico**, as they have for some seven centuries, much of the complex is now dedicated to the **Museo Civico** (daily Mar–Oct 10am–7pm, until 5.30pm or 6pm Nov–mid-Mar; charge), which displays some of the city's greatest treasures.

Siena's city council once met in the vast **Sala del Mappamondo**, although the huge map that then graced the walls has disappeared. What remains are two frescoes attributed to the medieval master Simone Martini: the majestic

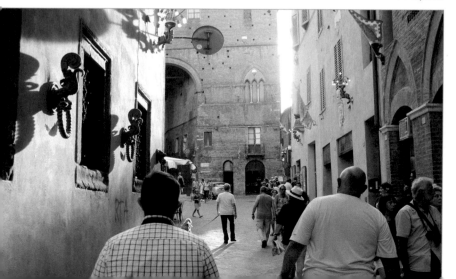

mounted figure of *Guidoriccio da Fogliano* and the *Maestà*. Martini's *Maestà*, a poetic evocation of the Madonna seated on a filigree throne, has a rich, tapestry-like quality. The muted blues, reds and ivory add a gauzy softness. Martini echoes Giotto's conception of perspective, yet clothes his Madonna in diaphanous robes, enhancing her spirituality in dazzling decoration.

Opposite is the iconic *Guidoriccio*, the haughty diamond-spangled *condottiero* (mercenary) reproduced on calendars and *panforte* boxes. But in recent years, despite Sienese denials, doubts have been cast on the authenticity of the fresco. Art historians maintain that a smaller painting uncovered below the huge panel is Martini's original, and the Guidoriccio we see was executed long after the artist's death.

In the next room is a genuine civic masterpiece, Ambrogio Lorenzetti's *Effects of Good and Bad Government*, painted in 1338 as an idealised tribute to the Council of the Nine. Its narrative realism and the vivid facial expressions used on this impressive painting give the allegory emotional resonance to observers. A wise old man symbolises the common good, while a patchwork of neat fields, tame boar and busy hoers suggests order and prosperity. By contrast, *Bad Government* is a desolate place, razed to the ground by a diabolical tyrant, the Sienese she-wolf at his feet.

The Cathedral

Exiting the Campo, turn left and head up the hill via one of the winding streets to the Piazza del Duomo. The **Duomo** ● (www.operaduomo.siena.it; Mon–Sat 10.30am–7-.30pm, Sun 1.30–6pm; combined ticket) is Siena's most controversial monument, either a symphony in black-and-white marble, or a tasteless iced cake, depending on your point of view. It began in 1220 as a round-arched Romanesque church, but soon acquired a Gothic façade festooned with pinnacles. Bands of black, white and green Tuscan marble were inlaid with pink stone and topped by Giovanni Pisano's naturalistic statues.

TIP

The Duomo's museum allows access to the parapets, which offer dazzling views of Siena – a more accessible alternative to the Torre del Mangia's panorama.

BELOW: Siena's ornate cathedral.

Turf Wars

The Palio horse race is the symbol of the Sienese's attachment to their city, and outsiders challenge it at their peril. One of the piazza's tight turns, the Curva di San Martino, set at a 95-degree angle, has often been the cause of fatalities among horses. Animal-rights activists have long protested against the event and Michele Brambilla, the Minister for Tourism, recently refused to allow the race to be put forward for Unesco World Heritage status. She said: "The shame of 48 horse deaths since 1970 marks the Palio of Siena, and a current investigation will shed light on accusations of doping in some horses. This damages the image of one of the most beautiful cities in the world." The Sienese beg to differ.

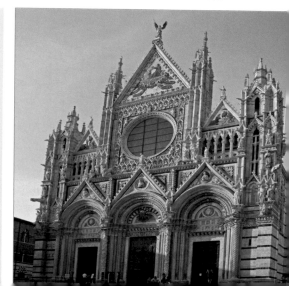

TIP

Siena is not the cheapest place to shop, but it is full of enticing shops, galleries and boutiques selling quality goods, often handmade. The main shopping streets are Via Banchi di Sopra and Via di Città. Opening hours are generally 9.30am–1pm and 3–7pm. Many shops close on Mondays.

BELOW: the fan-shaped Campo.

The Cathedral interior is creativity run riot – oriental abstraction, Byzantine formality, Gothic flight and Romanesque austerity. A giddy chiaroscuro effect is created by the black-and-white walls reaching up to the starry blue vaults.

The inlaid floor is even more inspiring, and the Duomo is at its best between August and October when the intricate marble-inlaid paving is on display. Outside these times, to preserve the well-restored floor, many of the most captivating scenes are hidden. Major Sienese craftsmen worked on the marble *pavimentazione* between 1372 and 1562. The finest scenes are Matteo di Giovanni's pensive sibyls and the marble mosaics by Beccafumi. Giorgio Vasari called these "the most beautiful pavements ever made".

Nicola Pisano's octagonal marble pulpit is a Gothic masterpiece: built in 1226, it is a dramatic and fluid progression from his solemn pulpit in Pisa Cathedral. Off the north aisle is the decorative **Libreria Piccolomini** (Mon–Sat 9am–7.30pm, Sun 1–7.30pm), built in 1495 to house the personal papers and books of Pope Pius II. The frescoes by Pinturicchio (1509) show scenes from the life of the influential Renaissance pope, a member of the noble Sienese Piccolomini family and founder of the town of Pienza.

The **Crypt** is an extraordinary discovery, with recently revealed frescoes attributed to Duccio's school. Because the frescoes were perfectly concealed for so long, the intensity of the colours shines through in a vivid array of blue, gold and red. Given that the frescoes date from 1280, the "modern" expressiveness is all the more remarkable.

In the unfinished eastern section of the Cathedral is the **Museo dell' Opera Metropolitana** (daily Mar–May and Sept–Oct 9.30am–7pm, June–Aug until 8pm, Nov–Feb 10am–5pm; combined ticket with Duomo) and Pisano's original statues for the facade. In a dramatically lit room above is Duccio's *Maestà*, the Virgin Enthroned, which graced the High Altar until 1506. Siena's best-loved work, the largest known medieval panel painting ever, was escorted from the artist's workshop to the Duomo in a torchlit procession in 1311. The biggest panel depicts the Madonna enthroned among saints and angels, and, since the separation of the painting, facing scenes from the Passion. Although Byzantine Gothic in style, the *Maestà* is suffused with melancholy charm. The delicate gold and red colouring is matched by Duccio's grace of line, which influenced Sienese painting for the next two centuries. The Sienese believe that Giotto copied Duccio but sacrificed beauty to naturalism. The small panels do reveal some of Giotto's truthfulness and sense of perspective.

Around the Cathedral

Opposite the cathedral on the piazza, **Santa Maria della Scala ⓔ** (www.santamariadellascala.com; daily mid-Mar–mid-Oct 10.30am–6.30pm, mid-Oct–mid-Mar 10.30am–4.30pm; charge) is often described as a city within a city. It began as a hospital a thousand years ago and continued as one until its reincarnation as a museum in the year 2000. The far-sighted foundation originally functioned as a pilgrims' hostel, a poorhouse, an orphanage and a hospital, but is now a magnificent museum complex, embracing frescoed churches, granaries and an archaeological museum. Symbolically, the hospital door never had a key, demonstrating its role as a sanctuary to all-comers. The Pilgrims Hall, depicting care for the sick, is frescoed by Siena's finest 15th-century artists. The scenes portrayed, of wet-nurses, alms-giving and abandoned children, reveal a human side of the city absent from the luminous sacred art. The complex is also a venue for major medieval and Renaissance art exhibitions.

The city's **Museo Archeologico** (times as above; combined ticket) is also here, with its significant collection of Etruscan and Roman remains. The vaulted, former granaries make a moody setting for the display of Etruscan treasures, including funerary urns and sarcophagi from Sarteano.

A set of steps behind the Duomo leads down to Piazza San Giovanni, a small square dominated by the **Battistero di San Giovanni** (times as

St Catherine, the daughter of a Sienese dyer, devoted her early life to the needs of the poor and sick. She then turned to politics and dedicated herself to reconciling anti-papal and papal forces; she was instrumental in the return of Pope Gregory XI, exiled in Avignon, to Rome. All the places she visited, from the day of her birth, have been consecrated.

BELOW: *contrada* procession in the Campo, by Vincenzo Rustici.

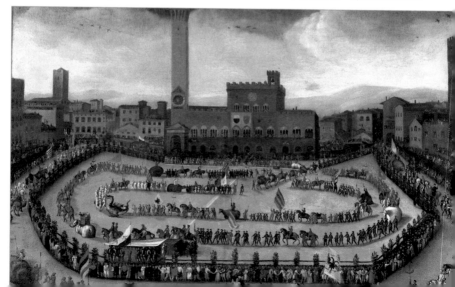

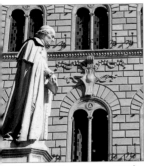

Statue of Sallustio Bandini, founder of Siena's library, on Piazza Salimbeni.

for the Museo dell'Opera del Duomo and Crypt; combined ticket), built beneath part of the Cathedral. Inside are frescoes and a beautiful baptismal font by Jacopo della Quercia.

Two art museums

There are two art museums in the vicinity of the Cathedral complex, at opposite ends of the scale of their content. The **Pinacoteca Nazionale ⑥** (Via San Pietro 29; Tue–Sat 8.15am–7.15pm, Sun and Mon until 1pm; charge) contains the finest collection of Sienese "Primitives" in the suitably Gothic Palazzo Buonsignori. The early rooms are full of Madonnas, apple-cheeked, pale, remote or warmly human. Matteo di Giovanni's stylised Madonnas shift to Lorenzetti's affectionate *Annunciation* and Ugolino di Neri's radiant *Madonna*. Neroccio di Bartolomeo's *Madonna* is as truthful as a Masaccio.

As a variant, the grisly deaths of obscure saints compete with a huge medieval crucifix with a naturalistic

spurt of blood. The famous landscapes and surreal Persian city attributed to Lorenzetti were probably painted by Sassetta around a century later. But his *Madonna dei Carmelitani* is a sweeping cavalcade of vibrant Sienese life.

Those suffering from a surfeit of medieval sacred art can visit the **Palazzo delle Papesse** (Via di Città 126; Tue–Sun noon–7pm; charge), a contemporary art gallery with changing exhibitions, which also offers a 360-degree view of Siena from its loggia.

For some outdoor space and greenery, turn left out of the gallery and head south to the **Orto Botanico ⑥** (Via P.A. Mattioli 4; Mon–Fri 8am–5.30pm, Sat 8am–noon), a small botanical garden just inside the city walls. Opposite the Orto Tolomei is another little garden, with a lovely view over the countryside and a sculpture that – although not obvious at first glance – outlines the shape of the city.

St Catherine trail

Slightly outside the historic centre, on Vicolo del Tiratoio, is the **Casa**

Sienese Sweets

Sienese pastries are so renowned that they even have their own saint watching over them, San Lorenzo. Exotic spices reached Siena along the Via Francigena pilgrimage route, and many find their way into the medieval recipes still used today. *Panforte*, a rich, filling cake, dates back to 1205, and is often eaten with sweet Vin Santo. The intense flavours are created by a mix of honey, almonds, hazelnuts, candied orange peel, and a secret blend of spices such as cinnamon and nutmeg. *Panpepato*, a spicier version, predates it. The delicacy was originally the preserve of Sienese nuns, who guarded their secret recipes, which were also a source of revenue. Such was *panforte*'s popularity that even in the 14th century, it was being exported. Originally a festive treat, *panforte* is now eaten all year round. *Ricciarelli*, small almond biscuits, are also typically Sienese, and far lighter.

The most famous place for *panforte* is **Nannini** (Banchi di Sopra 24), a bar and pastry shop, but **Pasticceria Bini** (Via Stalloreggi 91) is even more illustrious, occupying what was supposedly Duccio's workshop. Carved into the former stables of a patrician palace, **Antica Drogheria Manganelli** (Via di Citta 71) is another exotic shop for Sienese delights.

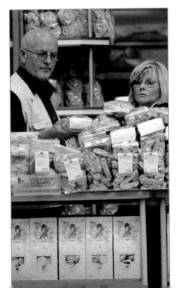

di Santa Caterina da Siena 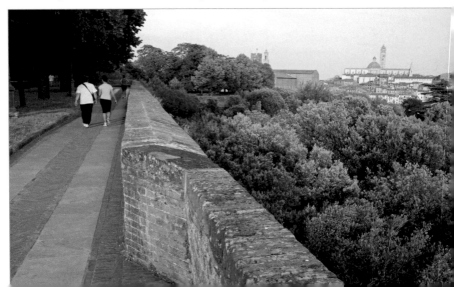 (Costa di Sant' Antonio; daily 9am–12.30pm, 3–6pm; free), the home of Catherine Benincase (1347–80), canonised in the 15th century by Pope Pius II and proclaimed Italy's patron saint in 1939, along with St Francis of Assisi. The house, garden and her father's dye-works now form the "Sanctuary of St Catherine". Although never taking holy orders, Catherine was an ascetic, and lived like a hermit in a cell, reputedly sleeping with a stone as her pillow. If it didn't sound too smug, the Sienese would admit to spiritual superiority. Apart from producing two saints and fine religious art, the city still venerates the Virgin.

Inside the nearby **Basilica di San Domenico** (Apr–Oct 7am–6.30pm, Nov–Mar 9am–6pm; free) – a huge fortress-like church founded by the Dominicans – a reliquary containing the saint's head is kept in the Cappella Santa Caterina. The chapel is decorated with frescoes depicting events in the saint's life, the majority completed by Il Sodoma in the early 16th century. The view from outside the Basilica across to the Duomo is spectacular.

The Fortress

From here it's a short walk to the Forte di Santa Barbara, also known as the **Fortezza Medicea**, built by Cosimo I after his defeat of Siena in 1560. The red-brick fortress now houses an open-air theatre, provides glorious views of the countryside and contains the **Enoteca Italiana** (tel: 0577-288 811; Mon–Sat noon–1am). The latter, a wine exhibition and shop, allows for guided tastings from a wide range of Tuscan wines. This is also the best place to study and savour Sienese wines, from Chianti Classico to Vino Nobile di Montepulciano, Brunello di Montalcino and Vernaccia di San Gimignano.

Via Banchi di Sopra, lined with fine medieval palazzi, is one of the three main arteries of the city centre (the other two being Via Banchi di Sotto and Via di Città). It links the Campo with the splendid **Piazza**

Sienese panforte.

BELOW: strolling the walls of Fortezza Medicea.

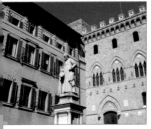

Statue of archdeacon Sallustio Bandini in Piazza Salimbeni.

Salimbeni at its northern end. The grand palazzi flanking the square are the head office of the Monte dei Paschi di Siena, one of the oldest banks in the world. Founded in 1472 and still an important employer, it is known as "the city father".

Basilica of St Francis

From the square, Via dei Rossi leads east to the **Basilica di San Francesco** (7am–noon, 3.30–7pm; free). Now housing part of the University, the vast church exhibits fragments of frescoes by Pietro and Ambrogio Lorenzetti. Next door, the 15th-century **Oratorio di San Bernardino** (mid-Mar–Oct 9.30am–7pm, Nov–Feb 10am–5pm; charge), dedicated to Siena's great preacher, contains frescoes by the artists Il Sodoma and Beccafumi.

Here, as at all its far reaches, the city has well-preserved walls and gateways. Siena's compactness makes these easy to explore, inviting you to wind through the sinuous medieval streets and stumble across secret courtyards, fountains and surprisingly rural views. This perfect, pink-tinged city is a delight to discover on foot, from the shell-shaped Campo to the galleries full of soft-eyed Sienese madonnas. In the backstreets, the city history is laid out before you, with noble coats of arms above doorways, or *contrada* animal symbols defining where their citizens belong. Everywhere leads back to the Campo, at its most theatrical in the late afternoon, after a day spent in the shadows of the city walls and inner courtyards.

But to escape the crowds, walk along the walls, or take the countrified lane of **Via del Fosso di Sant'Ansano**, which runs behind Santa Maria della Scala. Or stroll to **Santa Maria dei Servi** to lap up equally lovely views en route to a sublime church.

Given its impossibly narrow alleys threading between tall rose-brick palaces, Siena is mostly pedestrianised. Although the city is closed to traffic, visitors with hotel reservations are generally allowed to drive in, if only to park in a designated spot. ❑

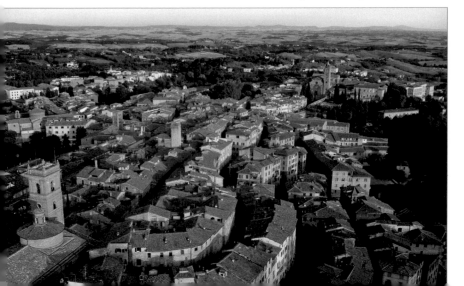

BEST RESTAURANTS, BARS AND CAFÉS

Restaurants

Prices for a three-course meal per person with a half-bottle of house wine:

€ = under €25
€€ = €25–40
€€€ = €40–60
€€€€ = over €60

Al Mangia
Piazza del Campo 42
Tel: 057-7281 121
www.almangia.it €€€–€€€€
In a great position on the Campo, this popular restaurant serves classic Tuscan cuisine. Seating outside in the summer. Closed Wed Nov–Feb.

Al Marsili
Via del Castoro 3
Tel: 057-7471 54
www.ristorantealmarsili.it €€–€€€
Elegant restaurant in an ancient building with wine cellars cut deep into the limestone. Sophisticated cuisine, including gnocchi in duck sauce. Closed Mon in winter.

Antica Trattoria Botteganova
Via Chiantigiana 29
Tel: 057-7284 230 €€€–€€€€
Refined restaurant serving fine Sienese cuisine. Specialities include local delicacies, fish and tasty puddings. Closed Sun, period in Jan, early Aug.

Certosa di Maggiano
Strada di Certosa 82
Tel: 057-7288 180
www.certosadimaggiano.com
€€€€
This converted Carthu-sian monastery, now a hotel, serves gourmet food in a magical setting: a courtyard overlooking Siena. Closed Tue.

Da Guido
Vicolo del Pettinaio 7
Tel: 0577-28004
www.ristorienteguido.com
€€–€€€
Veritable Sienese institution, set in medieval premises and popular with visiting VIPs. Traditional Sienese cuisine. Closed Wed and Jan.

Osteria del Castelvecchio
Via Castelvecchio 65
Tel: 0577-47093 €€
Converted from ancient stables, this perennially popular hostelry creates contemporary dishes with traditional flavours, including vegetarian dishes. Interesting wine list. Closed Tue.

Osteria Il Boccone del Prete
Via San Pietro 17
Tel: 0577-280 388
www.osteriaboccondelprete.it €
Family-run restaurant serving Sienese dishes in a pleasing setting. Closed Sun.

Osteria Il Carroccio
Via Casato di Sotto 32
Tel: 0577-41165 €
Well run, tiny trattoria serving local dishes. Closed Tue dinner, Wed, Feb and 1 week in Nov.

Osteria La Chiacchiera
Costa di San Antonio 4
Tel: 0577-280 631 €
Small, rustic inn offering Sienese fare – try the local pasta, *pici* (thick spaghetti), and the pork casserole. Dine outside in summer. Closed Tue.

Osteria La Taverna di San Giuseppe
Via G. Dupré 132
Tel: 0577-42286
www.tavernasangiuseppe.it €–€€
Delicious Tuscan fare in an atmospheric cavern with wooden furnishings. An antipasto is a must; delicious dishes using pecorino. Closed Sun.

Osteria Le Logge
Via del Porrione 33
Tel: 0577-48013 €€–€€€
Set in a 19th-century pharmacy, with authentic dark-wood and marble interior. One of a few gastronomic Siena eateries, it offers dishes such as ravioli with mint and pecorino, duck and fennel, or stuffed guinea fowl *(faraona)*. Montalcino wines from chef's estate. Closed Sun and Jan.

Pizzeria di Nonno Mede
Via Camporegio 21
Tel: 0577-247 966 €
Serves good pizza and great desserts. Splendid view of the Duomo, which is well lit in the evenings. Book ahead.

Trattoria Papei
Piazza del Mercato 6
Tel: 0577-280 894 €€
Ideal place for sampling genuine Sienese home cooking in large portions. Closed Mon (except public holidays) and end July.

Tre Cristi
Vicolo di Provenzano 1–7
Tel: 0577-280 608
www.trecristi.com €€–€€€
Elegant restaurant with frescoed walls and a contemporary Mediterranean menu. Booking advised. Closed Sun in Aug.

Bars and Cafés

Nannini's Conca d'Oro
(Banchi di Sopra) is an obligatory coffee stop on Siena's main shopping street. Opposite is **Caffè del Corso** – chic by day, boisterous by night. **Bar le Logge** (Via Rinaldini, at the end of Banchi di Sotto) is a non-touristic place to drink cappuccino. On Il Campo, to the left of the Palazzo Pubblico, **Gelateria Caribia** (Via Rinaldini) offers a multitude of ice-cream flavours. **The Tea Room** (Via Porta Giustizia; closed Mon) is cosy for tea and cake, or a cocktail with live jazz. **Fonte delle Delizie** (Costa di San Antonio, near Casa di Santa Caterina) makes delicious pastries. Further from the centre, **Il Masgalano** (Via del Camporegio, next to San Domenico) is a friendly place for coffees, light lunches or an *aperitivo*.

THE PASSION OF THE PALIO

In little more than a minute, the Campo is filled with unbearable happiness and irrational despair as centuries-old loyalties are put to the test

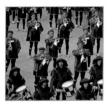

It is strange how a race that lasts just 90 seconds can require 12 months' planning, a lifetime's patience and the involvement of an entire city. But Siena's famous Palio does just that, as it has done since the 13th century, when an August Palio made its debut. At that time, the contest took the form of a bareback race the length of the city. The bareback race around Siena's main square, the Piazza del Campo, was introduced in the 17th century. Today the Palio is held twice a year, in early July and mid-August. The Palio, which has been run in times of war, famine and plague, stops for nothing. In the 1300s, criminals were released from jail to celebrate the festival. When the Fascists were gaining ground in 1919, Siena postponed council elections until after the Palio. In 1943, British soldiers in a Tunisian prisoner-of-war camp feared a riot when they banned Sienese prisoners from staging a Palio; Sienese fervour triumphed.

Although, as the Sienese say, *Il Palio corre tutto l'anno* ("The Palio runs all year"), the final preparations boil down to three days, during which there is the drawing by lots of the horse for each competing ward *(contrada)*, the choice of the "jockeys" and then the six trial races – the last of which is held on the morning of the Palio itself.

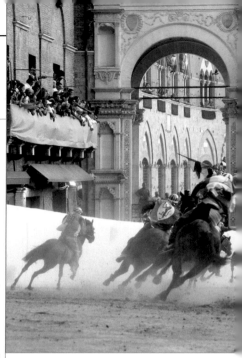

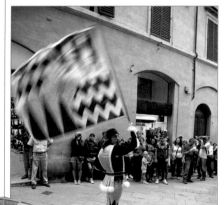

RIGHT: the words *"C'è terra in piazza"* ("There's earth in the Campo") are the signal to remove the colourful costumes from Siena's museums to feature in the great Historical Parade.

ABOVE: a highlight of the Palio pageantry is the spectacular display of the flag-wavers, famous throughout Italy for their elaborate manoeuvres.

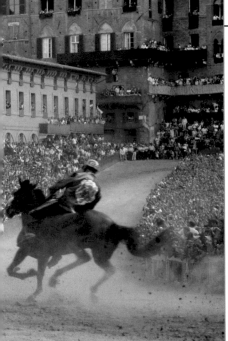

ABOVE: the ruthless race lurches around the Campo three times. If a riderless horse wins, the animal is almost deified: it is given the place of honour in the victory banquet and has its hooves painted gold.

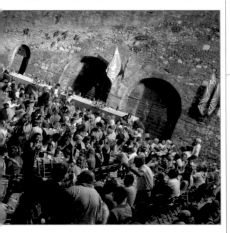

ABOVE: Siena's Campo becomes extremely crowded during the race so TV screens are set up in the *contrada* squares. After the race, feasts are held to celebrate, or to commiserate, the result.

THE POWER OF THE *CONTRADE*

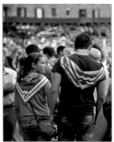

In Siena the *contrada* rules: ask a Sienese where he is from and he will say, *"Ma sono della Lupa"* ("But I'm from the Wolf *contrada*"). The first loyalty is to the city in the head, not to the city on the map.

Ten out of Siena's 17 *contrade* take part in each Palio: the seven who did not run in the previous race and three more who are selected by lot. Each *contrada* appoints a captain and two lieutenants to run their Palio campaign. In the Palio, the illegal becomes legal: bribery, kidnapping, plots and the doping of horses are all common occurrences.

Each *contrade* has its own standard, many of which are displayed around the city during the Palio and play an important role in the ceremonial aspect of the event.

Flags, or standards, are a central theme of the Palio event. In fact, the *palio* itself – the trophy of victory for which everyone is striving – is a standard: a silk flag emblazoned with the image of the Madonna and the coats of arms of the city, ironically referred to by the Sienese as the *cencio*, or rag. The *contrada* that wins the event retains possession of the prized *palio* standard until the next race takes place.

BELOW: the Historical Parade, which is staged in the run-up to the main race, retraces Siena's centuries of struggle against Florence, from the glorious victory against its rival in 1260 to the ghastly defeat in 1560.

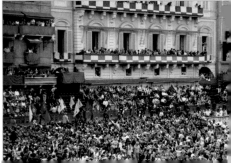

SOUTH OF SIENA

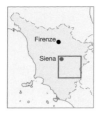

The route through the dramatic Crete region delivers you to the heart and soul of Tuscany. Pienza, Montalcino and Montepulciano are must-sees, but countless other lesser-known towns await discovery, while the hidden beauty of the Val d'Orcia river valley and the tortuous roads of Monte Amiata beckon the intrepid

The area just south of Siena is a primeval landscape of stark beauty. Appropriately called **Le Crete**, it is a moonscape of interlocking pale-clay hummocks and treeless gullies. In winter it is cold, bleak and even more crater-like. In summer the curvaceous terrain is softened by a deep green blanket. Sienese city dwellers love this barren landscape and are successfully discouraging local farmers from accepting European Union funds to flatten the land and grow wheat.

There is an extraordinary range of wildlife in the area: by day, wild deer roam beside the Ombrone River; by night, porcupines and foxes are about in the woods. If intrepid walkers venture out on a late autumn evening they may meet a strange character with a couple of dogs, a torch and a harness. He is a truffle hunter, sniffing out truffles in the dampest ditches. More legal are the Sardinian peasants selling cheese. Unlike many Tuscans, Sardinians are prepared to live in remote, infertile places.

The best route through the Crete is the SS438 to Asciano, and the SP451 to Monte Oliveto Maggiore – empty roads through a barren landscape, dotted with striking hilltop farmhouses and lone cypresses. Known as the Accona Desert in medieval times, it retains its spiritual remoteness.

Monte Oliveto Maggiore

After so much pale, undulating land, the red abbey of **Monte Oliveto Maggiore ❶** (daily 9am–noon, 3.15–6pm, winter until 5pm; free) is glimpsed through a wood of pines, oaks and olive trees. If the land appears to fall away from the abbey, it is not far from the truth: land erosion and frequent landslides provide a natural defence to the abbey's

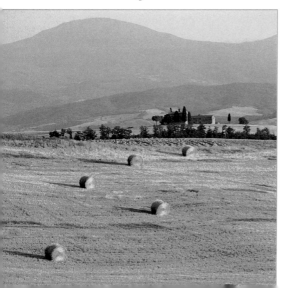

LEFT: a timeless Tuscan landscape.

mystical centre. In 1313 Tolomei, a wealthy Sienese, abandoned the law for a life of prayer in the wilderness, taking with him two fellow hermits. After a vision of white-robed monks, Tolomei established an Olivetan Order under Benedictine rule. The monks followed St Benedict's precept that "a real monk is one who lives by his own labour". Fortunately, a meagre diet, fervent prayer and lack of conversation stimulated the monks to artistic endeavour in the form of woodcarving, sculpture and manuscript design. As a noted artistic centre, the abbey invited Luca Signorelli and Il Sodoma to decorate the cloisters with scenes from St Benedict's life *(see box page 227)*.

The excitement of Il Sodoma aside, Monte Oliveto is a spiritual retreat. The austere refectory, the library cluttered with ancient manuscripts and books, the exquisite marquetry work of the choir stalls are as peaceful as the hidden walks deep into the woods. Today, there is a restaurant, and a lovely shop selling honey, oil and liqueurs made by the monks, as well as wine tasting in vaulted cellars.

The former monastic cells are also available for overnight visitors (tel: 0577-707 652; closed in winter).

Situated on a plain in the heart of the Crete, **Buonconvento** is worth a brief stop, if only to admire the imposing red 14th-century walls and massive medieval city gates of iron-bound wood. In 1366 Siena rebuilt the walls because, as a Sienese outpost, Buonconvento had been devastated. Today, the town is essentially a place for a leisurely introduction to truffles or game, or for a summer picnic in the peaceful gardens beside the town walls.

Pienza

Pienza ❷ is an exquisite Renaissance showpiece, slightly suffering from its over-popularity. Although created by a humanist pope, Pius II, Pienza is almost too perfect to be human and too precious to be spiritual. Every fountain, piazza and painting is harmonious. Model citizens walk through streets as romantic as their names – Via dell'Amore, Via del Bacio, Via della Fortuna – streets of "love", "kiss" and "fortune".

EAT

Vino Nobile is excellent with two local peasant dishes: *bruschetta*, a toasted garlic bread drenched in olive oil, or *panzanella*, a bread salad with herbs.

BELOW LEFT: sleepy street scene in Buonconvento.
BELOW RIGHT: a view of Pienza.

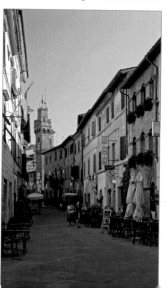

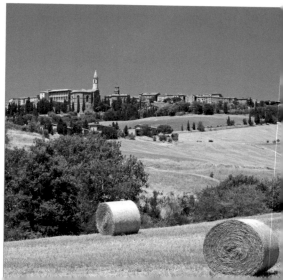

TIP

The pretty walled village of Monticchiello offers fine views of Pienza, just 4km (2.4 miles) away. It is also renowned for the Teatro Povero – an annual play written and starring the villagers about life in rural Tuscany.

Pienza's origins date back to 1458. When E.S. Piccolomini was elected pope, he could not resist playing God in his home village, Corsignano. He chose the noted Florentine architect Bernardo Rossellino to ennoble the hamlet in accordance with humanist principles. When the first masterpiece in modern town planning emerged late and over budget, the Pope reduced his fraudulent architect to tears with his words, "You did well, Bernardo, in lying to us about the expense involved in the work… Your deceit has built these glorious structures; which are praised by all except the few consumed with envy."

Bernardo Rossellino was rewarded with a scarlet robe, 100 ducats and some new commissions. The decision to build a cathedral enabled the pope to rechristen Corsignano the village as Pienza the city. The result is what locals call a *città d'autore*, a city inspired by one vision. After Pienza, other cities in Tuscany or elsewhere are liable to look chaotic.

Much of the symmetry lies in the cathedral square, **Piazza Pio II**, and the slightly listing Duomo adds to

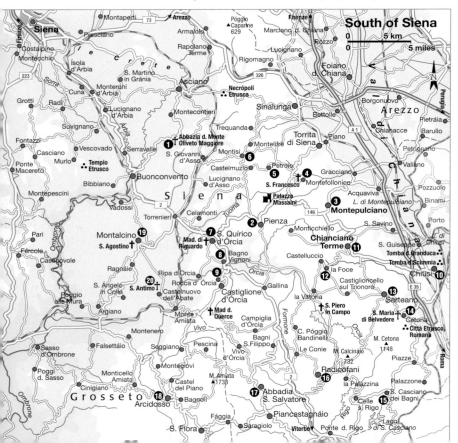

the charm. Despite a Renaissance facade, the interior is late Gothic and decorated with mystical paintings from the Sienese school. In one central alcove is a chilling *Assumption* by Vecchietta, in which St Agatha holds a cup containing her breasts, torn off by the executioner. The Duomo's facade, the gracious arches, the well and the Palazzo Piccolomini, the pope's home, are just as Pius left them when he set off to fight the Crusades, never to return.

Palazzo Piccolomini (Tue–Sun 10am–last entrance 6pm mid-Mar– mid-Oct, 4pm mid-Oct–mid-Mar; closed 7 Jan–mid-Feb and late Nov; guided tours only; charge), now a museum, is lined with both grand and homely treasures, including a library and arms collection. In the pope's bedroom, the intriguing bookholder, as cumbersome as a church lectern, is proof that the pope did not read in bed. The library opens on to a tranquil loggia with Etruscan urns, hanging gardens and a panorama stretching across the Orcia valley as far as Monte Amiata.

On the opposite side of the square,

the **Museo Diocesano** (Wed–Mon 10am–1pm, 3–6pm, Nov–mid-Mar Sat–Sun only; charge) has a rich collection of medieval paintings, tapestries, and ornate gold- and silverware.

Just outside Pienza is the **Pieve di Corsignano**, a simple but coherent Romanesque church where Pope Pius II was baptised.

Montepulciano

The winding road from Pienza up to **Montepulciano** ❸ – visible for miles around, with houses clustered on the sides of the hump of a hill on which it is built – is lined with *vendita diretta* signs, offering pecorino and wine. After Pienza, Montepulciano's asymmetrical design and spontaneous development give it the architectural tension that the earlier city lacks. If Pienza belongs to Rossellino, Montepulciano is Antonio da Sangallo's masterpiece.

Just outside and below the city walls, at the end of a long line of cypresses, lies Sangallo's **San Biagio**, the Renaissance church most at ease with its setting. The building's isolation focuses attention on the

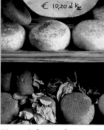

Pienza is famous for its home-made cheeses, especially pecorino and ricotta.

BELOW LEFT: one of the more spiritual aspects of the St Benedict frescoes.

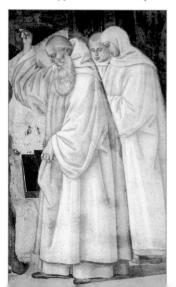

Il Sodoma's Frescoes

The main cloister of Monte Oliveto Maggiore *(see page 224–5)* is covered in frescoes dedicated to the *Life of St Benedict*, begun by Luca Signorelli in 1495 and completed by Il Sodoma from 1505. Of the two contemporaries, Signorelli had the more spiritual approach, but his loveliest work is a domestic scene portraying two monks being served by girls at an inn. In 1497, after only nine frescoes were completed, Signorelli left the rest for Il Sodoma to execute. Vasari adored Signorelli's spirituality as much as he loathed Il Sodoma's exuberance, hedonistic lifestyle and "licentious" fondness for "boys and beardless youths", which earned him his name. In one scene Il Sodoma portrays himself with his pet badgers looking like a pair of well-trained dogs. Il Sodoma's love of what Vasari called his Noah's Ark of "badgers, squirrels, apes, dwarf asses and Elba ponies" is often present, but his landscapes only come to life with the temptations of the flesh. His gaze rarely focuses on the main subject, but is deflected by the turn of an attractive leg, a mischievous smile, a perky badger or a soldier's buttocks. Needless to say, the inhibited monks preferred Signorelli's work to that of the man they labelled "Il Mataccio", the imbecile or madman.

TIP

Tuscany Pass (www.
tuscanypass.com) is a
reliable website that
offers an events
calendar and some of
the best day trips in
Tuscany. Choose from
day-long Tuscan cookery
courses to Vespa trips
to the wine country; or
arty walking tours.

honey-coloured travertine, the Greek Cross design, the dome and the purity of the line. Sangallo's design skills rival Bramante's, not just in the church, the elegant well and the porticoed Canon's House, but elsewhere in the city. The airy interior has a deeply classical feel, more akin to the Roman Pantheon than to a small Tuscan church.

Traffic is banned within the city walls, but you can park outside San Biagio, from where it's a short but steepish walk into town. Alternatively, park in one of the many car parks at Montepulciano's eastern end and enter through the Porta al Prato. Here, Piazza Savonarola is guarded by a statue of the Marzocco lion, the symbol of Florentine power. From here the princely Via di Gracciano nel Corso leads up to the main square. Its lower end is lined with noble palaces. The Renaissance **Palazzo Bucelli**, at no. 73, is decorated with a mosaic of Etruscan urns and pots, a reminder of the city's ancient origins. The road continues upwards to Piazza Grande, both the highest part of town and the highpoint culturally.

Florentine design has shaped the grand facades on Piazza Grande, but earlier Sienese Gothic touches are present in the interiors, double arches and doorways. Both styles reflect Montepulciano's buffeting between the two city-states and the eventual supremacy of Florence. On one side, the 15th-century **Palazzo Comunale** (Town Hall) has a Florentine Michelozzo facade adorning Sienese turrets. **The Tower** (Mon–Sat 10am–6pm; charge), modelled on that of Florence's Palazzo Vecchio, surveys the whole province: from Monte Amiata to Siena and across to Lake Trasimeno in Umbria.

Sangallo's **Palazzo Contucci** (Mon–Sat 8.30am–1.30pm), on the other side of the square, still belongs to the aristocratic Contucci family, who produce Vino Nobile. In the **Cantine Contucci** (wine cellars; Mon–Fri 8.30am–12.30pm, 2.30–6.30pm), Ginevra Contucci will be delighted to expand on the noble wine heritage of her family, the virtues of their silky *Riserva*, and the maze of secret tunnels underneath the palace. Vino Nobile, a smooth

BELOW: Montepulciano's Etruscan origins are evident everywhere.

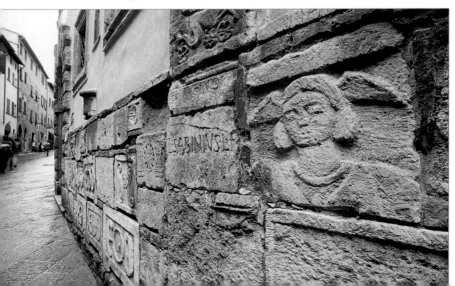

red wine with a hint of violets, was "ennobled" in 1549 when Pope Paul III's sommelier proclaimed it "a most perfect wine, a wine for lords".

Between the two grand palazzi, at the top of wide steps, stands the **Duomo** (daily 9am–noon, 4–6pm), which contains a masterpiece of the Siena school: the huge *Assumption* triptych by Taddeo di Bartolo (1401) shines out above the high altar in the vast, gloomy nave. If you need cheering up, call into the labyrinthine cellars of **Cantine del Redi** (Via Ricci), where part of the *Twilight* vampire series was filmed (*see box, page 196*).

A circular tour

Scattered among the rolling landscape of Siena province are some beautiful villages, each with a separate identity and architectural treasures espied almost incidentally over the brow of a hill. A circular itinerary from Montepulciano unites a group of tiny villages once ruled by the Cacciaconti barons.

Montefollonico ❹, 8km (5 miles) northwest of Montepulciano, has a 13th-century frescoed church and one of the best restaurants in Italy, La Chiusa (*see page 239*).

Petroio ❺, set on a rocky, wooded promontory, is a grand fortified village on an old pilgrim route. In recent years it has been undergoing a revival thanks to its terracotta – examples of which adorn the city walls, Palazzo Pretorio and the medieval towers. Look out for the Canon's House, which contains a remarkable *Madonna and Child* by Taddio di Bartolo. Near the village is the intact **Abbadia a Sicille**, built by the Knights Templar as a refuge for knights on the way to the Holy Land. The adjoining Romanesque church is decorated with two Maltese crosses, but an Olivetan coat of arms marks the abolition of the Templars.

Set among farmland and woods, **Castelmuzio** is a medieval village wrapped up in itself, its Museum of Sacred Art and its direct line to San Bernardo. Narrow shops in winding streets sell honey, salami and cheese made by an ageing population of churchgoers.

Once a Cacciaconti fortress, aristocratic **Montisi ❻** commands a

Pienza's reverence of Pope Pius is surpassed by Montepulciano's devotion to Poliziano. The renowned scholar, poet and resident tutor to Lorenzo de' Medici's children was named after the Latin term for the town – inhabitants of Montepulciano are called Poliziani. Poliziano eulogised the Montepulciano countryside in his Stanzas, which are thought to have inspired Botticelli's La Primavera.

BELOW: the Chiesa San Biagio in Montepulciano.

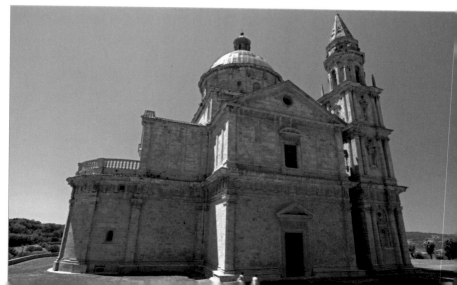

view over two valleys, a view that is even more stirring when seen from the basket of a hot-air balloon (www.balllooningintuscany.com). Even discounting the ballooning base in the village, Montisi offers lofty views, intriguing alleys, earthy inns, and two tiny Romanesque churches, one featuring a Scuola di Duccio crucifix. A few apparently stark, uninviting farmhouses conceal wonderful frescoes and the occasional private chapel so are worth investigating.

One can return to Montepulciano via **Sinalunga**, a dual-personality town with a hideous "low town" but a pleasant "old town". Its original name, Asinalunga, echoes its shape, "the long donkey". But in the lively market, pigs, not donkeys, are in evidence in the form of *porchetta*, the local speciality of roast pig flavoured with rosemary.

Val d'Orcia

The **Val d'Orcia** (*see whole page 232*) is a beguiling rural area south of Le Crete, but within sight of hulking Monte Amiata. Although these villages suffered from depopulation in the 1950s, today they are reaping the benefits of an intact urban and rural landscape. **San Quirico d'Orcia ❼** is a dignified valley town still waiting for its heyday. It survived both an attack by Cesare Borgia's troops in 1502 and a World War II bombardment.

The Romanesque **Collegiata**, made from sandstone and local travertine, has three remarkable portals and columns supported by two stony lionesses. The lovely park, the **Horti Leonini**, is a model 16th-century Italian garden, complete with geometric beds. Stern, 17th-century **Palazzo Chigi** has now opened its frescoed rooms for inspection (daily 8am–6.30pm; charge), and, round the corner, a bijou boutique hotel is flourishing. It seems that San Quirico might well be enjoying a belated renaissance.

Just south of San Quirico, off the SS2, **Bagno Vignoni ❽** is a tiny but lively spa station, at its most evocative at dusk. The steam rises from the hot springs, and the yellowish light of the lanterns dimly illuminates the stone facades of the buildings lining the square, which is in fact

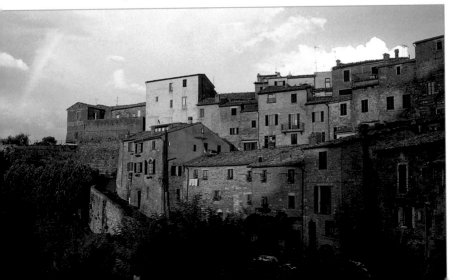

a stone pool of sulphurous water, where both Lorenzo de' Medici and St Catherine once bathed. The hot springs were used by the Romans but became public baths in medieval times. Bathing is now forbidden, but the baths of Hotel Posta Marcucci are open to non-residents for a fee, and are also open at night on summer weekends.

From the relaxation of the pool, all senses are fulfilled at once: outside the pool of light, the sound of sheep and crickets reverberates; the softness of the hot, chalky water dissolves tiredness; and the smell of sulphur evaporates into the night air. After a swim, a short *passeggiata* around the old baths shows the well-restored square at its most romantic.

In the vicinity are three medieval fortresses – Ripa d'Orcia, Rocca d'Orcia and Castiglione d'Orcia. After the turning to Bagno Vignoni, **Ripa d'Orcia**, an enchanted castle (now a hotel; tel: 0577-897 376; www.castelloripadorcia.com) set among cypress groves, comes into view.

Rocca d'Orcia ❾, a fortified village once owned by the warring Salimbeni clan, has an impressive castle open to visitors. **Castiglione d'Orcia** offers more of the same: an atmospheric, cobblestoned centre, a ruined fortress and wonderful views. The abbey of Sant'Antimo *(see page 238)* can be reached from here. The mountain roads in the area are tortuous but beautiful, as are the walks.

Chiusi

Although set among attractive low hills, **Chiusi** ❿ comes across as a rather unprepossessing town, somewhat devoid of Renaissance charm. The "low town" is a commercial centre and the shabby "high town" is endearing but overwhelmed by its glorious Etruscan past.

Then, as now, the Chiusini were farmers, merchants and craftsmen, a spirit that predominates over artistry. Yet, with a little Etruscan knowledge and much curiosity, the town is as fascinating as any in Tuscany. It boasts a complete underground city; an unrivalled collection of female cinerary urns; and the only tomb

The Strada del Vino Nobile di Montepulciano is an association that promotes the local wines. As well as organising tours of the local vineyards and cellars, it offers a range of cultural tours including visits to the Garden of Villa La Foce, the Montepulciano spa, and Siena's pottery workshops. Its office is on Piazza Grande (Mon–Sat 10am– 1pm, 3–6pm; tel: 0578-717 484; www. stradavinonobile.it)

BELOW: the thermal pool in Bagno Vignoni.

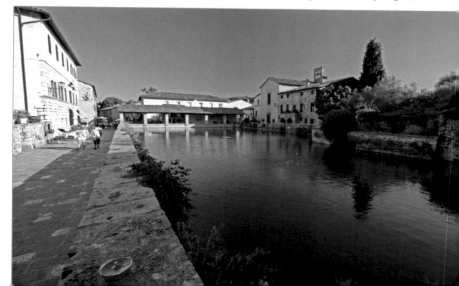

Val d'Orcia

The Val d'Orcia combines the most crowd-pleasing elements in one small valley: castles and country walks; spas and superb inns; iconic scenery and intoxicating settings.

The valley's prime location on the Via Francigena pilgrim route partially explains the surprisingly noble architecture and grandiose Romanesque churches; medieval insecurity accounts for the cluster of castles built to watch over the Orcia valley. But nothing quite explains why these elements come together so well.

Landscaped since time immemorial, the Val d'Orcia represents quintessential Tuscany: clusters of cypresses, ribbons of plane trees, sloping vineyards and farms perched on limestone ridges. But it was not this alone that won the area Unesco World Heritage status in 2004. It was as much to do with the harmonious relationship between the custodians and their landscape, a bond that has survived to the present day, leaving the countryside cultivated but unscathed. This harmony extends to the hilltop ham-

lets, the Romanesque churches, the isolated farmhouses and the contemplative abbeys. All entities are anchored in this mystical yet pragmatic patchwork: they serve a purpose yet transcend it. This happy partnership has produced an idealised landscape that is at once the continuation of the natural order and the best that man and nature can achieve in unison.

Partly boosted by its Unesco recognition, Pienza, in particular, has become very popular, almost as much for its superb pecorino cheeses as for its perfect architecture and splendid views of Monte Amiata.

But it's not a case of the valley selling its soul. If spas can be mystical, then Bagno Vignoni comes close, not just because St Catherine of Siena bathed there. The ancient abbey of Sant'Antimo continues to inspire visitors: the Romanesque church reels you in with its carved capitals, its Gregorian chant, its Cistercian spirit.

This soft mysticism extends to the landscape, where the rambles around Sant'Antimo are among the loveliest in Tuscany. A waymarked trail links the abbey with Montalcino on a gentle, 9.5km (6-mile) walk that unravels views over Monte Amiata and the whole of Val d'Orcia. A far more challenging 18km (11-mile) trail connects the abbey with Bagno Vignoni, via the medieval fortress of Ripa d'Orcia. En route are views of the Brunello vineyards, the soft hills around Pienza and the looming presence of Monte Amiata.

Alternatively, the so-called Nature Train (Treno Natura; www.trenonatura.terresiena. it) provides a similar atmosphere. This service runs through countryside, covering routes where towns are peripheral. The Nature Train generally does the Val d'Orcia run on Sundays in spring and autumn. At other times of the year, the train service focuses on quirky local festivals, including the olive-oil festival in San Quirico d'Orcia, or the pork festival in Vivo d'Orcia. During the autumn white truffle season, one special train travels round the Crete moonscape to San Giovanni d'Asso (www.museodeltartufo.it), culminating in truffle tasting over lunch. ❑

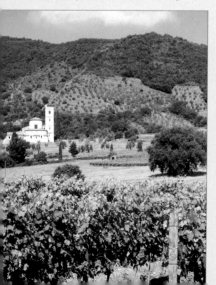

LEFT: vineyards below Sant'Antimo.

paintings in their original setting in all of Tuscany.

As one of the greatest city-states in the Etruscan League, Chiusi, or "Kamars", controlled the area from Lago di Trasimeno to Monte Amiata. After reaching its zenith as a trading centre in the 7th century BC, Etruscan Kamars became submerged by Roman Clusium and then by medieval Chiusi. The old city now survives on three levels of civilisation: the Etruscan necropolis beneath the city hills; the Roman street-grid system below the Cathedral; and the medieval city above it.

The **Museo Archeologico Nazionale** (tel: 0578-20177; daily 9am–8pm; charge) has one of the finest collections of its kind in Italy, which attests to the vitality of Kamars and shows a distinct bias in the outstanding female Canopic jars, cinerary urns and rounded *cippi* tombstones. The containers have Egyptian-style lids resembling human or animal heads. The Etruscans borrowed freely from the Greeks and Egyptians; the imitation Greek vases are less rational but more vigorous than the originals.

A speciality of Chiusi is *bucchero*, glossy black earthenware, often in the form of vases with figures in relief. This pottery has a sophisticated metallic finish that cannot be reproduced by modern craftsmen. Although much of the domestic pottery has a naturalness verging on the commonplace, the sarcophagi, the cinerary urns and the crouching sphinxes reveal an underlying obsession with death and the appeasement of shadowy spirits.

A visit to the **Etruscan tombs**, 3km (2 miles) outside town, can be arranged with the museum staff or pre-booked (tel: 0578-20177). The tombs contain sarcophagi, cinerary urns and, in the case of the **Tomb of the Monkey**, rare wall-paintings of athletic games and domestic scenes.

Three civilisations are visible at once in Chiusi's **Duomo**: the Romanesque Cathedral is built from Etruscan and Roman fragments. The **Museo della Cattedrale** (daily 10am–12.45pm, 4–6.30pm; charge) is of limited appeal, but your ticket entitles you to a tour of a fascinating labyrinth beneath the Cathedral. The recently excavated tunnels are part of an Etruscan water system cut into the rocks, which provided natural filtration. After being led through tunnels to a large Roman cistern dating from the 1st century BC, you emerge, blinking, at the bottom of the Cathedral bell tower. Climb to the top to gaze at Monte Amiata, the Val d'Orcia, and even Lake Trasimeno.

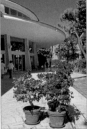

The entrance to Chianciano Terme.

Chianciano Terme

After underground Chiusi, **Chianciano Terme ⑪** is a breath of fresh air. Italians have flocked to this spa town since Roman times to enjoy the unique powers of Acqua Santa. The innovative **Terme Sensoriali** is just one of a new breed of swish thermal day spas that have appeared across Tuscany in recent years, replacing the more old-fashioned clinical baths.

BELOW: chapel in a golden field outside Pienza.

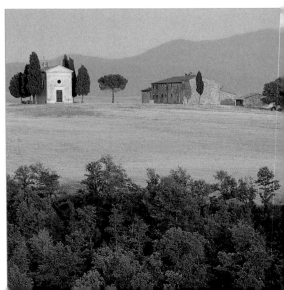

Although better known for its spa than for its culture, a new museum aims to put Chianciano on the artistic map. The **Museo d'Arte di Chianciano** (280 Viale della Liberta, 0578-60732; www.museodarte.org; charge) presents a collection by the Realists, Surrealists and Post-Impressionists, as well as staging international exhibitions.

Southern Siena province is positively bursting with Etruscan remains, and digging produces a continual flow of exciting finds. In Chianciano, well-marked walks lead to several recently discovered tombs and temples, and an excellent **Museo Etrusco** (tel: 0578-30471; Tue–Sun 10am–1pm, 4–7pm; charge) contains an intact monumental tomb of a princess, lined with bronze and adorned with gold and bronze artefacts. The museum also features the remains of a spa complex dating from the 1st century BC, which was discovered in Chianciano and is thought to be the sacred magic spring that cured Emperor Augustus in 23 BC from a life-threatening stomach ailment.

Around La Foce

Near the town are some of the loveliest walks and drives in Tuscany. Many walks start from **La Foce** ⑫, a 15th-century farmhouse that overlooks the fertile Val di Chiana and the desolate craters of the Val d'Orcia. The superb gardens here (Wed Apr–Sept 3–7pm, Oct–Mar 3–5pm; charge) were designed by the famous British landscape gardener Cecil Pinsent. There are views across an Etruscan site to Monte Amiata and Monte Cetona. Its excellent strategic position meant that its owners, the Anglo-Italian Origos *(see box, left)*, allowed it to be used as the partisans' refuge during World War II. Ongoing excavations on the property have uncovered some 200 Etruscan tombs. From here, a rough track leads to Petraporciana, the partisans' hidden headquarters, and to a primeval forest full of giant oaks, cyclamens, wild orchids or snowdrops: a perfect short spring or autumn walk.

Beside La Foce is **Castelluccio**, a castle – and summer concert venue – that commands the best-loved view in the province: a sinuous line of cypresses plotting an Etruscan

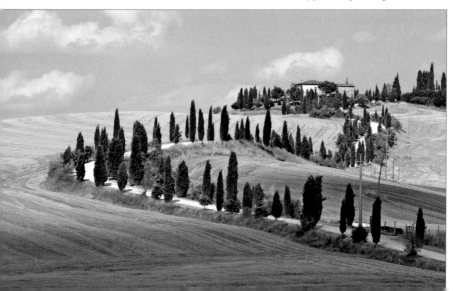

route across the craters. When Prince Charles stayed at La Foce, proud locals were not surprised to see him painting this view.

A short walk leads to **Pocce Lattaie** and prehistoric caves with dripping stalactites shaped like teats or nipples. These pagan caves were used in fertility rites and when propitiatory offerings were made to the gods. Be prepared to hire a guide (and a torch) from Chianciano.

Around Monte Cetona

From Chianciano, an idyllic rural drive leads via La Foce to Sarteano and Cetona, two small medieval and Etruscan towns. These views of desolate *crete*, fortified farmhouses and hazy Monte Amiata are captured by Paolo Busato in his celebrated photographs. It is worth sacrificing a hired car to the dirt roads, but the nervous can take the more direct route to Sarteano.

Castiglioncello sul Trionoro is a tiny village with a *castello* and a church containing a Trecento Madonna. The village is set amid vast expanses of abandoned countryside in which Etruscan remains are regularly uncovered.

Spilling over its double ring of city walls, **Sarteano 13** is a popular spa centre that has retained its traditional identity. The town offers Etruscan remains, a grandiose 13th-century Rocca and crumbling Renaissance palazzi built into the city walls. There is an interesting **Museo Etrusco** (tel: 0578-269 261; Tue–Sun 10.30am–12.30pm, 4–7pm; charge) but, contrary to rumours, the tomb of the Etruscan king Porsenna has never been discovered. In August each year, Sarteano holds a famous *Giostra* or jousting tournament.

Cetona 14 clings to a richly wooded hill. The grand 18th-century houses on the plains are a relic of past prosperity, but Cetona is a refreshingly authentic Tuscan community.

The broad traffic-free square is filled with locals going about their daily lives, free (as yet) of the quaint wine, food and craft shops that predominate in touristic towns such as Pienza. Although Cetona is noted for its textiles and copies of Etruscan vases, it now relies on *agriturismo* to keep its population from leaving. A short stay in a local farm with mountain walks, local cheeses and *bruschetti* drenched in olive oil is highly recommended.

A very scenic route, the Via della Montagna, goes from Cetona to the spa town of **San Casciano dei Bagni 15** (take the high road north out of town and follow signs to Mondo "X"). En route, it's worth stopping at the beautifully restored **Convento di San Francesco**. It now houses a rehabilitation centre (Mondo "X"), but if you ring the bell, one of the occupants of the *comunità* will be happy to show you round.

The **Fonteverde spa resort**, on the edge of San Casciano dei Bagni, is one of Tuscany's most alluring destination spas, with the Medici villa at the heart of the stylish resort. Fortunately, you can also use it as a day spa, and wallow

TIP

Monte Cetona (1,148 metres/3,800ft) is crisscrossed by woodland lanes and open tracks for walking, cycling and horse riding. A map of the network of mountain trails is available from the tourist offices of Cetona, San Casciano dei Bagni and Sarteano.

BELOW: a bather at Bagni San Filippo.

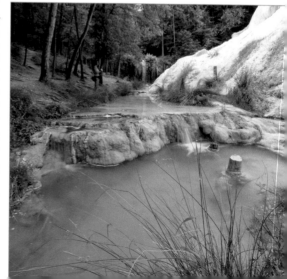

Radicofani is linked to the exploits of Ghino di Tacco, the "gentle outlaw" immortalised by Dante and Boccaccio. Exiled Ghino controlled the town from Radicofani Castle, built by Hadrian IV, the only English pope. A fierce basalt sculpture of Ghino stands in this forbidding town of low stone houses with external stairways, blind alleys and severe facades.

BELOW: the view towards Abbadia San Salvatore.

in the hot pools while gazing over a sea of greenery (www.fonteverdespa.com).

Routes up to Monte Amiata

The journey to Monte Amiata, southern Tuscany's highest peak, is at least as rewarding as the arrival. The fast Pienza to Abbadia San Salvatore route allows for a detour to the thermal baths at **Bagni San Filippo**, where you can float along on faded charm in a friendly, affordable time-warp spa, or dine in the good-value restaurant (www.termesanfilippo.it)

The alternative route, via Sarteano and **Radicofani** ⑯, was the one taken by both Dickens and Montaigne to a location second only to Volterra for natural drama. While the mountain villages have walking and food trails to thank for their revival, the villages on the edge of Amiata seem to be in permanent limbo, trapped rather than enhanced by a medieval identity. Dickens found Radicofani "as barren, as stony, and as wild as Cornwall, in England". Perched on a craggy basalt rock, it is the only place in Italy to possess a

triple Medicean wall. The town overlooks *"Il Mare di Sassi"*, the "Sea of Stones", suitable only for very hardy sheep. Although an 18th-century earthquake destroyed much of the town, enough atmosphere remains.

The drive from Radicofani up to **Abbadia San Salvatore** ⑰ is via Le Conie, a tortuous road known as "Amiata's sentry". For those not interested in skiing, mountain walks and disused mercury mines, Abbadia is best known for its overrated **Abbazia** (abbey) and its medieval "high town". The Romanesque **San Salvatore** (summer Mon–Sat 7am–6pm, Sun 10.30am–6pm, winter until 5pm; free) is all that remains of a once-magnificent abbey, but it has been clumsily restored. A 12th-century *Crucifix* and the crypt with 36 columns remain relatively unspoilt. Geometric symbols, grapes, palm leaves, animals and Gordian knots decorate the pillars.

From Abbadia, a winding road with sharp bends and sheer drops leads to the top of **Monte Amiata**, 1,738 metres (5,700ft) high. The wooded area around the extinct volcano has

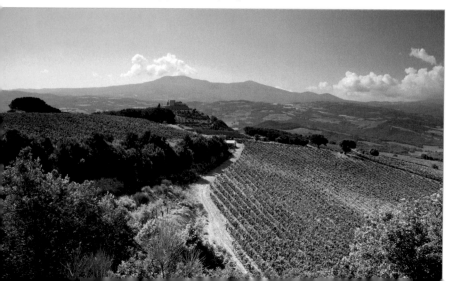

attractive walks. The Fosso della Cocca, a leafy tunnel, is the best place to spot unusual wildlife and vegetation.

Castel del Piano, set among pine forests and wild raspberries, is the oldest settlement in the area, but **Piancastagnaio** is a better base. Perched among chestnut groves, the town has a newly restored Rocca and Franciscan monastery.

Arcidosso ⑱ was the birthplace of David Lazzaretti, "The Prophet of the Amiata". In the 19th century, Lazzaretti created a revolutionary social and religious movement with its headquarters on **Monte Labro**, a lonely peak. Now a nature reserve where deer, chamois and wolves roam, the park is best visited in autumn, when the crowds have left and the wild mushrooms appear.

Santa Fiora is particularly delightful, and has fine works of art in the 12th-century Santa Fiora and Santa Lucilla churches, including some della Robbia ceramics.

Montalcino

In both temperament and identity, **Montalcino** ⑲ is certainly the most Sienese town in the province. In essence, its history is a microcosm of Sienese history. From a distance, Montalcino even looks like a Sienese Trecento painting: the landscape could be a background to a saint's life; in the foreground would be the fortress and scenes of rejoicing and celebration after a historic victory.

Montalcino has been known as "the last rock of communal freedom" since its time as the Sienese capital-in-exile between 1555 and 1559. After the fall of Siena, exiles gathered around Piero Strozzi and the Sienese flag. As a reward, Montalcinesi standard-bearers have the place of honour in the procession preceding the Palio in Siena.

The magnificent 14th-century **Fortezza** (Apr–Oct daily 9am–8pm, Nov–Mar Tue–Sun 9am–6pm; free) is the key to Montalcino's pride. The approach is through olive groves and the slopes famous for Brunello wine. But the asymmetrical fortress, astride a spur of land, dominates the landscape. From its gardens, there is a sense of boundless space and absolute freedom. In winter, the wind howls over

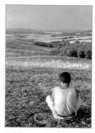

A Sienese shepherd.

BELOW LEFT: within the walls of the Fortezza, Montalcino. **BELOW RIGHT:** a view of Montalcino.

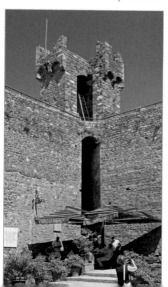

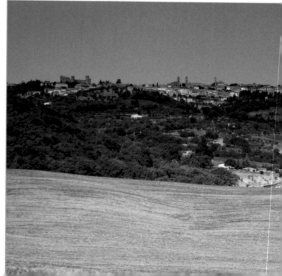

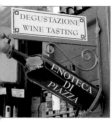

Brunello di Montalcino is one of Italy's best wines. Opportunities abound to taste and buy Brunello and the younger Rosso di Montalcino.

the massive walls and drives visitors to a different type of fortification in the *Enoteca* bar inside. This "National Wine Library" naturally serves Brunello, a magnificent wine whose reputation is slightly tarnished after some producers were charged with illegally blending it with other grapes.

Architecturally, Montalcino offers a neoclassical cathedral, a Gothic loggia, a Romanesque church and myriad intriguing alleys. The Duccio and della Robbia schools are well served by the Civic and Sacred museums. Most significant is the Palazzo Comunale, a mass of *Fiorentinità* finished off by a Sienese tower to prove that the Sienese always surpass the Florentines.

In spring, the area is very green, but yellow rapeseed, poppies, sunflowers and grapes soon take over. Before leaving, try *pici*, home-made spaghetti, in the Grappolo Blu *(see page 239)* or sweet *sospiri* ("sighs") in a *fin-de-siècle* bar.

Sant'Antimo

Nearby is **Sant'Antimo** ⑳ (daily 10am–12.30, 3–6.30pm; free), the remains of a Romanesque abbey founded by Charlemagne, set amidst cypress trees in a peaceful valley. Designed in the French and Lombard style, the abbey is built from local travertine, which resembles alabaster or onyx. The interior has a translucent quality that, as the light changes, turns luminous shades of gold, white and brown.

The community of Augustinian monks who tend the church sing the Gregorian chant at Mass every Sunday afternoon throughout the year. From here there are several superb marked trails through timeless countryside.

Not far away, **Sant'Angelo in Colle**, a fortified hilltop village, once cast a dramatic shadow over Grosseto and other enemies. Until 1265, it was a Sienese outpost, but the tower is all that remains. Today it is a quiet medieval village.

Modern Siena province ends just there. As a frontier castle, Sant' Angelo looked down on to the plain that falls into Grosseto. After Siena province, Grosseto can look deceptively flat.   ❏

BELOW: the Romanesque abbey of Sant'Antimo.

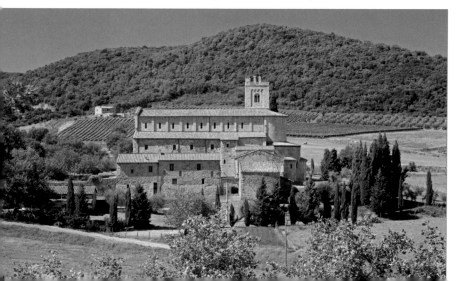

BEST RESTAURANTS

Restaurants

Prices for a three-course meal per person with a half-bottle of house wine:

€ = under €25
€€ = €25–40
€€€ = €40–60
€€€€ = over €60

Montalcino

Osteria di Porta al Cassero

Via Ricasoli 32
Tel: 0577-847 196 €
This is a local favourite. Be sure to try the restaurant's polenta with wild-boar sauce, a regional speciality.

Taverna Il Grappolo Blu

Via Scale di Moglio 1
Tel: 0577-847 150 €€–€€€
Intimate, well-run inn with a rustic atmosphere, charming service and excellent cuisine that spans the full range of Tuscan dishes. Typical dishes include filling soups, rabbit dishes and pasta with porcini. Excellent wine list. Reserve.

Trattoria L'Angolo

Via Ricasoli, 9
Tel: 0577-848 017 €
Among the pricey restaurants of Montalcino, this well-known trattoria remains a down-to-earth and fairly priced option. Particulary good is the bean soup and home-made pasta. Closed Tue.

Montefollonico

La Chiusa

Via Madonnina 88
Tel: 0577-669 668
www.ristorantelachiusa.it €€€€
One of Tuscany's fanciest restaurants, set in an old oil mill on the outskirts of Montefollonico, with glorious views of the countryside. Seasonal dishes are lovingly prepared according to traditional recipes, using locally sourced ingredients and vegetables grown in the adjoining kitchen garden. Dine on duck with wild fennel or tagliatelle with truffles. 15 rooms to rent. Come here for a special occasion. Closed Tue.

Monte Oliveto

La Torre

Monte Oliveto Maggiore
Tel: 0577-707 022 €€
Tourists fill every table on the lovely shaded terrace of this restaurant beside the Benedictine abbey, but the food is surprisingly good. Service is brusque but efficient. Picnic tables nearby. Closed Tue.

Montepulciano

Caffè Poliziano

Via di Voltaia nel Corso, 27
Tel: 0578-758 615
www.caffepoliziano.it €–€€
Lovingly restored Art Nouveau café-restaurant in the historic heart of Montepulciano. It's a landmark, often full, but worth trying to get a table, even just for a coffee. Glorious panoramic balcony.

La Grotta

Località San Biagio 16
Tel: 0578-757 607 €€€
Once the home of architect Sangallo, and right next to his stunningly positioned church of San Biagio. Rustic Tuscan dishes, with French influences. Alfresco dining in summer. This is where locals go for a special occasion. Closed Wed and Jan–Feb.

Osteria Acquacheta

Via del Teatro 22
Tel: 0578-717 086
www.acquacheta.eu €–€€
Authentic osteria serving uncomplicated but tasty dishes such as pici (the chunky local pasta) with wild boar ragù and tagliatelle with white truffles. Wine is sloshed into glass tumblers and your bill will be scribbled on the tablecloth. Excellent value, but book or be prepared to wait.

Monticchiello

La Porta

Via del Piano, 1
Tel/fax: 0578-755 163
www.osterialaporta.it €€
Pleasant inn just outside the walled town of Monticchiello. Stop here for the sweeping views, a glass of wine and a choice of both traditional and more inventive dishes. Closed Thur, most of Jan.

Pienza

La Buca delle Fate

Corso il Rossellino, 38/a
Tel: 0578-748 272 €
Simple trattoria and bar in the lovely 16th-century Palazzo Gonzaga, on the main thoroughfare through town. One of the best of Pienza's many eateries. Closed Mon.

Proceno

La Fondue

Localita Fosso Acquaviva
Tel/Fax: 0763-710 163 €€
After running restaurants in Atlantic City and Moscow, Neapolitan chef Francesco has chosen this scruffy hideaway beside the border with Lazio as his latest experiment. The food is simple but prepared with southern, Italian flair. Check out the photo gallery of celebrities he has fed.

Sinalunga

Le Coccole dell'Amorosa

Località l'Amorosa 2km (1 mile) south.
Tel: 0577-677 211
www.amorosa.it €€€–€€€€
Superb restaurant, romantically set in the stables of a medieval estate. The food is a mix of traditional and new, with a good choice. There is no better place to eat a bistecca chianina (farmed locally). Book well in advance. Closed Mon and Tue lunch.

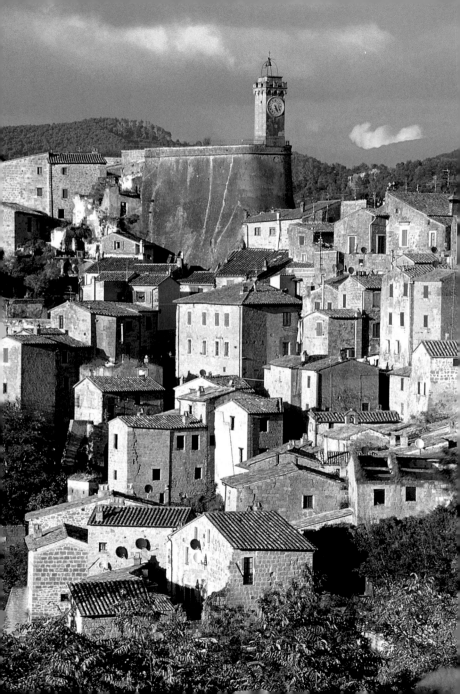

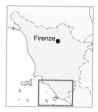
THE MAREMMA AND MONTE ARGENTARIO

Grosseto province has some of the most beautiful
stretches of coast and wilderness areas in the region.
The Maremma, "the marsh by the sea", is Tuscany's
Wild West, where cowboys and long-horned cattle
roam. Inland, the marshy plains give way to densely
wooded hills, where towns seem to grow from the tufa

T uscany's southwestern corner offers a wonderfully varied landscape, ranging from the flat coastal plains to the wooded, snow-capped peak of Monte Amiata, or to the gentle hills bordering Siena province. The coastline has an unrivalled mix of Mediterranean flora and fauna, but the region is dominated by the marshy plain of the Maremma, stretching from the Piombino headland to Tuscany's border with Lazio. Backed by striking hills, this coastal marshland is famous for its horse-breeding, wild-boar hunting, Etruscan sites and austere inland villages, not to mention its rich cuisine.

Abundant remains reveal that the Etruscans thrived in this area, cultivating the land and exploiting the mineral wealth on Elba. However, while the Romans continued to mine Elba for the iron they needed to make swords, they allowed the drainage and irrigation systems the Etruscans had put in place on the mainland to decay. By the Middle Ages, the Maremma had become a malarial swamp and the population had migrated to the hills. It wasn't until the mid-19th century, with the draining of the swamps and land reclamation, that the revival of these evocative lowlands began, spear-headed by the return of the *butteri* (Tuscany's tough cowboys) with their herds of long-horned cattle.

Grosseto

The provincial capital, **Grosseto ❶**, is a commercial and administrative centre, with little to recommend it, unless you are passing through and have an interest in things Roman and Etruscan. The **Museo Archeologico e d'Arte della Maremma** (Piazza Baccarini 3; July–Sept Tue–Sat 10am–

Main attractions
ROSELLE
PARCO DELLA MAREMMA
MONTE ARGENTARIO
GIGLIO
COSA
SCANSANO
SATURNIA
PITIGLIANO
SOVANO

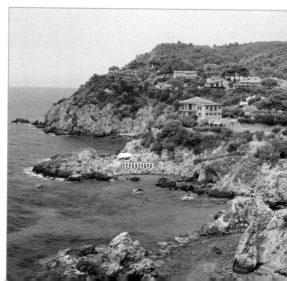

LEFT: the tufa town of Sorano. **RIGHT:** the harbour at Porto Ercole.

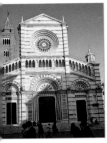

The pink-and-white candy-striped facade of Grosseto's Cathedral overlooks Piazza Dante, the hub of the town.

8pm, Sun 10am–1pm, 5–8pm, other periods Tue–Sat 10am–7pm, Sun 10am–1pm, 4–7pm; charge) is one of the richest museums in the area. It has a fine collection of pre-Etruscan, Etruscan and Roman artefacts from the archaeological sites of Roselle, Vetulonia, Talamone, Pitigliano and Saturnia to the south.

The excavations at **Roselle** ❷ (daily 8.30am–6pm, May–Aug until 7pm; charge; follow signs to the ruins, not the town of Roselle), about 10km (6 miles) northeast of Grosseto, reveal one of the most important Etruscan cities in northern Etruria. The paved streets, ruins of Etruscan taverns and workshops, and the nearly intact circuit of Romano-Etruscan walls, as well as the outlines of the Roman forum and amphitheatre, are all very evocative. Most of the finds are on display in Grosseto's archaeological museum.

On the other side of the old Roman Via Aurelia (also less romantically known as the N1), about 20km (12 miles) north of Grosseto, the hilltop village of **Vetulonia** ❸ lies above another ancient Etruscan city, Vetluna. The small excavated area (the *Scavi Città*) is more Roman than Etruscan. More interesting are the tombs (summer 10.15am–6.45pm, winter 9.15am–4pm; archaeological park same hours; free), 3km (2 miles) from the *Scavi Città*.

The coast

This stretch of coast ranges from the mundane to the magical, often with little in between. South of the rural delights of the Maremma reserve, the decidedly chic Monte Argentario peninsula is dotted with charming coves and small beaches. Instead, north of Castiglione della Pescaia, the Gulf of Follonica represents tawdry, cheap-and-cheerful tourism aimed at the local market. Ignore the unprepossessing **Marina di Grosseto** in favour of the old fishing village of

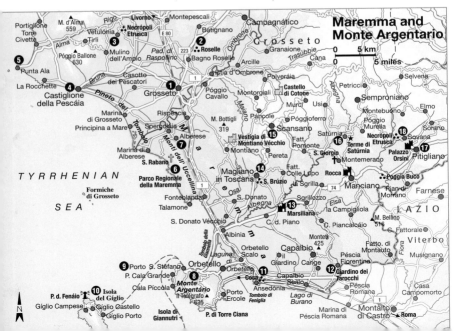

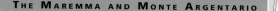

Castiglione della Pescaia ❹.

The boat-lined harbour is believed to be the Etruscan Hasta, or Portus Traianus in Roman times. Overlooking the port is the Rocca Aragonese, with its walls and towers dating back to the 14th century. This low-key resort has pleasant, family-friendly hotels tucked away in the pine groves bordering the beach.

The coastal stretch from Castiglione della Pescaia south to the Parco della Maremma is bordered by a magnificent forest of umbrella pines known as the **Pineta del Tombolo**. You can leave your car by the roadside and take any of the footpaths through the umbrella pines to the lovely beach.

From here the road leads north to the brash Gulf of Follonica. The gulf's southern promontory is occupied by **Punta Ala** ❺, an elite summer resort with a flashy marina, upmarket hotels, golf clubs, horse riding and polo facilities. It's an attractive spot, and offers an amusing window on the lemming-like habits of moneyed Italians at leisure.

If you are in Bay of Follonica area and yearning for the seaside, **Cala Violino** is a quiet bay just before the resort. Alternatively, there are some good beaches between Follonico and Piombino. Otherwise, at this point you're better off heading inland to **Massa Marittima** (see page 194), or back south to the beautiful Parco della Maremma.

Parco Regionale della Maremma

Also known as the Parco dell' Uccellina, the **Parco Regionale della Maremma** ❻ covers an area of around 60 sq km (150 sq miles), including about 20km (12 miles) of coastline.

Evidence of human settlement here can be seen in the remains of a castle, the Benedictine monastery of **San Rabano**, and lookout towers used for the unfortunate soldiers posted here to watch for Saracen pirates and Spanish galleons.

The main entrance to the park is at **Alberese** ❼, where you have to leave your car. The helpful visitor centre (tel: 0564-407 098; www.parcomaremma. it; and www.naturalmentetoscana.it; daily

The Maremma's increasing reputation as a centre for wine-making and gastronomy has been endorsed by high-profile French chef Alain Ducasse. He has transformed a former ducal residence near Castiglione della Pescaia into an elegant hotel with a superb restaurant. Wine and olive oil are produced by the estate, which is surrounded by ancient olive groves and vineyards.

BELOW: beach at Castiglione della Pescaia, with Rocca Aragonese above.

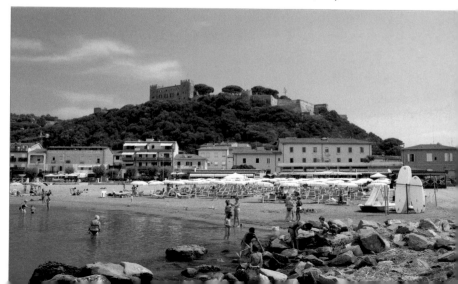

TIP

The beaches within the Parco dell'Uccellina are among the most beautiful and unspoilt in Tuscany. To preserve this wilderness, the number of visitors is limited during the summer, and apart from the road to Marina di Alberese, cars are not permitted in the park. Transport from Alberese is arranged on buses. Visiting in the height of summer is ill-advised, as the weather becomes hot and humid, and there are tiny insects, *serafiche*, whose bite is painful.

8am–8.30pm; charge to park), where you buy your entrance ticket, is full of information on the flora and fauna, and activities within the park. With your ticket you'll be given a map of clearly explained waymarked trails you can follow, of various levels of difficulty and duration, from gentle two-hour walks to day-long treks. Shuttle buses into the park leave from outside the visitor centre at regular intervals, but be sure to check the time of the last bus back down.

Activities within the nature park include canoeing on the Ombrone River, sailing along the coast, riding across the mountains, birdwatching beside the salt marshes, and visiting the noble ruins of San Rabano and other towers strung out along the mountain tops and overlooking the sea, each with its story of marauding pirates and hidden treasures, going back to the times of the Saracens and the Spanish galleons.

If time is limited or you'd rather not walk, you can take the one access road (you still need a ticket) from Alberese to **Marina di Alberese**, a 6km (4-mile) stretch of beach.

Just outside the southern boundaries of the park is the walled village of **Talamone** (18km/11 miles from Alberese), a low-key resort with decent hotels and restaurants. You can gain access to local trails around here from nearby Caprarecce.

Monte Argentario

It's a short drive from Talamone along the Aurelia-Etrusca (Grosseto–Rome highway) to **Monte Argentario** ❽, a craggy peninsula that was once an island, thought to have been occupied by Roman money lenders in the 4th century – *argentarius* in Latin is money lender. From 1556 until 1815, Argentario existed as a separate state from the Grand Duchy of Tuscany, under Spanish rule. This kingdom encompassed the whole promontory and the existing ports of Orbetello, Talamone and Porto Azzurro, on the island of Elba. The Spanish legacy lingers on in the medieval watchtowers that still hug the coast.

Monte Argentario gradually became attached to the land by two long sandbanks: Tòmbolo della Giannella and **Tòmbolo di Feniglia**. Both

Parco della Maremma

As the last virgin coast on the Italian peninsula, Tuscany's most beguiling park is extraordinarily precious and thus well cared for. The landscape ranges from salt marshes, sand dunes and open plains to rocky mountains, sheer cliffs, pine forests and Mediterranean maquis – dense scrubland characterised by rosemary, broom, sea lavender and holm oaks. Wild deer, boar and small mammals thrive in the undergrowth, while it is incredibly rich in birdlife. Wading birds flock to the marshes around the mouth of the Ombrone River, and birds of prey circle the hills. The park is also an important resting place for birds migrating between Europe and Africa. Depending on the habitat and the season, you can see flamingoes, falcons, ospreys, herons and black-winged stilts.

Down on the open fields and low-lying

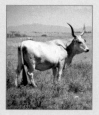

olive groves, herds of long-horned cattle and horses graze. They are reared by *butteri*, the tough Tuscan cowboys who settled in the region in the 19th century, after the swamps were drained and the land could be used for cattle grazing.

One of the loveliest marked routes leads to a high cliff overlooking a forest of umbrella pines cascading all the way down to a sea, and beach, that looks almost Caribbean.

The park headquarters in Alberese (Via del Bersagliere, tel: 0564-407 098, www. parco-maremma.it) has recently launched new itineraries, as well as opening a tasting zone where visitors can try selected local produce for free, including wine, honey and cheeses. (Naturalmente Toscana, tel: 39-33710 65079, www. natutralmentetoscana.it).

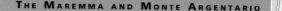
have fine beaches, but while Giannella is backed by a main road, Feniglia is traffic-free and backed by protected pine forest. It's a 7km (4-mile) walk or bike ride to the mainland.

Like two outstretched arms holding on to the mainland, the sandbanks embrace a lagoon, an important wintering spot for migrating birds. The lagoon is cut in half by a central causeway that links Argentario to the town of **Orbetello**, which juts into the lagoon. The town's Baroque architecture reflects its history as a 16th-century Spanish garrison, where the sea laps the city walls. Visitors come from afar for the excellent fish restaurants found here and on Monte Argentario.

The rugged peninsula rises to a height of 635 metres (2,000ft) and is cloaked in Mediterranean maquis, olive groves and vineyards. Apart from **Porto Santo Stefano ⑨**, the mountain has been spared from the property developers, but the exclusive villas outside the port towns remain the preserve of the rich. Sadly, most of this delightful coastline is inaccessible, unless, of course, you are the owner of a yacht. The best way to enjoy Argentario is to stay in a hotel with a private beach. Otherwise, of the few beaches with public access, the nicest are Le Cannelle (roughly opposite Isola Rossa) and the beach to the left of the luxury hotel Il Pellicano, near Porto Ercole.

Porto Santo Stefano's busy harbour is crowded with fishing boats and yachts. It is an atmospheric town, lined with upmarket boutiques, bars and fish restaurants. For a breathtaking and often hair-raising drive, the scenic coastal road from here (follow signs to La Panoramica) takes you along the clifftops.

Porto Ercole is Santo Stefano's smaller, more exclusive sister, but what was once a quiet fishing village is often overwhelmed by all the traffic that converges on it from sea and land. Its main attractions for land-lubbers are the *centro storico* and the 16th-century Spanish fortress overlooking the harbour.

Island excursions

Santo Stefano has ferry connections with Giannutri and Giglio, two of

Umbrella pines line many of the long, straight roads through the Maremman plains.

BELOW: the harbour at Porto Ercole.

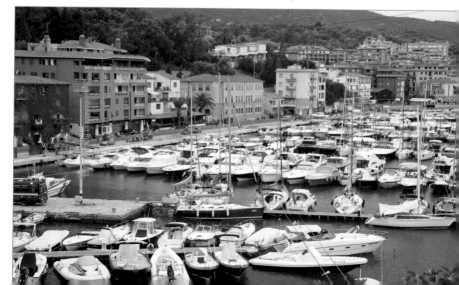

BELOW: Porto Santo Stefano.

the seven islands in the Arcipelago Toscano (*see page 186*). The archipelago was declared a nature reserve in 1996 – not that all the regulations are interpreted as strictly as one might imagine. Crescent-shaped **Giannutri** is a tiny, flat, virtually uninhabited island 22km (14 miles) away, where day-trippers go to visit the ruins of a Roman villa – columns, mosaics, baths and a private pier.

Giglio ❿, an hour's sail from Porto Santo Stefano, has more to offer. It is a playground for sailors and divers, and the second-largest island in Tuscany after Elba. It has an almost impenetrable coastline, with only one easily accessible port, Giglio Porto. A rocky road uphill leads to Giglio Castello, which dominates the landscape. Set among vineyards (which produce grapes for the very strong, distinctive local wine, Ansonica), it is a picturesque settlement, with archways, alleyways and stairs carved from the rock. Giglio abounds in sandy beaches on its western side and is covered in typical Mediterranean vegetation: aromatic herbs and plants, and orange and lemon groves.

Cosa to Capalbio

Back on the mainland coast, across the Aurelia from the town of **Ansedonia** are the important Roman remains of **Cosa** ⓫ (daily May–Sept 9am–7pm, Oct–Apr 9am–5pm; free) built on top of an Etruscan settlement. Excavations have revealed a main street, a forum, a walled acropolis and *capitolium* with magnificent views out to sea, but the site is somewhat overgrown and has a melancholy air.

Below the promontory is the silted-up Roman port and the Tagliata Etrusca, the Etruscan Cut – a canal in fact built by the Romans to drain the **Lago di Burano** reserve.

Inland lies **Capalbio**, one of the first towns on the hills bordering Lazio. Capalbio is a fashionable, foodie haunt among wealthy Italians. Nearby is the magical **Giardino dei Tarocchi** ⓬, or Tarot Garden (daily, summer 2.30–7.30pm, winter 9am–1pm; charge), created by French sculptor Niki de Saint-Phalle, who died in 2002, and inspired by the arcane symbolism of the Tarot. The park displays 22 fantastic, brightly coloured sculptures covered in mirror and mosaic,

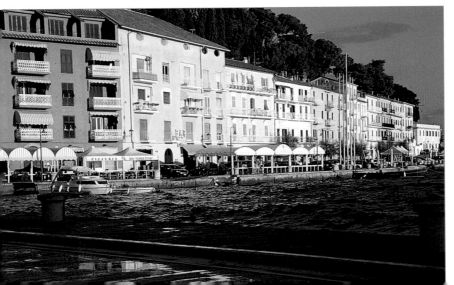

glinting in the sun among the flowers and fountains.

Fortified towns

Across the densely wooded hills north of Capalbio is the drained Albegna plain, which leads to the castle of **Marsiliana** , once an Etruscan town and now the only property left belonging to the Corsini family, who originally owned the entire area. Most of these swamps were expropriated by the state, drained and then distributed to small landowners.

North of here lies **Magliano in Toscana** , a fortified medieval village perched above olive groves. Both civil and religious architecture shows a strong Romanesque influence, with Gothic and Renaissance additions. A perfect example of the blend of styles is San Giovanni Battista, a Romanesque church with Gothic side windows and a Renaissance facade.

A few kilometres further inland, **Scansano** , a breezy hill village with a fortified section (*oppido*), was once the summer capital of the province, when the administrative powers were moved from malarial Grosseto during the hot season. Now famous for the fine wine Morellino di Scansano, there are several *cantine* for wine tasting.

Spa resort

Travelling eastwards across hills and moors inhabited by *butteri* (cowboys) and Maremman cattle, you come to Montemerano, another typically Tuscan walled town, with 15th-century fortifications. From here you can head to the ancient Roman spa centre of **Saturnia** . On the approach to the town, around a sharp curve, you will glimpse the **Cascate del Gorello**, a steaming waterfall where you can bathe in hot sulphur springs. Alternatively, soak car-weary limbs in the upmarket thermal swimming pools of Terme di Saturnia *(see page 301)*. Saturnia, drowsy under the weight of its Etruscan and Roman past, is centred around a large oak-ringed piazza with one or two notable trattorias.

Tufa towns

Pitigliano, Sovana and Sorano are three southern Tuscan jewels situated above dramatic cliffs of soft, porous tufa covered in a thick jungle

It's always worth packing a pair of binoculars. Apart from being useful for close inspection of frescoes, in this area they will be handy for some rewarding birdwatching. The Orbetello lagoon and Parco dell'Uccellina are among the few places along the Italian coast that provide refuge for a wide variety of native and migratory birds.

BELOW: bathing in the Cascate del Gorello.

Spa therapy

Tuscany has an ancient spa tradition. Etruscans worshipped water and were believers in water rituals and herbal cures, but it was the Romans who perfected water cures, pioneering the virtues of moving between the hot and cold of the *caldarium*, *tepidarium* and *frigidarium*. The steaming thermal waters that gush from the ground are channelled into spa pools. These waters stimulate, remineralise, relax and revive the body, with sodium and magnesium nourishing bones, while the therapeutic mud is collected at the source of the spring and used in natural face and body treatments. The top Tuscan spas are pampering as well as curative. *(For a list of Tuscany's best spas, see page 301).*

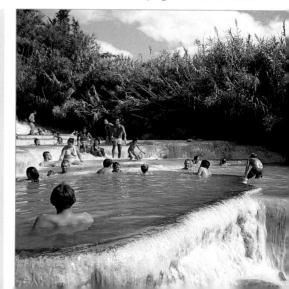

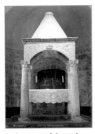

Ciborium of the 8th or 9th century inside Sovana's exquisite Romanesque church of Santa Maria.

of fern, ivy and evergreen trees. The roads here, hewn out of the hills, are an experience in themselves. The winding stretch between Sovana and Pitigliano, which rises spectacularly above it, is particularly memorable.

In the middle of the 18th century, **Pitigliano** ⓱ was one of the most important settlements in southern Tuscany. This majestic town is built on a hill of volcanic tufa and straddles a vast aqueduct with wine and olive-oil cellars carved out of the hillside below. The town is centred around a magnificent medieval citadel built by the Orsini. Laid out around two parallel streets, Pitigliano is crossed by countless atmospheric alleys.

Pitigliano used to be called "little Jerusalem", as it was a refuge for Jews fleeing from religious persecution in the Papal states. Even today, the Jewish quarter of the city, which has the oldest Italian synagogue, remains distinct. It is one of the few places in Italy where you can find kosher cakes, from a Jewish bakery no less. The **Museo Ebraico** (**Jewish Museum**) (via Zuccarelli; Tue–Sun 10am–12.30, 4–7pm, winter until 5pm; charge) is

utterly compelling. Although resident in the former ghetto, Pitigliano's Jewish community were never persecuted. Before leaving town, dip into a Slow Food inn and enjoy a glass of Bianco di Pitigliano from the tufa wine cellars.

Sovana ⓲, situated a few kilometres away, is a perfectly formed one-street village with two outstanding proto-Romanesque churches. The surrounding area is scattered with Etruscan tombs, hidden in the woods, as well as evocative Etruscan streets, carved, like deep gorges, into the rock. These are best seen with a guide (tel: 0564-633 099; www.leviecave.it).

Situated above a deep ravine with a roaring stream and waterfall is medieval **Sorano**, which is also built on a tufa outcrop.

Visible from all corners of the Maremma on a clear day, is **Monte Amiata** *(see page 236)*, the highest peak in Tuscany south of Florence. It is a dormant volcano, with hot geysers and underground waters that supply the spa at Saturnia. Monte Amiata is a refreshing escape during the summer months and a ski resort in winter. ❏

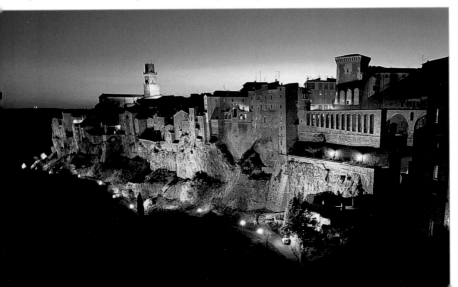

BEST RESTAURANTS

Restaurants

Prices for a three-course meal per person with a half-bottle of house wine:
€ = under €25
€€ = €25–40
€€€ = €40–60
€€€€ = over €60

Capalbio

Il Fontanile dei Caprai
7km (4½ miles) from Capalbio on the Marsiliana road
Tel: 0564-896 526 €€
This country restaurant and its jovial owner are full of Tuscan rustic charm. Tasty Maremman dishes made from locally sourced ingredients are lovingly prepared and served. Weekends for lunch and dinner, and from mid-June–mid-Sept, 26 Dec–8 Jan in the evenings, too.

Castiglione della Pescaia

La Griglia
Via delle Rocchette
Tel: 0564-941 402
www.lagriglia.org €€
A modest but reliable trattoria that offers customers its fantastic speciality – a mixed platter of fresh and tasty grilled-fish.
La Terrazza
Corso Della Libertà 49
Tel: 0564-934 617 €
Reliable restaurant and pizzeria. Spring and summer only.

Grosseto

Il Canto del Gallo
Via Mazzini 29
Tel: 0564-414 589 €€
A tiny trattoria set in the old town walls that favours organic, local produce for its dishes. Closed Sun and two weeks in Feb.

Montemerano

Da Caino
Via della Chiesa, 4
Tel: 0564-602 817
www.dacaino.it €€€€
One of the best restaurants in all of Tuscany. Serves exquisite and creative food, specialising in wild mushrooms and truffles. Booking essential. Closed Wed, Thur lunch, late Jan–late Feb and 2 weeks in July.

Orbetello

Osteria dell Lupacante
Corso Italia 103
Tel: 0564-867 618 €€€
This is one of Orbetello's many good fish restaurants. It serves delicious and creative dishes to customers alla siciliana. Closed Wed Sept–June.
Osteria Il Nocchino
Via Lenzi 64
Tel: 0564-860 329 €€
Squeeze yourself into this tiny fish restaurant and enjoy tucking into such dishes as salt cod and chickpeas or the

seafood risotto. Open in the evenings only. Closed Tue and weekend lunchtimes during winter.

Pitigliano

Osteria Il Ceccottino
Piazza San Gregorio V11, 64
Tel: 0564-614 273
www.ceccottino.com €€
Set on a lovely square in the old town, this Slow Food inn lives up to its good reputation. In summer, dine on the terrace, sipping a chilled glass of Bianco di Pitigliano. On the seasonal menu are dishes including pumpkin ravioli, Florentine steak, pasta with porcini or truffles, and apple-and-cinnamon tart.
Trattoria del Grillo
Via Cavour, 18
Tel: 0564-615 202 €
Authentic trattoria, beside the aqueduct, mixing Tuscan classics with local flourishes. So you might follow good old bruschetta or pici, with escalopes in Pitigliano wine. Honestly priced and packed with locals. Closed Tue.

Porto Santo Stefano

Il Moletto
Via del Molo
Tel: 0564-813 636
www.moletto.it €€
The last in a long line of fish restaurants along the marina's main drag.

Share a seafood platter while watching the port activity. Closed Wed.

Saturnia

Due Cippi-da Michele
Piazza Vittorio Veneto 26/A
Tel: 0564-601 074
www.iduecippi.com €€–€€€
Better known simply as Da Michele, this is an inn serving Maremman dishes in a patrician palazzo. Tasty Tuscan dishes are offered across the board, from steaks to pasta and the range of antipasti. Closed Tue.

Sovana

Taverna Etrusca
Piazza del Pretorio 16
Tel: 0564-616 183
www.tavernaetrusca.info €€
The best restaurant in town, and not just for the quality of the local specialities on offer. Meals are served in an atmospheric medieval dining room with exposed beams and a terracotta floor. Closed Wed and July.

Scilla

Via del Duomo
Tel: 0564-616 531
www.albergoscilla.net €€
This bright and elegant hotel/restaurant has a more contemporary feel than the Taverna Etrusca in Sovana (above) and offers a vegetarian menu. Closed Tue.

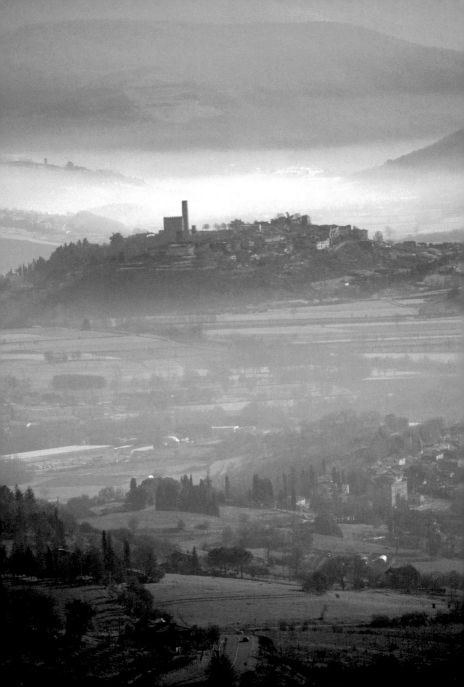

AREZZO AND EASTERN TUSCANY

Known for its gold, art and antiques, Arezzo can feel removed from tourism. The province is also blessed with prosperous farms, castles and abbeys tucked into deep woods. For all its wealth, there is a spirituality in the air that feels more akin to mystical Umbria

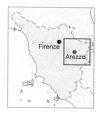

rezzo province is rugged, with steep, thickly wooded valleys that shield its towns and villages from view. The source of the Arno is here, too, in an area of great natural beauty known as the Casentino. This remote, northern area of chestnut woods, vineyards and monasteries leads to the farms of the fertile Val di Chiana. To the west, across the Pratomagno ridge, lies the Arno valley. At the heart of the province, its capital, Arezzo, was one of the most important towns in the Etruscan federation, thanks to its strategic position on a hill at the meeting point of three valleys. Today, it is one of Tuscany's wealthiest cities, as witnessed by the proliferation of jewellers, goldsmiths and antique shops on the city's streets.

Arezzo city

Arezzo ❶ abounds in monuments and works of art from all eras, but tourism is mostly muted. The old, hilly part of the city is the most picturesque, with its massive main square, the **Piazza Grande Ⓐ**, barely on an even keel. On the first Sunday of every month, this square welcomes an antiques market, the largest of its kind in Italy. Stalls

cover the square, run around the base of the Duomo, and spill into the cobbled **Corso Italia**, the city's main shopping street. After being tempted by the jewellery shops, linger over a leisurely lunch around Piazza Grande, ideally at **La Torre** (Piaggia di San Martino, tel: 0575-352 035), a rustic inn serving salami, cheese platters and stuffed pasta (*see page 263*).

Spiritual duties await in one of the loveliest Romanesque churches in Tuscany. Rising from the southern

Main attractions

PIERO DELLA FRANCESCA FRESCOES, SAN FRANCESCO, AREZZO
SANSEPOLCRO
MONTERCHI
THE CASENTINO COUNTRYSIDE
MONASTERO DI CAMALDOLI
CASTELLO DEI CONTI GUIDI, POPPI
LUCIGNANO
CITYSCAPE, CORTONA
MUSEO DIOCESANO, CORTONA

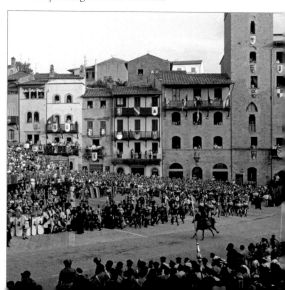

LEFT: view of Poppi. **RIGHT:** Giostra del Saracino, Arezzo.

side of the square, sitting on the Corso, is the **Santa Maria della Pieve** **Ⓑ** (daily 8am–1pm, 3–7pm; free), with its "tower of a hundred holes", so named because of the filigree pattern of arches that pierces the belfry.

A spiritual trail

Just west stands the cavernous church of **San Francesco** **Ⓒ** (Mon–Fri 9am–6.30pm, Sat until 5.30pm, Sun 1–5.30pm; free) which contains Piero della Francesca's restored *Legend of the True Cross* (1452–66) (advance booking necessary; tel: 0575-352 727; charge). This haunting fresco cycle weaves together a complex story in which the wood of the *Tree of Knowledge* (from which Adam and Eve ate the apple) becomes the wood of the cross on which Christ died, and which was later discovered by the Empress Helena, mother of the Emperor Constantine the Great, who converted to Christianity and made it the state reli-

gion of the Roman Empire, AD 313. What matters more is the spirituality that suffuses his art, a transcendent quality that elevates his work beyond the mere mastery of perspective and space. Look for his graceful figures framed by idealised depictions of Arezzo and Sansepolcro.

Medieval monuments cluster together in the northern part of the city, where you will find the **Duomo** **Ⓓ** (daily 6.30am–noon, 3–6.30pm; free), sheltered by the encircling walls of the Grand Duke Cosimo's 16th-century Fortezza, now a park with fine views of the town and the Casentino beyond. The lofty Duomo, dating from the late 13th century, boasts a Gothic bell tower but still feels stranded on its hilltop site. Inside you can see 16th-century stained-glass windows and the 14th-century tomb of Guido Tarlati, which flanks the *St Mary Magdalene* fresco by Piero della Francesca. This work can be contemplated in

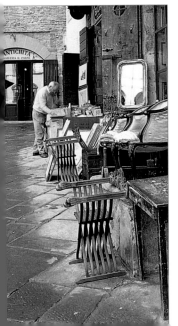

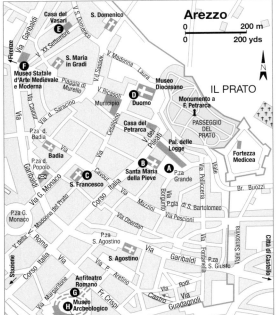

comparative peace, unlike the frescoes in San Francesco. The **Museo Diocesano** (Thur–Sat 10am–noon; charge), behind the Cathedral, contains medieval crucifixes and some Vasari frescoes.

Vasari trail

Further west is the **Casa del Vasari** 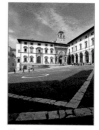 (Mon, Wed–Sat 9am–7pm, Sun 9am–1pm; charge), the attractive house that Giorgio Vasari – Mannerist painter, architect and author of *The Lives of the Artists* (1550) – built for himself and decorated with frescoes painted by the artists he most admired. The 500th anniversary of his birth was celebrated with much pomp in Arezzo in 2011, including the painstaking restoration of a Vasari altarpiece before visitors' very eyes.

Close by is the **Museo Statale d'Arte Medioevale e Moderna** (Tue–Sun 8.30am–7.30pm; charge), housed in the 15th-century Palazzo Bruni. Its varied collection includes an excellent display of majolica pottery, a selection of frescoes and fine examples of the Arezzo goldsmiths'

work, featured alongside paintings by Vasari and modern works by local artists.

Roman Arezzo

Last but not least, in the flat southern part of the city, you will find the **Anfiteatro Romano** (daily 8.30am–7.30pm, request to be accompanied by museum custodian; charge). The Roman Arretium was originally an Etruscan city, but in 294 BC it became a Roman settlement, a convenient resting post on the Via Cassia between Rome and Florence. The site was later plundered to build the city walls and churches, and the perimeter wall is all that remains.

A section of the amphitheatre walls was incorporated into an Olivetan monastery (near the station), now occupied by the excellent **Museo Archeologico** (daily 8.30am–7.30pm; charge). This museum features the Aretine ware for which Arezzo has long been famous. This Roman pottery once competed with the more famous Samian ware as the crockery

Piazza Grande is the scene of the Giostra del Saracino, a historic jousting tournament held twice a year, in June and September.

BELOW: the Corso.

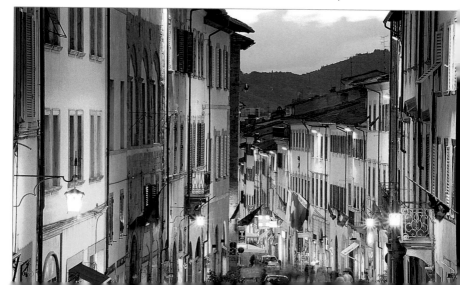

*Piero della Francesca's
1463 masterpiece,
The Resurrection,
was hailed by Aldous
Huxley as "the best
picture in the world".*

of choice on the dinner tables of
Roman aristocrats.

Piero della Francesca trail

East of Arezzo, the Upper Tiber valley
is tightly enclosed at its northern end
by the Alpe di Catenaia and the Alpe
della Luna. Two important towns
for Piero della Francesca enthusiasts
are here. **Sansepolcro** ❷ is famous
for two things: as the town where
Buitoni pasta is produced; and as the
birthplace of the great Renaissance
artist. The old town, huddled behind
crumbling ramparts, is an important
artistic centre. The quiet, narrow

streets are linked by four ancient
gates, the best preserved of which is
the Porta Fiorentina.

In the town centre, at the junc-
tion of Piazza Torre di Berta and
Via Matteotti, is the **Duomo** (daily
8am–12.30pm, 3–6.30pm; free).
Dedicated to St John the Evangelist,
it began life in the 11th century as
a monastic abbey. A wide range of
excellent artworks cover the walls of
the interior, including a tabernacle by
the della Robbia school. Perugino's
Ascension of Jesus is also here.

However, the reason most people
make the pilgrimage here is to see

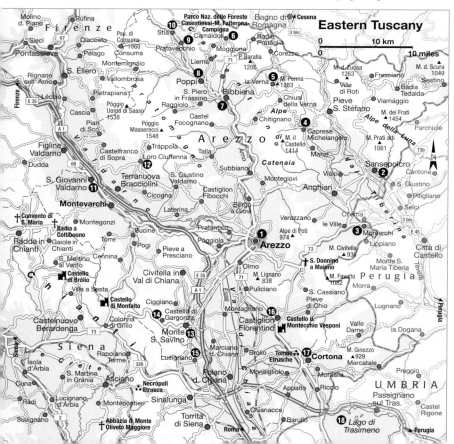

Piero della Francesca's greatest work, *The Resurrection*. The fresco, created in 1463, was nearly destroyed by the Allies during World War II as they bombarded Sansepolcro, believing the Germans were still occupying the town. The fresco was thankfully saved from destruction by the villagers, who surrounded it with sandbags. Today, this intense, brooding work is displayed in the **Museo Civico** (daily June–Sept 9am–1pm, 2.30–7.30pm, Oct–May 9.30am–1pm, 2.30–6pm; charge), in Via degli Aggiunti, alongside the *Madonna della Misericordia*, another Piero della Francesca masterpiece.

Also stop to admire the 16th-century Palazzo delle Laudi (the Town Hall) and the Gothic Palazzo Gherardi, both in Via Matteotti, and the Palazzo Pretorio opposite Piazza Garibaldi.

From Sansepolcro, the Piero della Francesca trail leads south to **Monterchi ❸**, where a former schoolhouse displays his striking *Madonna del Parto* in the **Museo Madonna del Parto** (Tue–Sun 9am–1pm, 2–7pm, winter until 5pm; charge). The Madonna, heavily pregnant and aching, has unbuttoned the front of her dress for relief, while above, two angels hold up the entrance to the tent in which she stands.

Michelangelo's birthplace

Northwest of Sansepolcro, on a steep slope above the Tiber, is the hamlet of **Caprese Michelangelo ❹**, birthplace of Michelangelo. Protected by an almost complete set of walls, this cluster of rustic buildings – which includes the Buonarroti house, the old town hall where Michelangelo's father was the Florentine governor, and the tiny chapel in which Michelangelo was baptised – are interesting more for their connections than for their contents. The views over Alpine countryside explain why Michelangelo attributed his good brains to the mountain air he breathed as a child.

The Casentino

The Casentino is the name given to the little-known region of the Upper Arno valley that runs from the eastern side of the Consuma Pass down

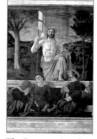

The Resurrection, *by Piero della Francesca.*

Bed, Borghi and Wine

Tuscany excels at rescuing medieval hamlets *(borghi)* and turning them into country retreats, often with a castle or wine estate attached. Set in the hills near Arezzo, **Il Borro** (www.ilborro.it) is part of a patchwork of cypresses, sunflowers, olive groves and vineyards that once inspired Leonardo da Vinci. The setting may feature in fashion shoots, but the Ferragamo fashion dynasty are serious hoteliers and wine producers. As Salvatore Ferragamo says, "It's a wine estate, not Disneyland. The medieval village was in ruins after the war but my father and I had a vision of turning it into a rural resort and wine estate for trailblazing Super Tuscans rather than traditional Chianti Classico." Formerly owned by the Savoia, Italy's former royal dynasty, the estate is unstarry, with craft workshops set up for a goldsmith, carpenter, ceramicist, glassmaker and, of course, a cobbler, a reminder of Ferragamo's shoemaking heritage.

Set in the Val d'Orcia, **Castiglion del Bosco** (www.castigliondelbosco.com) is another medieval *borgo* converted into a chic country estate, as smooth as its Brunello vintages. **Castello del Nero** (www.castellodelnero.com) represents rural luxury, with frescoed, vaulted suites and views of vineyards and olive groves. **Laticastelli** (www.laticastelli.it) is a simpler affair, set in a fortified hamlet outside Rapolano. In the Chianti, **Castel Monastero** (www.castelmonastero.com) boasts frescoed bedrooms, superb wines and cookery courses in a former monastery. Just north, **Borgo di Vescine** (www.vescine.it) is a medieval hamlet converted into a Chianti wine estate and country resort. Near Colle di Val d'Elsa, the latest boutique bolthole is **Castello di Casole** (www.castellodicasole.com), combining castle suites with farmhouse hideaways.

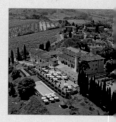

BELOW: in Tuscany, shop decoration is an art form.

to the source of the river just north of Arezzo. It is an area of great natural beauty, enclosed by high mountains, cloaked in fir, chestnut and beech woods, and concealing ancient monasteries and farming villages. The narrow, winding, rural roads are slow going, and with views at every turn, the temptation to stop and admire them is hard to resist.

At its remoter edges, this region is rooted in the 13th century, when St Francis took to a desolate crag on the wooded slopes of **Monte Penna at La Verna** ⑤, using a niche between two huge boulders as a hermitage. On this spot in 1224, St Francis is supposed to have received the stigmata while he was praying. Today, in the middle of the ancient forest, a Franciscan sanctuary still occupies the rock. Assembled around a tiny piazza is a collection of monastic buildings, including one large church containing yet more examples of della Robbia terracotta sculptures.

Sixteen kilometres (10 miles) northeast of La Verna, high in the spectacular woodland cut by moun-tain streams and waterfalls, is another more ancient monastery, **Camáldoli** ⑥ (daily 9am–1pm, 2.30–7pm; summer until 7.30pm; tel: 0575-556 012; www.camaldoli.it; free). It was founded in 1012 by San Romualdo (St Rumbold), a former member of the Benedictine Order, who founded a strict community of hermits. The monastery is still inhabited, and the monks run a welcoming café here. The old cloister pharmacy (9am–12.30pm, 2.30–6pm), with its mortars and crucibles, now sells soaps and liqueurs made by the monks.

Another 300 metres (1,000ft) up the mountain (a beautiful hour-long walk), above the monastery, is the **Eremo**, a hermitage comprising a small Baroque church and 10 cells, each surrounded by a high wall and a tiny kitchen garden. Here the hermits still live in solitude and silent contemplation. The church and St Rumbold's cell are open to visitors (daily 8.30–11.30am, 2.30–6.30pm; tel: 0575-556 021), but access to the monks' quarters is closed.

After the silence and isolation of Camáldoli, noisy **Bibbiena** ⑦ will bring you sharply back to the modern world. Although hidden by urban sprawl and best known for its tobacco industry and salty salami, Bibbiena is still a typical Tuscan hill town at heart. Buildings of note in the historic centre include the church of **San Lorenzo** (daily 8am–6pm), which has some richly decorated della Robbia panels, and the church of **Sant' Ippolito Martire** (daily 8am–7pm), which has a fine triptych by Bicci di Lorenzo.

Nearby is the Renaissance Palazzo Dovizi, home of Cardinal Dovizi, who, as Cardinal Bibbiena, became the secretary of Pope Leo X. Bibbiena's central piazza offers distant views to Camáldoli and Poppi – the latter is the gateway to an interesting area for castles and fortified towns.

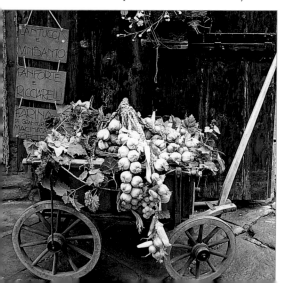

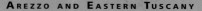

Casentino castles

This region was continually fought over by the Guelf Florentines and the Ghibelline Aretines. A decisive battle in 1289, which firmly established the dominance of the former over the latter, is marked by a column on a site called Campaldino, just between Castel San Niccolò and Poppi.

Poppi ❽ surveys the surrounding countryside from its hilltop perch, dominated by the brooding **Castello dei Conti Guidi** (daily 10am–6pm, winter until 5pm; www.buonconte. com; free), the most important medieval monument in the Casentino. Built in the 13th century for the ruling Guidi counts, the castle's design was inspired by the Palazzo Vecchio in Florence, and it is thought likely that Arnolfo di Cambio was the architect. The courtyard and stairway are impressive, and the Florentine frescoes may be viewed on request. The ancient streets of this quiet town are lined with arcades linked by steep steps and decorated with finely carved capitals and stone seats. There is a Romanesque church and a few shops here selling locally made copper pots.

Off in the distance, on a hill above the village of **Pratovecchio ❾**, birthplace of Paolo Uccello, is the 11th-century **Castello di Romena** (open in summer or by appointment; tel: 0575-520 516; free), another Guidi castle. The noble family gave refuge to Dante here after his expulsion from Florence at the beginning of the 14th century. Of the 14 towers that Dante would have seen at the castle, only three remain.

Standing on a lonely slope, a stone's throw from the castle, **Pieve di Romena** (visits by appointment with the custodian; tel: 0575-583 725; free) is one of the most important Romanesque churches in Tuscany. Beneath its apse, which dates from 1152, excavations have revealed the remains of an Etruscan building as well as two earlier churches. The finely carved capitals atop the gigantic granite columns in the nave make reference to the four Evangelists and to St Peter.

Back down in Pratovecchio, you'll find the headquarters of the **Parco**

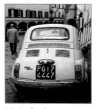

Fiat's classic Cinquecento "Bambino" is still a much-loved runaround, perfect for the narrow streets of small towns such as Poppi.

BELOW: the view across Poppi from the Palazzo Pretorio.

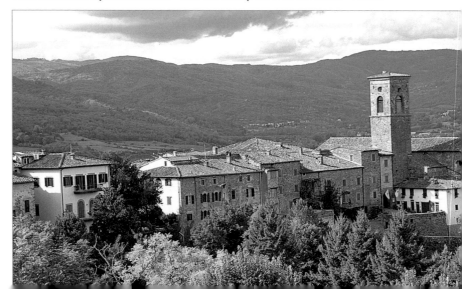

TIP

East of the Arno, and skirting the western edge of the high Pratomagno ridge, is the panoramic road known as the Strada dei Sette Ponti, or Road of the Seven Bridges. The winding route passes through several medieval towns, including Castelfranco di Sopra, and Loro Ciuffena to the south and the abbey at Vallombrosa to the north.

BELOW: the white Chianina cattle are prized for their beef.

Nazionale delle Foreste Casentinesi (Casentino national park) (Via G. Brocchi 7; tel: 0575-50301; www.parco-forestecasentinesi.it; free; see tip p256).

To the north and guarding the source of the Arno (Monte Falterona) is the medieval town of **Stia** ⑩, with a pretty porticoed piazza. Here stand the ruins of the **Castello di Porciano** (mid-May–mid-Oct Sun 10am–noon, 4–7pm, or by appointment; tel: 0575-582 635; free), another Guidi stronghold that once watched over the Arno valley.

The **Castello di Romena** is visible from up here. Whereas most monuments are easily accessible, the fortified remains at Castel Castagnaia, with the nearby ruined Roman temple, both to the west of Stia, are harder to reach. The road peters out, and they can only be reached on foot through rough, stony countryside.

Remains of yet another Guidi castle can be seen in the tiny village of Montemignaio. There's not much left to see, but the village church does have Ghirlandaio's *Virgin and Child with the Four Church Elders*.

On the slope of the forested Pratomagno ridge, south of Bibbiena, is the restored castle at **Chitignano.** The medieval remains were rebuilt in the 18th century. There are other ruined castles located at Talla and Subbiano.

The Valdarno

The most scenic route to Florence skirts the Pratomagno ridge on the eastern side of the Arno. It's full of twists and turns, but the views are rewarding. In the Middle Ages, the Valdarno was bitterly fought over by the Ghibellines and the Guelfs. At the close of the 13th century pressure was exerted on the Florentines by the warlike Aretine bishops, who controlled powerful strongholds in the Arno valley. In an effort to resist them, the Florentines built three fortresses, which were really fortified towns, at San Giovanni Valdarno, Terranuova and Castelfranco di Sopra.

Halfway between Florence and Arezzo, **San Giovanni Valdarno** ⑪ was fortified as a bulwark against the Aretines, but little evidence remains

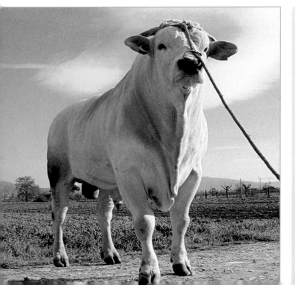

Val di Chiana Cattle

The Val di Chiana, the most extensive valley in the Apennine range, is rich farmland mainly used for cattle-rearing. Here graze herds of one of Italy's most prized breeds of beef cattle – the Chianina, which is native to Tuscany. (Its only rival is the Razza Piemontese from Piedmont.) The cream-coloured Chianina cow grows quickly to a large size, so that it is butchered when the steer is a grown calf. The meat is firm and tasty, with a distinctive flavour. For any beef-loving Italian, *bistecca alla Fiorentina* – a huge, tender Val di Chiana T-bone steak, grilled over an open fire and seasoned with nothing more than crushed peppercorns, salt, and a hint of garlic and olive oil, served very rare – is the ultimate steak.

of its former military function. The central piazza and arcaded **Palazzo Comunale** were designed by Arnolfo di Cambio. The nearby church of **Santa Maria della Grazia** (daily; free) contains a *Virgin and Child with the Four Saints* by Masaccio, who was born here in 1401. Just outside the town, the Renaissance monastery of Montecarlo houses an *Annunciation* by Fra Angelico.

In prehistoric times, the Arno basin was one big lake, and farmers today frequently dig up fossil remains and bones of long-extinct animals. At **Montevarchi**, south of San Giovanni Valdarno, is a castle housing the **Accademia Valdarnese** (closed for restoration until 2013), an important museum of prehistory. It will be home to an impressive collection of fossilised remains of the Pliocene period discovered in this stretch of the Arno valley.

Unlike San Giovanni Valdarno, **Castelfranco di Sopra**, across the Arno (also fortified for the Florentines by Arnolfo di Cambio), retains its military character: the Porta Fiorentina gate is as forbidding as it ever was, and

many of the 14th-century streets and buildings have survived.

About 10km (6 miles) south of Castelfranco, on the scenic **Strada dei Sette Ponti** (Road of the Seven Bridges), is **Loro Ciuffenna** ⑫, a medieval village positioned on a chasm cut by the Ciuffenna river. A couple of kilometres away is the rural Romanesque church of Gropina, dating from the early 13th century, noted for the carvings of animals, figures and geometrical patterns on the pulpit and columns. From here the picturesque route to Talla, where you'll find another ruined castle, crosses into the Casentino.

Val di Chiana

Surrounded by hills and charming towns, the fertile **Val di Chiana** plains south of Arezzo supply Florentine restaurants with the raw ingredient of *bistecca alla Fiorentina* (see box, page 258). **Monte San Savino** ⑬, on the edge of the Val di Chiana, has been a citadel since Etruscan times, although the existing fortifications date from the Middle Ages. In 1325 the inhabitants were unable

The church and square in Lucignano, known for its unique concentric street plan.

BELOW: Piazza Collegiata, Lucignano.

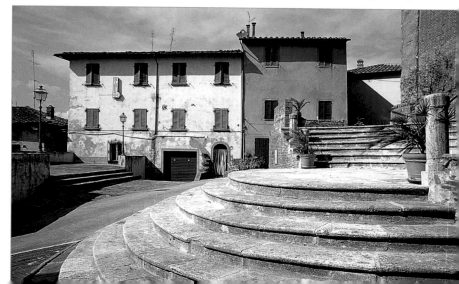

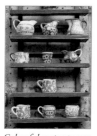

Colourful contemporary ceramics can be found in and around Cortona.

to fend off a ruthless Aretine mob, who razed the town as punishment for their Guelf sympathies. It was subsequently rebuilt. Its once large Jewish community was wiped out – many were burnt at the stake – for resisting the French army in 1799. "Progress" has hardly touched Monte San Savino; it retains medieval and Renaissance houses, of which the **Palazzo Comunale**, with a facade by Antonio da Sangallo the Elder and a fine museum (Nov–Mar Wed–Fri 9am–1pm, Sat–Sun also afternoons 4–7pm, Apr–Oct Wed–Fri 9am–1pm, 4–7pm, Sat–Sun until 7.30pm, Tue am only), is the most important.

Other important landmarks here include the Loggia del Mercato by Sansovino, and the churches of Santa Chiara and Sant'Agostino.

The wild hills northwest of the town shelter a feudal retreat, the **Castello di Gargonza ⓮**. This 13th-century *borgo*, or walled village, on the western slope of Monte Palazzuolo dominates the Chiana valley and is the centre of a vast wooded estate producing oil and wine. The walled settlement has been converted into a

hotel and restaurant complex (www.gargonza.it). The adapted cottages, tiny cobbled streets, a chapel, a baronial tower, attractive gardens and a magnificent view down to the Chiana all make Gargonza a very pleasant retreat.

South of Monte San Savino is **Lucignano ⓯**. Originally an Etruscan stronghold, the concentric arrangement of streets around a fortress make it unique among Tuscan hill towns. With a few exceptions, Lucignano's buildings (13th–18th-century) are perfectly preserved, as is the Gothic church of San Francesco. The 14th-century **Palazzo Comunale** (Tue–Sun 10am–1pm, 2–6pm, winter until 5pm; charge) contains frescoes from the Sienese and Aretine schools, as well as some examples of finely worked gold ornaments for which the province of Arezzo has long been famous, including the beautiful 14th-century *Tree of Lucignano*, richly embellished with jewels.

Fortified villages

Marciano della Chiana 6km (4 miles) northeast, another tiny village

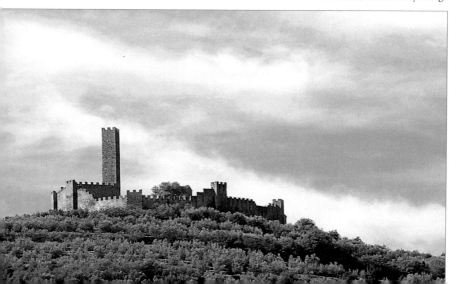

of great character, was also fortified in the Middle Ages. Much of the castle remains intact, as do the walls and a gateway that has a clock tower built into it. Three kilometres (2 miles) to the southeast is the octagonal chapel of Santa Vittoria, designed by Ammannati to mark the spot where the Florentines defeated the Sienese in battle in 1554.

Foiano della Chiana clings prettily to the side of the hill. Much of it dates from the 15th–16th centuries, though traces of medieval defences can be seen around the edge of the town. At **Cisternella**, about 3km (2 miles) to the northeast of the centre, are the remains of what is believed to have been a Roman bathhouse.

From here, looming large in the distance, is the fortified village of **Castiglion Fiorentino** ⑯, bounded by thick walls and dominated by the **Cassero Fortress** (Tue–Sun 10am–12.30pm, 4–6pm, weekends until 7pm; charge). This well-preserved medieval settlement has an unusually high number of churches. The oldest of these, the **Pieve Vecchia** (the oldest church), has a Signorelli fresco of the *Deposition of Christ* (1451), and the 13th-century church of San Francesco also contains a sculpted version.

Other sacred works and gold, and silverware from the surrounding churches can be seen in the **Pinacoteca Comunale** (Tue–Sun 10am–12.30pm, 4–6pm, until 7pm Sat–Sun; charge). On the old market square Vasari's famous loggias can be found. Their stone arches frame a fine vista of the rooftops and surrounding countryside.

Just outside the village is the fine octagonal temple of **Santa Maria della Consolazione**. Looming beyond the village, and visible from the Cassero Fortress, are the battlements of the **Castello di Montecchio** (tel: 0575-651 272; www.castellodi montecchiovesponi.it). This crenellated

medieval castle once belonged to the legendary English *condottiero* John Hawkwood *(see page 33)*.

Cortona

Close to the Umbrian border, 30km (18 miles) south of Arezzo, **Cortona** ⑰ is one of the most enchanting hill towns in Tuscany. It was founded by the Etruscans, colonised by the Romans, and, after being sold to the Florentines in 1409, thrived under the Grand Duchy of Tuscany. The success of the celebrity-studded Tuscan Sun festival, and the book by Frances Mayes, mean that Cortona's quaintly crooked, cobbled streets can be awash with summer visitors.

Cortona is perched majestically on a ridge of Monte Sant'Egidio, dominating the Val di Chiana. The approach road winds its way through terraced olive groves and vineyards, past villas, farms and monasteries. But Cortona's main attraction lies in the steepness of its crooked streets, linked by stone staircases, which work their way painfully to the Medici fortress at the top.

The town is entered from the relatively flat Piazza Garibaldi and

Frances Mayes' books, Bella Tuscany *and* Under the Tuscan Sun *(now a lavishly shot film), have elevated Cortona, where she lives, to celebrity status.*

BELOW: the lofty heights of Cortona.

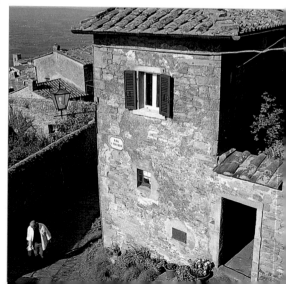

One of a number of celebrated artists from Cortona, Luca Signorelli (1450–1523) produced frescoes for Orvieto Cathedral, and was summoned to the Vatican to complete frescoes in the Sistine Chapel. In a tiny courtyard below the Medici Fortress, the church of San Niccolò houses his wonderful standard of the Deposition.

Via Nazionale, which lead to Piazza Signorelli, with its 13th-century **Palazzo Comunale** (Town Hall) and the **Museo dell'Accademia Etrusca** (summer daily 10am–7pm, winter Tue–Sun until 5pm; charge). The highlights are the lovely fresco of Polymnia, generally considered to be a fine Roman painting of the *Muse of Song* until recent research proved it to be an 18th-century forgery; and a genuine Etruscan chandelier dating from 300 BC.

At the bottom of the hill, a new archeological park, the **Parco Archeologico del Sodo**, showcases the Etruscan Sodo Tombs, including a sculpted sacrificial altar.

West of the piazza is the 16th-century Cathedral and its companion, the **Museo Diocesano** (summer daily 10am–7pm, winter Tue–Sun until 5pm; charge), which contains some rare masterpieces by Fra Angelico, Lorenzetti and Luca Signorelli.

Before leaving town, seek out **Via Janelli** for its row of brick buildings with overhanging upper storeys – some of Tuscany's oldest surviving medieval houses. Other picturesque streets include the Via Ghibellina and

Via Guelfa. It's a steep climb up to the **Basilica di Santa Margherita**, dedicated to the local saint and follower of St Francis. The citizens of Cortona still make pilgrimages up the winding stone-flagged streets to her tomb to offer her prayers during hard times. The **Medici Fortress** above is overgrown and rarely open, but the views from up here are splendid, and it's a fine spot to stop for a picnic.

One side of Cortona's public gardens opens to a belvedere with sweeping views south, enveloping the **Lago di Trasimeno** ⑱, Italy's fourth-largest lake, which lies in neighbouring Umbria. Its shallow waters are surprisingly clean and popular with swimmers, boaters and windsurfers. There was a day, though, in 217 BC, when the lake waters ran red with the blood of the Roman legions, more than 16,000 of whom were slaughtered by Hannibal's troops.

Today, the scene is considerably more peaceful, especially on the southern shore, with Castiglione del Lago the place to toast farewell to underrated Arezzo province over a lakeside fish feast. ❑

BELOW: the domed church of Santa Maria della Grazia, below Cortona.

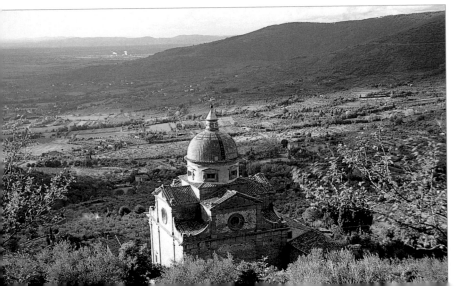

BEST RESTAURANTS

Restaurants

Prices for a three-course meal per person with a half-bottle of house wine:

€ = under €25
€€ = €25–40
€€€ = €40–60
€€€€ = over €60

Arezzo

Antica Osteria L'Agania
Via Mazzini 10
Tel: 0575-295 381 €–€€
Very pleasant and hugely popular family-run trattoria serving good, homely Tuscan fare, including the *Chianina* steak. Excellent value. Closed Mon, except June–Aug.

Buca di San Francesco
Via San Francesco 1
Tel/fax: 0575-23271
www.bucadisanfrancesco.it €€
A famous cellar restaurant adjoining San Francesco church, with trecento frescoes and a Roman-Etruscan pavement. The medieval atmosphere is matched by rustic cuisine. Closed Mon evening and Tue.

Il Cantuccio
Via Madonna del Prato 76
Tel/fax: 0575-26830 €€
Vaulted basement restaurant run by the Volpi family, who produce their own wine and olive oil. Try the *bistecca*, perhaps with deep-fried *porcini*

mushrooms. Closed Wed.

Il Torrino
Strada dei Due Mari 1
Tel: 0575-360 649
www.iltorrino.com €€
Eight km (5 miles) along the San Sepolcro road, this restaurant is worth seeking out for the good food and view. Truffles in season. Closed Mon.

La Lancia d'Oro
Piazza Grande 18/19
Tel: 0575-21033 €€–€€€
Excellent Arezzo cuisine features in this pleasing, central restaurant. In summer you can dine alfresco. Closed Sun evening, all day Mon and 5–25 Nov.

La Torre di Gnicche
Piaggia San Martino 8
Tel: 0575-352 035
www.latorredignicche.it €
Just off the northern corner of the main square, this tiny wine bar is an excellent choice for a cheap and simple meal – a hearty *ribollita* soup or a cheese platter – and some wine from its long and excellent selection. Popular with the antique-dealing fraternity. Closed Wed.

Cortona

Il Falconiere
Loc. San Martino 370 (4km/ 2½ miles north of Cortona)
Tel: 0575-612 679
www.ilfalconiere.it €€€€
In a lovely setting in the

hills, this hotel makes you feel as though time stands still. The imaginative cuisine includes fish and meat dishes, and the service is excellent. Lovely panoramic terrace. Reserve in advance.

La Grotta
Piazzetta Baldelli 3
Tel: 0575-630 271
www.trattorialagrotta.it €€
A well-established family-run trattoria with local food and a warm welcome. Alfresco dining in summer. Popular with tourists. Closed Tue.

Osteria del Teatro
Via Maffei 2
Tel: 0575-630 556
www.osteria-del-teatro.it €€–€€€
Simple but delicious food, located in a 15th-century palazzo, and friendly serv-

ice. One of Cortona's nicest eateries. Closed Wed.

Lucignano

Osteria da Totò
Piazza del tribunale 6
Tel: 0575-836 763
www.trattoriatoto.it €–€€
Run by well-known chef Lorenzo Totò, dishes are inspired by traditional Italian cooking. Closed Tue.

Mercatale di Cortona

Mimmi
Via Pietro della Cortona 29
Tel: 0575-619 029 €
A wonderful experience: arrive early to enjoy plentiful home-made Tuscan cuisine, cooked in a wood-fired oven. Vegetables from the kitchen garden and local wines. Closed 1 week in Nov.

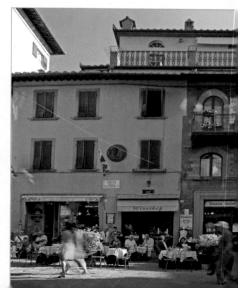

RIGHT: restaurants on Piazza della Repubblica, Cortona.

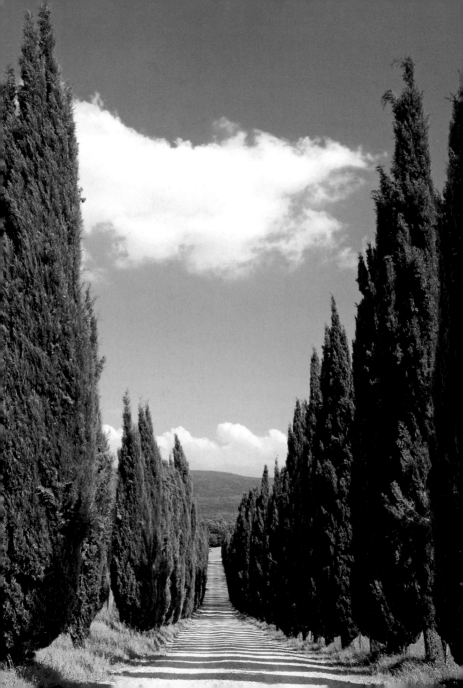

INSIGHT GUIDES **TRAVEL TIPS**
TUSCANY

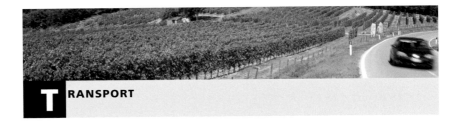

TRANSPORT

GETTING THERE AND GETTING AROUND

GETTING THERE

By Air

From the UK, low-cost airlines such as Ryanair and easyJet operate from many of Italy's smaller provincial airports, making travel between the UK and Italy easy, as well as opening up Italian routes to greater competition.

In addition to the national airline, Alitalia, many major scheduled airlines run direct flights to Italy, as well as charter flights, which tend to offer lower fares and often fly to more convenient provincial airports.

From the US, the main carriers are Alitalia, Delta, United and US Airways, which fly to Rome, Milan and Venice. European airlines such as British Airways and Air France also fly to Italy, with a stopover.

The country has two airports designed for intercontinental flights: **Roma Leonardo da Vinci** (known as Fiumicino) and **Milano Malpensa**.

Pisa's Galileo Galilei Airport is the usual airport for most international visitors to Florence. Getting from Pisa to Florence is easy and cheap *(see page 267).*

Florence's Peretola-Florence Airport (also known as Amerigo Vespucci) is 4km (2 miles) north-

west of the city centre. Some international flights land here, but these tend to be more expensive than flights to Pisa. Meridiana operates regular flights between Florence and the UK (www.meridiana.it). CityJet airlines have introduced a direct flight from London City Airport to Florence (www.cityjet.com). **Bologna Airport** is a further alternative; it is conveniently located for Florence and Tuscany (there's a direct train to Florence and Arezzo).

By Rail

Rail travel is a slow but scenic option, although Italy has improved the speed and quality of its inter-city trains in recent years. (Florence is now only 37 minutes from Bologna and 1 hour 45 minutes from Milan). And the rise of "slow travel" makes rail an appealing option, travelling through Alpine scenery, avoiding the airports, and arriving in the heart of the city. It's both civilised and eco-friendly.

For those under 26, travel is far cheaper if you sign up to the Inter-Rail scheme (providing a month's unlimited rail travel in Europe). When travelling from Great Britain via Paris (the usual route when travelling to Florence), it is necessary to change in Paris (from Gare du Nord to Gare de Lyon).

ES (Eurostar), EC (EuroCity), IC (Inter City) and TEE (Trans Europe

Express) trains are top-of-the-range, running between the main Italian and European cities. A supplement is charged and seat reservation is obligatory. You can check your route or book tickets online on the official Italian railway website: www.trenitalia.it.

In the UK, consider booking through **Railbookers** (tel: 020-7065 7728; www.railbookers.com). A week's break includes an independent rail tour staying in Florence, Siena and Lucca.

Alternatively, for train bookings, contact **Rail Europe** tel: 08448-484 064; visit the ticket office at 1 Regent Street, London W1, Mon–Fri 10am–6pm, Sat until 5pm; or consult www.raileurope.co.uk.

Visitors from the US and Canada can also buy tickets and passes in advance through Rail Europe, or holidays through Railbookers *(for details see above).* Visit www.raileurope.com or tel: 08708-302 008.

By Road

When calculating the cost of travelling to Italy by car, allow for the price of motorway tolls as well as accommodation en route and petrol. The quickest cross-Channel car ferries are from Dover to Calais. The Channel Tunnel transports cars on the train between Folkestone and Calais (Eurotunnel, tel: 08443-353 535; www.euro tunnel.com). The usual route from France to Italy is via Paris and the Mont Blanc Tunnel (between Chamonix and Courmayeur), or from Switzerland through the Gran San Bernardo Tunnel (between Bourg St-Pierre and Aosta). Some of the Alpine passes are seasonal, so check the viability of your route with the tourist board or a motoring organisation before setting off.

To take your car into Italy, you will need your current driving licence, your vehicle registration document and insurance certificate. You are also required to carry a warning triangle in case of breakdown. Headlights should be illuminated at all times. Some petrol stations require payment in cash, not credit card. Keep cash handy for autostrada tolls, too. The AA and RAC in the UK give up-to-date advice on Channel crossings, with or without a car, and also driving on the Continent.

In the US, the AAA provides information on travel in Italy.

By Coach

Travelling to Italy from the UK by coach is not much cheaper than flying. National Express Eurolines runs coaches from London Victoria, via Paris and Mont Blanc, to Aosta, Turin, Genoa, Milan, Venice, Bologna, Florence and Rome. To book from London, contact: National Express (www.nationalexpress.co.uk).

GETTING AROUND

On Arrival

Pisa Airport: The international airport, Galileo Gallilei (tel: 050-849 111) has its own railway station. Trains take five minutes into Pisa Centrale and one hour for the 80km (50 miles) to Florence (www. trenitalia.com). A CPT bus (www.cpt.pisa. it) also links the airport with Pisa Centrale rail station. You can pre-book on the 70-minute coach transfer between the airport

(departing outside Arrivals) and Florence's Santa Maria Novella train station (tel: 050-260 8034; www.terravision.eu). Car hire is available from the airport, and so are taxis. A toll-free superstrada links Pisa airport with Florence. **Peretola (Amerigo Vespucci) International Airport** (tel: 055-306 1700) in northwest Florence is also connected by Terravision bus (15-minute transfer) to central Florence.

By Air

Alitalia offers a huge range of internal flights from Florence and Pisa airports. These are supplemented by Meridiana's domestic services, which are usually a bit cheaper.

By Rail

For information, visit www.trenitalia.it. The state-subsidised railway network is a relatively cheap and convenient form of transport for travelling between major cities in Tuscany. The principal Rome–Milan line is convenient for Bologna (37 minutes), Florence and Arezzo, while the Rome–Genoa line serves Pisa, Livorno and Grosseto. The Florence–Siena route is much faster by coach than by train.

Note that Pisa and Florence both have several train stations: **Pisa Centrale** station serves Pisa city, while **Pisa Aeroporto** serves the airport. In Florence, **Santa Maria Novella** is the main station for the city, although the second station, **Rifredi**, is served by several Eurostar trains. In Florence, a controversial additional station for high-speed routes is being built by Norman Foster and opens in 2014.

Categories of Trains

Eurocity: these trains link major Italian cities with other European cities – in Germany and Switzerland, for instance. A supplement is payable on top of the rail fare. **Eurostar Italia and Alta Velocità**: these swish, high-speed trains have first- and second-class carriages (supplements payable).

Intercity: this fast service links major Italian cities. Intercity Plus is the latest fleet of plush, new fast trains. A supplement is payable; reservations required. **Interregionali**: these inter-regional trains link cities within different regions (eg Tuscany and Umbria) and stop fairly frequently. **Regionali**: these trains link towns within the same region and stop at every station.

Tickets
Booking
Reservations are mandatory for superior trains (such as Eurostar and Eurocity) and tickets should be purchased in advance. Other tickets with compulsory supplements should be purchased at least three hours in advance. You must date-stamp (convalidare) your rail ticket before beginning the journey at one of the small machines at the head of the platforms, or you may be fined. If you wish to upgrade to first class or a couchette, you can pay the conductor the difference.

To avoid long lines for tickets at major stations, book online with Trenitalia or, for a small charge, buy from local travel agencies. There are automatic ticket machines at major stations, although these are often out of order. Payment can be made either by cash or by credit card.

Wagons Lits/Carrozze Letto (sleeper cars) are found on long-distance trains within Italy, as well as on trains to France, Austria, Germany, and Switzerland. Reservations are essential.
Special Offers
There are a wide variety of train tickets and special offers available, which vary constantly and with the season. Some of the more established are:

The Trenitalia Pass: available for foreign visitors, it allows between 3 and 10 days unlimited travel on the Italian State Railway network, within a two-month period. **Group fares**: groups of between 6 and 24 people can benefit from a 20 percent discount. **Youth fares**: students aged between 12 and 26 can buy a yearly Carta Verde – "green card". This season ticket entitles them to a 10 percent discount on national trains and a 20 percent discount on international trips.

Children's fares: children under four travel free; children aged between 4 – 12 are eligible for a 50 percent discount on all trains but must pay the full supplement for Intercity and Eurocity trains.

Pensioners' fares: the over-60s can buy a Carta d'Argento. Valid for a year, this "silver card" entitles them to a 15 percent discount on all train tickets.

Railway Stations

The main railway stations are open 24 hours a day and are integrated with road and sea transport. They provide numerous services, including telecommunications, left luggage, food and drink, tourist information and porters (luggage trolleys are hard to find).

Florence: The train information office at Santa Maria Novella station is next to the waiting room. The train reservation office is just inside the building (daily 6am – 10pm). There is a left-luggage counter, where pieces of luggage are left at your own risk. The station also has an air terminal where you can check in for Pisa airport. There are bars and a pharmacy in the main hall, and shops on the lower level.

Siena: The railway station has an information office, counter for left luggage (and bicycles), and restaurant. Immediately outside the station is a bus ticket office and a tourist office. However, Siena's railway station is outside the town centre. More useful, and with faster services and a greater range of local destinations, is the coach service, with coaches leaving from Piazza San Domenico to Florence and various other Tuscan towns.

By Coach

Coaches are very comfortable and often quicker than trains. Especially convenient is the Rapida bus to Siena, running several times a

day. Provincial bus companies include (websites in Italian only):

CPT, Pisa; tel: 0508-84111 or free phone line: 800-012 773; www.cpt. pisa.it (for travel in Pisa Province).

CAP, Piazza Duomo 18, Prato; tel: 0574-6081; www.capautolinee.it (for travel in Tuscany and elsewhere).

Lazzi, Piazza Stazione 3r, Florence; tel: 055-215 155; www.lazzi.it (for travel in Tuscany).

Sita, Via S. Caterina da Siena 15, Florence; tel: 800-001 311; www.sitabus.it (for travel in Tuscany and Italy in general).

SENA, Sottopassaggio (Underpass) la Lizza, Siena; tel: 0577-283 203; www.sena.it (travel to and from Tuscany, great for Siena – Rome).

Tuscan Island Ferries

Numerous ferries ply the waters between the mainland and the islands of the Tuscan archipelago (Elba, Giglio, Capraia, Gorgona and Pianosa). Services from Piombino to Elba are regular throughout the day – every half-hour in the summer – but during the peak months, especially August, you should book in advance. At other times you can turn up and buy your ticket direct from the harbour office. The journey time for the car ferry is under an hour. Hydrofoil services for foot passengers only are less frequent but take around 35 minutes.

The biggest operator is **Toremar**, which connects Piombino to Portoferraio, Porto Azzurro, Rio Marina and Cavo. For information and online bookings, go to www.toremar.it (in Italian only) and see www.elba.org. Alternatively, book Toremar services through www.traghetti-toremar.com; tel: 0565-31100 (Piombino office); the website is in various languages. **Moby Lines**, the other main operator, runs a regular service between Piombino and Portoferraio. For information and bookings, see: www.moby.it.

If you are booking from the UK, or you want to compare the two main ferry operators to Elba, consult www.ferrysavers.com, tel: (UK only) 0844 371 8021. Toremar also

operates services from Livorno to Capraia and Gorgona, from Piombino to Pianosa, and from Santo Stefano on the Argentario peninsula to the island of Giglio.

City Transport

Local Buses/Trams

Buses within each province are cheap and plentiful. Tickets can be bought at designated offices, tobacconists, bars and newspaper stands. They are purchased in booklets or as singles, and have to be stamped by a machine on the bus at the start of a journey. Failure to do so risks a fine. All provincial bus services are routed past the railway station in every town.

In **Florence**, a range of tickets for the city's buses and new tram system is available from the ATAF office (Piazza Stazione; tel: 800-424 800). One of the handiest options is the three-day Firenze Card (see page 92), which includes museum access and public transport on buses and trams, including the new tram to the Cascine Park and Scandicci.

Rather confusingly for English-speakers, **Siena's** city/regional bus service is called TRA-IN.

Pisa province bus times are displayed on a board in Pisa's APT office on Piazza Garibaldi. Just outside Pisa Centrale Station, on the left, is a window for bus tickets.

Sightseeing Buses

Numerous sightseeing tours are offered in all the main cities.

Florence: **City Sightseeing Italy** (Piazza Stazione 1; tel: 055-290 451; www.city-sightseeing.it) offers a tour to Fiesole and a tour to Piazzale Michelangelo, both with multilingual commentary. Given the gradual pedestrianisation of parts of the city, the route is subject to change. Tickets are valid for 24 hours, allowing you to hop on and off at numerous points around the city. However, far more interesting are the thematic Florence walking tours booked through the Link guiding service (see 95).

Taxis

Taxis are plentiful in all towns and tourist resorts. They wait in special ranks at railway stations and main parts of the city but can be contacted by telephone. If you book one by phone, the cost of the journey begins then. (In Florence, tel: 055-4242, 055-4390 or 055-200 1326). Meters display fares: the fixed starting charge varies and extra charges are payable for night service, Sunday service and public holidays, luggage and journeys outside the town area. In Florence, there are taxi ranks in Via Pellicceria, Piazza di San Marco and Piazza Santa Trinità, and outside Stazione di Santa Maria Novella.

Cycling and Mopeds

Mopeds and bicycles are the most efficient way to get around the narrow streets of Florence, Siena and Lucca. They can be hired in the main cities. Try to find one with good brakes and a stand. You may have to leave an identity card or passport as security.

Florence: The brand new **Bike Sharing** initiative allows cyclists to borrow bikes from 50 distribution points 300 metres away from one another. Or you can rent a bike from Florence by Bike, Via San Zanobi 120r; tel: 055-488 992; www.florencebybike.it.

Siena: Perozzi, Via del Romitorio 5 (near the Lizza park); tel: 0577-223 157; www.perozzi.it. Amici della Bicicletta di Siena, c/o Public Assistance, Viale Mazzini 95; tel: 0577-45159; www.adbsiena.it.

Lucca: Barbetti, Via Anfiteatro 23; tel: 0583-954 444; Cicli Bizzarri, Piazza S. Maria, 32; tel: 0583-496 031.

Driving

To ease traffic, many city centres are closed to most vehicles. Since cities such as Florence, Montepulciano and Pistoia have introduced partial or complete city-centre driving bans (at least for non-residents), it makes sense to leave the car in the car parks on the edge of the historic centre. Florence, in particular, is extending its pedestrianised areas to include Via de Tornabuoni, the Palazzo Pitti area and parts of the Oltrano.

State highways in Tuscany include the No. 1 "Aurelia", which runs north–south, to the west of Pisa. National motorways *(auto-strade)*: the A11, the "Firenze-mare", and the A12, the "Sestri Levante–Livorno". Both of these are toll roads. The two *superstrade* (Florence–Siena and the Florence–Pisa–Livorno) are toll-free.

Car Hire

The major rental companies (Hertz, Avis, Europcar, etc.) have representation in most cities and resorts. The smaller local firms offer cheaper rates but cars can only be booked on the spot. Booking online, or in advance, often as part of a fly-drive package, is usually cheaper than hiring on arrival.

Rates normally allow unlimited mileage and include breakdown service. Basic insurance is included but additional cover is available at fixed rates. Most firms require a deposit and often take and hold a credit-card payment until the car is returned. You will usually be asked to return the car with a full tank; do so, as if the rental company has to fill it, they charge a premium for the petrol.

Licences and Insurance

Licences: Drivers must have a driving licence issued by a nation with a reciprocal agreement with Italy. The pink EU licence does not need an Italian translation. All other licences do need a translation, obtainable (free) from motoring organisations and Italian tourist offices. You are legally required to keep documents related to the car and driver on you.

Insurance: If you are bringing your own vehicle, check that your insurance covers Italy. A Green Card, obtainable from your insurance company, is not obligatory within the EU and does not provide extra cover, but it is internationally recognised, which may be useful if you have an accident.

Rules of the Road

Italy drives on the right. Road signs are international, with a few local differences:

Road signs: ALT is a stop line on the road for road junctions; STOP is for a pedestrian crossing.

Precedence: At crossroads, motorists must give precedence to vehicles on their right, except on recently built roundabouts, when those already on the roundabout have priority. If a motorist approaching a crossroads finds a precedence sign (a triangle with the point downwards) or a Stop sign, he/she must give precedence to all vehicles coming from both the right and left.

Parking: Outside cities and towns, parking on the right-hand side of the road is allowed, except on motorways, at crossroads, on curves and near any hilly ground not having full visibility. Illegally parked vehicles will be towed away, and incur a hefty fine. To understand the parking options in Florence, look at the clear advice and map on www.visitflorence.com. To find a car park in an Italian town online, look on www.parcheggi.it; for Florence go to www.firenzeparcheggi.it. There is a *"parcheggio scambiatore"* in Viale Europa (south Florence) – drivers can park their cars here and get a bus, hire a bike or take part in the car-sharing scheme to get into the centre. Special "tourist" rates (24 hours and nightly tickets) are available at the "Parterre" (Piazza della Libertà), "Oltrarno" (Porta Romana), and "Beccaria" garages.

Breakdowns and accidents: In case of a breakdown, dial 116. On motorways, telephones are 2km (1 mile) apart, with buttons to call for the police and medical assistance. Both have to be contacted if an accident involves an injury.

Motorways

Access signs to the motorways, unlike in other European countries, are in green, not blue. Motorway tolls can be high. There is rarely a hard shoulder on motorways, and often there are only two lanes. Accidents are frequent, so take care.

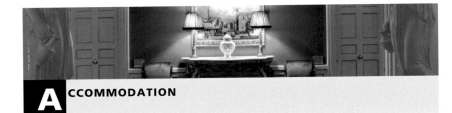

ACCOMMODATION

WHERE TO STAY

Choosing a Hotel

The quality and choice of accommodation in Tuscany is extremely varied. Visitors can choose between a city palazzo, grand country villa, or a historic family-run hotel, a rented apartment or villa, a bucolic farm-stay holiday (*agriturismo*) or even, in the most popular cities, a private home stay. (This is not known as bed and breakfast since breakfast is not usually provided.)

Hotel rooms generally need to be booked well in advance in Florence and Siena. During local summer festivals, particularly the Sienese Palio and Arezzo's Giostra, it can become very difficult to find a room.

Attractive accommodation in the centre of Volterra and San Gimignano is popular, so early booking is advisable.

There is a huge variation in what you get for your money. A moderately priced hotel in Florence may be somewhat underwhelming, whereas the same money could buy you a luxurious 4-star room in a grand country house off the tourist track.

Generally speaking, "high season" in Tuscany is May to September. However, in towns this does not necessarily include August. In Florence, for instance, many of the more expensive

hotels reduce their prices during this month. It can sometimes pay to bargain.

Many hotels with restaurants insist on a half- or full-board arrangement, especially in the high season. This ploy is particularly prevalent on the islands (eg Elba), in seaside resorts (eg Forte dei Marmi), in spa resorts (eg Montecatini Terme and Chianciano Terme), and where accommodation is in short supply.

Hotel Listing

The hotel recommendations listed on pages 273–288 are grouped to correspond to the Places chapters. The towns and hotels within each section are listed alphabetically.

In the case of Florence and Siena, where so many hotels are available, the listing is subdivided into price categories. Other cities' hotels have price indicators at the end of their descriptions. These refer to the cost of a standard double room for one night during high season, usually including breakfast; the ranges are as follows:

€ = under €100
€€ = €100–200
€€€ = €200–300
€€€€ = over €300

Private Home Stays

This is a fairly new development in Tuscany, but it is a good way of meeting the locals while paying modest prices. In Florence and Siena, the homes are carefully graded from simple to luxurious.

In Florence, contact www.firenze alloggio.com for B&B accommodation booked online directly with the owners, and no booking charge. For B&B accommodation in Florence, Lucca, Pisa and Siena, book online through the reliable American website: www. bedandbreakfast.com. Also try **APABB** (Associazione Provinciale Affittacamere Bed & Breakfast Firenze): www.apabb.it – apabb@libero.it; tel: 055-553 5141.

In Siena, request the *Affittacamere* (private lodgings) booklet of addresses from the tourist office (APT, Piazza Campo 56, Siena; tel: 0577-280 551). The list includes private accommodation in the whole of Siena Province, including San Gimignano, Montalcino and the Sienese Chianti.

Agriturismo

Farm stays (*agriturismo*) are an excellent way of experiencing the Tuscan countryside while staying on a farm or a wine estate. Standards vary widely from simple, rustic accommodation at low prices to relatively luxurious surroundings, complete with swimming pool. Before booking, check the website if they have one, or insist on a description or a photo, since many may be modern and fail to match up to the visitor's romantic image of Tuscany. Some farms, however, are genuine 16th-century wine and oil estates. There is usually the opportunity to buy local produce on site and meals are sometimes provided. For obvious reasons, you will normally need a car to make the most of a farm stay.

Reservations: During peak season, it is best to book in advance. Official accommodation tends to be booked for a minimum of one week, but individual arrangements for weekends and overnight stays are often possible, especially during mid- and low season.

Every local tourist authority produces farm-stay booklets. Or you can browse the following websites: www.agriturismo.com; www.agriturismo.net; and www.agriturist.it (Italian only). Also try **Terranostra**, tel: 06-4899 3209; www.terranostra.it; and www.toscana.campagnamica.it.

Rural Stays

These overlap with farm stays but can include country houses or even entire restored medieval villages (such as Sovicille, near Siena). In general, there is a working farm attached to the accommodation, or at least the opportunity to sample or buy wine, oil and local produce grown on the estate. As with farm stays, the accommodation offered can vary from simple rooms to self-contained apartments. The owners often use the profits from letting to reinvest in the restoration of the family estate or village. With rural stays, the emphasis is on country living in traditional buildings rather than in luxurious villa accommodation.

Many of the owners may speak basic English, French or German, but at least a smattering of Italian is appreciated. Always request detailed descriptions and directions.

Local tourist offices are a good source for recommendations (see page 307). Extensive listings, supported by images, can also be found on www.agriturismo.com and www.agriturismo.net. The following are some typical examples of rural stays, but are just a handful among countless options:

La Ripolina, Località Pieve di Piana, 53022 Buonconvento, Siena Province; tel: 0577-282 280; www.laripolina.it. Most of the holiday apartments are in converted farmhouses; one is in a fortified abbey with a 10th-century wall. Fresh farm produce available.

Agriturismo Podere San Lorenzo, Via Allori 80, 56048 Volterra, Pisa; tel: 0588-39080; www.agriturismo-volterra.it. Podere San Lorenzo is a working olive farm that has nine guest apartments in the farmhouse. Organic produce from its garden is used in the preparation of delicious meals served in an old Franciscan chapel. Cooking classes are available and there is a chemical-free swimming pool.

San Savino, Val di Chio, Località Santa Lucia 89/a, 52043 Castiglion Fiorentino, Arezzo province; tel: 0575-651 000; www.agriturismo-sansavino.it. This restored 11th-century monastery overlooks a lake, olive groves and woods and offers several apartments (plus pool and stables).

Villa Igea, Torre Alta, 55060 Ponte del Giglio, Lucca province; tel: 0583-353 122; www.villa-igea.biz. This charming traditional Tuscan villa and cottage is set among woodland and olive groves overlooking a valley. Home-produced extra-virgin olive oils and tastings.

La Parrina, km 146 Via Aurelia, Località Parrina, 58010 Albinia, Grosseto province; tel: 0564-862 636; www.parrina.it. This long-established agricultural estate is set among vineyards, olive groves and orchards. The rooms and dining rooms are decorated with an unfussy elegance that makes you feel right at home. To prove you're on a working farm, you may be woken early by the sound of tractors. Rooms and apartments; swimming pool; chapel; farm shop; restaurant and wine tasting; and bicycles.

Villa and Apartment Rentals

One of the most popular ways of visiting Tuscany is to stay in a rented villa or apartment. They do not come cheap, but you have the benefit of independence, and the freedom to cook for yourself using delicious fresh Tuscan produce. Prices vary enormously, depending on the season and the luxuriousness of the accommodation. The following agencies deal with rentals:

To Tuscany: UK: (44) 0844 488 1063. US: (toll-free) 888 768-4401; email: dick@to-tuscany.com, www.to-tuscany.com. This recommended, well-established company is well known for its customer service. Specialising in the Chianti, it offers cottages, villas with pool and entire estates, and has both a US and a (main) UK office.

The Best in Italy, tel: (+39) 055-223 064; www.thebestinitaly.com. A Florence-based lettings agency offering luxurious villas and palazzi with pools, tennis courts, stables, domestic staff and other such luxuries.

Caffelletto, tel: (+39) 049-663 980; www.caffelletto.it. This Italian company offers a selection of villas, castles, stylish country manors and city apartments, some on a bed-and-breakfast basis, others self-catering.

Cottages to Castles, tel: (+44) 01622-775 236; www.cottagestocastles.com. UK-based and established.

Cuendet, tel: (+39) 041-251 6100; www.cuendet.com. A good selection of Tuscan villas and apartments.

Hello Italy, tel: (+44) 01483-419

964; www.helloitaly.co.uk: recommended for the Lunigiana region.
Casa Glyn, Cotto, Lunigiana, tel: (+44) 020-3326 1213; www.merrioncharles.com. From €1,600 (£1,356) a week. Lovely setting with striking views of the Apuan Alps and the Carrara hills. A tempting base for walks in the Apennines and foodie forays to Lucca. Unwind in a modest family retreat with great character and comfort. Pizza oven, pool, gardens and south-facing terrace.
Humilis Caellaccia: Val d'Orcia, tel: (+44) 01886 853 920; www.globalartichoke.co.uk. From £5,700 a week. Restored farm sleeps 19 in contemporary style. A lovely pool and great kitchen where local cook Marcella Libertini can be hired. She supposedly inspired the late River Café founder Rose Gray. Foodie forays to Pienza for pecorino cheese and oil, and Montalcino and Montepulciano for red wines.
Villa Rignana: Via di Rignana 7, Greve in Chianti, Chianti; tel: (+44) 055-852 137; www.villarignana.com. From €12,000 (£10,000) a week. Set among vineyards, this former monastery is now a villa retreat with the air of a minor stately home, dotted with heirlooms. Sleeps 20, with a chapel that makes it popular for wedding parties.

Castles and Monasteries

Accommodation is available in a variety of castles and palaces. Standards will vary from very simple to luxurious. Many convents, monasteries and other religious institutions offer simple accommodation for tourists and pilgrims. Monte Oliveto Maggiore is just one example (see page bhth9). Each provincial tourist office should be able to supply you with a full list.

Youth Hostels

A list of youth hostels is available from ENIT (Italian National Tourist Offices (see page 306) and places can be booked through them or through local Tuscan tourist offices. Alternatively, contact the Associazione Italiana Alberghi per la Gioventù, Via Cavour 44, 00184 Rome; tel: 06-487 1152; www.aighostels.com. The main city youth hostels in Tuscany are:

Cortona

San Marco, Via Maffei 57; tel: 0575-601 392; www.aighostels.com

Florence

Archi Rossi, Via Faenza 94r; tel: 055-290 804; www.hostelarchirossi.com
Ostello Villa Camerata, Viale Augusto Righi 2–4; tel: 055-601 451; www.aighostels.com
Santa Monaca Hostel, Via Santa Monaca 6; tel: 055-268 338; www.ostello.it
Sette Santi, Viale dei Mille 11; tel: 055-504 8452; www.7santi.com
Youth Hostel Firenze 2000, Viale R. Sanzio 16; tel: 055-233 5558 www.hostels.com
Youth Hostel Tavernelle Val di Pesa, Via Roma 137; tel 055-805 0265; www.aighostels.com

Lucca

Ostello San Frediano, Via della Cavallerizza 12; tel: 0583-469 957; www.aighostels.com
Near Piazza Anfiteatro, in the centre of town.

Marina di Massa

Ostello Apuano, Via della Pineta 237; tel: 0585-780 034; www.aighostels.com

Pistoia – Abetone

Ostello Renzo Bizzarri, Tel: 0573-60117; www.aighostels.com.

Siena – Cetona

Ostello La Cocciara, Tel: 0578-237 104; www.aighostels.com

Camping

For a free list of campsites, contact the Federazione Italiana Campeggiatore, Via Vittorio Emanuele II, 50041 Calenzano, Firenze; tel: 055-882 391; www.federcampeggio.it.

Florence

Michelangelo, Viale Michelangelo 80; tel: 055-681 1977. Apr–Oct, crowded in high season. No. 13 bus from station. Good facilities; 320 pitches.
Camping Panoramico, Via Peramonda 1, Fiesole; tel: 055-599 069; www.florencecamping.com. Terraced site in Fiesole, outside Florence. All year.
Ostello Villa Camerata, Via Augusto Righi 2–4; tel: 055-601 451. Next door to the hostel is a campsite, Villa Camerata, which is also open all year round. No. 17B bus from station.

Pisa

Campeggio Torre Pendente, Viale delle Cascine 86; tel: 050-561 704; www.campingtorrependente.it. Apr–mid-Oct. No. 5 bus from the station.
Camping Internazionale, Via Litoranea 7, Marina di Pisa; tel: 050-35211. Facilities include a private beach, bar and pizzeria.

Siena

Campeggio "Siena Colleverde", Strada di Scacciapensieri 47; tel: 0577-332 545; www.campingcolleverde.com. End Mar–end Oct; 2km (1 mile) from the city; No. 8 bus.
There are also companies that organise camping holidays in Tuscany. In the UK, these include:
Eurocamp Travel, Hartford Manor, Greenbank Lane, Northwich, Cheshire CW8 1HW; tel: 0844-406 0402; www.eurocamp.co.uk.
Keycamp, Hartford Manor, Greenbank Lane, Northwich, Cheshire CW8 1HW; tel: 0844-406 0200; www.keycamp.co.uk.

Caravan and Camper Hire

In Tuscany, caravans and camper vans are available for hire from **Caravanmec**, Via della Cupola 281, Peretola, Florence; tel: 055-315 101; www.caravanmec.it, although there are other companies, too.

FLORENCE

In Florence, at the top end, there's a surfeit of new or revamped luxury hotels compared with most other Italian cities. It's ultimately a choice between the style of hotel you prefer: grand, palatial and historic in the city centre; a grand villa hotel on the outskirts; or a charming, often contemporary boutique hotel in the centre of town. Among mid-range hotels, there is also an increasingly wide range of quirky boutique hotels. For peace and privacy, don't exclude the villa-rental option either (*see page 271*).

Alessandra
Borgo SS Apostoli 17
Tel: 055-283 438
www.hotelalessandra.com
An old-fashioned, simple hotel conveniently situated near the Ponte Vecchio. Many of the 25 spacious rooms are furnished with antiques. **€€**

Annalena
Via Romana 34
Tel: 055-222 402
www.hotelannalena.it
A discreet spot in a 15th-century palazzo, originally built as a refuge for widows of the Florentine nobility. Opposite the rear entrance to the Boboli Gardens. Some rooms have balconies looking on to the horticultural centre. **€€**

Aprile
Via della Scala 6
Tel: 055-216 237
www.hotelaprile.it
Much more appealing than most hotels near the station, this is an ex-Medici palace complete with frescoes, a pleasant breakfast room and garden. Rooms range from simple to reasonably grand. **€€**

Astoria
Via del Giglio 9
Tel: 055-239 8095
www.boscolohotels.com
Completely refurbished hotel near the station, with grand dimensions and elaborate decor. **€€€**

Beacci Tornabuoni
Via de' Tornabuoni 3
Tel: 055-212 645
www.hoteltornabuoni.it
Ever-popular de-luxe guesthouse, comfortable and very welcoming, although some rooms are on the small side. Flower-filled rooftop terrace for breakfast and drinks. Half-board terms compulsory. **€€€**

Botticelli
Via Taddea 8
Tel: 055-290 905
www.hotelbotticelli.it
Close to the central San Lorenzo market, this 3-star hotel is both comfortable and appealing, with all the mod cons you could want but also well-preserved 16th-century features, including vaulted ceilings and frescoes. Friendly staff. **€€€**

Brunelleschi Hotel
Via de' Calzaiuoli, Piazza Santa Elisabetta 3
Tel: 055-273 7487
www.hotelbrunelleschi.it
Set in a Byzantine tower and a medieval church with a view of the Duomo or of Via dei Calzaiuoli – one of the city's favourite shopping streets. There's a reasonable restaurant. Look out for the museum with the remains of a Roman caldarium (early sauna). **€€**

Casci
Via Cavour 13
Tel: 055-211 686
www.hotelcasci.com
Frescoed quattrocento palazzo, family-run and with a welcoming atmosphere. Five minutes' walk north of the Duomo. **€€**

Classic Hotel
Viale Machiavelli 25
Tel: 055-229 351
www.classichotel.it
Elegant villa, washed in pink, with lovely rooms, a conservatory and pretty gardens, situated on a tree-lined avenue just above the Porta Romana. Excellent value. **€€**

Continentale
Vicolo dell'Oro 6r
Tel: 055-27262
www.lungarnohotels.com
Chic hotel in the Ferragamo group. The shades of pink and pistachio in the lobby set the tone for the fabulous retro-style interiors. Ideal location near the Ponte Vecchio, with rooms overlooking the Arno. The chic bar, the Sky Lounge, offers spectacular views across the Florentine skyline. **€€€–€€€€**

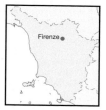

Davanzati
Via Porta Rossa 5
Tel: 055-286 666
www.hoteldavanzati.it
Centrally located, this tastefully refurbished hotel has 21 quiet rooms all with a laptop and internet connection. Clean rooms and helpful service. **€€**

Fiorino
Via Osteria del Guanto 6
Tel: 055-210 579
www.hotelfiorino.it
Located in the centre of the city, this unpretentious hotel has a pleasant family atmosphere. **€€**

Four Seasons Florence
Borgo Pinti 99
Tel: 055-26261
www.fourseasons.com/florence
This frescoed Renaissance palazzo is now the city's top hotel, with Il Conventino acting as a "hotel within a hotel".

PRICE CATEGORIES

These refer to the cost of a standard double room during high season, usually including breakfast:
€ = under €100
€€ = €100–200
€€€ = €200–300
€€€€ = over €300

This arty city sanctuary is adorned with original frescoes and sculptured reliefs. Superb suites. The secluded gardens are dotted with follies. €€€€

Gallery Hotel Art
Vicolo dell'Oro 5
Tel: 055-27263
www.lungarnohotels.com
Another classy boutique hotel in the Ferragamo stable. Sleek decor and central location. The lobby and trendy Fusion Bar host regular photography and contemporary-art exhibitions. €€€–€€€€

Giada
Canto de'Nelli 2
Tel: 055-215 317
www.hotelgiada.it
Friendly *pensione* near San Lorenzo market. Some rooms overlook the Medici Chapels. €€

Grand Hotel Villa Cora
Viale Machiavelli 18
Tel: 055-228 790
www.whythebesthotels.com
Newly revamped historic hotel in landscaped grounds near the Boboli. It's situated in three 19th-century mansions, with the main one home to a chic spa. Outdoor heated swimming pool overlooking the gardens. Gourmet restaurant. €€€€

Grand Hotel Villa Medici
Via II Prato 42
Tel: 055-277 171
www.villamedicihotel.com
Convenient hotel near the train station, with a pool, gym, gardens and large airy rooms. €€€€

Helvetia & Bristol
Via dei Pescioni 2
Tel: 055-26651
www.royaldemeure.com
One of the best of the luxury small hotels in the city, with many illustrious

names numbered among its former guests. Supremely comfortable rooms and suites; excellent restaurant. Delightful winter garden. €€€€

Hermitage
Vic. Marzio 1, Piazza del Pesce
Tel: 055-287 216
www.hermitagehotel.com
Charming hotel behind the Ponte Vecchio. Personal attention from staff. Lovely roof garden views. €€€

The J&J
Via di Mezzo 20
Tel: 055-26312
www.jandjhotel.net
The setting of this small hotel – in a modest street near Santa Croce – belies the luxury within. It's in a former convent near Sant'Ambrogio, highly individual, romantic and chic. Lovely old cloister for summer breakfasts and evening drinks. €€€

JK Place
Piazza Santa Maria Novella
Tel: 055-264 5181
www.jkplace.com
This stylish town house and fashionable boutique hotel combines contemporary chic and welcoming service. A lovely rooftop terrace and views over Santa Croce itself. €€€–€€€€

Liana
Via Alfieri 18
Tel: 055-245 303
www.hotelliana.com
Lovely hotel some way north of the centre in the former British Embassy, but not far from Santa Croce. Rooms vary from simple to elegant, with frescoed ceilings and original floors. Good breakfast and pretty garden. Private car park. €€

Loggiato dei Serviti
Piazza della SS Annunziata 3
Tel: 055-289 592

www.loggiatodeiservitihotel.it
Atmospheric hotel facing the Innocenti hospital across a traffic-free piazza. Sangallo's 16th-century palazzo now has 38 rooms and suites and an annexe, all tastefully furnished. This is one of the city's best-loved and most refined hotels. No garden. €€€

Marignolle Relais & Charme
Via di San Quirichino 16
Tel: 055-228 6910
www.marignolle.com
A few minutes to the south of Florence, this charming hotel with pool is comfortable and handy for exploring the surrounding area. €€€

Monna Lisa
Borgo Pinti 27
Tel: 055-247 9751
www.monnalisa.it
This Renaissance palazzo, furnished with antiques, drawings and sculpture, is a popular choice. There is a delightful garden and private parking. €€€

Morandi alla Crocetta
Via Laura 50
Tel: 055-234 4747
www.hotelmorandi.it
Tiny hotel tucked away in a backstreet near the university, in a former convent. Antiques, par-

quet flooring and colourful rugs; 10 bedrooms, two with private terraces. Book well in advance. €€€

Orto de'Medici
Via San Gallo 30
Tel: 055-483 427
www.ortodeimedici.it
Attractive little neoclassical palazzo near Piazza San Marco, with grand public rooms. Simpler bedrooms, most with private baths; lovely breakfast room leading on to a terrace. €€

Palazzo Benci
Piazza Madonna degli Aldobrandini 3
Tel: 055-213 848
www.palazzobenci.com
Patrician palazzo, traditionally the seat of the Benci family, recently restored but retaining original features. €€

Palazzo dal Borgo
Via della Scala 6
Tel: 055-278 686
www.arshotels.com
Every bedroom is different in this gorgeous 15th-century palazzo, with some rooms frescoed or overlooking the inner courtyard or the cloisters of Santa Maria Novella. The rooms on the lower floor have more character, but the top floor has the views. €€€

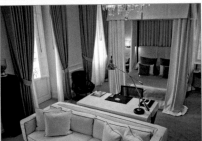

BELOW: Master Room at JK Place.

Plaza Lucchesi
Lungarno della Zecca
Vecchia 38
Tel: 055-26236
www.plazalucchesi.it
This tranquil, charmingly dated hotel on the River Arno boasts superb views of Santa Croce on one side and San Miniato on the other: it's like living in a Renaissance time capsule. Good restaurant and friendly service. **€€**

Regency
Piazza d'Azeglio 3
Tel: 055-245 247
www.regency-hotel.com
Luxurious hotel in an elegantly converted Florentine palazzo situated in a quiet, leafy square, a short walk from the main sights. Rooms are welcoming and comfortable. Cool, shady garden. Good restaurant. **€€€€**

Relais Cavalcanti
Via Pellicceria 2
Tel: 055-210 962
www.relaiscavalcanti.com
Simple guesthouse near the Palazzo Davanzati, where the rooms are clean, nicely decorated and cheap. Staff are helpful, although not always present. In high season it enters the next price bracket. **€**

Relais del Duomo B&B
Piazza dell'Olio 2
Tel: 055-210 147
www.relaisdelduomo.it
Four-roomed B&B just a stone's throw from the Duomo. Rooms are clean and all have private bath and TV. Can be noisy at times, but it's a good deal for Florence, especially during low season. **€**

Relais Santa Croce
Via Ghibellina 87
Tel: 055-234 2230
www.relaisantacroce.com
Recently restored by the

stylish Baglioni group, this is a brooding, intimate palazzo for dangerous liaisons, matched by a noted restaurant, and featuring a special dining package with Enoteca Pinchiorri next door, the city's most sought-after restaurant. **€€€–€€€€**

Residenza Johanna 1
Via Bonifacio Lupi 14
Tel: 055-481 896
www.johanna.it
The cheapest of a group of four great-value-for-money residences across the city. Rooms are clean and comfortable, even though there are few mod cons and breakfasts are do-it-yourself. In an unmarked building in a quiet street near Piazza Libertà. **€**

Residenze Johlea and Antica Johlea
Via San Gallo 80/76
Tel: 055-463 3292
www.johanna.it
These two residences are located in a nice area around San Marco. They retain an authentic Tuscan feel, but are equipped with more modern conveniences than their cheaper sister residence (Johanna 1) near San Lorenzo (see below). **€€**

Hotel Rivoli
Via della Scala 33
Tel: 055-278 686
www.hotelrivoli.it
Conveniently close to Santa Maria Novella, this former Franciscan friary is now an elegant family-owned hotel, with rooms overlooking the former cloisters, and an excellent restaurant. (For other hotels in the group, see www.arshotels.it). **€€**

The St Regis Florence
Piazza Ognissanti 1,

50123 Florence
Tel: 055-27161
www.stregisflorence.com
Formerly the Grand Hotel, but now revamped as the St Regis. Expect River Arno views and an equally grand style, from crystal chandeliers to suites adorned with coffered ceilings, frescoes and brocades. hotel pays homage to Florentine history. **€€€€**

Savoy
Piazza della Repubblica 7
Tel: 055-27351
www.hotelsavoy.it
Elegant Rocco Forte luxury hotel in the heart of the city, close to historic cafés and the main museums, galleries and fashion houses. Stylish, spacious rooms with contemporary Italian decor. **€€€€**

Silla
Via de'Renai 5
Tel: 055-234 2888
www.hotelsilla.it
An elegant arched courtyard leads to this first-floor hotel in a quiet, relatively leafy area south of and overlooking the Arno. **€€**

Torre di Bellosguardo
Via Roti Michelozzi 2
Tel: 055-229 8145
www.torrebellosguardo.com
Bellosguardo ("beautiful view"), the hill on which this Renaissance villa was built, is only 15 minutes' walk up from Porta Romana, but a world away. This quiet, roomy hotel has frescoed reception rooms and charmingly decorated bedrooms, dotted with antiques and quirky details. Secluded swimming pool and delightful grounds with lily pond. **€€€€**

Torre Guelfa
Borgo SS Apostoli 8
Tel: 055-239 6338
www.hoteltorreguelfa.com
Elegant, recently refurbished hotel with a grand "salon", pastel-shaded bedrooms, a sunny breakfast room and the tallest privately owned tower in the city. **€€**

Villa Azalee
Viale Fratelli Rosselli 44
Tel: 055-214 242
www.villa-azalee.it
Pleasant, 19th-century villa near the station, with the feel of a private house, set in a garden full of azaleas and camellias. Private garage; bicycles for hire. **€€**

Villa Belvedere
Via Benedetto Castelli 3
Tel: 055-222 501
www.villabelvederefirenze.it
Exceptionally friendly and modern hotel, south of the city, above Porta Romana. Sunny rooms, a pretty garden and lovely views across Florence. Pool and tennis court. You can take the bus into town. **€€**

Villa la Vedetta
Viale Michelangelo 78
Tel: 055-681 631
www.villalavedettahotel.com
Elegant hotel in a panoramic position near Piazzale Michelangelo. Rooms are elegant and well equipped; Michelin-starred restaurant. **€€€€**

PRICE CATEGORIES

These refer to the cost of a standard double room during high season, usually including breakfast:
€ = under €100
€€ = €100–200
€€€ = €200–300
€€€€ = over €300

AROUND FLORENCE

Artimino

Paggeria Medicea
Viale Papa Giovanni XXIII 1
Tel: 055-875 141
www.artimino.com
Grand hotel in the former stables of a restored Medici villa, nestling between glorious olive groves and vineyards near Carmignano, 24km (15 miles) west of Florence. Very good restaurant and a farm shop selling local produce and wine. There are also a number of apartments available for weekly rental. **€€€**

Candeli

Villa La Massa
Via La Massa 24
Tel: 055-62611
www.villalamassa.com
Some 7km (4 miles) north of Florence, this cluster of beautifully converted 17th-century villas radiates elegance. Riverside restaurant; swimming and tennis. Free shuttle service provided for guests from the hotel to the Ponte Vecchio. **€€€€**

Fiesole

Demidoff Country Resort
Via della Lupaia, 1556, Pratolino Firenze
Tel: 055-505 641
www.hotel-demidoff.it
Recently refurbished resort close to Fiesole and Florence, with a view of the Duomo in the distance. The elegant 1556 restaurant serves haute cuisine,

indoors and on the charming terrace. **€€€**

Pensione Bencistà
Via Benedetto da Maiano 4
Tel: 055-59163
www.bencista.com
Delightful but over-popular 14th-century villa, decorated with antiques and rustic furnishings. Reliable restaurant; half-board is compulsory. Flower-decked terrace with panoramic views over Florence. **€€**

Villa Fiesole
Via Beato Angelico 35
Tel: 055-597 252
www.villafiesole.it
Comfortable but chic hotel with frescoes, panoramic views and a pool. Full wheelchair access. **€€**

Villa San Michele
Via Doccia 4
Tel: 055-567 8200
www.villasanmichele.com
One of the finest and most expensive hotels in Tuscany. Supposedly designed by Michelangelo, this former Franciscan monastery enjoys harmonious lines and heavenly views of the city, particularly from the loggia and restaurant. Spacious grounds; pool; piano bar. The plush suites have jacuzzis. **€€€€**

Galluzzo

La Fattoressa
Via Volterrana 58
Tel: 055-204 8418
www.lafattoressa.it
Old farmhouse converted into simple but comfortable bed-and-breakfast accommodation with double and tri-

ple rooms. Dinner prepared on request. Very friendly and family-run place just southwest of Florence and conveniently situated for access to the *autostrada*. **€€**

Impruneta

Villa Cesi
Via delle Terre Bianche
Tel: 055-231 101
www.villacesi.it
A stone's throw from Impruneta's main square, this pleasant, modern hotel has a swimming pool, a restaurant, and regular food and wine tastings. Friendly staff (who speak very little English). **€€**

Molino del Piano

Hotel il Trebbiolo Relais
Via del Trebbiolo 8, Località Olmo
Tel: 055-830 0098
www.iltrebbiolo.it
Delightful 3-star hotel 14km (9 miles) from Florence. The villa is set amid olive groves, with cosy little rooms and an annexe with cooking facilities. The hotel restaurant offers solid Tuscan cuisine. **€€**

Poggio a Caiano

Hotel Hermitage
Via Ginepraia 112
Tel: 055-877 7085
www.hotelhermitageprato.it
Nice, if businesslike hotel set on a hill, close to the Medici Villa; handy for exploring the surrounding area. Members receive dis-

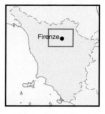

count at Le Pavoniere golf course, near Prato. Restaurant; swimming pool in summer. Good value. **€-€€**

Prato

Villa Rucellai
Via di Canneto 16
Tel: 0574-460 392
www.villarucellai.it
This mellow, medieval villa northeast of the town is an oasis in Prato's industrial landscape. A relaxed yet elegant B&B with a family atmosphere. Swimming pool, chapel and garden. Very good value for money. **€**

Sesto Fiorentino

Villa Villoresi
Via Campi 2, Colonnata di Sesto Fiorentino
Tel: 055-443 212
www.villavilloresi.it
A pleasant villa that feels a world away from the ugly industrial suburb of Sesto that surrounds it. Complete with chandeliers and frescoes, plus the longest loggia in Tuscany. There's also a restaurant and pool. **€€**

Trespiano

Villa Le Rondini
Via Bolognese Vecchia 224
Tel: 055-400 081

www.villalerondini.it
This is a secluded villa in a wonderful setting, overlooking the Arno valley just 4km (2 miles) from Florence. Lovely views over the city from the swimming pool, set in an olive grove. Restaurant. Bus link to the city. €€€

Vicchio

Villa Campestri
Via di Campestri 19
Tel: 055-849 0107
www.villacampestri.it
Imposing Renaissance villa in a wonderful, rural setting in the Mugello, 35km (25 miles) north of Florence. Impressive public rooms, excellent food and a relaxed atmosphere. Bedrooms in the main villa are quite grand; those in the annexe less so. Pool and horse riding available. €€–€€€

LUCCA AND PISTOIA

Abetone

Bellavista
Via Brennero 383
Tel: 0573-60028
www.bellavista-abetone.it
Typical wood-and-stone mountain building with panoramic views, close to the centre of Abetone and ski lifts. Comfortable and spacious rooms. Seasonal opening. €€

Regina
Via Uccelliera 5
Tel: 0573-60257
www.albergoregina.com
Pleasant 19th-century villa within an attractive setting. 3-star. €–€€

Lucca

Albergo Villa Marta
Via del Ponte Guasperini, 873 San Lorenzo a Vaccoli
Tel: 0583-370 101
www.albergovillamarta.it
Set in the Lucca countryside en route to Pisa, this boutique villa-hotel is a popular hideaway for Italian celebrities. Bedrooms are cosy and cosseting, while the Botton d'Oro is a noted gastronomic restaurant, focusing on Tuscan recipes. Bicycles are available to explore the surrounding countryside. €€€

Alla Corte degli Angeli
Via Degli Angeli 23
Tel: 0583-469 204
www.allacortedegliangeli.com
A sister hotel to the San Martino (see below), this delightful tiny hotel is also within the city walls, close to the Piazza dell'Anfiteatro. Each of the six rooms has a flower theme and affords splendid views over the city roofs. €€

Antico Casale Toscano
Località Piaggia 10
Tel: 340-360 0646
www.anticocasaletoscano.com
This charming, typical Tuscan farmhouse is set in the hills above Lucca among olive groves on a working farm. Rooms are available on a nightly basis from Nov–Mar and on a weekly basis Apr–Oct. Teresa organises special free cookery evenings including tastings of her own extra-virgin olive oil during the summer. €

Diana
Via del Molinetto 11
Tel: 0583-492 202
www.albergodiana.com
Centrally located hotel off Piazza San Martino; a pleasant budget option. €

Hotel Carignano
Via di Sant'Alessio, 3680 Carignano (5km/3 miles outside Lucca)
Tel: 0583-329 618
www.hotelcarignano.it
This family-run hotel is set in a quiet, hilly location outside Lucca, within easy reach of the sea and mountains. Rooms are large and bright. €–€€

Hotel Ilaria e Residenza dell'Alba
Via del Fosso 26
Tel: 0583-47615
www.hotelilaria.com
Ideally located in the historic centre and set in splendid grounds, this very stylish hotel is dedicated to comfort and good service. The annexe, Residenza dell'Alba, is located in the former medieval church of the Annunziata. Large bedrooms but a period feel. €€–€€€

La Luna
Via Fillungo Corte Compagni 12
Tel: 0583-493 634
www.hotellaluna.com
Family-run hotel in the historic centre just a stone's throw from the Piazza dell'Anfiteatro. €€

La Romea (B&B)
Vicolo delle Ventaglie 2 (corner of Via S. Andrea)
Tel: 0583-464 175
www.laromea.com
Small, very pleasing establishment on the first floor of a medieval palazzo in the historic centre. The two young hosts, Giulio and Gaia, are most helpful. Five rooms all with private bathrooms and air-

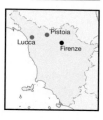

conditioning. Generous breakfast. €€

Piccolo Hotel Puccini
Via di Poggio 9
Tel: 0583-55421
www.hotelpuccini.com
A small and very popular three-star hotel just around the corner from Puccini's birthplace, crammed with mementos of the maestro. Excellent value. €

San Martino
Via della Dogana 9
Tel: 0583-469 181
www.albergosanmartino.it
Warm, welcoming little hotel in a quiet location, within the city walls, a stone's throw from the Duomo. Nearby private car parking organised by

PRICE CATEGORIES

These refer to the cost of a standard double room during high season, usually including breakfast:
€ = under €100
€€ = €100–200
€€€ = €200–300
€€€€ = over €300

the hotel. Excellent value. **€–€€**

Stipino
Via Romana 95
Tel: 0583-495 077
www.hotelstipino.com
Simply decorated, 2-star hotel graced with a personal touch. **€**

Villa Rinascimento
Loc. Santa Maria del Giudice, Via del Cimitero 532b
Tel: 0583-378 292
www.villarinascimento.it
Rustic villa with a lovely garden and swimming pool, on a hillside 9km (5 miles) west of Lucca. **€€**

Monsummano Terme

Grotta Giusti Spa Resort
Tel: 0572-90771
www.grottagiustispa.com
A short hop from Monte-catini Golf Course, this historic spa resort appeals to couples keen to improve their swing while sampling some of the most innovative spa treatments in Tuscany. Spread around a hand-some villa, the resort is proud of its steamy but restorative spa caverns and its award-winning head barman. The steamy grottoes were dubbed "the eighth won-der of the world" by the composer Giuseppe

Verdi. **€€€**

La Speranza
Via Grotta Giusti 62
Tel: 0572-51313
Basic hotel with well-maintained garden. Good option if you're passing through and all you want is a bed for the night. **€**

Montecatini Terme

Florio
Via Montebello 41
Tel: 0572-78343
Montecatini Terme is overrun with hotels. This one, with its own garden, is a good mod-erately priced option. **€**

Grand Hotel Plaza e Locanda Maggiore
Piazza del Popolo 7
Tel: 0572-75831
www.hotelplaza.it
Grand hotel with good facilities including a pool. Special deals for families. **€€**

Torretta
Viale Bustichini 63
Tel: 0572-70305
www.hoteltorretta.it
A modern, family-run hotel with a pool; spe-cial diets catered for. **€**

Pescia

Azienda Agricola Marzalla
Via Collecchio 1

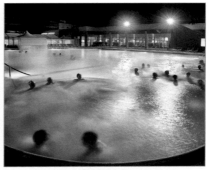

ABOVE: pool at Grotta Giusti Spa Resort.

Tel: 0572-490 751
Unpretentious, family-run *agriturismo* in the hills. With a pool, and a pleasant *trattoria* nearby. Weekly basis only in high season. **€**

Pistoia

Il Convento
Via San Quirico 33
Tel: 0573-452 651/2
www.ilconventohotel.com
Tranquil hotel, formerly a Franciscan monastery. The dining room was once the monks' refec-tory and the bedrooms their cells; some have a terrace. Breakfast is served in the cloister in fine weather. Includes a lovely garden sur-rounded by woodland, a

pool, a good restaurant and a chapel. Five kilo-metres (3 miles) from town. **€€**

Hotel Patria
Via Crispi 8
Tel: 0573-358 800
www.patriahotel.com
Welcoming small hotel in the city's historic cen-tre. Parking permits available. **€**

Villa Vannini
Villa di Pitecchio
Tel: 0573-42031
www.villavannini.it
Delightful villa some 6km (4 miles) north of Pistoia, with the atmos-phere of a private house. Stylish and comfortable bedrooms; fine food; wonderful walks in the woods. Good value.
€–€€

VERSILIA, GARFAGNANA AND LUNIGIANA

PRICE CATEGORIES

These refer to the cost of a standard double room during high season, usually including breakfast:
€ = under €100
€€ = €100–200
€€€ = €200–300
€€€€ = over €300

Bagni di Lucca

Azienda Agriturismo La Torre
La Torre, Fornoli
Tel: 0583-805 297
www.latorreagriturismo.com
Set among olive and chestnut groves, this delightful farmhouse can accommodate up

to 15 people in six apartments. It is simply furnished in traditional Tuscan style and offers lovely views over the rolling countryside. An added bonus is the good home cooking offered and there is also a swimming pool.
€–€€

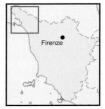
Firenze

TRANSPORT

Barga

Alpino
Via G. Pascoli 1
Tel: 0583-723 336
This 3-star hotel in the lower, busier half of town has been offering a warm welcome to its guests for over 100 years. There are seven rooms and two suites, which have all been recently refurbished. Restaurant. €€

Castelnuovo di Garfagnana

La Lanterna
(1km/half a mile east at Monache-Piano Pieve)
Tel: 0583-639 364
www.hotellalanterna.com
Set in a peaceful, green location, with 22 plain but comfortable rooms and a large restaurant. This is a good base for exploring the Garfagnana. €

Fivizzano

L'Albergo Ristorante Pieve San Paolo
Località Pieve San Paolo
Tel: 0585-949 800
This is a small, family-run albergo in the heart of magnificent mountain scenery. Very welcoming. €€€

Hotel Terme
Via Noce Verde (Equi Terme)
Tel: 0585-97830
A 3-star hotel set in the beautiful Parco Naturale delle Alpi Apuane. The scenery makes up for the somewhat dated decor. There are 60 bedrooms and two swimming pools, plus spa treatments. €€€

Il Giardinetto
Via Roma 151
Tel: 0585-92060
A rather eccentric hotel/restaurant, full of character and characters. Traditional Tuscan food. €

Il Mulino di Posara
Via del Mulino 12-20, Localita Posara, 54013 Fivizzano
Tel (UK): +44 020-7193 6246
www.watermill.net
Called "the Watermill at Posara" in English, this is a retreat for painting holidays, creative writing, and excursions into the hills, mountains and olive groves. Transfers from Pisa are organised, and week-long courses include all meals and a sightseeing tour to Lucca. €€

Forte dei Marmi

Hotel Byron
Viale Morin 46
Tel: 0584-787 052

www.softlivingplaces.com
A seductive luxury hotel on the most chic stretch of the Forte dei Marmi promenade. This patrician villa is now a discreet boutique hotel popular with Italian celebrities in summer. You can also dine on the summer terrace of La Magnolia, the gourmet restaurant. Nearby are parks, tennis courts, riding stables and the Versilia Golf Club (4km/2.5 miles away). €€€€

Licciana Nardi

Del Pino
Via Bastia 37, Lunigiana
Tel: 0187-475 041
A quiet, comfortable and modern pensione in a mountain village, surrounded by pine trees. €

Pontremoli

Hotel Napoleon
Piazza Italia, 2bis
Tel: 0187-830 544
www.hotelnapoleon.net
Set in the heart of Pontremoli, this family-run hotel offers its guests lovely views of the Apennines. There is also a very sophisticated restaurant. €

Viareggio

London
Viale Manin 16
Tel: 0584-49841
www.hotellondon.it
Very pleasant family-run hotel in a former Liberty-style palazzo. There are good-sized public rooms and 33 very comfortable bedrooms. €€

Locanda le Monache
Piazza XXIX Maggio 36, Camaiore (10km/6 miles from Viareggio)
Tel: 0584-989 258
www.lemonache.com
This is a traditional Tuscan restaurant, which also has 15 rooms, in a former monastery. The rooms are of a good size, albeit simply furnished. €

Hotel Plaza e de Russie
Piazza D'Azeglio, 1
Tel: 0584-44449
www.softlivingplaces.com
Set on the seafront, a short hop from the beach and the Art Nouveau promenade, this is Viareggio's most historic luxury hotel. It was built in 1871 to cater to Grand Tourists, especially Russians. Lovely view of the seafront from the rooftop restaurant. €€€–€€€€

ACCOMMODATION
ACTIVITIES
A – Z

PISA AND THE ETRUSCAN RIVIERA

Casale Marittimo

Il Poggio
Località Il Poggio
Tel: 0586-652 308
www.ilpoggio.org
Agriturismo on the road from Bibbona offering small apartments. Ideal base for exploring the area, especially for fam-

ilies with children. €

Livorno

Gran Duca
Piazza Micheli 16
Tel: 0586-891 024
www.granduca.it
Attractive hotel (for Livorno) on the seafront with views over the old

harbour. A good place to stay if you are catching an early ferry. Fitness centre with pool, spa and sauna. €€

Massa Pisana

Villa La Principessa
Via Nuova per Pisa, 1616
Tel: 0583-370 037

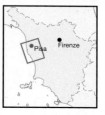

LANGUAGE

Exclusive 4-star mansion open Apr–Oct. Old-fashioned elegance; modern comforts. Swimming pool, lovely garden. €€€

Montenero

La Vedetta
Via della Lecceta 5
Tel: 0586-579 957
www.hotellavedetta.it
Modern hotel in Livorno hills. Basic rooms but sweeping views. Near the sanctuary of Madonna di Montenero. €

Palaia

Borgo di Colleoli
Palaia
Tel: 0587-622 524
www.ilpalazzocolleoli.com
Combination of hotel and self-catering accommodation. Rooms are spacious and the "hamlet" enjoys a gorgeous setting in well-manicured grounds surrounded by rolling hills. Pisa is a short drive away; the coast about an hour and a half. Good for families. Two swimming pools. €€–€€€

Pisa

Albergo Helvetia
Via Don Gaetano Boschi 31
Tel: 050-553 084
This small budget hotel is situated in a particularly quiet area and yet it's right on the Piazza dei Miracoli's doorstep. Only half of the 29 rooms have private bathrooms. Pleasant courtyard garden. Plain but cheap. €

Ariston
Via Cardinale Maffi 42
Tel: 050-561 834

www.hotelariston.pisa.it
The best thing about this hotel is its position, literally in the shadow of the Leaning Tower. The rooms are of an acceptable standard, but the service can be unfriendly. €€

Grand Hotel Duomo
Via Santa Maria 94
Tel: 050-561 894
www.grandhotelduomo.it
Comfortable, business-like hotel, close to the Piazza dei Miracoli. Restaurant; private garage. €€€

Hotel Locanda La Lanterna
Via S. Maria 113
Tel: 050-830 305
www.locandalalanterna.com
Pleasant, no-frills bed-and-breakfast hotel, close to the Leaning Tower. Very good value for money. €

Hotel Novecento
Via Roma 37
Tel: 050-500 323
www.hotelnovecento.pisa.it
Elegant hotel in the historic heart of Pisa, a 10-minute walk from the Leaning Tower. Rooms are stylish and the little garden is a peaceful retreat.

Hotel Relais dell'Orologio
Via della Faggiola 12/14
Tel: 050-830 361
www.hotelrelaisorologio.com
Conveniently located between the Campo dei Miracoli and Piazza dei Cavalieri, this gracious 14th-century manor house has been transformed into a stylish and elegant boutique hotel with just 21 individually decorated rooms. Romantic courtyard garden. A luxurious treat. €€€€

Royal Victoria
Lungarno Pacinotti 12

Tel: 050-940 111
www.royalvictoriahotel.it
The most characterful hotel in the city opened in 1842 and played host to Dickens and other Grand Tourists. It has been in the same family for generations. The current custodians have retained its authentic, old-fashioned atmosphere and charm. Rooms overlooking the Arno are in great demand, though they can be noisy. Garage. Bikes for hire. €€

Touring
Via Puccini 24
Tel: 050-46374
www.hoteltouringpisa.it
Well run, if dowdy hotel across the Arno from the main sights, but near the station. €€

Villa Kinzica
Piazza Arcivescovado 2
Tel: 050-560 419
www.hotelvillakinzica.it
Remarkably positioned hotel, two minutes' walk from the Leaning Tower. Many original features remain, though some rooms need attention and service can be brusque. Own restaurant/pizzeria. €–€€

San Giuliano Terme

Corliano
Strada Statale Abetone 50
Tel: 050-818 193
www.corliano.it
Faded villa of grand dimensions, halfway between Pisa and Lucca. Informal, with plenty of atmosphere. A good find. Restaurant attached. €€

Villa C Bagni di Pisa
San Giuliano Terme
Tel: 050-88501

www.bagnidipisa.com
Convenient for Pisa and Lucca, this atmospheric 18th-century spa resort has been sensitively restored as a romantic retreat (with private hammam). Enjoy distant views of the Leaning Tower while tucking into superb Pisan steak, Tuscan bouillabaisse *(cacciucco)*, truffled pasta and Antinori wines. €€€–€€€€

Sassetta

Campo di Carlo
Via Campagna Nord 62
Tel: 0565-794 257
www.campodicarlo.it
Child-friendly guest-house in the heart of the country, not far from Sassetta and within easy reach of the sea. Six lovely rooms. €

Tirrenia

Bristol
Via delle Felci 38
Tel: 050-37161
www.bristol.it
Three-star, unpretentious and comfortable hotel with pool and tennis court. €€

Green Park Resort
Via dei Tulipani 1,
Calambrone 56018
Tel: 050-313 5711
www.softlivingplaces.com
This modern resort is spread out in villas and apartments in spacious grounds just behind the dunes and seafront. Facilities include a spa, outdoor swimming pool and open-air summer bar, as well as two restaurants. Lunasia is romantic and targeted at couples, while Le Ginestre is more for families. Both are excellent, with charming staff. €€€

ISOLA D'ELBA

Capo Sant'Andrea

Hotel Ilio
Via Sant'Andrea 5
Tel: 0565-908 018
www.hotelilio.com
This welcoming 19-room hotel is a hidden gem among the many small establishments stacked up on the hillside around Capo Sant'Andrea. As with many of the Elban hotels, half-board is obligatory, but the restaurant is excellent and pre-dinner cocktails on the terrace add an extra touch. Mountain bikes are also available for rent. **€€€**

Marciana

Bel Tramonto
Località Patresi
Tel: 0565-908 027
www.valverdehotel.it
Modern hotel with lovely swimming pool and grounds. Most rooms have balconies overlooking the sea. **€**

Portoferraio

La Hermitage
Località Biodola
Tel: 0565-9740
www.hotelhermitage.it
Large and lively resort hotel, founded in the 1950s. **€€€**
Hotel Mare
Località Magazzini

Tel: 0565-933 069
www.elba-on-line.com
This peaceful hotel, located just across the bay from Portoferraio, is part of a tiny village with its own marina. Excellent restaurant and friendly hotel staff. Rooms are simple and clean. **€**
Hotel Scoglio Bianco
Località Viticcio
Tel: 0565-939 036
www.scogliobianco.it
Low-key whitewashed hotel in one of Elba's quieter corners. You can get great sunset views from the terraces. Half-board is obligatory, but still represents good value for money. **€**

Villa Ottone
Località Ottone
Tel: 0565-933 042
www.villaottone.com
Refined hotel in a gleaming white 19th-century villa located just east of Portoferraio. Beautifully tended grounds and a poolside restaurant. **€€**

VOLTERRA AND MASSA MARITTIMA

Massa Marittima

Albergo il Sole
Corso della Libertà 43
Tel: 0566-901 959
Simple hotel in an old palazzo in the medieval heart of the town. **€**
La Fenice Park Hotel
C. Diaz 63
Tel: 0566-903 941
www.lafeniceparkhotel.com
One of the best in town, this charming hotel occupies a mansion convenient for the city sights. Individualistic suites are matched by Carrara-marble bathrooms and a pleasant garden where you can enjoy a delicious breakfast during the summer. There is also a small swimming pool and Ayurveda massage is offered in the small spa. **€€–€€€**

Volterra

San Lino
Via San Lino 26
Tel: 0588-85250
www.hotelsanlino.com
Monastic building whose original austerity has been softened by a successful conversion into a 4-star hotel. Swimming pool and garage available to guests. **€**
Villa Nencini
Borgo Santo Stefano 55
Tel: 0588-86386
www.villanencini.it
Pleasant stone villa situated just outside Volterra's old town walls, with a garden and a pool, as well as a restaurant and *enoteca*. **€€**
Villa Palagione
Località Palagione
Tel: 0588-39014

www.villa-palagione.com
Aristocratic villa, 7km (4 miles) from Volterra, converted into a hotel and cultural centre specialising in group activities (cooking, wine tasting, painting, horse riding, walking, language courses, etc), but individual guests are welcome. Beautiful frescoed rooms. Bicycles can also be hired. **€€**
Villa Rioddi
Strada Provinciale Monte Volterrano
Tel: 0588-88053
www.hotelvillarioddi.it
This family-run 15th-century villa sits on a hillside 2km (1 mile) from the centre of Volterra. The 15 rooms are simply furnished; garden and swimming pool with views over the

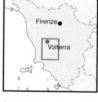

Cecina valley. The staff are ultra-friendly and the breakfasts delicious, making this a charming rural retreat. **€–€€**

SAN GIMIGNANO AND CHIANTI COUNTRY

Casole d'Elsa

Hotel Castello di Casole
Località Querceto
Tel: 0577-967 511
www.castellodicasole.com
Owned by Timber resorts, this vast (4,200-acre/1,700-hectare) private estate northwest of Siena features a meticulously restored 12th-century castle that has just opened as an all-suite hotel. It blends grand style with rustic Tuscan furnishings. The rest of the estate is dotted with villas which can be rented or even acquired on a Fractional basis. **€€€–€€€€**

Castellina in Chianti

Belvedere di San Leonino
Località San Leonino
Tel: 0577-740 887
www.hotelsanleonino.com

Imposing 15th-century country house surrounded by olive trees and vineyards. Swimming pool. **€€**

Colle Etrusco Salivolpi
Via Fiorentina 89
Tel: 0577-740 484
www.hotelsalivolpi.com
Well-restored farmhouse with an appealing garden and uncontrived rustic decor of original beams, whitewashed walls, terracotta tiles and decorative ironwork. **€**

Collelungo
Località Castellina in Chianti
Tel: 0577-740 489
www.collelungo.com
Lovingly restored stone farmhouse divided into comfortable apartments (named after the Siena *contrade*) for 2–4 people. Barbecue and pool. Minimum stay: three nights. **€€**

Le Piazze
Località Le Piazze
Tel: 0577-743 190
www.locandalepiazze.it

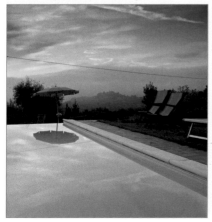
BELOW: hotel pool view in San Gimignano.

Converted 17th-century farmhouse with terraces and gardens. Rustic furnishings and luxurious bathrooms. Meals on request. **€€**

Tenuta di Ricavo
Località Ricavo 4
Tel: 0577-740 221
www.ricavo.com
A highly rated hotel occupying a series of rustic houses in a medieval hamlet, 5km (3 miles) from Castellina. Pool; good quality restaurant. Apr–Oct. **€€**

Villa Casalecchi
Località Casalecchi
Tel: 0577-740 240
www.villacasalecchi.it
Mid-range hotel in a 19th-century villa, surrounded by oak trees. Pool, tennis courts, restaurant. Mar–Oct. **€€**

Certaldo Alto

Osteria del Vicario
Via Rivellino 3
Tel: 0571-668 228
www.osteriadelvicario.it
A former monastery converted into a noted restaurant serving dishes inspired by ancient Tuscan recipes, and set in the former cloisters. Charming rooms (ex-monastic cells) in a pretty hilltop town. **€€**

Colle di Val d'Elsa

Hotel Arnolfo
Via F. Campana 8
Tel: 0577-922 020
www.hotelarnolfo.it
Occupies a 15th-century palazzo in a commanding position at the top of town, though rooms are basic. **€**

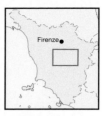

Villa Belvedere
Via Senese
Tel: 0577-920 966
www.villabelvedere.com
Delightful 18th-century villa surrounded by a large park. Excellent restaurant. **€€**

Gaiole in Chianti

Castello di Spaltenna
Via Spaltenna 13
Tel: 0577-749 483
www.spaltenna.it
Formidable fortified monastery, now a luxurious hotel with an excellent restaurant, indoor and outdoor pools, gym, steam room, sauna and tennis court. Supremely comfortable, individually designed rooms. **€€€**

L'Ultimo Mulino
Localita La Ripresa di Vistarenni
Tel: 0577-738 520
www.ultimomulino.it
Atmospheric hotel in a converted mill. An ideal setting for exploring Chianti; pool. **€€**

Greve in Chianti

Albergo del Chianti
Piazza Matteotti 86
Tel: 055-853 763
www.albergodelchianti.it
Small, pleasant hotel with pool, garden and a friendly atmosphere. **€€**

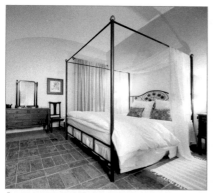

ABOVE: a room at the Laticastelli Resort.

Monastero d'Ombrone

Castel Monastero
Tel: 0577-570 001
www.castelmonastero.com
Set just east of Siena and convenient for the Chianti, this is a romantic castle retreat with an exceptional restaurant. Occasional cooking classes with celebrity chef Gordon Ramsey, as well as photography and other courses.
€€€–€€€€

Monteriggioni

Hotel Monteriggioni
Via 1 Maggio 4
Tel: 0577-305 009
www.hotelmonteriggioni.net
A couple of village houses converted into an elegant hotel with a garden and swimming pool, in a pretty walled town 10km (6 miles) north of Siena. €€€

Il Piccolo Castello
Via Colligiana, 8
Tel: 0577-307 300
www.ilpiccolocastello.com
This well-designed modern resort is close to historic Monteriggioni and the Chianti

hills. Facilities include a pool, spa and Tuscan restaurant. Horse riding, archery and cookery classes are easily arranged. €€€

Panzano in Chianti

I Fagiolari
Case Sparse
Tel: 055-852 351
Mobile: 335-612 4988
www.fagiolari.it
This small, restored Tuscan farmhouse is surrounded by olive trees and forest. The friendly owner, Giulietta, gives cooking classes and can prepare meals for guests. All four rooms have a private bath and cosy decor. There's also a separate cottage for rent. Swimming pool. €€

Villa Le Barone
Via San Leolino 19
Tel: 055-852 621
www.villalebarone.com
Patrician villa in the Chianti hills filled with family antiques, giving the feel of a private house. Some rooms have their own terrace. Facilities include swimming pool,

tennis court and a good restaurant. Half-board rates. €€–€€€

Villa San Giovese
Piazza Bucciarelli 5
Tel: 055-852 461
www.villasangiovese.it
Well-restored villa in the Florentine Chianti, with rooms in a converted traditional farmhouse. Noted restaurant and wines. €€

Radda in Chianti

Relais Fattoria Vignale
Via Pianigiani 9
Tel: 0577-738 300
www.vignale.it
Discreetly elegant old manor house with a relaxed atmosphere. Excellent wine produced on site; bar and restaurant in the old wine cellars; pool. €€€

Rapolano Terme

Laticastelli Resort
53040 Rapolano Terme
Tel: 0577-724 419
www.laticastelli.com
This is a *borgo*, a fortified castle-hamlet dating from the 12th century. It was one of several fortresses built to protect Siena from the south. Panoramic views. Dine on typical Tuscan antipasti (cheese, cold cuts and bruschetta) on a charming terrace. €€–€€€

San Casciano Val di Pesa

Il Borghetto
Via Collina 23, Montefiridolfi
Tel: 055-824 4442
www.borghetto.org
Very welcoming *agriturismo* with homely rooms and apartments, part of a working wine and olive-oil estate. Swim-

ming pool; cookery classes. €€

San Gimignano

L'Antico Pozzo
Via San Matteo 87
Tel: 0577-942 014
www.anticopozzo.com
Charming old house in the heart of the medieval town, carefully restored and simply but tastefully furnished. €€

Hotel La Cisterna
Piazza della Cisterna 23
Tel: 0577-940 328
www.hotelcisterna.it
Medieval palazzo with a fine restaurant. The best rooms have views of the main piazza or across the valley. One of the most atmospheric and popular hotels in town. €€

Hotel Pescille
Località Pescille
Tel: 0577-940 186
www.pescille.it
Converted manor house 3km (2 miles) southwest of San Gimignano. Some rooms have a balcony with views of the medieval towers. Swimming pool; tennis. €€

Villa San Paolo
Strada per Certaldo
Tel: 0577-955 100
A 19th-century hillside villa, 5km (3 miles) from San Gimignano, with attractive rooms, terraced grounds and a fitness centre. €€€

PRICE CATEGORIES

These refer to the cost of a standard double room during high season, usually including breakfast:
€ = under €100
€€ = €100–200
€€€ = €200–300
€€€€ = over €300

TRANSPORT

ACCOMMODATION

ACTIVITIES

A – Z

LANGUAGE

SIENA

Albergo Centrale
C. Angiolieri 26
Tel: 0577-280 379
www.hotelcentralesiena.it
A clean and spacious budget hotel that is situated just a stone's throw from the Campo.
€

Antica Torre
Via Fiera Vecchia 7
Tel: 0577-222 255
www.anticatorresiena.it
A tiny, atmospheric hotel, essentially a conversion of a 17th-century tower, with a small garden and private car park. Only 12 rooms, so booking early is essential.
€€

Certosa di Maggiano
Strada di Certosa 82
Tel: 0577-288 180
www.certosadimaggiano.com
Just outside Siena, this 14th-century Carthusian monastery – the oldest in Tuscany – has been converted into a 5-star hotel furnished with antiques. Set in olive groves with an outdoor pool, tennis courts, a prestigious restaurant and stunning original features.
€€€€

Continental
Banchi di Sopra 85
Tel: 0577-56011
www.royaldemeure.com
This majestic hotel, recently restored with fine frescoed interiors, is in the heart of Siena. Covered courtyard, restaurant and wine bar.
€€€€

Duomo
Via Stalloreggi 38
Tel: 0577-289 088
www.hotelduomo.it
Situated at the heart of the historic centre, this 18th-century palazzo has a cloistered, intimate atmosphere. Some rooms have views of the cathedral and the surrounding Sienese hills. **€€**

Garden
Via Custoza 25
Tel: 0577-567 111
www.gardenhotel.it
Just north of Siena, this 16th-century patrician villa is now a prestigious hotel with a formal, Italian garden and a pool. Four-star rooms available, too. Good for families. Drops a price bracket in low season.**€€€**

Grand Hotel
Palazzo Ravizza
Pian dei Mantellini 34
Tel: 0577-280 462
www.palazzoravizza.it
A historic town house with frescoed ceilings and lovely gardens with views over the Tuscan hills. There are well-chosen antiques in the bedrooms, with the first-floor "noble rooms" particularly desirable. It also has welcoming public rooms. **€€**

Piccolo Hotel Etruria
Via delle Donzelle 3
Tel: 0577-288 088
www.hoteletruria.com
Friendly, family-orientated hotel with simple

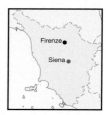

but clean rooms divided between two town houses. Good value for money.**€€**

Santa Caterina
Via Enea Silvio Piccolomini 7
Tel: 0577-221 105
www.hscsiena.it
Friendly three-star hotel set in a garden just outside the city walls, near Porta Romana, about a 15-minute walk to the centre. Breakfast is served on a lovely veranda with views across the Sienese hills. Be aware that roadside rooms can be noisy. **€€**

Tre Donzelle
Via delle Donzelle 5
Tel: 0577-280 358
www.tredonzelle.carbonmade.com
Facilities at this hotel are limited and the rooms are basic but clean and comfortable. For a hotel so near the Campo however, it's still excellent value for money. **€**

Villa Scacciapensieri
Via Scacciapensieri 10
Tel: 0577-41441
www.villascacciapensieri.it
Supremely elegant villa hotel located in lovely grounds 3km (1½ miles) north of the city. Sophisticated interior, bedrooms with rural views, and a panoramic city view from the restaurant terrace. **€€€**

BELOW: ballroom at the Grand Hotel Continental.

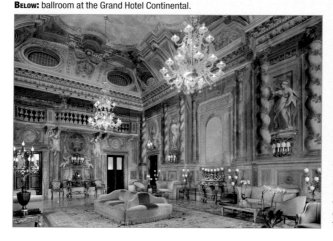

SOUTH OF SIENA

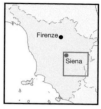

Castiglione d'Orcia

Agriturismo Le Case
Tel: 0577-888 983
www.agriturismolecase.com
A delightful hilltop farmhouse overlooking the Val d'Orcia, close to Castiglione d'Orcia and the spa centres of Bagno San Filippo and Bagno Vignoni. Convenient for the wine routes, too. This extremely good-value rural B&B is run by a charming English-speaking couple and has five double rooms, each with its own private bathroom. **€**

Cetona

Locanda di Anita
Piazza Balestrieri 5
Tel: 0578-237 075
www.locandadicetona.com
Charming little inn and bar set back from the main square. Guests are given a special pass for access to the luxury Fonteverde spa in San Casciano dei Bagni (see page 286). **€€**

Chianciano Terme

Hotel Niagara
Via dei Colli 57
Tel: 0578-64693
Set close to the spa establishments of Terme di Silene and Terme di Sant'Elena, it is also convenient for the contemporary spa, the swish Terme Sensoriali, and the old town centre. Tuscan fare in the restaurant. Free shuttle service to and from Chiusi-Chianciano railway station. Free use of

the Olimpus Sports Centre nearby. **€€**

Montalcino

Castiglione del Bosco
Tel: 0577-191 3001
www.castigliondelbosco.it
This is a sprawling 800-year-old country estate in the heart of Val d'Orcia, outside Montalcino. The Ferragamo's 4,000-acre (1,600 hectare) estate was once a private club but is now a resort offering antique-studded villas or suites. The estate comprises two restaurants, a cookery school, a spa, a herb garden, golf course, outdoor infinity pool and a winery. **€€€€**

Il Giglio
Via Saloni 5
Tel: 0577-846 577
www.gigliohotel.com
Small family-run hotel suspended above the city walls. Its 12 rooms all offer fabulous views over the lush Val d'Orcia. **€€**

Il Marzocco
Piazza Savonarola 18
Tel: 0578-757 262
www.albergoilmarzocco.it
Medieval palazzo with fine, if old-fashioned, rooms, some of which have balconies with fine valley views. **€**

Montepulciano

Albergo di San Biagio
Via San Bartolomeo 2
Tel: 0578-717 233
This modern, family-run hotel is set below historic Montepulciano but still enjoys lovely views over San Biagio and the countryside. Comfortable rooms. It's a

10-minute walk into town but there's also a shuttle bus and plenty of parking. **€–€€**

Il Borghetto
Via Borgo Buio 7
Tel: 0578-757 535
www.ilborghetto.it
Three 16th-century palazzi in the heart of town, converted into a hotel. Rooms are small but comfortable. Be sure to request one with views over the valley. Cosy sitting room with a big fireplace and resident cat. The owner is also a tour guide. **€€**

Palazzo Contucci
Pizza Grande 13
Tel: 0578-757 006
www.residenzecontucci.it
This palatial 16th-century building designed by Sangallo still belongs to the aristocratic Contucci family. The Contessa rents out an apartment above the wine cellars. **€€**

Pienza

Antica Locanda
Corso Il Rossellino 72
Tel: 0578-493 110
www.anticalocandapienza.com
Small but comfortable bed and breakfast, with some rooms overlooking the valley. **€**

Il Chiostro di Pienza
Corso Il Rosellino 26
Tel: 0578-748 400
www.relaisilchiostrodipienza.com
Beautifully converted medieval convent, with a quiet cloister, in the heart of Pienza. Charming, highly idiosyncratic rooms. Also runs an excellent restaurant. Very welcoming. **€€–€€€€**

Piccolo Hotel
Via Circonvallazione 7

Tel: 0578-749 402
www.piccolohotellavalle.it
Popular, comfortable spot with balconies offering fine panoramic views of the Val d'Orcia. **€–€€**

Ripa d'Orcia

Castello di Ripa d'Orcia
Località Castiglione d'Orcia
Tel: 0577-897 376
www.castelloripadorcia.com
Peaceful medieval hamlet, dominated by a tower, parts of which have been converted into hotel rooms and apartments. Trattoria with panoramic terrace views. Closed Dec–Feb. **€€**

Hotel Palazzuolo
Via Santa Caterina 43
Tel: 0577-897 080
www.hotelpalazzuolo.it
Surrounded by lush countryside, with terrace and swimming pool; Tuscan cuisine. Free use of mountain bikes. **€**

PRICE CATEGORIES

These refer to the cost of a standard double room during high season, usually including breakfast:
€ = under €100
€€ = €100–200
€€€ = €200–300
€€€€ = over €300

TRANSPORT

ACCOMMODATION

ACTIVITIES

A – Z

LANGUAGE

San Casciano dei Bagni

Fonteverde Natural Spa Resort
Tel: 0578-57241
www.fonteverdespa.com
Tuscany's most beguiling destination spa and a favoured hideaway for Italian celebrities who lap up the laid-back luxury, rolling hills, and seemingly remote setting. Strong in Mediterranean and oriental treatments. One of the best spas in Italy.
€€€–€€€€

San Quirico d'Orcia

Adler Thermae Spa
San Quirico d'Orcia 53027

Tel: 0577-889 001
www.adler-thermae.com
Set in rolling hills in Tuscany's prettiest province, this is a romantic, perfectly groomed destination spa, with inclusive t'ai chi, yoga and Pilates. It is also a very child-friendly resort, with kids' clubs and pools to entertain youngsters while parents indulge in the pampering treatments on offer or Tuscan gastronomy.
€€–€€€

Sinalunga

Locanda dell'Amorosa
Località l'Amorosa
Tel: 0577-677 211
www.amorosa.it

Renaissance hamlet, complete with chapel, now converted into a first-class hotel. Romantic setting with a superb "destination" restaurant, with menu prices to match.
€€€–€€€€

Sovicille

Borgo Pretale
Tel: 0577-345 401
www.borgopretale.it
A beautifully restored hamlet with homely apartments and restaurant. €€€

Val d'Orcia

Bagni di San Filippo
Bagni San Filippo 53023
Tel: 0577-872 982

www.termesanfilippo.it
Set in the heart of the Val d'Orcia, this is an affordable, time-warp spa that works. Friendly service, low-key bedrooms and hearty Tuscan cuisine – plus a range of restorative water and mud treatments. €–€€

La Locanda del Loggiato
Piazza del Moretto 30
Tel: 0577-888 925
www.loggiato.it
This romantic six-roomed B&B in the Val d'Orcia is a perfect place for couples to stay if wine tasting in the nearby villages in the region. Has its own wine bar. No children.
€€

THE MAREMMA AND MONTE ARGENTARIO

Albinia

La Parrina
Km 146 Via Aurelia
Tel: 0564-862 626
www.parrina.it
Genuine *agriturismo* set among vineyards, olive groves and orchards on the Maremman plains. It has retained the traditional decor of a country estate. Excellent buffet breakfast on garden terrace. Swimming pool, chapel,

farm shop and bicycles.
€€–€€€

Castiglione della Pescaia

Albergo Tirreno
Via Ansedonia 69
Tel: 0564-933 796
www.hoteltirrenocastiglione.it
Clean hotel with 12 rooms. Tariff includes room and board – tasty meals at the restaurant on the premises. €
L'Andana
Tenuta La Badiola
Tel: 0564-944 800
www.andana.it
The former estate of Tuscan Grand Duke Leopold II has been transformed into a supremely refined hotel with an excellent restaurant, serving French creative cuisine by one of France's most celebrated chefs, Alain

Ducasse, who has also set up his own winery here. The height of luxury. €€€€

Isola del Giglio

Pardini's Hermitage
Cala degli Alberi,
Giglio Porto
Tel: 0564-809 034
www.hermit.it
Pleasant, secluded island retreat with 12 small rooms and well-tended gardens. Accessible by boat from Giglio Porto. Relaxed atmosphere, friendly welcome and good facilities. Half-board only. €€

Montemerano

Villa Acquaviva
Strada Scansanese 10 Nord
(2km/1 mile from Montemerano)
Tel: 0564-602 890

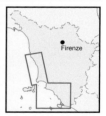

www.relaisvillaacquaviva.com
Family-run villa near Saturnia with a lovely garden and comfortable rooms. Mountain bikes available for hire. Swimming pool. €€

Piombino

Poggio all'Agnello
Localita Poggio all'Agnello 31
Tel: 0565-29618
www.poggioallagnello.it
This is a countryside and beach resort on the Costa degli Etruschi,

not far from Livorno. On offer are self-catering apartments tucked between the sea and the pine groves; shuttle bus to the private beach. Several outdoor pools, sports centre, spa and children's club. €€–€€€

Porto Ercole

Don Pedro
Via Panoramica 7
Tel: 0564-833 914
www.hoteldonpedro.it
Long-established family-run hotel with views over the port below. The decor is rather old-fashioned, but it is well positioned. Half-board preferred. Easter–Sept. €€

Hotel Il Pellicano
Località o Sbarcatello
Tel: 0564-858 111
www.pellicanohotel.com
Chic hotel for the celebrity set in summer. It enjoys a superb, isolated clifftop position. Bedrooms are located in various buildings; terraces lead down to the private beach. Tennis courts and swimming pool. Weekly barbecues in summer. An expensive treat.
€€€€

Porto Sants Stefano

Torre Di Cala Piccola
8km (5 miles) from Porto Santo Stefano on the Strada Panoramica, Argentario
Tel: 0564-825 111
www.torredicalapiccola.com
Charming clifftop hotel, built around a 17th-century Spanish lookout tower. Rooms and apartments with private beach and superb sea views. Mar–Oct. €€€€

Punta Ala

Hotel Cala del Porto
Via del Pozzo
Tel: 0564-922 455
www.hotelcaladelporto.com
This chic Baglioni-owned hotel overlooks the lovely bay of Cala del Porto and Punta Ala, with Elba in the distance. Highlights are the Pagoda beachside restaurant and the Belvedere gourmet restaurant, set on a terrace. Equally appealing is the private sandy beach and the Punta Ala golf club. €€€€

Saturnia

Terme di Saturnia Spa & Golf Resort
Via della Follonata

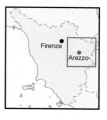

ABOVE: beach at Hotel Cala del Porto.

Tel: 0564-600 111
www.termedisaturnia.it
Set in the Maremma, and fed by historic springs, this sophisticated, luxury spa resort is a contrast to the rugged Etruscan countryside beyond. The pampering spa boasts a lovely authentic hot-springs pool, and an indoor recreation of Ancient Roman baths. Fine dining, elegant suites and an 18-hole golf course make it great for sophisticates. The thermal pool and treatment centre is open to non-residents. €€€€

Hotel Villa Clodia
Via Italia 43
Tel: 0564-601 212
www.hotelvillaclodia.com
Centrally located mid-range hotel with lovely view and swimming pool, within walking distance of the spa. Good value. €

Sovana

Albergo Ristorante Taverna Etrusca
Piazza del Pretorio 16
Tel: 0564-616 183
Comfortable rooms with the best small restaurant in town. €

La Scilla
Via R. Siviero 3
Tel: 0564-616 531
www.scilla-sovana.it
Eight bright and elegant rooms in a pretty tufa-built hotel. €€

Talamone

Hotel Capo d'Uomo
Via Cala di Forno 7
Tel: 0564-887 077
www.hotelcapoduomo.com
Clifftop hotel with balconies overlooking the sea and access to a private rocky beach. Within easy reach of the wilds of the Parco della Maremma, also known as Parco'Uccellina. €€

AREZZO AND EASTERN TUSCANY

Arezzo

Continentale
Piazza G. Monaco 7
Tel: 0575-20251
www.hotelcontinentale.com
A centrally located 3-star hotel, with good facilities, comfortable rooms and a lovely roof terrace. Popular among business travellers. €€

Graziella Patio Hotel
Via Cavour 23
Tel: 0575-401 962
www.hotelpatio.it
Innovative hotel in an old palazzo in the historic heart of Arezzo, not far from San Francesco. The colourful decor of each of the seven rooms was inspired by the writings of widely travelled novelist Bruce Chatwin. €€

Val di Colle
Località Bagnoro, Scopeto
Tel: 0575-365 167
www.dimorastoricavaldicolle.it
A meticulously restored 14th-century house, sitting on a hilltop 4km

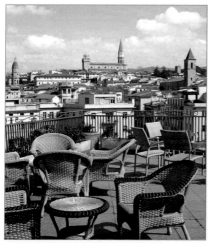

ABOVE: roof-terrrace view from the Continentale, Arezzo.

(2½ miles) from the centre of Arezzo. There are eight elegant bedrooms decorated with a rustic theme. Antique furniture sits harmoniously alongside the modern art. Golfers can use the driving range and 9-hole putting green on the premises. **€€€**

Bibbiena

Albergo Borgo Antico
Via Cappucci 2
Tel: 0575-536 445
www.brami.com
Welcoming hotel-restaurant in the centre of Bibbiena, with comfortable, if nondescript, bedrooms. Good base for exploring the Casentino area. **€**

Castiglion Fiorentino

Villa Schiatti
Località Montecchio 131
Tel: 0575-651 440
www.villaschiatti.it

Situated in the hills between Arezzo and Siena, and equipped with pool, restaurant and terrace offering splendid views over the Tuscan countryside. **€–€€**

Cortona

Il Falconiere
Località San Martino.
Tel: 0575-612 679
www.ilfalconiere.it
Luxurious country retreat set in olive groves 3km (2 miles) above Cortona. First-class restaurant. **€€€**

Rugapiana Vacanze
Via Nazionale 63
Tel: 0575-630 712
www.rugapianavacanze.com
Rooms and apartments for short or longer stays, in central Cortona. Guests can use the facilities at an *agriturismo* just outside town. **€€**

San Michele
Via Guelfa 15
Tel: 0575-604 348
www.hotelsanmichele.net

Centrally situated, comfortable hotel in an impressively restored Renaissance palace. **€€**

Foiano della Chiana

La Lodola
Via Piana 19
Tel: 0575-649 660
www.lalodola.com
Bed and breakfast in an 18th-century farmhouse. The rooms are lovingly decorated by the antique-dealer owners – some of the furniture is for sale. **€€**

Gargonza

Castello di Gargonza
Monte San Savino
Tel: 0575-847 021
www.gargonza.it
Attractive fortified village near Arezzo, with a frescoed chapel and castle walls, converted into a hotel with separate apartments. The 13th-century buildings overlook the Val di Chiana. The restaurant, with large terrace, specialises in game. **€€**

Loro Ciuffenna

Villa Cassia di Baccano
Via Setteponti Levante 132
Tel: 055-977 2310
www.villacassiadibaccano.it
Stylishly converted villa 17km (11 miles) from Arezzo, offering comfortable, airy apartments on a weekly basis, and suites on a daily basis. Numerous services and a swimming pool. Lovely views. **€€–€€€**

Monterchi

B&B Il Colle
Località. Il Colle 4b

Tel: 0575-709 856
www.bedandbreakfastilcolle.com
Former farmhouse that has been well converted into a homely bed and breakfast. Living room, terrace and kitchen available to guests. Open fire makes it cosy in colder weather. **€€**

Regello

Villa Rigacci
Via Manzoni 75
Tel: 055-865 6718
www.villarigacci.it
Country-house hotel in a pleasant setting, off the scenic "Road of the Seven Bridges" and handy for easy access to the Rome–Florence motorway. Sophisticated Mediterranean food, extensive grounds and a swimming pool. Good base for designer-outlet shopping – there are malls in nearby Leccio and Montevarchi. **€€**

Sansepolcro

Relais Oroscopo
Via Togliatti 68
Tel: 0575-734 875
www.relaisoroscopo.com
Located on the outskirts of Sansepolcro, this mid-range hotel offers individually decorated bedrooms and a renowned restaurant. **€–€€**

PRICE CATEGORIES

These refer to the cost of a standard double room during high season, usually including breakfast:
€ = under €100
€€ = €100–200
€€€ = €200–300
€€€€ = over €300

ACTIVITIES

THE ARTS, NIGHTLIFE, FESTIVALS, SPORTS AND SHOPPING

THE ARTS

Archaeological Sites

There are various places of archaeological interest in Tuscany. These include **Etruscan** (8th–2nd century BC) sites at Volterra, Fiesole, Arezzo, Chiusi, Vetulonia and on the island of Elba. There is an archaeological museum in Florence, and other museums in Volterra, Chiusi, Cortona, Asciano, Grosseto and Massa Marittima.

Notable **Roman** (8th century BC–5th century AD) remains can be seen at Fiesole, Cosa, Roselle, Volterra and Arezzo.

Art and Architecture

Art

Renaissance art is, of course, what Tuscany is most famous for. The most outstanding Renaissance collections are in Florence, in the Uffizi Gallery, the Pitti Palace and the San Marco Museum.

Works of art from the late Renaissance and Mannerist periods, the Baroque, the neoclassical and Romantic, and also the 21st century are exhibited at most galleries and museums in the main cities of the region.

The exciting La Strozzina gallery, in the restored cellars of the Palazzo Strozzi, has finally put Florence on the contemporary-art map. The Palazzo Strozzi itself is a major exhibition site focusing on high-profile art exhibitions *(see page 96).*

Architecture

Tuscany is a treasure trove of architectural history *(see feature on pages 60–5).*

Churches and civil buildings from the Romanesque period can be found at Pisa, Florence, Lucca, Siena, Pistoia and Arezzo. The most important Gothic buildings are in Florence, Siena, Pisa, Pistoia and Arezzo. Tuscany also abounds in religious and secular Renaissance buildings, Florence being the most important centre.

Sightseeing

Details of important museums and art galleries are in the Places section of this book. Be sure to take advantage of multi-entrance tickets, especially in Florence.

Florence

There are stands in shops and cafés where free leaflets detailing events and exhibitions can be picked up.

The Friends of Florentine Museums Association (Via degli Alfani 39; tel: 055-293 007) arranges museum visits 9–11pm in the summer, with orchestral recitals.

If you plan to visit a lot of museums in Florence, consider a membership to Amici degli Uffizi, which allows free entrances and no queues. *(See tip on page 11 and also www.amicidegliuffizi.it)*

It is advisable to reserve Uffizi and Accademia tickets in advance, or face lengthy queuing *(see pages 110 and 118).*

The new **Firenze Card** covers three days of museums and public transport *(see tip on page 92).* Entry prices for museums and galleries vary greatly, with the Uffizi the most expensive. State museums are closed on Monday, while most other museums close on Tuesday or Wednesday. Most museums also close on 1 May.

Every year, in the spring, Florence has a "culture week" *(La Settimana di Beni Culturali),* when all the state museums are free. Enquire at the tourist office for more information.

Florence on foot: Walking tours are an excellent way to gain more insight into the city. **Link** (tel: 055-218 191, and (+39) 338-390 3070; www.linkfirenze.it) is a Florentine-based guiding service that covers personalised thematic tours, ranging from arty walking tours to nature rambles and gastro-tours that visit the markets and Chianti wine estates. All the guides can be recommended, with Guido perfect for art and history, and Silvia the best for foodie experiences.

Florence by rickshaw: Tre Rote; tel: (+39) 338-638 9245; www.pedicabfirenze.it

Florence by Segway: www.segway.it

Florence by horse-drawn carriage: from Piazza Duomo or Piazza della Signoria.

Florence by Vespa: Tuscany Pass (www.tuscanypass.com), which also offers Vespa trips to the Chianti, as well as walking tours and cookery courses.

Pisa

The main sites can be easily visited on foot or by local bus. Buy a joint ticket to see all the sights on the Campo dei Miracoli. A horse-and-carriage ride is a pleasant introduction to the city; prices are negotiable.

Siena

The tourist office can provide a list of authorised guides. With one week's notice, you can visit any of the *Contrada* (district) museums that celebrate the Palio and the ancient city traditions: the numbers are available on www.paliodisiena.biz.

Themed Tours

ABTOI, the Association of British Tour Operators to Italy (www.loveitaly.co.uk) is a good place to start when planning holidays to Italy, and for booking unusual themed itineraries ranging from art trails to adventures, such as foodie, wine and walking trails.

Sapori + Saperi (UK tel: +44 (0)7768-474 610; Italy tel: +39 339-763 6321; wwwi.sapori-e-saperi.com) specialises in Slow Travel and Slow Food in Northern Tuscany. These are culinary adventures to meet the local wine and food producers and get a taste of their lives, far from Chiantishire stereotypes.

Tuscany Pass (www.tuscanypass.

com) is a reliable website that offers an events calendar and some of the best day trips in Tuscany. Choose from day-long Tuscan cookery courses to Vespa trips to the wine-growing Chianti; arty Florentine walking tours; designer shopping excursions; or even quad-biking to Lucca.

Link (tel: 055-218 191, and 338-390 3070; www.linkfirenze.it): Tuscan tours *(as above)*

Wine & Cookery Courses

Italy abounds in foodie courses but these are two of the best, which remain small, authentic, professional and memorable:

Camilla in Cucina (tel: 055-461 381; 348-279 3443, email: smaccari@iol.it). Tour the Florentine food markets with chef-guide Silvia Maccari before cooking up a storm in her Florentine home. The experience includes tasting cheese, balsamic vinegar and olive oil, as well as learning about the cultural and historical traditions that are so tightly intertwined with Italian food.

Cucina Giuseppina (tel: 0571-650 242; www.cucinagiuseppina.com) is a warm yet authentic cookery school in medieval Certaldo, not far from San Gimignano. The chef, helped by her wine-specialist son, guides you through regional recipes. The school also offers wine appreciation and truffle-hunting experiences.

Listings

The Florentine is the city's free bi-weekly English-language newspaper. Issues can be found around town or downloaded from its website (www.theflorentine.net). Articles cover current events in Florence and event listings. The monthly publication, *Firenze Spettacolo*, also has complete listings of city events; although in Italian, the listings are usually straightforward. Also check the entertainment pages of *La Nazione*, the regional newspaper, or the Tuesday edition of the national, *La*

Repubblica. Also see the city website: www.comune.fi.it.

Music, Ballet and Opera

Florence

The **Maggio Musicale** music festival (www.maggiofiorentino.com), held from mid-May to the end of June, is a big event with top names in music, ballet and opera performing in various venues throughout the city. Major performances will then be staged in **the Nuovo Teatro del Maggio**, Florence's new opera house and auditorium. This opens in early 2012, close to the existing **Teatro Comunale**, where tickets are still available (Corso Italia 16; tel: 055-211 158). In summer, concerts are also given in cloisters, piazzas and the Boboli Gardens. Louder (and free) rock concerts are held in **Le Cascine park**.

During the **Estate Fiesolana** – Fiesole's summer festival – concerts, opera, ballet and plays are presented in the **Roman amphitheatre**, and in many city churches.

The **Estate Fiorentina** summer music festival, held in July and August, takes over the newly restored **Ampitheatre** at Le Cascine park; the new contemporary space at **Le Murate**; as well as city squares, courtyards of major palaces and churches. Rock concerts are relegated to Le Cascine park, while Le Murate becomes an open-air cinema.

Chamber music is often performed in **Teatro della Pergola**, Via della Pergola (tel: 055-226 4335; www.pergola.firenze.it), a superb example of a 17th-century theatre (inaugurated in 1656). Concerts are generally given at weekends, and are well publicised.

The **Fiesole Music School** in San Domenico also gives a concert series (tel: 055-597 8527; www.scuolamusica.fiesole.fi.it) and the Orchestra Regionale Toscana's lively concert series runs December–May.

Florence's **Teatro Verdi**, Via Ghibellina 99 (tel: 055-212 320; www.teatroverdifirenze.it) is the venue for light opera, ballet, jazz and rock concerts.

Teatro del Maggio: a new era for the opera company in its new location (see left).

The **Orchestra da Camera Fiorentina** gives bi-monthly classical concerts in the Bargello and the church of Orsanmichele. Their schedule is available at www.orcafi.it.

The **Florence Dance Festival**, held in late June/early July, features well-known national and international names along with up-and-coming dancers and choreographers (tel: 055-289 276; www.florencedance.org for information).

Lucca

Lucca's summer festival in July attracts big-name international artists to a range of venues.

"Puccini e la sua Lucca" is a permanent festival dedicated to Giacomo Puccini, with concerts in the Basilica di San Giovanni. Tickets available at the church on performance days from 6pm; www.puccinielasualucca.com. (See Puccini panel, page 137.)

Pisa

Pisa's opera season runs at the Teatro Verdi from October to February. Tel: 050-941 111 or visit www.teatrodipisa.pi.it.

Pistoia

Held every July, the Pistoia Blues Festival hosts big-name blues, jazz and rock artists for three days of concerts.

Siena

Public performances of rare, unpublished and new music are held in August each year during the Sienese Music Week.

Arezzo

Every July, the Arezzo Wave Love Festival brings a variety of Italian and world-famous musicians to Tuscany to perform free

concerts in a five-day music fest.

Theatre

In addition to the main theatres, Teatro della Pergola (see left) and Teatro Verdi (Via Ghibellina 99; tel: 055-212 320; www.teatroverdi firenze.it), there are numerous smaller companies performing regularly in Florence, but most productions are in Italian.

Ticket Sales

Useful ticket agencies in Florence are Agenzia Box Office, Via Alamanni 39; tel: 055-210 804 (Mon 3.30–7.30pm, Tue–Sat 10am–7.30pm); Rinascente, 4th Floor, Piazza della Repubblica; tel: 055-292 508 (Tue–Sat 1.30–7.30pm).

Cinema

Almost all films are dubbed into Italian, but there are a few cinemas that occasionally show original versions, screenings by organisations such as the British Institute, and the odd film festival or special season that will use subtitles rather than dubbing. The main cinema for foreigners is the **Odeon** (Piazza Strozzi; tel: 055-

BELOW: the entrance to the Odeon.

214 068), which shows recent films in English and is packed with foreign students and expatriates. During the summer, a number of films are shown in the open air, including at Le Murate.

NIGHTLIFE

Tuscany's cities offer a wide variety of music and entertainment, especially in the summer when there are any number of festivals around the region. In Florence, bars and clubs are set up in the warm weather in several piazzas, often with live music. There are a number of late-night bars and clubs dotted around town, but most of the bigger clubs are on the outskirts. Nightclubs come and go, so it's best to ask around for recommendations. The following places are all in Florence. Elsewhere, your hotel or local tourist office may advise about clubs, bars and events. Note that most clubs close on Monday; and very few get going before 10pm on other nights.

Bars and Live Music

Astor
Piazza del Duomo 20r; tel: 055-

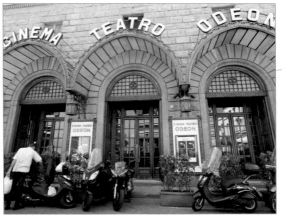

284 305. Cocktail bar with dance floor, frequented by Americans.

Be Bop
Via dei Servi 76r; tel: 055-218 799. Cocktail bar with live music: country, blues and jazz.

Il Caffè
Piazza Pitti 9; tel: 055-239 6241. Chic and refined: a cosy spot to chat to friends, day or evening.

Caffè Cibreo
Via del Verrocchio 8r; tel: 055-234 1100. Atmospheric annexe to the famous restaurant, ideal for anything from a morning coffee to a late-night *digestivo*. Closed Sun and Mon.

Cantinetta dei Verrazzano
Via dei Tavolini 18r; tel: 055-268 590, www.verrazzano.com. Old-fashioned wine bar serving rustic lunch snacks and wines from the owners' Chianti estate; closed 9pm.

Café Giacosa
Via della Spada 10; tel: 055-277 6328, www.cavalliclub.com. Historic café given a hip makeover by designer Roberto Cavalli, whose own estate wines are served there.

Dei Frescobaldi
Via de' Maggazini 2r; tel: 055-284 724, www.deifrescobaldi.it. Snack on Tuscan antipasti (salami, cheeses, salads) in this new wine bar founded by the famous Frescobaldi wine dynasty. Their adjoining restaurant is more elegant.

Dolce Vita
Piazza del Carmine 6r; tel: 055-284 595; www.dolcevitaflorence.com. Arty, full-on, fashion-conscious bar in the bohemian Oltrarno quarter that appeals to the Happy Hour and late-night crowd.

Fusion Bar
Vicolo dell'Oro 3; tel: 055-27263, www.lungarnocollection.com. Swanky bar in the Gallery Hotel Art, perfect for tea, cocktails, sushi and showing off.

Jazz Club
Via Nuova dei Caccini 3; tel: 055-247 9700. Relaxed basement bar with live music daily. Small charge to become a member.

Moyo
Via dei Benci 23r; tel: 055-247

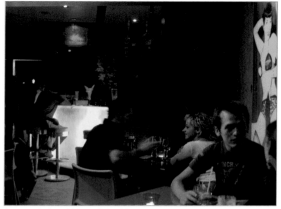

ABOVE: enjoying drinks at Dolce Vita.

9738. Smart cocktail bar in the Santa Croce area with outside seating and delicious cocktails.

Opera del Gusto
Via della Scala 17r; tel: 055-288 190, www.operadelgusto.com. Eclectic new dining club where you can listen to opera or jazz while dining.

Slowly
Via Porta Rossa 63r; tel: 055-264 5354. Trendy cocktail bar with a great aperitif buffet.

Teatro del Sale
Via de Macci 111r; tel: 055-200 1492, www.teatrodelsale.com. Hedonistic dining club run by celebrity chef Fabio Picchi. A Tuscan buffet before live blues, jazz or theatre; membership essential but cheap, as is the good-value buffet dinner.

I Visacci
Borgo Albizi 80r; tel: 055-200 1956. Pleasant arty café with friendly staff, relaxed music and a good selection of wines and cocktails.

Le Volpi e le Uva
Piazza de Rossi 1r; tel: 055-239 8132. Elegant but friendly wine bar for a light supper of superb wines, cheeses, cold cuts and bruschetta; closes 9pm.

Zoe
Via dei Renai 13; tel: 055-243 111. All day (and late-night) arty, contemporary café in trendy Oltrarno that takes you from

brunch to cocktails and beyond.

Nightclubs

Cavalli Club
Piazza del Carmine 7r; tel: 055-211 650, www.cavalliclub.com. Flashy club, restaurant and disco bar founded by Florentine fashion supremo, Roberto Cavalli.

Central Park
Via del Fosso Macinante 1, Parco delle Cascine; tel: 055-359 942. Dinner, disco, House music. Tue–Sat.

Dolce Zucchero
Via de Pandolfini 36/38r; tel: 055-247 7894. One of the few clubs in the city centre, it operates a drinks card whereby you pay on exit. Tue–Sun.

Doris
Via de' Pandolfini 36r; tel: 055-233 7783. Centrally located, multi-level club with music ranging from soft and romantic to high-energy. Wed–Sat.

Meccanò
Viale degli Olmi 10; tel: 055-331 371. One of Florence's oldest and most famous discos. Vast dance floor, bar and lounge areas. Thur–Sat.

Tenax
Via Pratese 46; tel: 055-308 160. Popular club and live-music venue. Fri–Sat.

YAB
Via Sassetti 5r; tel: 055-215 160; www.yab.it. Established disco-pub.

FESTIVALS

Arezzo

Last Sunday in June and first Sunday in September: Giostra del Saracino – Jousting match in which mounted knights attack a wooden effigy of a Turk.

Chianciano Terme

September: The Chianciano Biennale is a celebration of contemporary art, staged in uneven years (www.museodarte.org)

Cortona

July/August: The Tuscan Sun Festival features concerts, stars, wine and food events, and art exhibitions (www.tuscansunfestival.com).
15 August: Sagra della Bistecca – "Feast of the Beefsteak".
September (first half of the month): antiques fair.

Florence

Easter Day: Scoppio del Carro, the Explosion of the "Carriage" (actually fireworks on a float). Colourful musical processions.
Ascension Day: Festa del Grillo, Festival of the Crickets in the Cascine park. Sale of crickets and sweets.
End of April: Flower Show, Parterre, near Piazza Libertà – a riot of colour.
May and June: Maggio Musicale Fiorentino – performances of opera, ballet and classical music.
Saturday in late June: Notte Bianca in Oltrarno – all-night festivities, music and food in and around Piazza Santo Spirito.
July-August: Estate Fiorentina – Florence's summer festival *(see Listings above)*
June–September: Estate Fiesolana in Fiesole (just outside

Florence) – music, dance, opera, cinema and theatre.
24 June: San Giovanni – Florence's patron saint's day, with a holiday in the city and an evening firework display near Piazzale Michelangelo.
June–July: Calcio in costume (Calcio Fiorentino) – football in medieval costume in Piazza Santa Croce.
7 September: night festival of the Rificolona (lanterns) – procession of carts, lanterns and singers.
First three weeks of December: German Christmas Market – Piazza Santa Croce becomes a festive German market with decorations, mulled wine, sausage and beer, and other German specialities. For Florence events, see www.comune.fi.it.

Lucca

July: One of Tuscany's best festivals – with big-name international bands in Piazza Anfiteatro and a range of venues around town.
September – first weekend. Festival of Flowers.
September: Luminaria di Santa Croce – a religious procession.

Lucignano

Last two Sundays in May: Maggiolata Lucignanese festival that includes a procession of carts decorated with allegorical scenes in flowers.

Massa Marittima

Sunday following May 20 and the second Sunday in August: Balestro del Girifalco – crossbow competition.

Montalcino

Last Sunday in October: Sagra del Tordo – Thrush Festival. Pageant, costume ball, banquet and archery at the fortress.

Monticchiello

Last fortnight of July: Il Teatro

Povero – "The Poor Theatre" presents a performance written by locals about locals.

Pienza

First Sunday of September: Fiera del Cacio – a fair devoted to Pienza's famous cheese.

Pisa

May and June: concerts at various annual festivals and fairs, especially during the Gioco del Ponte on the last Sunday of June.
16–17 June: Luminaria di San Ranieri – thousands of candles light up buildings along the Arno. Boat race in the evening of the second day.
Last Sunday in June: Gioco del Ponte.
Mid-September to end October: The annual Anima Mundi International Festival of Sacred Music takes place in Pisa Cathedral. Tel: 050-387 2229/2210; www.opapisa.it.

Pistoia

25 July: Giostra dell'Orso – a mock battle between a wooden bear and 12 knights in costume on Piazza del Duomo.

San Gimignano

July–September: Summer Fair, Estate Sangimignanese – varied programme of events, including ballet, concerts and cinema.

Siena

28–30 April: Feast of St Catherine.
2 July and 16 August: Il Palio traditional horse race. For tickets and hotel bookings, plan six months in advance (www.ilpalio.org).
Mid-July–August: Incontri in Terra di Siena – chamber-music festival featuring top-quality concerts held in stunning settings south of Siena.
August: Sienese Music Week –

performances of opera, symphonies and chamber music.

13 December: Festa di Santa Lucia – ceramics festival.

Torre del Lago

July and August: Puccini Opera Festival, Torre del Lago, near the composer's villa on Lake Massaciuccoli (www.puccinifestival.it).

Viareggio

February: Carnevale – one of the best carnivals in Italy.

Volterra

First Sunday in September: Torneo di Tiro con la Balestra – crossbow tournament.

OUTDOOR ACTIVITIES

Sources of Information
For information about green tourism and outdoor activities, contact the nearest office of ENIT, the Italian national tourist board (see page 306). Also check the Tuscan Regional Tourism website, www.turismo.intoscana.it. As the individual Tuscan APT tourist offices are being dissolved and reorganised, this should be your first port of call.

In English, the most comprehensive guide to green tourism is *Wild Italy* (by Tim Jepson, Sheldrake Press, 2005).

Hiking

Hiking (usually called "trekking" in Italian) is a popular activity in Tuscany. The region is well served by tough, long-distance trails for serious hikers. But more casual (or less-experienced) hikers should be wary of embarking on any trail without fully researching it, especially given the idiosyncrasies of some Tuscan signposting and maps. At the easy end of the spectrum, the region abounds in short walks,

whether along the Versilia seafront or in regional parks, such as the Maremma. The middle spectrum of mixed-ability walkers, those wishing for a walking holiday of at least several days, softened by great scenery, food and wine, are better served by a dedicated walking-tour operator.

Specialist UK tour operators

Whether opting for a self-guided or accompanied walking holiday, booking through a specialist often ensures a better deal, along with tried-and-tested routes, not subject to the vagaries of regional maps or to "lost in translation" itineraries. These tours follow the operator's wonderfully detailed route, and generally include the transporting of your luggage to the following hotel, which can be luxurious, or a simple farm-stay.

Make the most of walks that combine hills, history and cosy inns by booking through a specialist offering a portfolio of Tuscan trails:
Collett's (tel: +44 01763-289 660; www.colletts.co.uk)
Gusto tours (www.gustocycling.com)
Inntravel (tel: +44 01653-617 001; www.inntravel.co.uk)
Headwater (tel: +44 01606-720 199; www.headwater.com)
Hedonistic Hiking (tel: +44 0845-680 1948; www.hedonistic hiking.com.au)

Long-distance hiking: Serious hikers can follow the Italian Alpine Club (CAI or Club Alpino Italiano: www.cai.it) paths, which crisscross the region. There is a branch of the CAI in Florence (tel: 055-612 0467; www.caifirenze.it).

Two long-distance paths, Apuane Trekking (a four-day trek) and the Grande Escursione Apenninica (GEA, taking 25 days, end to end, along the ridges of the Apennines), have well-marked trails and can be joined at various points. Shorter waymarked trails (such as those in the Maremma or Chianti regions) tend to be less well signposted, so take good

local maps (such as those produced by CAI).

All walkers should bear in mind that there is no public right of way across private property. Be particularly vigilant during the hunting season, especially on Sundays. If travelling without a car, forward planning is required. City-to-city transport is generally fine (often quicker by bus than train), but rural transport is poor: either of the "two buses a day" variety, or simply nonexistent.

Areas to Explore

The following are guidelines to some of the more accessible areas of natural beauty. Also see: www.parks.it (Italian Parks and Nature Reserves).
Abetone and the Tuscan-Emilian border
Abetone makes a good base for exploring this forested mountain region, also known as the Alto Appennino. The town has a profusion of Swiss chalet-style hotels. The picturesque medieval centres of Fiumalbo and Cutigliano make good alternative bases but have fewer facilities and lack Abetone's more dramatic Alpine views.
Transport: by public transport, it is quicker to reach Abetone by bus from Modena (in Emilia-Romagna) than by other routes.
Apuan Alps (Alpi Apuane)
Maps and information on mountain refuges are available from Massa, Carrara and most coastal tourist offices. Numerous one-day hikes are available through the Alps, with typical starting points being the villages of Stazzema and Levigliano on the western flanks of the mountains. Almost as appealing is a car journey along the winding mountain roads towards the interior.
Arezzo/Pratovecchio
The Parco delle Foreste Casentinesi (www.parks.it) straddles Tuscany and Emilia-Romagna. The park headquarters is at Pratovecchio, Via G. Brocchi 7; tel: 0575-50301. Alternatively, contact the Arezzo tourist office for more information.

Lunigiana and Garfagnana

Serious hikers should request the Trekking in Lunigiana map, with long-distance trails beginning in Aulla, Fosdinovo, Frignoli and Sassalbo. To appreciate the rural atmosphere, avoid staying in such fashionable coastal resorts as Forte dei Marmi. Instead, choose the Garfagnana hinterland, where Castelnuovo di Garfagnana is picturesque, and Barga, the main town, makes a gorgeous base. Both are convenient for **Parco dell'Orecchiella**, the national park, 15km (9 miles) north of Castelnuovo di Garfagnana. San Pellegrino in Alpe, 16km (9½ miles) northeast of Castelnuovo, is appealing in summer and winter. **Transport:** coastal transport is good, with transport into the Garfagnana hinterland less so. If you are planning to explore Garfagnana and Lunigiana by train or bicycle, a small branch line connects Lucca with Aulla and allows bicycles on the train.

The Maremma

If you want to be by the sea, stay in Santo Stefano, Talamone, Orbetello or Castiglione della Pescaia. Otherwise, opt for a ranch or farm near the park. **Transport:** visitors using public transport should go to Orbetello (by bus or train) or to Monte Argentario (by bus from Grosseto). To visit the nature reserve is trickier: by train to Alberese station (only a couple of trains a day, from Grosseto), then a taxi.

The Mugello

The best website is www.mugello toscana.it. Avoid staying in Borgo San Lorenzo, the main town, which is not very attractive, or in the semi-industrialised valleys. Instead, choose the countryside or such villages as Vicchio. **Transport:** for those who wish to explore the Mugello by train or bicycle, the Faenza–Florence train service stops at stations along the Apennine ridge (Vicchio, Marradi, Ronta), ideal places to begin trekking.

The Val d'Orcia, Montalcino,

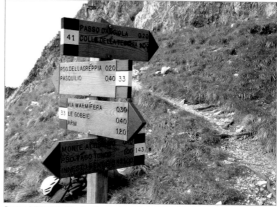

ABOVE: hiking trail in the Apuan Alps.

San Gimignano, Volterra

Expect a range of dreamy trails in the Val d'Orcia that combine rolling hills and fortified villages with a mystical atmosphere. Hiking trails linking San Gimignano and Volterra are superb, including several by Headwater (www.headwater.com).

The Via Francigena pilgrimage route passes through some of the loveliest areas, including the Chianti, Lucca, and the Sienese countryside around Montalcino – en route to Rome and Canterbury (www.viafrancigena.com).

Green Sites

These include nature reserves, caves, botanical gardens and museums of rural life. The classification of Italian conservation areas is chaotic and confusing. (See: www.parks.it, the website of Italian Parks and Nature Reserves).

Abetone

On the Tuscan-Emilian border, Abetone is the main ski and summer resort in the northern Apennines (*see page 145*). It is also the centre for information on GEA long-distance trails and shorter botanical rambles. For details, contact the Abetone tourist office.

The Apuan Alps and Lunigiana

The Frignoli Botanical Gardens, near Sassalbo (tel: 0187-422 598) have an arboretum and display the full range of plants grown in the Apuan Alps. In Aulla, in Lunigiana, there is an interesting natural-history museum and ecological centre set in historic Brunella castle (daily summer 9am–noon, 4–7pm, winter 9am–noon, 3–6pm; charge; tel: 0187-400 252), as well as neighbouring botanical gardens. From Aulla, visitors can organise tours of glacial moraines, karst gorges and caves.

Garfagnana

Here, **Parco dell'Orecchiella**, 15km (9 miles) north of Castelnuovo di Garfagnana, is the chief regional park in the Lucca stretch of the Apennines. The main entry point is Corfino. There are also botanical gardens nearby, at Villa Collemandina, Pania di Corfino (tel: 0584-644 911). The local visitors' centre (tel: 0583-619 002) includes a civilised mountain refuge and nature trails. Contact the Comunità Montana Garfagnana (tel: 0583-644 911) or the tourist office in Barga, the region's main town. The Orrido dei Bottri reserve is a narrow gorge with sheer cliff faces that can be crossed by serious hikers.

The Maremma

In the Maremma region, the Centro Visite Parco della Maremma (tel: 0564-407 098) is closed to traffic. Entry points are Marina di Alberese (the coast and lovely beach) or Alberese (the landward side, with the park ticket office, shuttle bus, guiding service and free tasting of local produce and wine). The Alberese entrance provides access to the park on foot or by means of the park shuttle bus. In addition to short trails, there are longer trails of 5 or 4km (3 or 2½ miles, lasting about three hours). The way-marked paths are not wholly reliable. It is advisable to take drinking water and a picnic. In Alberese, canoes can be hired to explore the canals, and horse riding is also available.

The Mugello

In the Mugello, the hamlet of Grezzano has Casa d'Erci, which is a farmhouse converted into a museum of rural life and peasant culture. Check opening times on tel: 055-92519.

Cycling

Cycling is increasingly popular in Tuscany, especially on the Chianti route, and in key cities such as Florence, Pisa and Lucca, where bike hire is easy.

Cycling in the city

Lucca: Hire a bike at one of the two tourist offices, one at the East Gate and the other at the West Gate. Also see the advice in the chapter on Lucca (see page 141).

Florence: there are cycle rental points at the main railway station, as well as on Piazza Santa Croce and Piazza Annigoni (Sant'Ambrogio market). Contact: **Alinari**, via San Zanobi 38R; tel: (+39) 055-280 500; www.alinari rental.com.

Gusto tours (www.gustocycling. com) rents bicycles, including racers, to villas, hotels, and individual holiday-makers anywhere in Tuscany.

Cycle routes

These are great for families as an alternative to a day on the beach.

Viareggio: from Parco di Migliarino and Torre del Lago, where Giacomo Puccini lived.

Viareggio to Marina di Massa: an easy 23km cycle along the seafront.

Viareggio seafront to Lido di Camaiore, Marina di Pietrasanta and Forte dei Marmi.

Pisa (a harder ride): from the seafront to the top of Monte Serra, crossing nature reserves and passing Etruscan sites and medieval castles (www.pisaturismo.it).

In the Maremma, see www. naturalmentetoscana.it and www. maremmabike.it.

Wildlife-watching

In theory, the Arcipelago Toscano (Tuscan Archipelago, including Elba and the other islands) is a marine park, but in reality much remains unprotected. Illegal hunting continues in the larger parks. The best-run sanctuaries tend to be the smallest, often those administered by the Worldwide Fund for Nature (WWF, www.wwf.it/ oasi) or by LIPU, the Italian bird protection society (for which there is a great need). For more information on parks, see *Wild Tuscany* chapter and *A Walk in the Park*, pages 70–1.

Dolphin-watching: dolphins live in the waters off Versilia. Between April and September visitors can join research groups that look for dolphins and whales. Contact the CETUS centre in Viareggio (www. cetusresearch.org) and Versilia tourist office (www.aptversilia.it)

Wildlife sanctuary: the **Oasi di Bolgheri** is the best bird and wildlife sanctuary, a mixture of scrub, lakes and marshy grasslands. This WWF reserve is home to native and migratory birds and small mammals such as wild boar. The reserve lies 10km (6 miles) south of Cecina and is reached by train to Bolgheri. Contact Marina di Cecina or Livorno provincial tourist offices

for details.

Bird-watching: Bottaccio Wood, outside Castelvecchio di Compito, in Lucca province, is a marshland nature reserve good for birds and best visited in spring (tel: 0583-65008).

The lakeside habitat at **Lago di Massaciuccoli** is home to migratory and wintering wildfowl as well as native species, including flamingoes, geese, ducks, cranes and tern. The region's lone surviving lagoon has suffered from intensive shooting but survives nonetheless. For details of opening times and tours, contact Pisa provincial tourist office.

Lago di Burano (tel: 0564 898 829) in the Maremma, south of Alberese, offers one of the best bird-watching opportunities in Tuscany. This is the southernmost of two lagoons beside the peninsula of Monte Argentario. This WWF lagoon is home to falcons, cormorants, the black-winged stilt, purple and grey herons, with peregrines, ospreys and marsh harriers using the lagoons as feeding grounds. (By road, the reserve is at the Capalbio Scalo exit on the SS1; by rail, travel to the small Capalbio station.) For details of opening times, contact the Parco della Maremma (as above).

Horse riding

There are over 40 centres belonging to the National Association of Equestrian Tourism (Fitetrecante; Piazza A. Mancini 4, 00196 Rome; tel: 06-326 50230; www. fitetrecante.it) or to the Federazione Italiana Sport Equestri (Viale Tiziano 74, Rome; tel: 06-323 3826; www.fise.it).

Here are some suggestions for riding near Tuscany's main cities:

Maneggio Belvedere, Località. Filetta 58010 Sorano (Grosseto province); tel: 0564-615 465; www.maneggiobelvedere.it.

Club Ippico Senese, Località Pian del Lago, Siena; tel: 0577-318 677; www.clubippicosenese.it.

In the Mugello, north of Florence: **Nonna Aida,** Via Nazionale, 88, Localita Le Maschere, Barberino di Mugello; mobile tel: (+39) 340-783 9670; www.nonnaaida.net

Equestrian Escapes (tel: +44 01829-781 123; www.equestrianescapes.com) offers tailor-made riding holidays on the Tuscan–Umbrian border.

For horse-riding centres elsewhere in Tuscany, call the **Centro Ippico Toscano,** Via Vespucci 5r, Florence; tel: 055-315 621.

Fishing

For freshwater fishing,foreigners need a temporary membership of FIPS (Federazione Italiana della Pesca Sportiva) and a government licence issued by the Provincial Administration. Sport fishing can be practised both from the shore and from a boat. In some ports, a special permit is required from the Harbourmaster's Office.

Golf

There are some decent courses, often with spas attached; the best include:

Golf Club Ugolino, Via Chiantigiana, Grassina; tel: 055-230 1009; www.golfugolino.it

Montecatini Golf and Country Club (18 holes), Via dei Brogi 32, Località Pievaccia, Monsummano Terme; tel: 0572-62218; www.montecatinigolf.com

Cosmopolitan Golf and Country Club, Viale Pisorno 60, Tirrenia-Pisa; tel: 050-33633; www.cosmopolitangolf.it

Golf Club Punta Ala; tel: 0564-922 121; www.puntaala.net/golf

Skiing

Tuscany has a major ski resort at Abetone in the Apennines, north of Pistoia, extending over four valleys with 30km (19 miles) of trails. For information on ski passes and pistes, call Abetone tourist office; tel: 0573-630 145.

Watersports and Diving

At all Tuscan sea resorts it is possible to water-ski and row with hired boats. Yacht-chartering facilities are also available in the resorts of Marina di Pisa and Tirrenia, and Porto Azzurro, **Elba** (www.aptelba.it).

Diving is very popular in Tuscany, the best areas being around the Argentario on the southern coast, and the islands Giglio, Giannutri, Elba and Capraia. There is red coral, a huge variety of Mediterranean underwater flora, and even a couple of wrecks off Giannutri. Many of the seaside ports have diving clubs that take boats out regularly.

Elba Diving Centre, Marciana Marina; tel: 0565-904 256; www.elbadiving.it

Giglio Diving Club, Via della Torre Campese; tel: 0564-804 065; www.geocities.com/gigliodiving.

Swimming Pools

Many Tuscan hotels, villas and agriturismo (farm-stay) places have pools, and there are public pools in most towns, although these often have limited opening hours.
Public swimming pools in Florence:

BELOW: cyclists on the Chianti route.

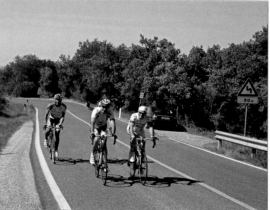

Piscina Le Pavoniere, Viale della Catena 2; tel: 055-362 233. During the summer. There is also a bar and pizzeria here.
Piscina Nannini, Lungarno Aldo Moro 6; tel: 055-677 521. Olympic-size pool that is open-air during the summer months.

Siena has its own Piscina Comunale, Piazza Amendola; tel: 0577-47496.

Spectator Sports

Football is the national sport. Almost every city and village has a team and the most important national championship is the "Serie A" (Premiership), the winner of which is eligible to play in the Champions League, against other top European teams. The season runs from September to May. Florence usually does well but has fierce battles with Juventus, its loathed rival. Matches here tend to be safe, family affairs. If you want to see a game, ask your hotel concierge to help.

Horse racing is also popular and there is a racecourse in Florence's Cascine park: Ippodromo le Cascine; tel: 055-226 076.

For tickets to any sporting event, consult the local tourist office or, alternatively, buy the pink *Gazzetta dello Sport* newspaper, which gives the lowdown.

SHOPPING

What to Buy

The quality is exceptionally high, especially in terms of craftsmanship, but prices are generally reasonable. Suggested buys are:
Fashion: dresses, suits, hats, gloves, linen, silk ties and shirts, scarves, knitwear, designer labels (*see outlet shopping, below*) and jewellery.
Leather goods: prices are not rock-bottom but the quality is often excellent and the designs appealing. Shoes and handbags are particularly good buys, but there are also boxes and belts, luggage, briefcases and wallets.
Fabrics: silk, linen, wool and cotton.
Handicrafts: lace and tablecloths; pottery, ceramics and porcelain; gold- and silverware; alabaster and marble objects; woodwork; straw and raffia goods; glass and crystal work; art books and reproductions; marbled paper; rustic household goods; prints; antiques; reproduction furniture.
Alcohol: regional wines – along with the well-known Chianti, Montalcino and Montepulciano, wines from the coastal Maremma such as Sassicaia and Ornellaia are celebrated Super Tuscans; also try Vin Santo, Tuscan dessert wine.
Food: extra-virgin olive oil, herbs, locally made pasta, farmhouse cheeses, bottled vegetables, truffles, dried mushrooms, cured ham, salami etc.

Shopping Hours

Food stores and general shops open 8.30am–1pm and 3.30 or 4–7.30pm. They stay open a little later in the summer. Many of the bigger supermarkets stay open through lunch and close at

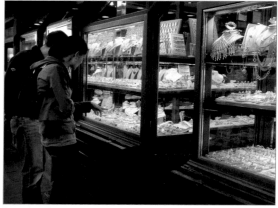
ABOVE: jewellery shop on Ponte Vecchio.

around 8pm. Department stores and other shops in bigger cities stay open all day (9.30am–7.30/8pm), and there is now limited Sunday trading in some places. Many clothes shops are closed on Monday mornings.

Where to Shop

Chain stores such as Oviesse and Standa can be found in most towns in Tuscany, and the upmarket Rinascente is in Florence.
Open-air markets are held once or twice a week in almost all tourist resorts and towns.
Supermarkets are found in most big centres but are otherwise more scarce.
Tobacconists (called *tabacchi*) sell bus tickets, stamps, cigarettes and tobacco.

Outlet Shopping

The Arno Valley is the cradle of many clothes factories for some of Italy's top designer labels. They tend to be located between Pontassieve and Incisa Val d'Arno, and have retail outlets with huge discounts. Avoid weekends. The best retail outlets, within easy reach of Florence and Arezzo, include:
The Mall, Via Europe 8, Leccio Regello; tel: 055-865 7775; www.

themall.it. Gucci, Cavalli, Giorgio Armani, Sergio Rossi, Yves Saint Laurent, Bottega Veneta, Loro Piana, Agnona, Tod's, Hogan, La Perla, Salvatore Ferragamo, Ungaro, Ermenegildo Zegna, Valentino, Alexander McQueen, Balenciaga, Burberry, Fendi, Stella McCartney, Yohji Yamamoto. Best for bags and shoes. Take the free shuttle from your hotel.
Fendi, Via Pian dell'Isola 66, Rignano sull'Arno; tel: 055-834 981. Best for accessories.
Barberino, Via Meucci snc, Barberino del Mugello; tel: 055-842 161, www.mcarthurglen.it/barberino. Outlet of over 100 stores including designer fashion: Bottega Verde, Bruno Magli, Coccinelle, D&G, Furla, Guess, Missoni, Prada, Puma.
Dolce e Gabbana, Via Santa Maddalena 49, Santa Maria Maddalena; tel: 055-833 1300. Everything from accessories and clothes to household designer goods.
Prada, Località Levanella, Montevarchi; tel: 055-978 9481. A limited selection, but great for bags, shoes and accessories – if you get there early, or queue.

For more information on outlet shopping, go to www.outlet-firenze. com. Dedicated fashionistas may consider investing in a copy of *Lo Scopri Occasioni* (published in English as *Designer Bargains in Italy*), which has over 1,000 outlet addresses. Visit www.scoprioccasioni.it.

Shopping in Florence

Despite tourism, consumerism and high labour costs, Florence still has a reputation as a city with high standards of craftsmanship, from silver jewellery to marbled paper. If you wish to visit craftsmen at work, check the craft list on www.turismo.intoscana.it or request the leaflet from the tourist office. It lists the main craftspeople, including the Santa Croce leather school, on Piazza Santa Croce, a popular place to watch skilled Florentine leatherworkers.

Most artisan workshops can be found in the Oltrarno neighbourhood, near the Pitti Palace and Piazza Santo Spirito.

Antiques

There are two main areas for antiques shops: Via Maggio and the surrounding streets in the Oltrarno and Borgo Ognissanti, west of the centre. There is a wide choice of goods, but you are unlikely to find a bargain.

Books

Edison, Piazza della Repubblica 27; tel: 055-213 110; www.libreria edison.it. Large bookshop with an extensive range of language books and guidebooks. Until midnight.
Feltrinelli Internazionale, Via Cavour 12/20r; tel: 055-292 2196. The best bookshop in Florence, with a range of foreign-language books and guides.
Seeber-Melbookstore, Via Cerretani 16; tel: 055-287 339; www.melbookstore.it. A range of books and music as well as a café.
The Paperback Exchange, Via delle Oche 4r; tel: 055-293 460; www.papex.it. Just south of the Duomo, this is no ordinary bookshop: it stocks just about every book ever written on Florence. It

also has a vast stock of quality second-hand English and American paperbacks.

Boutiques

Florence is full of top designer boutiques. The most elegant street is the newly pedestrianised Via de' Tornabuoni where Gucci, Valentino and other big names in fashion have their outlets. Other exclusive streets are the Via Calzaiuoli and Via Roma (for leather goods), Via della Vigna Nuova and Via del Parione.

The top designer shops are: **Giorgio Armani**, Via Tornabuoni 48r; tel: 055-219 041. For a more affordable Armani, visit Emporio Armani, Piazza Strozzi 14–16r; tel: 055-284 315.
Cavalli, Via de' Tornabuoni 83r; tel: 055-239 6226. The Florentine designer's store, with a stylish café, Giàcosa.
Dolce e Gabbana, Via della Vigna Nuova 27r; tel: 055-281 003. Sexy, stylish, often outrageous.
Enrico Coveri, Lungarno Guicciardini 19; tel: 055-287 676. Flamboyant, colourful.
Ferragamo, Via de' Tornabuoni 2; tel: 055-271 121. The famous Florentine shoemakers have now branched out into accessories and clothes. Upstairs, the Ferragamo Museum (Wed–Mon 10am–6pm) hosts various historical shoe exhibitions.
Gucci, Via de' Tornabuoni 73r; tel: 055-264 011. The range has expanded, but belts and handbags remain its trademark.
Prada, Via de' Tornabuoni 51–55r and 67r; tel: 055-283 439. Gorgeous accessories and shoes.
Emilio Pucci, Via de' Tornabuoni 20–22r; tel: 055-265 8082. Famous for its retro prints, beautiful scarves and dresses.
Raspini, Via Roma 25r; tel: 055-213 077. Upscale boutique carrying top brands.
Valentino, Via dei Tosinghi 52r; tel: 055-293 143.
Versace, Via de' Tornabuoni 13r; tel: 055-296 167. Haute couture by Donatella.

Also worth checking out are:
Ethic, Borgo Albizi 37; tel: 055-234 4413. One of few fashionable boutiques to offer clothing at reasonable prices.
Christian Dior, Via de' Tornabuoni 57r; tel: 055-266 911.
Hogan, Via de' Tornabuoni 97r; tel: 055-274 1013.
Trussardi, Via de' Tornabuoni 34/36; tel: 055-219 9023.

Ceramics

Sbigoli Terracotte, Via Sant' Egidio 4r; tel: 055-247 9713. Good choice of hand-painted ceramics in traditional and contemporary designs.

Fabrics

Antico Setificio, Via L. Bartolini 4; tel: 055-213 861; www.antico setificiofiorentino.com. Fabrics made traditionally, above all silk, still woven on 18th-century looms.
Casa dei Tessuti, Via de' Pecori 20–24; tel: 055-217 385. Fine silks, linens and woollens in a historic Florentine store.

Gloves

Madova, Via Guicciardini 1r; tel: 055-210 204. Every kind of gorgeous glove imaginable.

Jewellery

There is still a flourishing jewellery trade in Florence (particularly on the Ponte Vecchio and in Oltrarno, on the south side of the river), though most gold jewellery is now made in Arezzo. The following traditional goldsmiths and silversmiths remain:

Brandimarte, Viale Ariosto 11; tel: 055-230 411. Hand-crafted silver and jewellery.
Donato Zaccaro, Sdrucciolo de' Pitti 12r; tel: 055-212 243.
Gatto Bianco, Borgo SS Apostoli 12r; tel: 055-282 989. Contemporary designs in gold and silver.
Maurizio Casprini, Via Rosso Fiorentino 2a; tel: 055-710 008. Silversmith.
Exclusive Jewellery
If you can afford to push the boat out, these are some major names:
Buccellati, Via della Vigna Nuova

71/2; tel: 055-239 6579.
Bulgari, Via de' Tornabuoni 56r;
tel: 055-218 012.
Torrini, Piazza del Duomo 10r;
tel: 055-230 2401.

Leather

Quality ranges from hand-tooled
creations to shoddy goods aimed
at undiscerning tourists. For top-
of-the-range quality (and prices),
start with the designer boutiques in the Via de' Tornabuoni
or in streets around the Piazza
della Repubblica. Try the following outlets:

Il Bisonte, Via del Parione 31r;
tel: 055-216 232. Leather goods
at high prices.

Furla, Via della Vigna Nuova 47r;
tel: 055-282 779. Bags and
accessories in contemporary
designs.

Raspini, Via Roma 25–29; tel:
055-213 077. Superb leather
bags and coats.

For more down-to-earth prices,
head for the San Lorenzo market
northwest of the Duomo, where
numerous street stalls sell shoes,
bags, belts and wallets; you can
also try the Santa Croce area.

Marbled Paper

Marbled paper is very closely
associated with Florence and
many of the designs echo
ancient themes or Medici crests.
With their beautiful colours,
vibrant patterns and particular
smells, the shops are a joy to
visit.

Giulio Giannini e Figlio, Piazza
Pitti 37r; tel: 055-212 621. Florence's longest-established mar-
bled-paper shop.

Il Papiro, Via Cavour 55r; tel:
055-215 262; Piazza del Duomo
27r; tel: 055-281 628.

Il Torchio, Via de' Bardi 17; tel:
055-234 2862. Cheaper than
some other shops, you also see
the artisans at work.

Markets

Many neighbourhoods have a
weekly market. Try the following:
Straw Market (Mercato del Porcellino): hand-embroidered work,

Florentine straw, leather goods,
wooden objects and scarves; the
most touristic market.

Flea Market (Mercato delle Pulci,
Piazza dei Ciompi): basically junk,
but great fun.

Sant'Ambrogio (Piazza Ghiberti):
food, fruit and vegetables
(cheaper than San Lorenzo).

San Lorenzo Market (Mercato di
San Lorenzo, Piazza San Lorenzo):
the fascinating covered market
sells vegetables, fruit, meat and
cheeses etc, while the surrounding streets are filled with stalls
selling clothes, shoes, leather
goods and jewellery.

Cascine Market (Mercato delle
Cascine, Tuesday mornings only):
fresh produce, household goods
and clothing.

Artisan Market (Piazza Santo
Spirito, 2nd Sun of the month,
Sept–June): craft market with
some organic food.

Pharmacy

**Officina Profumo Farmaceu-
tica di Santa Maria Novella**, Via
della Scala 16; tel: 055-436
8316. Housed in a frescoed
chapel, this fascinating perfumery and herbalist was founded by
monks in 1612. It sells herbal
remedies and beautifully pack-
aged perfumes.

Shoes

Florence is still a good place to
buy shoes at reasonable prices.
Cresti, Via Roma 9r; tel: 055-214
150. Beautiful shoes at much
lower prices than at Ferragamo.
Ferragamo, Via de' Tornabuoni
16r; tel: 055-292 123. Italy's
most prestigious shoemaker,
providing hand-tooled shoes and
beautifully crafted ready-to-wear
collections.

The roads leading from the
Duomo to Santa Maria Novella
station have a good range of
slightly cheaper shoe shops.

Shopping in Siena

Clothes and Shoes

The main shopping streets in

Siena are Banchi di Sopra and
Via di Città. They are lined with
chain stores and individual
stores selling a range of clothes
and footwear.

Crafts

A wide choice of wrought-iron
and copper, ceramics, crystal
and stained glass. **Giogi Leonardo & Co**, at Antica Siena,
Piazza del Campo 28 (tel: 0577-
46496) sells beautiful blue and
yellow porcelain, while **Il Papiro**
(Via di Città) sells handmade
paper and gifts. **Acquarelli Orig-
inali** (Via Monna Agnese
14–16), a tiny store near the
Duomo, sells hand-painted
watercolours.

Food and Wine

Siena is known for its pastries
and cakes, particularly *panforte*,
which is made from a sweet
dough, flavoured with vanilla and
full of candied citrus fruits. The
most famous maker of such specialities is **Nannini**, at Piazza Matteotti 32 and Piazza del Monte
95/99, and **Bar Pasticceria
Nannini** at Via Banchi di Sopra 24
(www.grupponannini.it).

Siena Province produces
superb wines including Chianti,
Brunello di Montalcino and Vino
Nobile di Montepulciano. The
Fortezza Medicea (tel: 0577-
228 811; www.enoteca-italiana.it)
displays and sells regional wines
in the fortress (Mon–Sat until
1am). **Gino Cacino**, Piazza Mercato 31 (tel: 0577-223 076)
sells superb cheeses, salami
and hams.

Shopping in Volterra

Crafts

Ali, Piazza Martiri della Liberta;
tel: 0588-86078; www.alialabastro.
it. This is one of the oldest and
best alabaster workshops in
town. Admire the wide range of
picture frames, chess pieces,
mosaics, vases, table lamps and
sculptures – all made by local
craftsmen.

OTHER ACTIVITIES

Children

Tuscany has much to offer children of all ages, from medieval castles to ice creams galore and plenty of child-friendly restaurants. There are several good parks, nature reserves and numerous opportunities for horse riding, cycling and swimming. Much of the coast of Tuscany, particularly the well-equipped resorts near Viareggio and the beaches on islands such as Elba, is also great for children.

Tuscan festivals can be fun, especially the Lenten carnivals, the horse races, the jousting, boat pageants, and all the tiny food festivals that take place throughout the region. To find out what's on, check the listings in *La Repubblica* or *La Nazione*, as well as enquiring at the tourist offices. If you read Italian, buy *Firenze Spettacolo*, which has a good children's section: *Città & Ragazzi*.

Some of the suitable places in Tuscany for children are:
The Boboli Gardens (Giardini di Boboli) in Florence are fun for children to clamber around. There is an amphitheatre, strange statues and grottoes, and a handy café.

The **Museo dei Ragazzi in Palazzo Vecchio** offers special children-friendly tours of the Palace led by actors in costume, as well as activities and workshops.

The Cascine, Florence's other main park with a tiny zoo.

Giardino dei Tarrocchi (tel: 0564-895 700, near Capalbio) is a bizarre garden full of Niki de Saint-Phalle's colourful fantasy figures.

Ludoteca Centrale, Via Fibbiai 2, Florence; tel: 055-247 8386, is a fun children's centre with games, music and audiovisual equipment for the under-sixes.

Pinocchio Park (Parco di Pinocchio) at Collodi, near Pisa, is an obvious, if old-fashioned choice for children (tel: 0572-429 364; www.pinocchio.it; 8.30am–sunset).

Pistoia Zoo, Via Pieve a Celle, Pistoia; tel: 0573-911 219; www.zoodipistoia.it. Compact zoo, but one of the region's best.

Zoo Fauna Europa, just south of Poppi; tel: 0575-529 079. A conservation centre for such breeds as the lynx and the Apennine wolf. 8am–sunset.

Spas

Tuscany has a large number of authentic thermal spas, offering a range of health and beauty treatments from mud baths to hydromassage, or just the opportunity to relax in hot springs. Check www.turismo.intoscana.it (look at the Terme e Golf section). The Consorzio Terme di Toscana, presso Terme di Montecatini (Via Manzoni 5; tel: 0572-910 357; www.termeditoscana.com) also provides information.

Here is a list of Tuscany's top thermal spas:
Bagni di Pisa, San Giuliano Terme; tel: 050-88501; www.bagnidipisa.com. Atmospheric spa resort, with distant views of the Leaning Tower – a romantic retreat.

Grotta Giusti Spa Resort, Monsummano Terme; tel: 0572-90771; www.grottagiustispa.com. Historic spa resort around an elegant villa that is proud of its restorative spa caverns and innovative treatments; golf course nearby.

Fonteverde Natural Spa Resort, San Casciano dei Bagni; tel: 0578 57241; www.fonteverdespa.com. A lovely rural setting. The spa is equally strong on Mediterranean and oriental treatments. One of the best spas in the country.

Petriolo Spa & Resort, Pari-Civitella Paganico; tel: 0564-9091; www.atahotels.it/petriolo. Timeless resort near Siena, offering everything from an Ayurvedic massage to sweating in a dry-ice cave.

Terme di Saturnia Spa & Golf Resort, Saturnia; tel: 0564-600 111; www.termedisaturnia.it. Fed by historic springs, this exclusive pampering resort boasts a peaceful setting in the Maremma. The sulphurous spa boasts hot springs, waterfalls and a recreation of Ancient Roman baths. Elegant suites and an 18-hole golf course.

Terme Sensoriali, Parco Acqua Santa, Chianciano Terme; tel: 0578-68480; www.termesensoriali.it. Innovative spa with an eclectic approach, from classic treatments based on the healing powers of the thermal springs to therapies inspired by Ayurveda.

BELOW: thermal pools at Bagni San Filippo.

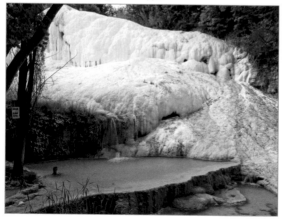

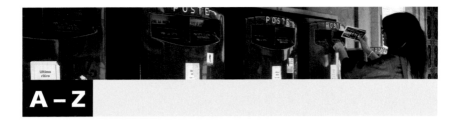

A – Z

An Alphabetical Summary of Practical Information

C limate

The Tuscan climate is pleasantly mild in the spring and autumn, cool and wet in the winter, and very hot near the sea and on low-lying land in the summer, with a pleasant warmth in the hills. There is very little wind except for on the Tyrrhenian coastline around Marina di Pisa and Tirrenia, but surprise storms can be very heavy at any time of the year, and flooding in a number of places has caused severe damage in the past. The rainfall in Tuscany is generally higher than in most other parts of Italy. The temperature is slightly lower than in other areas, making it more agreeable in summer but somewhat colder in winter.

The weather in Florence can be extreme. The city is situated in a bowl, surrounded by hills, with the Arno cutting through it, and this accounts for the high degree of humidity that is often a feature of midsummer. The worst of the humidity is likely to occur between mid-July and mid-August, with temperatures climbing well into the 30s Celsius (90s Fahrenheit).

Crime and Safety

Although violent crime is rare, in recent years, much crime in the north has tended to be gang- or drug-related. With increasing numbers of immigrants in Italy, the harassment of so-called "foreigners" (essentially immigrants from former Yugoslavia, Eastern Europe, Albania or Africa) is unfortunately on the increase in a country traditionally unused to dealing with immigrants.

The main problem for tourists is petty crime, from pick-pocketing and bag-snatching to the theft of objects left unattended in cars; it is wise to have insurance coverage against this and to take basic, sensible precautions against theft. If driving, lock your car and never leave luggage, cameras or other valuables inside. This applies particularly in major cities.

If you are the victim of a crime (or suffer a loss) and wish to claim against your insurance, it is essential to make a report at the nearest police station as soon as possible and get documentation to support your claim. When you need a policeman, dial **113** (or **112** for the *Carabinieri*, the national police force). Or, in Florence, call the Tourist Aid Police, 055-203 911.

CLIMATE CHART

Tuscany

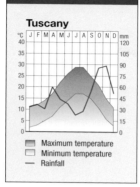

☐ Maximum temperature
☐ Minimum temperature
— Rainfall

Customs Regulations

Examination of luggage, passports, currency and hand baggage may take place on both entering and leaving Italy at airports, ports and borders. Formalities may also be carried out on trains. Registered luggage may be sent to towns with Customs Offices: examination takes place at the destination.

It is no longer possible to buy duty-free or tax-free goods on journeys within the EU; VAT and duty are included in the purchase price. Shops at ports and airports will sell goods duty- and tax-paid to those travelling within the EU; in practice, many shops have chosen not to pass on price increases since the sale of duty-free goods within the EU was abolished.

There are no longer any limits on how much you can buy on journeys within the EU, provided it's for your own personal use. But there are suggested limits, and if you exceed them Customs may seize your goods if you can't prove they are for your own use. The guidance levels are:

• 3,200 cigarettes or 400 cigarillos or 200 cigars or 1 kg of smoking tobacco;
• 10 litres of spirits; 20 litres of fortified wine; 90 litres of wine; 110 litres of beer.

Duty-frees are still available to those travelling outside the EU.

Professional photographers must carry an ata Carnet (issued in the UK through the London Chamber of Commerce, 33 Queen Street, London EC4R 1AP; tel: 020-7248 4444) for temporary importation of equipment.

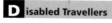 isabled Travellers

Despite difficult cobbled streets and poor wheelchair access to many tourist attractions and hotels, many people with disabilities visit Florence and Tuscany every year.

However, unaccompanied visitors will usually experience some difficulty, so it is best to travel with a companion.

Conditions and disability awareness are improving slowly in Tuscany (as well as in Italy in general), although the situation is certainly not ideal, and access is not always easy. More museums now have lifts, ramps and adapted toilets; newer trains and buses are accessible (although wheelchair users may need help when boarding); and recent laws require restaurants, bars and hotels to provide the relevant facilities. These laws, however, do not always cover access to those facilities. In 2004, Siena became the first Italian city to have an itinerary for the deaf. The brochure, *Siena in Lingua dei Segni*, is available from the tourist information centre, as is information about the facilities offered at sights and museums.

The Accessible Guide to Florence, by Cornelia Danielson, provides very detailed information on museums, restaurants, hotels and more for disabled travellers to Florence.

For drivers with disabilities, there are plenty of reserved park-

BELOW: policewoman in Florence helping a tourist.

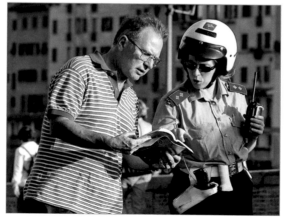

EMERGENCY NUMBERS

Fire Brigade: 115.
Medical Aid/Ambulance: 118.
Police Immediate Action: 112.
General Emergency: Fire, Police or Ambulance (replies are in foreign languages in the main cities): 113.
Automobile Club d'Italia (ACI):
• 24-hour breakdown: 803-116.
• 24-hour information line: 1518.

ing places in towns, and these are free.

In the UK, you can obtain further information from Radar, 12 City Forum, 250 City Road, London EC1V 8AF; tel: 020-7250 3222; www.radar.org.uk. In the US, contact Sath, 5th Avenue, Suite 610, NY 10016; tel: 212-447 7284; www.sath.org.

E lectricity

Italy uses 220v and two-pin plugs. Adaptors for British three-pin appliances can be purchased from airports or department stores in the city. You will need a transformer to use 100–120 volt appliances.

Embassies

Australian Embassy: Via Antonio Bosio 5, 00161 Roma; tel: 06-852 721.
UK Embassy: Via XX Settembre 80a, 00187 Roma; tel: 06-4220 0001.
UK Consulate: Lungarno Corsini 2, 50123 Firenze; tel: 055-284 133.
US Embassy: Via Vittorio Veneto 119a, 00187 Roma; tel: 06-46741.
US Consulate: Lungarno A. Vespucci 38, 50123 Firenze; tel: 055-266 951.

Emergencies

Useful Florence Contacts

Ambulances (Misericordia) – tel: 118
Specialist Mobile Units for medical assistance – Via del Sansovino 176; tel: 055-717 745; and Viale del Mille 32; tel: or 055-500 500, including for the most urgent cases.
Tourist Medical Service (Guardia Medica Turistica), with English-, German- or French-speaking doctors: Piazza del Duomo; tel 055-212 221, no need to book if 8am–8pm (normal cases) or call any time for emergencies.

Lost Property, Via Circondaria 19; tel: 055-328 3942/43; but first report to the Police (Questura, tel 055-49771).
Automobile Club d'Italia (aci) tel: 055-24861.
Car breakdown, call ACI Road Serve, tel: 116.
Car pound – if your car is towed away – tel: 055-422 4142.
Police Headquarters (Questura) – the place to visit in the event of thefts, stolen cars, lost passports, etc., Via Zara 2; tel: 055-49771 and 055-497 7602.
Tourist Police (Polizia Assistenza Turistica) are at Via Pietrapiana 50r (Piazza dei Ciompi); tel: 055-203 911, and have interpreters on hand to assist.
Associazione Volontari Ospedalieri, Florence; tel: 055-234 4567. This group of volunteers will translate (free) for foreign patients.

Useful Siena Contacts

Siena Hospital Nuovo Policlinico di Siena, Località le Scotte, Viale Bracci; tel: 0577-585 111.
Police Station (Questura), Via del Castoro 6; tel: 0577-201 111 – 24 hours a day.
Pronto Soccorso (Misericordia), Via del Porrione 49; tel: 0577-21011, or dial 118 in an emergency.
Lost Property Via Casato di Sotto 23; tel: 0577-292 230.
Associazione Volontari Ospedalieri; tel: 0577-247 869.
See the Siena Town Hall website for all key numbers: www.comune.siena.it

Etiquette

Tuscans are generally friendly and will appreciate efforts to speak the language. Any attempt to rush or pressurise them, however, will be regarded as the height of bad taste, and whatever you want will take longer. Almost everything is done on the basis of personal favours or contacts, so any personal recommendations you can

muster will always come in useful.

H ealth and Medical Care

UK visitors are entitled to medical treatment in Italy provided they have a European Health Insurance Card (tel: 0845-606 2030; visit www.nhs.co.uk; or obtain an application form from the post office). There are similar arrangements for citizens of other European Union countries. As few Italians have faith in their own state health service, it may be advisable to take out insurance for private treatment in case of accident.

Visitors from outside the EU are strongly advised to take out adequate holiday and medical insurance to provide full cover during their stay abroad.

In high summer, the weather can be very hot; sunscreen, shady hats and mosquito repellent are recommended.

Medical Services

Pharmacies: The staff in chemists *(farmacie)* are usually very knowledgeable about common illnesses and sell far more medicines without prescription than in some other countries (even so, most drugs still require a prescription). Pharmacies are identified by a cross, often red or green and usually in neon.

Normal pharmacy opening hours are Mon–Fri 9am–1pm and 4pm–7pm. Every *farmacia* posts a list of the local chemists who are on emergency duty in their window. The following are chemists that are open 24 hours in Florence:
Farmacia Comunale 13, in Florence station; tel: 055-216 761.
Farmacia Molteni, Via Calzaiuoli 7r; tel: 055-215 472.
Farmacia all'Insegna del Moro, Piazza San Giovanni 20r; tel: 055-211 343.
In addition, you can call 800-420 707 to find out which chemists are on the night rota.
First Aid Service *(Pronto Soc-*

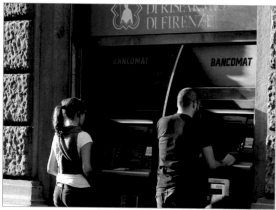

Above: Bancomat in Florence.

corso) with a doctor is found at airports, railway stations and in all hospitals. See box on page 303 for numbers to call in an emergency.

Internet

Most large hotels offer internet, email and fax facilities. There are numerous internet cafés around Florence, and most other cities, including the chain Internet Train, which allows you to connect using its computers or your own laptop. Most main post offices, travel agencies and hotels have fax facilities.

Maps

Touring Club Italiano does a good fold-out map of the Tuscany region showing major and minor roads. The Siena and Florence tourist offices supply reasonable city maps. *Insight Guide Fleximaps* are also available for Florence and Tuscany.

Media

Each large Italian town has its own newspaper. The centre-right *Il Corriere della Sera*, and the centre-left *La Repubblica* also have a national following. *La Nazione* is the paper favoured by most Tuscans for regional matters.

Television is deregulated in Italy. In addition to the state network, rai (which offers three channels), there are about 1,000 channels, of which the main ones are Canale 5, Rete 4, Italia 1 and Telemontecarlo.

There are several useful publications for visitors to Tuscany, including *The Florentine*, a bi-weekly English-language paper focusing on current events and city life, *and Firenze Spettacolo*, a monthly listings magazine in Italian (with some listings also in English), focusing on nightlife, clubs, bars and the live arts in Florence.

Money

In common with the other euro-zone countries of the EU, Italy's monetary unit is the euro (€), which is divided into 100 cents. The currency is available in 500, 200, 100, 50, 20, 10 and 5 euro notes, and 2-euro, 1-euro, 50-cent, 20-cent, 10-cent, 5-cent, 2-cent and 1-cent coins.

Italy is a society that prefers cash to credit cards, except for large purchases, or, for instance, hotel bills. In the case of petrol stations, more modest restaurants and smaller shops, it is usual to pay in cash. Check beforehand if there is any doubt. Most shopkeepers and restaurateurs will not change money, so it is best to change a limited amount at the airport when you arrive, especially if it is the weekend, when banks are closed. Try to avoid changing money in hotels, where the commission tends to be higher than in banks.

Traveller's Cheques

Although traveller's cheques are being replaced by credit cards, euro, dollar or sterling traveller's cheques are easy to cash, subject to a commission, but remember that you will be required to present your passport. In some cases they can be used in exchange for goods and services in shops and hotels.

Cash Machines and Credit Cards

Given the long queues for money-changing in Italy, it is simplest to get cash from cashpoint machines. Most main cards work in Italian machines, with your normal PIN number, though you may sometimes have to look for particular "Bancomats" (cashpoint machines) that take your card.

In cities, many restaurants, hotels, shops and stores will take major credit cards, but in rural areas especially, you may be able to pay only in cash.

Banks

Banks offer the best exchange rates (small exchange booths often charge up to 3 percent commission) and are normally open Mon–Fri 8.30am–1.30pm. Some banks also open in the afternoon, 2.30pm–4.30pm. Outside these hours and at weekends you can use automatic exchange machines to change cash, which helps to avoid bank queues. There is a high concentration of banks in Florence, including foreign banks, to the west of Piazza della Repubblica, around Via de'Tornabuoni.

TRANSPORT

ACCOMMODATION

ACTIVITIES

A – Z

LANGUAGE

Florence
American Express, Via Dante Alighieri 22r.
Banca d'Italia, Via dell'Oriuolo 37/39.
Banca Toscana, Corso 6.
Credito Italiano, Via Vecchietti 11.
Cassa di Risparmio di Firenze, Via Bufalini 6.

Siena
Banca Nazionale del Lavoro, Via Vittorio Veneto 43.
Banca di Roma, Via dei Termini 37.
Cassa di Risparmio di Firenze, Piazza Tolomei 11.
Monte dei Paschi di Siena, Via Banchi di Sopra 84.

Exchange Offices
Florence
Change Underground, Piazza Stazione 14, Int. 37 (under the station).

Siena
Viaggi Seti (Piazza del Campo 56) – changes notes and traveller's cheques.
Forexchange (Via di Città 80-82)

PUBLIC HOLIDAYS

1 January – *Capodanno* (New Year's Day).
6 January – La Befana (Epiphany)
Easter – *Pasqua.*
Easter Monday – *Pasquetta.*
25 April – *Anniversario della Liberazione* (Liberation Day).
1 May – *Festa del Lavoro* (Labour Day).
24 June – *San Giovanni* (St John the Baptist) – in Florence only.
15 August – *Ferragosto* (Assumption of the Virgin Mary).
1 November – *Ognissanti* (All Saints' Day).
8 December – *Immacolata Concezione* (Immaculate Conception).
25 December – *Natale* (Christmas Day).
26 December – *Santo Stefano* (Boxing Day).

– changes notes and traveller's cheques and processes Western Union transfers.

O pening Hours

Shops in the main cities open Monday to Friday 8.30am–1pm and 3.30–7.30pm. The majority open on Saturday, and several are open on Sunday, too, especially in high season. Some shops in coastal resorts and tourist centres now stay open all day throughout the summer and have Saturday and Sunday opening. Stores in most cities will close for at least two weeks around the *Ferragosto* holiday on 15 August. This is especially true of smaller cities not on the coastline.

Food shops are closed on Wednesday afternoons in winter and Saturday afternoons in summer. Clothes shops are closed on Monday mornings.

Offices are usually open 8am–1pm and 2–4pm, although many have more extensive opening hours.

On Italian national holidays, all shops and offices are closed.

P ostal Services

Main post offices in major towns are open all day; otherwise the hours are 8am–1.30pm (12.30pm Saturday). Stamps are sold at post offices and tobacconists *(tabacchi)*.

There is also a courier service for sending important documents worldwide in 24/48 hours. This service is only available at major post offices. In Florence, these are at Via Pellicceria 3 (main post office) and Via Alamanni 20r (by the station).

T elephones

Public telephones are now virtually nonexistent as Italy has the highest ownership of mobile phones in Europe. Annoyingly, many people, including small companies, only use their mobile phone, thus making calls to

them more expensive. To keep costs down, it's worth getting an Italian SIM card while there, or keeping a second mobile for this purpose. For long-distance calls, the cheapest time to telephone is between 10pm and 8am Monday to Saturday, and all day Sunday.

For directory enquiries, dial 12. For international enquiries, call 176, and to make a reverse charges (collect) call, dial 170.

When dialling Italy from abroad, dial the country code (0039) and the area code **including** the initial zero. In Italy, when calling numbers either inside or outside your area, dialling must always be preceded by the area code including the zero. Key area codes are: Florence (055); Pisa (050) and Siena (0577).

Tipping

Most Italian restaurants levy a *coperto* of around €2 per person – a cover charge for linen, bread and service – and so tipping isn't as common as in other countries. However, in pricier places, a tip of around 10 percent is an appropriate indication of appreciation of good service. Only in the finest hotels, and for lengthy stays, is it customary to tip bellboys, maids and head waiters. You may wish to note that according to Italian law, you should keep the bill with you until you are at least 100 metres (300ft) from the restaurant.

Tourist Board

The Italian State Tourist Board, known as ENIT (Ente Nazionale per il Turismo), provides tourist information. ENIT's headquarters are in Via Marghera 2/6 Rome (tel: 06-49711; www.enit.it).
In the UK, ENIT, 1 Princes Street, London W1R 2AY; tel: 020-7408 1254; fax: 020-399 3517.
In the US, ENIT, Suite 1565, 630 Fifth Avenue, New York, NY 10111; tel: 212-245 4822; fax: 212-586 5618. There are also

CALLING HOME

To call abroad from Italy, dial 00, followed by:

Australia	61
Canada	1
Ireland	353
New Zealand	64
UK	44
USA	1

Then dial the number, omitting the initial "0" if there is one.

offices in Chicago, Los Angeles and Canada.

The (woefully inadequate) ENIT website for all offices worldwide is: www.enit.it.

ABOVE: tipping in Italy is not as common as in other countries.

Tourist Offices

The Tuscan tourism system is currently being restructured and the transitional period may last some time. Local tourist offices, known as APTs (Aziende di Promozione Turistica) were dissolved in early 2012, with responsibility for tourism passing to each individual province. While certain offices may be closed, and all offices renamed, it is to be hoped that most survive in some shape or form, including their useful websites.

The current office details are listed below. If you are unable to contact them, consult www.turismo.intoscana.it, Tuscany's official tourism website, which should list all the new contact details for each province as they emerge. This umbrella website also contains useful information about the region, offered in several languages.

In addition to the institutional tourist offices, there are also dynamic tourism consortia that act as tourist offices in many destinations. The best are also listed throughout the book, as here below.

Arezzo Province

Arezzo: Piazza Risorgimento 116, Arezzo; tel: 0575-23952; Piazza della Repubblica 28; tel:

0575-377 678.
Cortona: Via Nazionale 42; tel: 0575-630 352. www.apt.arezzo.it

Florence Province

Florence: Via Manzoni 16, 50121 Firenze; tel: 055-23320; Via Cavour 1r; tel: 055-290 832; Borgo Santa Croce 29r; tel: 055-234 0444; and Piazza della Stazione 4; tel: 055-212 245. www.firenzeturismo.it
Fiesole: Via Portigiani 3/5; tel: 055-598 720.

Grosseto Province (including the Maremma)

Grosseto: Viale Monterosa 206; tel: 0564-462 611. www.lamaremmafabene.it www.turismoinmaremma.it
Maremma park (Parco della Maremma):
Alberese: 0564-407 269; www.naturalmentetoscana.it

Livorno Province (and Etruscan Coast with Elba)

Livorno: Piazza Cavour 6, 57100; tel: 0586-204 611. There is also the Harbour Information Office, Porto Mediceo; tel: 0586-895 320. www.costadeglietruschi.it
Elba: Calata Italia 26, Portoferraio; tel: 0565-914 671. www.aptelba.it.

Lucca Province (Lucca, Garfagnana and Versilia Coast)

Lucca: Piazza Guidiccioni 2; tel: 0583-91991; Piazza Santa Maria 35; tel: 0583-919 931; Vecchia Porta San Donato, Piazzale Verdi; tel: 0583-442 944. www.luccatourist.it
Bagni di Lucca: Via E. Wipple; tel: 0583-804 557.
Viareggio: Viale Carducci 10; tel: 0584-962 233

Versilia (including the Viareggio and Forte dei Marmi coast)

Viale Carducci 10, Viareggio; tel: 0584-962 233
www.aptversilia.it and www.turismo.provincia.lucca.it

Massa-Carrara Province

Marina di Massa: Lungomare Vespucci 24; tel: 0585-240 046.
Marina di Carrara: Via Garibaldi 41d; tel: 0585-632 519. www.aptmassacarrara.it

Pisa Province

Pisa: Via Matteucci; tel: 050-929 777; Piazza Arcivescovado 8; tel: 050-560 464; www.pisaunicaterra.it
Volterra: Piazza dei Priori 20; tel: 0588-87257; www.volterratur.it.

Pistoia Province

Pistoia: Piazza del Duomo 1; tel: 0573-21622.

TRANSPORT
ACCOMMODATION
ACTIVITIES
A – Z
LANGUAGE

TIME ZONE

Italy works on GMT + 1 and switches to DST – daylight saving time, GMT + 2 – at the same time as the rest of Europe.

Montecatini Terme
tel: 0572-772 244; www.monte-catini.turismo.it
San Marcello Pistoiese: Via Marconi 70; tel: 0573-630 145. www.pistoia.turismo.toscana.it

Prato Province

Prato: Piazza Santa Maria delle Carceri 15; tel: 0574-24112. www.pratoturismo.it

Siena Province

Siena: Piazza del Campo 56, 53100; tel: 0577-280 551. www.terresiena.it

Chianciano Terme (and Val d'Orcia area)

Piazza Italia; tel: 0584-962 233. www.chiancianotermeinfo.it

V isas and Passports

Citizens of European Union countries require either a passport or a Visitor's Identification Card to enter Italy. A visa is not required. Holders of passports from most other countries do not require visas for stays of less than three months, except for nationals of Eastern European countries, who need to obtain visas from the Italian Embassy in their own country.

Police Registration

A person may stay in Italy for three months as a tourist, but police registration is required within three days of entering Italy. If staying at a hotel, the management will attend to the formality.

You are legally obliged to carry a form of identification (passport, driving licence, etc.) with you at all times. This rule is often flouted but bear in mind that it would be unwise to call the police or attempt to report a problem (eg theft) unless you are carrying appropriate identification.

W ebsites

Useful websites are given above and throughout the book. The following is just a selection of the many additional sites on Italy, Florence and Tuscany that are available on the web:
Tuscany Tourist Information: www.turismo.intoscana.it.
Database on all Italian museums: www.museionline.com
Florence: www.firenzemusei.it; www.polomuseale.firenze.it.
Best routes in Italy: www.auto-strade.it; www.rac.co.uk; www.theaa.com. Plan your journey from one Italian destination to another.
Information plus hotels and restaurants: www.firenzeturismo.it.
Agriturismi **(farm-stays) in Tuscany**: **www.turismo.intoscana.it**
Events: www.firenzespettacolo.it; www.theflorentine.net

Weights and Measures

The metric system is used for weights and measures.
Multiply by the following:

Centimetres to inches	0.4
Metres to feet	3.3
Metres to yards	1.1
Kilometres to miles	0.6
Kilograms to pounds	2.2

Italians refer to 100 grams (about a quarter of a pound) as *un etto;* 200 grams are therefore *due etti.*

Liquid measurements are in litres. One litre is 1.75 pints.

Temperatures are given in Celsius (Centigrade).

What to Bring

Towns such as Florence, Lucca and Siena are sophisticated, so take something smart for shopping or dining out, although ties are rarely required for men. It can rain unexpectedly wherever you are, so a raincoat is handy.

Decent dress is required when visiting religious buildings: men and women are expected to have their arms covered, and shorts are frowned upon. Women often carry a headscarf as a head covering.

Sunhats are also recommended as protection.

Shoes need to be sturdy but comfortable and suitable for walking – especially on cobbled streets and for climbing steps.

Binoculars are a good idea if you are going on a nature trail and for viewing architectural details and frescoes.

BELOW: respectful dress in San Biagio church, Montepulciano.

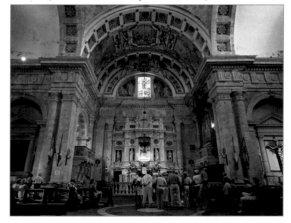

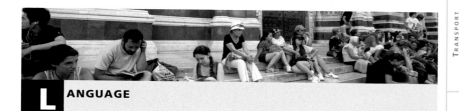

L ANGUAGE

UNDERSTANDING ITALIAN

Language Tips

In Tuscany, everyone speaks the Italian language but regional dialects and accents survive. The Tuscan accent features a strongly aspirated "h", much like in Spanish. In major centres, many people speak English, French or German. It is well worth buying a good phrase book or dictionary, but the following will help you to get started. Since this glossary is aimed at non-linguists, we have opted for the simplest options rather than the most elegant Italian.

Pronunciation and Grammar Tips

Italian speakers claim that pronunciation is straightforward: you pronounce it as it is written. This is approximately true but there are a couple of important rules for English speakers to bear in mind: c before e or i is pronounced "ch", eg *ciao, mi dispiace, coincidenza.* Ch before i or e is pronounced as "k", eg *la chiesa.* Likewise, sci or sce are pronounced as in "sheep" or "shed". Gn in Italian is rather like the sound in "onion", while gl is softened to resemble the sound in "bullion".

Nouns are either masculine (il, plural i) or feminine (la, plural le). Plurals of nouns are most often formed by changing an o to an i and an a to an e, eg *il panino, i panini; la chiesa, le chiese.* Words are stressed on the penultimate syllable unless an accent indicates otherwise, generally speaking.

Like many languages, Italian has formal and informal words for "You". In the singular, *Tu* is informal while *Lei* is more polite. For visitors, it is simplest and most respectful to use the formal form unless invited to do otherwise. There is, of course, rather more to the language than that, but you can get a surprisingly long way towards making friends with a few phrases.

Basic Communication

Yes *Sì*
No *No*
Thank you *Grazie*
You're welcome *Prego*
Alright/OK/That is fine *Va bene*
Please *Per favore* or *per cortesia*
Excuse me (to get attention) *Scusi* (singular), *Scusate* (plural)
Excuse me (to get through a crowd) *Permesso*
Excuse me (to attract attention, eg of a waiter) *Senta!*
Excuse me (sorry) *Mi scusi*
Could you help me? (formal) *Potrebbe aiutarmi?*
Certainly *Ma, certo*

Can I help you? (formal) *Posso aiutarLa?*
I need … *Ho bisogno di …*
I'm sorry *Mi dispiace*
I don't know *Non lo so*
I don't understand *Non capisco*
Could you speak more slowly, please? *Può parlare piu lentamente, per favore?*
Could you repeat that please? *Può ripetere, per piacere?*
What? *Quale/come?*
When/why/where? *Quando/perchè/dove?*
Where is the lavatory? *Dov'è il bagno?*

Greetings

Hello (Good day) *Buon giorno*
Good afternoon/evening *Buona sera*
Good night *Buona notte*
Goodbye *Arrivederci*
Hello/Hi/Goodbye (familiar) *Ciao*
Mr/Mrs/Miss *Signor/Signora/Signorina*
Pleased to meet you (formal) *Piacere di conoscerLa*
Do you speak English? *Parla inglese?*
I am English/American *Sono inglese/americano*
Canadian/Australian *canadese/australiano*
How are you (formal/informal)? *Come sta/come stai?*
Fine thanks *Bene, grazie*

Telephone Calls

the area code *il prefisso*
May I use your telephone, please? *Posso usare il telefono?*
Hello (on the telephone) *Pronto*
My name's *Mi chiamo/Sono*
Could I speak to...? *Posso parlare con...?*
Can you speak up please? *Può parlare più forte, per favore?*

In the Hotel

Do you have any vacant rooms? *Avete camere libere?*
I have a reservation *Ho fatto una prenotazione*
I'd like... *Vorrei...*
a room with twin beds *una camera a due letti*
a single/double room (with a double bed) *una camera singola/doppia (con letto matrimoniale)*
a room with a bath/shower *una camera con bagno/doccia*
for one night *per una notte*
for two nights *per due notti*
How much is it? *Quanto costa?*
Is breakfast included? *E compresa la prima colazione?*
half/full board *mezza pensione/ pensione completa*
Do you have a room with a balcony/view of the sea? *C'è una camera con balcone/con una vista del mare?*
Is it a quiet room? *E una stanza tranquilla?*
Can I see the room? *Posso vedere la camera?*
Can I have the bill, please? *Posso avere il conto, per favore?*
Can you call me a taxi, please? *Può chiamarmi un tassi/taxi, per favore?*

Eating Out

Bar snacks and drinks

I'd like... *Vorrei...*
coffee *un caffè* (espresso: small, strong and black)
un caffellatte (like café au lait in France)
un caffè lungo (weak, served in a tall glass)
un corretto (laced with alcohol, probably brandy or grappa)
tea *un tè*
herbal tea *una tisana*
hot chocolate *una cioccolata calda*
orange/lemon juice (bottled) *un succo d'arancia/di limone*
fizzy/still mineral water *acqua minerale gassata/naturale*
with/without ice *con/senza ghiaccio*
red/white wine *vino rosso/ bianco*
beer *una birra*
milk *latte*
a (half) litre *un (mezzo) litro*
ice cream *un gelato*
sandwich *un tramezzino*
roll *un panino*
Cheers *Salute*

In a Restaurant

I'd like to book a table *Vorrei riservare una tavola*
Have you got a table for...? *Avete una tavola per ...?*
I have a reservation *Ho fatto una prenotazione*
lunch/supper *il pranzo/la cena*
I'm a vegetarian *Sono vegetariano/a*
Is there a vegetarian dish? *C'è un piatto vegetariano?*
May we have the menu? *Ci dia la carta?*
wine list *la lista dei vini*
home-made *fatto in casa*
What would you like? *Che cosa prende?*
What would you recommend? *Che cosa ci raccomanda?*
home-made *fatto in casa*
What would you like as a main course/dessert? *Che cosa prende di secondo/di dolce?*
What would you like to drink? *Che cosa desidera da bere?*
a carafe of red/white wine *una caraffa di vino rosso/bianco*
the dish of the day *il piatto del giorno*
cover charge *il coperto/pane e coperto*
The bill, please *Il conto per favore*
Is service included? *Il servizio è incluso?*

Menu Decoder

Antipasti (hors d'oeuvres)

antipasto misto **mixed hors d'œuvres** (including cold cuts, possibly cheeses and roast vegetables)
buffet freddo **cold buffet**
caponata **mixed aubergine, olives and tomatoes**
insalata caprese **tomato and mozzarella salad**
insalata di mare **seafood salad**
insalata mista/verde **mixed/ green salad**
melanzane alla parmigiana **fried or baked aubergine** (with parmesan cheese and tomato)
mortadella/salame **salami**
peperonata **grilled peppers** (drenched in olive oil)

Primi (first courses)

Typical first courses include soup, or numerous varieties of pasta in a wide range of sauces.
il brodetto **fish soup**
i crespolini **savoury pancakes**
gli gnocchi **dumplings**
la minestra **soup**
il minestrone **thick vegetable soup**
pasta e fagioli **pasta and bean soup**

EMERGENCIES

Help! *Aiuto!*
Stop! *Fermate!*
I've had an accident *Ho avuto un incidente*
Watch out! *Attenzione!*
Call a doctor *Per favore, chiama un medico*
Call an ambulance *Chiama un'ambulanza*
Call the police *Chiama la Polizia/i Carabinieri*
Call the fire brigade *Chiama i pompieri*
Where is the telephone? *Dov'è il telefono?*
Where is the nearest hospital? *Dov'è l'ospedale più vicino?*
I would like to report a theft *Voglio denunciare un furto*

il prosciutto (cotto/crudo) **ham** (cooked/cured)
i tartufi **truffles**
la zuppa **soup**

Secondi (main courses)

Typical main courses are fish-, seafood- or meat-based, with accompaniments *(contorni)* like beans, spinach or roast vegetables.

La carne (meat)
allo spiedo **on the spit**
arrosto **roast meat**
al ferro **grilled without oil**
al forno **baked**
al girarrosto **spit-roasted**
alla griglia **grilled**
stufato **braised, stewed**
ben cotto **well-done** (steak, etc.)
al puntino **medium** (steak, etc.)
al sangue **rare** (steak, etc.)
l'agnello **lamb**
il bresaolo **dried salted beef**
la bistecca **steak**
il maiale **pork**
il manzo **beef**
l'ossobuco **shin of veal**
il pollo **chicken**
la salsiccia **sausage**
saltimbocca (alla romana) **veal escalopes with ham**
le scaloppine **escalopes**
lo stufato **stew**
il sugo **sauce**

Frutti di mare (seafood)
Beware the word *"surgelati"*, meaning frozen rather than fresh.
affumicato **smoked**
alle brace **charcoal grilled/barbecued**
alla griglia **grilled**
fritto **fried**
ripieno **stuffed**
al vapore **steamed**
le acciughe **anchovies**
l'aragosta **lobster**
il branzino **sea bass**
i calamari **squid**
i calamaretti **baby squid**
i crostacei **shellfish**
le cozze **mussels**
il fritto misto **mixed fried fish**
i gamberi **prawns**
i gamberetti **shrimps**
il granchio **crab**
il merluzzo **cod**
le ostriche **oysters**

il pesce **fish**
il pesce spada **swordfish**
il polipo **octopus**
il risotto di mare **seafood risotto**
le sarde **sardines**
la sogliola **sole**
le seppie **cuttlefish**
la triglia **red mullet**
la trota **trout**
il tonno **tuna**
le vongole **clams**

I legumi/la verdura (vegetables)
a scelta **of your choice**
i contorni **accompaniments**
ripieno **stuffed**
gli asparagi **asparagus**
la bietola **similar to spinach**
il carciofo **artichoke**
le carote **carrots**
i carciofini **artichoke hearts**
il cavolo **cabbage**
la cicoria **chicory**
la cipolla **onion**
i funghi **mushrooms**
i funghi porcini ceps **best mushrooms**
i fagioli **beans**
i fagiolini **green beans**
le fave **broad beans**
il finocchio **fennel**
l'insalata mista **mixed salad**
l'insalata verde **green salad**
la melanzana **aubergine**
le patate **potatoes**
le patatine fritte **French fries**
i peperoni **peppers**
i piselli **peas**
i pomodori **tomatoes**
le primizie **spring vegetables**
il radicchio **red lettuce**
la rughetta **rocket**
i ravanelli **radishes**
gli spinaci **spinach**
la verdura **green vegetables**
la zucca **pumpkin/squash**
gli zucchini **courgettes**

I dolci (desserts)

al carrello **(desserts) from the trolley**
un semifreddo **semi-frozen dessert (many types)**
la bavarese **mousse**
un gelato **ice cream**
una granita **water ice**
una macedonia di frutta **fruit salad**

il tartufo (nero) **(chocolate) ice cream dessert**
il tiramisù **cold, creamy rum and coffee dessert**
la torta **cake/tart**
lo zabaglione **dessert made with eggs and Marsala wine**
lo zuccotto **ice-cream liqueur**
la zuppa inglese **trifle**

La frutta (fruit)

le albicocche **apricots**
le arance **oranges**
le banane **bananas**
il cocomero **watermelon**
le ciliege **cherries**
i fichi **figs**
le fragole **strawberries**
i frutti di bosco **fruits of the forest**
i lamponi **raspberries**
la mela **apple**
il melone **melon**
la pesca **peach**
la pera **pear**
il pompelmo **grapefruit**
le uve **grapes**

Basic foods

l'aceto **vinegar**
l'aglio **garlic**
il burro **butter**
il formaggio **cheese**
la frittata **omelette**
la grana **Parmesan cheese**
i grissini **bread sticks**
l'olio **oil**
la marmellata **jam**
il pane **bread**
il pane integrale **wholemeal bread**
il parmigiano **Parmesan cheese**
il pepe **pepper**
il riso **rice**
il sale **salt**
le uova **eggs**
lo zucchero **sugar**

Si può visitare? *Can one visit?*
Suonare il campanello **ring the bell**
aperto/a **open**
chiuso/a **closed**
chiuso per la festa **closed for the festival**
chiuso per ferie **closed for the holidays**
chiuso per restauro **closed for restoration**

Is it possible to see the church?
E possibile visitare la chiesa?
Where can I find the custo-dian/sacristan/key? *Dove posso trovare il custode/il sacris-tano/la chiave?*

At the Shops

What time do you open/close?
A che ora apre/chiude?
Closed for the holidays (typical sign) *Chiuso per ferie*
Pull/push (sign on doors) *Tirare/spingere*
Entrance/exit *Entrata/uscita*
Can I help you? (formal) *Posso aiutarLa?*
What would you like? *Che cosa desidera?*
I'm just looking *Sto soltanto guardando*
How much does it cost?
Quant'è, per favore?
Do you take credit cards? *Accet-tate carte di credito?*
I'd like... *Vorrei...*
this one/that one *questo/quello*
I'd like that one, please *Vorrei quello lì, per cortesia*
Have you got ...? *Avete ...?*
We haven't got (any) *... Non (ne) abbiamo...*
Can I try it on? *Posso provare?*
the size (for clothes) *la taglia*
What size do you take? *Qual'è Sua taglia?*
the size (for shoes) *il numero*
expensive/cheap *caro/econom-ico*
It's too small/big *E troppo piccolo/grande*
I (don't) **like it** *(Non) mi piace*
I'll take it/I'll leave it *Lo prendo/Lo lascio*
This is faulty. Can I have a replacement/refund? *C'è un difetto. Me lo potrebbe cambiare/rimborsare?*
Anything else? *Altro?*
Give me some of those *Mi dia alcuni di quelli lì*
a (half) kilo *un (mezzo) chilo*
100 grams *un etto*
200 grams *due etti*
more/less *più/meno*
with/without *con/senza*
a little *un pocchino*
That's enough *Basta così*

Types of shops

bank *la banca*
bureau de change *il cambio*
chemist's *la farmacia*
food shop *l'alimentari*
leather shop *la pelletteria*
market *il mercato*
news-stand *l'edicola*
post office *l'ufficio postale*
supermarket *il supermercato*
tobacconist *il tabaccaio*
travel agency *l'agenzia di viaggi*

Travelling

Transport

airport *l'aeroporto*
arrivals/departures *arrivi/partenze*
boat *la barca*
bus *l'autobus/il Pullman*
bus station *l'autostazione*
car *la macchina*
ferry *il traghetto*
first/second class *prima/seconda classe*
flight *il volo*
left luggage office *il deposito bagagli*
motorway *l'autostrada*
no smoking *vietato fumare*
platform *il binario*
railway station *la stazione (ferroviaria)*
stop *la fermata*

At the station

Can you help me please? *Mi può aiutare, per favore?*
Where can I buy tickets? *Dove posso fare i biglietti?*
at the ticket office/at the counter *alla biglietteria/allo sportello*
What time does the train leave? *A che ora parte il treno?*
What time does the train arrive? *A che ora arriva il treno?*
Can I book a seat? *Posso preno-tare un posto?*
Is this seat free/taken? *E libero/occupato questo posto?*
I'm afraid this is my seat *E il mio posto, mi dispiace*
You'll have to pay a supplement *Deve pagare un supplemento*
Do I have to change? *Devo cambiare?*

Where does it stop? *Dove si ferma?*
You need to change in Firenze *Bisogna cambiare a Florence*
Which platform does the train leave from? *Da quale binario parte il treno?*
The train leaves from platform one *Il treno parte dal binario uno*
When is the next train/bus/ferry for Pisa? *Quando parte il prossimo treno/Pullman/traghetto per Pisa?*
How long does the crossing take? *Quanto dura la traversata?*
What time does the bus leave for Siena? *Quando parte l'autobus per Siena?*
Next stop please *La prossima fermata per favore*
Is this the right stop? *E la fermata giusta?*
The train is late *Il treno è in ritardo*
Can you tell me where to get off? *Mi può dire dove devo scendere?*

Directions

right/left *a destra/a sinistra*
first left/second right *la prima a sinistra/la seconda a destra*
Turn to the right/left *Gira a destra/sinistra*
Go straight on *Va sempre diritto*
Go straight on until the lights *Va sempre diritto fino al semaforo*
opposite/next to *di fronte/accanto a*
up/down *su/giù*
traffic lights *il semaforo*
Where is ...? *Dov'è ...?*
Where are ...? *Dove sono ...?*
How do I get there? *Come si può andare?* (or: *Come faccio per arri-vare a ...?*)

On the Road

petrol *la benzina*
petrol station/garage *la stazi-one servizio*
oil *l'olio*
Fill it up please *Faccia il pieno, per favore*
lead free/unleaded/diesel *senza piombo/benzina verde/diesel*
My car won't start *La mia macchina non s'accende*
My car has broken down *La macchina è guasta*

FURTHER READING

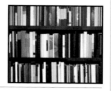

Art and History

The Architecture of the Italian Renaissance, by Peter Murray. Thames & Hudson.
Autobiography, by Benvenuto Cellini. Penguin Classics.
Catherine de' Medici: a Biography by Leonie Frieda. Phoenix
A Concise Encyclopedia of the Italian Renaissance, edited by J.R. Hale. Thames & Hudson.
Etruscan Places, by D.H. Lawrence. Olive Press.
The Florentine Renaissance and *The Flowering of the Renaissance*, by Vincent Cronin. Fontana.
The High Renaissance and *The Late Renaissance and Mannerism*, by Linda Murray. Thames & Hudson.
The Italian Painters of the Renaissance, by Bernard Berenson. Phaidon Press.
Lives of the Artists, vols. 1 & 2, by Giorgio Vasari. Penguin Classics.
Machiavelli, by Anglo Sydney. Paladin.
The Merchant of Prato, by Iris Origo. Penguin.
Painter's Florence, by Barbara Whelpton Johnson.
The Rise and Fall of the House of Medici, by Christopher Hibbert. Penguin.
Siena: A City and its History, by Judith Hook. Hamish Hamilton.
Silvio Berlusconi: Television, Power and Patrimony, by Paul Ginsborg. Verso Books.

Travel Companions

A Room with a View, by E.M. Forster. Penguin.
The Italians, by Luigi Barzini. Hamish Hamilton.

Italian Hours, by Henry James. Century Hutchinson.
Love and War in the Apennines, by Eric Newby. Picador.
The Love of Italy, by Jonathan Keates. Octopus.
Pictures from Italy, by Charles Dickens. Granville Publishing.
The Stones of Florence, by Mary McCarthy. Penguin.
The Villas of Tuscany, by Harold Acton. Thames & Hudson.
The Birth of Venus, by Sarah Dunant. Random House.

SEND US YOUR THOUGHTS

We do our best to ensure the information in our books is as accurate and up-to-date as possible. The books are updated on a regular basis using local contacts, who painstakingly add, amend and correct as required. However, some details (such as telephone numbers and opening times) are liable to change, and we are ultimately reliant on our readers to put us in the picture.

We welcome your feedback, especially your experience of using the book "on the road". Maybe we recommended a hotel that you liked (or another that you didn't), or you came across a great bar or new attraction we missed.

We will acknowledge all contributions, and we'll offer an Insight Guide to the best letters received.

Please write to us at:
Insight Guides
PO Box 7910
London SE1 1WE
Or email us at:
insight@apaguide.co.uk

Summer's Lease, by John Mortimer. Penguin.
Death in Springtime, by Magdalen Nabb. Heinemann.
Under the Tuscan Sun and two sequels, by Frances Mayes. Bantam.

Other Insight Guides

Europe is comprehensively covered by over 400 books published by Apa Publications. They come in a variety of series, each tailored to suit different needs.
Insight Guides, the main series of guides that Apa publishes, provide the reader with a cultural background, plus comprehensive travel coverage linked to photography and maps. The series includes titles on Italy, the Italian Lakes, Sicily, and Sardinia.
Italian destinations in Insight's detailed and colourful **City Guides** series include Rome, Florence and Siena, and Venice.
The itinerary-based **Insight Step by Step Guides**, written by local hosts, come complete with a pull-out map. Titles include Naples and the Amalfi Coast, the Italian Lakes, Venice, Florence, and Rome.
Insight Smart Guides give you the facts about a destination in a very digestible form and feature Italian titles such as Venice and Rome.
Insight Select Guide to Rome offers new insights into the city for informed and experienced travellers.

TRANSPORT · ACCOMMODATION · ACTIVITIES · A – Z · LANGUAGE

ART AND PHOTO CREDITS

PHOTO FEATURES

INDEX